Clinical
Heart Disease

By

SAMUEL A. LEVINE, M.D., F.A.C.P.

Clinical Professor of Medicine, Harvard Medical School
Physician, the Peter Bent Brigham Hospital, Boston
Consultant Cardiologist, Newton-Wellesley Hospital
Physician, New England Baptist Hospital

FIFTH EDITION, ILLUSTRATED

W. B. SAUNDERS COMPANY
Philadelphia and London

TO MY SON

Herbert

Preface to the Fifth Edition

The main advance that has taken place in the past six years, since the last edition of this book appeared, is in surgery of the heart. Rheumatic mitral stenosis is now amenable to surgery and involves a rapidly decreasing operative risk. Surgical correction of other acquired valvular lesions is being attempted with varying degrees of success. It is no longer sufficient simply to diagnose mitral or aortic disease or mitral stenosis or insufficiency. We are now challenged to estimate the degree of stenosis or incompetency of a particular valve, a task that has become very important and at times rather difficult.

Surgery for various forms of congenital heart disease continues to expand. New methods of anesthesia, new operative techniques, and new diagnostic procedures have broadened the field of congenital heart disease that is amenable to surgical correction. Because of the growing importance of this aspect of heart disease, the chapter on congenital heart disease has been completely revised. For this I am greatly indebted to Dr. Alexander Nadas, Cardiologist of the Children's Hospital, Boston, and Assistant Clinical Professor of Pediatrics, Harvard Medical School. He has been in charge of the Cardiac Clinic there and has been carrying on the medical studies in collaboration with Dr. Robert E. Gross in surgical cases in that hospital.

Some advance has been made in the field of electrocardiography, and also vectorcardiography is being further explored. Newer information in these fields is incorporated in the chapter "Clinical Electrocardiography," written by Dr. Harold D. Levine, who is now in charge of that work at the Peter Bent Brigham Hospital, Boston.

A striking illustration of the fruitful advances that may come from the correlation of laboratory and clinical studies is the development of modern surgery of the heart. After the early but unsatisfactory attempts of Cutler and Levine in operations for mitral stenosis in 1923, there was a lapse of about twenty-five years before D. E. Harken and C. P. Bailey, working independently, attacked the problem again, with what has since proved to be phenomenal success. Even before this R. E. Gross had pioneered in this new era of cardiac surgery by achieving the first surgical cure of patent ductus arteriosus in 1938. Since then progress has been rapid. Crafoord of Stockholm, Brock of London, Blalock and Taussig of Baltimore, and Potts of Chicago all have contributed brilliantly to this new development. In all this work the clinicians must not lose sight of the role played by the physiologist and by other workers in the laboratory. Suffice it to recall the indispensable aid given by catheterization of the heart and the various instruments employed in this work.

I shall ever remain grateful to Dr. C. Sidney Burwell, Dr. Lewis Dexter, and Dr. Walter Goodale, for the help they have given me in the field of cardiac dynamics and cardiopulmonary relationships, derived, as often happens amongst medical colleagues, from numerous interesting conversations and discussions.

Some additions and elaborations in this edition are the result of aid obtained from Dr. Gerald Whipple, in the preparation of the vectorcardiograms, and from Dr. Paul Zoll, in the management of heart block.

I am also greatly indebted to Dr. Bernard Lown for reviewing the manuscript and for his comments concerning its contents, and to Dr. Egon Riss for his painstaking work in constructing an adequate index. Finally, I want to thank the publishers, W. B. Saunders Company, for their sustained interest and cooperation in the printing of several editions of this book.

The preface to the First Edition has been reprinted unchanged, partly for historical reasons, but mainly because it contains some general philosophical notes that have not lost any validity that they may have had twenty years ago.

SAMUEL A. LEVINE

Boston, Massachusetts

Preface to the First Edition

The purpose of this book is to present in a simple form the important aspects of the diagnosis, prognosis and treatment of heart disease. It is meant to appeal to the general practitioner, and in so far as the information or the points of view that it contains are applicable at the bedside and available to any intelligent physician, just so far will it be useful. No attempt has been made to cover in detail the entire field of cardiovascular disease. Larger textbooks have appeared recently that have done this adequately. Nor does it contain any bibliographic references. For the most part opinions have been adopted that are shared by present-day authorities on the subject. When apparently unorthodox views are presented, I alone must bear the blame for error, if time proves these views to be incorrect. Where questions of opinion or speculations are involved, I have tried to draw the distinction between fact and surmise. This should not detract but rather add to the interest of a medical treatise, for unproved impressions often precede by years established dogma.

It cannot be said that the arrangement of the chapters follows any usual plan. Each chapter may be regarded as distinct in itself and as a brief treatise on that subject. The advantage of this is that they can be read independently. In fact, many of the chapters represent the essence of individual papers that I have published in the past twenty years with the help of various men working at the Peter Bent Brigham Hospital and reflect, therefore, the results of personal intensive study of the problems involved.

After the introductory chapter the various important types of heart disease are considered. When specific or peculiar modes of treatment arise, they are taken up as they come along, reserving the general subject of the treatment of congestive heart failure for the end. Special topics that concern the practitioner, which merit emphasis, are discussed separately. For example, because systolic murmurs are present in many forms of functional and organic heart disease and in fact even in normal individuals, a special chapter is devoted to their clinical significance. Similarly, acute cardiovascular emergencies arise under a variety of circumstances with and without organic heart disease and so, rather than discuss them in each chapter dealing with the respective type of heart disease, a special one is given over to this topic. In this way the reader can review all the types of cardiovascular emergencies for which a physician may be hurriedly called. Although the chapter on Clinical Electrocardiography was inserted at the very end, it may prove more useful to many to read it first.

Some repetition has seemed necessary and advisable in order to spare the reader from referring too frequently to one part of the book while reading another. In discussing rheumatic heart disease, auricular fibrillation, for example, has to be considered. It also is taken up as a complication of acute coronary thrombosis, hyperthyroidism and other conditions. Nevertheless, when it is reviewed in the chapter on Clinical Electrocardiography, a brief summary is made of all the conditions in which auricular fibrillation is likely to occur. Apart from avoiding this necessity of constant reference to different chapters, such a method has an added advantage. It helps to give the reader two different modes of approach in medical diagnosis. One may start from a given known finding, like a certain irregularity of the heart or clubbing of the fingers, and review what the various causes may be, or begin with a known disease such as coronary thrombosis and predict what kind of complications may arise. Such repetitions, therefore, can only serve a useful purpose.

The hope is that this volume will prove practical. By this is meant that it will be easily understood and useful. It may seem that certain parts receive more than their proper share of space and emphasis. In general, points have been emphasized if they were simple, applicable at the bedside and of direct value to the patient. Little time needs to be spent in a discussion of those subjects or phases of medicine that are already well understood. A consultant with any extensive experience quickly finds out what is known and what is overlooked by the general practitioner. From this experience he can readily sense the type of emphasis that is needed in teaching.

If I may be permitted to digress a bit, I should like to express some views about our current methods of pedagogy in American Medical Schools. Inasmuch as the main purpose of our schools is to train men to go out into the active practice of medicine, we should keep constantly in mind that type of teaching that is practical and useful. The minority of our students, who are to become teachers and investigators, must and do receive postgraduate training in their respective fields. The initial undergraduate course, however, should be the same for all. This curriculum seems to lack a proper distribution of time with insufficient attention to that type of teaching that is most useful. For example, many hours are given to discussions concerning a subject like cancer of the pancreas which is entirely irremediable and too little to tumors of the spinal cord which are often completely curable. The former of course is more common, but the latter is more important because it is amenable to effective treatment. Granted that a medical student cannot be taught all we know about medicine in four or six years, it is more important, when he goes out into practice, that he should not overlook a case of spinal cord tumor with paralysis that has been diagnosed amyotrophic lateral sclerosis or multiple sclerosis than to recognize a malignant growth of the tail of the pancreas. Likewise, it is much more important that a physician should be able to recognize the thyrocardiacs who are masked as heart patients and suffer invalidism that can be so readily prevented, than to be able to make an early diagnosis of sub-acute bacterial endocarditis. Until more is known about chronic arthritis and chronic nephritis it might be well to spend less time in our teaching of these subjects and more time with a rare condition like hyperpara-thyroidism, because the limb pains, renal insufficiency and other disa-bilities due to the latter can be readily eradicated or prevented by appro-priate treatment. In a word, the first purpose in teaching is that the practicing physician should acquire that information which is directly helpful in the care of the patient. This does not mean that clinical investi-gations and laboratory research concerning the unsolved problems should be discontinued. A certain part of our profession must be constantly engaged in such effort.

Another aspect of medical education pertains to the simplification of medical diagnosis. In teaching hospitals and medical centers elaborate laboratory facilities are readily available for diagnostic purposes. After an extensive *constructive differential diagnosis* has been built up, one pos-sibility after another is eliminated by various tests. When that same house officer or student goes out into practice, he recalls the numerous possibilities involved in a given set of circumstances, but he no longer has the x-ray to rule out tuberculosis, a Wassermann test to eliminate syphilis and a blood culture to dismiss the diagnosis of septicemia. What simple clinical bedside methods remain to enable him to establish a temporary working diagnosis? In other words, how is he to disentangle the complicated differential diagnosis without putting the patient to great expense? This type of clinical teaching has been neglected, for there are simple methods that can be used in what might be called the *destructive differential diagnosis*, which the older or more experienced physicians have learned and which they are really practicing, con-sciously or unconsciously. A physician finds that a patient has a pal-pable spleen and fever. Among the various conditions to be considered is subacute bacterial endocarditis. He learned in his hospital training that a positive blood culture would establish the diagnosis, but that a negative one does not eliminate it. He has not been taught, however, that if there are no murmurs whatever, he can with assurance dismiss the diagnosis of subacute bacterial endocarditis. This finding he can obtain in one minute and with no expense to the patient. This merely illustrates one example, of which there are many, where simple methods enable one to rule out possible diagnoses. It would be desirable if our medical teachers paid more attention to this type of instruction.

A further difficulty in our teaching concerns the completeness or thoroughness of the examination. There are numberless tests and signs for various diseases. The practitioner cannot perform them all every time he sees a new patient. There is not enough time nor can the public afford the necessary expense. Therefore, we must not only teach these various procedures, but we should emphasize more than we do in our schools when these procedures should be carried out. For example, a systolic thrill in the aortic area is an extremely important sign of aortic stenosis, and yet this sign is often overlooked. It can be missed when it is slight, because then it has to be detected by a special technic, i.e., placing the palm over the upper sternum with the patient upright and holding a deep expiration. Physicians cannot and need not go through this procedure with all patients, but should be urged to do so only if there is also a fairly loud basal systolic murmur. Similarly determining the visual fields is a specialized examination and will not be performed by most practitioners. However, it can be emphasized that, if there is some reason to suspect a pituitary tumor, a simple test for bitemporal hemianopsia can be performed in one minute by any physician. Moving a pencil on each side of the patient while he is looking forward and ascertaining when he begins to notice its movements will serve as a gross test of bitemporal hemianopsia. A further example is coarctation of the aorta. We must not only teach what the condition is, but under what circumstances it should be particularly sought. If a routine x-ray examination were made of the chest in all adult cases it would not be overlooked. This is impracticable. We can emphasize that it needs to be thought of in all those who have hypertension, particularly in younger individuals, and if pulsations of the abdominal aorta or femoral arteries are diminished or absent, then further search for the evidence for or against this diagnosis should be made, even including the x-ray. In other words teachers need to emphasize and simplify more than has been done, those sets of circumstances in which special procedures either simple or complicated need to be carried out.

I want to take this opportunity to express my lasting gratitude to Dr. J. H. Pratt, who first excited in me an interest in heart disease while I was an undergraduate student. I also wish to thank Dr. A. E. Cohn of the Rockefeller Hospital for first teaching me the experimental method as it might be applied to the study of cardiac problems. All this would not have been sufficient if my chief, Dr. Henry A. Christian, had not afforded me every opportunity during the subsequent years for developing these interests. I well recall the early days in 1913 and 1914 when Dr. Christian first set up the electrocardiograph in the Peter Bent Brigham Hospital, having no one to turn to when this part or the other would not function. After giving me my earliest instruction concerning this new apparatus and the subject of electrocardiography, he set me off on my own. From then on I have remained constantly in debt to him for his stimulus and guidance in my work.

Much of the joy and stimulus has come from the undergraduate students, whose insatiable curiosity and perplexing questions must ever keep the teacher's interest alive, and from the many house officers and resident physicians of the Peter Bent Brigham Hospital who have helped me in these studies during the past fifteen years. We little realize the constant acquisition in knowledge that we experience from the casual and more spirited conversations with our intimate colleagues and medical friends. This is one of the most characteristic and laudable aspects of our great profession. Among a host of such friends I cannot refrain from acknowledging my enduring gratitude to Dr. Frank N. Wilson of Ann Arbor, Dr. Tinsley R. Harrison of Nashville, Drs. Paul D. White and Soma Weiss of Boston, Dr. R. W. Scott of Cleveland and Sir Thomas Lewis of London. From all I have learned a great deal.

I also wish to thank Dr. F. Van Nuys of Weston, Massachusetts and Dr. W. D. Stroud of Philadelphia for their help in reviewing the manuscript and giving me the benefit of their criticism.

Considerable time and effort have been saved by the kindly services of Miss Bertha I. Barker, who has done all the technical work in electrocardiography at the Peter Bent Brigham Hospital these past twenty years. I also wish to acknowledge my obligations to the Oxford University Press for permitting me to use some of the figures in Chapter XX that were previously published in their System of Medicine.

SAMUEL A. LEVINE

Contents

CHAPTER 1

Introductory Considerations

Considerable knowledge has been gained since the turn of the century concerning the normal and abnormal changes that occur in the heart and the peripheral part of the circulation. One may ask whether or not this knowledge has improved the methods of treatment in actual practice. This question is often put with the inference that therapy has remained at a standstill and that progress in our understanding, although interesting to physiologists and teachers and somewhat tedious to students, has merely made the subject matter clearer and has put diagnosis on a more positive basis. Even if the latter alone were true and heart conditions could now be diagnosed more accurately, a distinct advance of a practical nature would have been made. However, as will be demonstrated, prognostication, although still difficult, has become much more definite and, in certain respects, treatment more efficacious. There are now patients suffering from certain heart affections who are treated effectively, for whom improvement may be expected and, in some instances, health completely restored, whereas little more than a generation ago similar conditions were entirely overlooked or were improperly understood and utterly beyond the help of any therapy that was then available. It will become clear in subsequent chapters that even the ablest clinician of not so long ago was helpless before some of the problems that have since responded dramatically to treatment.

These advances have resulted from the more careful clinical study of patients, utilizing the common bedside methods of observation, the pathologic study of autopsy material, and the newer data available to us from the laboratory. With respect to the latter type of knowledge, we owe a great deal to the pioneer investigators, such as Mackenzie, Wenckebach, Einthoven, and Lewis, who established modern cardiography on a scientific basis as a result of the introduction of the polygraph and the electrocardiograph. The determination of basal metabolism in clinical work has also materially helped our therapy. These and other laboratory procedures have fortified our knowledge so that, as a result of their use, we are now successfully treating patients suffering from certain conditions that previously were regarded as hopeless. Reference is made at this point to the improvement of our knowledge and to the means by which the advance was obtained, to combat the view

1

that seems to prevail in the minds of many that laboratory methods have come to occupy too prominent a position in our medical study. An understanding of both the purely clinical and the more intricate laboratory aspects of disease is absolutely necessary for a proper approach to the diagnosis, prognosis, and treatment of heart disease, and the slighting of one method or undue emphasis of the other will diminish the accuracy and value of our work.

AIMS IN THE TREATMENT OF HEART DISEASE

At the outset, the proper aims in the treatment of heart disease must be appreciated. Unlike other conditions in medicine, most sufferers from heart disease cannot be cured. The disease generally is a chronic one, and the purpose of intelligent care is the prolongation of life, the diminution of suffering, and the increase of mental and physical efficiency of the patient. If the difference between correct and incorrect advice given to a patient with early heart failure is a matter of two to five additional years of life, then proper treatment renders much more aid than most of the unhappy sufferers of cancer obtain from the thousands of surgical operations that are performed for their relief. In addition, there is an increasingly large group of heart patients who present problems in which knowledge of the proper treatment saves life and effects complete restoration of health, whereas, with lack of that specific knowledge, fatalities occur. To be sure, such instances are still not common but are increasing in number. To the few who must inevitably succumb it is little comfort that these conditions are rare, and therefore we should be ready to render this invaluable service when the occasion arises.

There is a further aim to strive for in accurate study of heart disease which results purely from correct diagnosis. I have reference to distinguishing organic from functional heart disease. Many patients have been thought to have structural heart disease because of certain signs or symptoms that we now know are benign. Such error results in great and unnecessary economic loss and unhappiness and frequently in the perpetuation, aggravation, or actual production of a cardiac neurosis which might have been cured or prevented at the outset if the condition were properly understood. In other words, many patients with functional heart disease owe their disability to the inaccurate diagnosis made by some physician and to the effect produced by the fear and worry which such diagnosis engenders.

A final purpose that one hopes will be even more important in the future is the possible prevention or diminution in the incidence of heart disease which may follow a sound understanding of its problems. To be sure, the cry of prevention is constantly heard from the lay public and the medical profession. It seems that, with our limited available information, too much is being promised by our medical brethren with regard to the prevention of heart disease. Although much is being said, too little that is effective has as yet been accomplished, but the great importance of the subject warrants the tremendous agitation that is current.

NORMAL CIRCULATION

Before taking up the discussion of heart disease, it may be well to review briefly some of the simple events upon which a normal circulation depends. The main functions of the circulation are the distribution of oxygen and other nutrient and essential constituents through the capillaries to the tissues throughout the body, and the elimination of noxious products mainly through the lungs and kidneys. Let us at this point trace the different steps in the flow of blood within the body. The venous blood returning from the periphery enters the right auricle through the superior and inferior venae cavae. After an appropriate interval of diastolic filling of the auricle, during most of which time the tricuspid valve between the right auricle and right ventricle is open, the auricle contracts, and slightly less than one-fifth of a second later the ventricle contracts. It must be appreciated that most of the blood, in fact about seven-eighths of it, goes from auricles to ventricles during diastole before the auricles contract, merely because of differences in pressure in the two chambers and the effect of gravity. Only a last bit of blood is ejected by auricular systole, which gives the ventricle its final stretching before it contracts. When the right ventricle contracts, the tricuspid valve closes and the pulmonary valve opens. Blood is thereby sent through the pulmonary artery to the lung capillaries. There the essential change is the liberation of carbon dioxide and the absorption of oxygen in the alveoli of the lung, i.e., the venous blood becomes arterial. The blood then returns by way of the pulmonary veins to the left auricle. The same movement of blood is going on in the left side of the heart that was described above as taking place in the right side, from left auricle through the mitral valve to the left ventricle, only in the one case the blood is venous and in the other it is arterial. When the ventricles contract, the mitral valve closes, the aortic valve opens, and the arterial blood leaves the left ventricle through the aorta to enter the systemic circulation and to nourish the various organs of the body. The blood returns from the capillaries through the veins back to the heart, only to start the cycle all over again. The flow of blood is essentially a dynamic phenomenon and results from differences of pressure in one part of the system as compared with another.

The above events recur with a rhythmic regularity under normal conditions at about the rate of seventy times a minute. The disturbances in this rhythm that occur in certain normal and abnormal states are taken up in Chapter 21, familiarity with which is essential to a precise understanding of the treatment of heart disease. These events produce two heart sounds, the first and second heart sounds, that may well be described as lub-dub. The first heart sound is essentially the result of the contraction of the ventricles and the closure of the mitral and tricuspid valves; the second sound is the result of the closure of the semilunar valves (the aortic and pulmonary). It has been maintained by some investigators, notably Dock, that the first sound is entirely valvular and that the contracting muscle itself produces no sound. The

mitral + tricuspid close @ start of systole (1st sound),
Semilunar   "   " end " " " (2nd sound).

interval between the first and second heart sounds coincides with systole, and that between the second and first sounds with diastole. The
length of the former is approximately two-thirds that of the latter.
It will be seen later that in some cases, in order to avoid overlooking
important findings in the heart which are to be heard by auscultation,
it will be necessary for the physician to train himself to listen to one of
the four features independently of the others. With a little training it
is not difficult to dissociate from one's mind everything except the
quality of the first or the second heart sound. Likewise, certain murmurs that occur in systole or diastole will be heard only if the mind is
concentrated for a given length of time on the interval between the
first and second heart sounds or on that between the second and first
sounds. I have emphasized this particular point because important diagnoses have frequently been overlooked as a result of aimless and more
casual auscultation instead of concentrating attention upon a single
element at a time while listening to the heart.

FORMS OF HEART DISEASE

Before taking up any discussion of heart disease, it would be well
to classify the general paths along which a heart may be diseased and
the varying ways by which such disease may become manifest. A very
common affection of the heart results from deformation of the valves.
Such abnormalities may produce a regurgitation of blood through valves
at a time when they should be closed or a constriction of the valves
impeding the free flow of blood from one chamber to another at a time
when they should be wide open. The point of view I should like to emphasize at this time is that damage to valves is of great importance in
undermining the efficiency of the circulation apart from the health of
the heart muscle. To express this somewhat differently: if we assume the
valves to be seriously injured at a time when the heart muscle is normal, progressive heart disease and failure of the circulation may yet take
place because of the mechanical embarrassment that exists.

A second form of disorder develops from changes in the musculature
of the heart entirely apart from the integrity of the valves. Here, as a
result of alterations in the coronary blood vessels or of more diffuse
damage to the heart muscle from toxins or certain poisonous substances
circulating in the body, heart failure may result. Good examples of this
are coronary thrombosis or diphtheritic heart disease. Furthermore, the
heart muscle may fail functionally, even when it is not significantly diseased, if there is marked hypertrophy. In this event the blood supply
to the heart may be relatively insufficient for the thick muscle fibers.
An entirely different form of heart disease occurs when bacteria start
growing on the valves of the heart. Here the heart muscle may be
normal and efficient and the mechanical embarrassment to the circulation as a result of the valvular deformations may be of trivial importance. The victim is nevertheless suffering from an affection of the heart
which is always extremely grave. It must be clear, however, that in this

condition the disease presents itself with the picture of infection and sepsis and not as circulatory failure, whereas in ordinary myocardial or valvular disease the patients are apt to complain of varying degrees of shortness of the breath or chest pain.

Disease of the pericardium may embarrass the circulation either as the direct result of the inflammation that is present in acute pericarditis or by the mechanical impediment to the normal free movements of the heart that follows a pericardial effusion or pericardial adhesions. In much the same way extracardiac conditions such as thoracic tumors that produce pressure on the heart or great vessels or emphysema that produces increased pressure in the pulmonary circulation may affect the heart.

Another form of heart disease, which is comparatively rare, is that which results from congenital abnormalities. Here, as a rule, the musculature is essentially normal but the chambers of the heart, its valves or partitions, or the large blood vessels are improperly constructed. The result is either an impediment to the flow of blood in the normal manner or an admixture of venous and arterial blood because of defects in the septa that divide the right and left sides of the heart.

Apart from the foregoing structural changes that account for most forms of heart disease there are disturbances in the mechanism of the beat itself which present distinct problems in diagnosis and treatment. Such disturbances occur in normal people as well as in patients who also have structural disease of the heart. For example, a perfectly normal individual may suddenly develop a paroxysm of tachycardia under such circumstances that very disastrous results may ensue. Here the mere acceleration in rate enfeebles the circulation although there is no disease of the heart muscle or valves and no infection. A similar situation may develop in a patient who already has mitral stenosis. Then the embarrassment of the circulation may be more serious and develop more quickly. Such abnormalities in the mechanism of the heart may properly be regarded as functional and will be taken up in detail later.

A final condition which goes by a variety of terms also deserves consideration. I have reference to functional heart disease and cardiac neurosis. These conditions were very prevalent during the First World War and were known by one or another of the following names: soldier's heart, effort syndrome, disorderly action of the heart (D.A.H.), neurocirculatory asthenia (N.C.A.), irritable heart, functional heart, or nervous heart.

The disability of which the patient will complain in one form of myocardial disease may be quite different from that in another. Dyspnea is generally the most prominent symptom of cardiac failure whether it occurs in a patient with valvular or with myocardial disease; however, when there is localized coronary artery disease producing angina pectoris, there may be no dyspnea whatever and only chest pain. Likewise, the heart may be intoxicated as a result of hyperthyroidism without any dyspnea. Here the heart is actually hyperactive, and the primary complaint may be palpitation. The inference from all this is that there can be no single method of testing the health of the heart. This explains why the various functional tests of the heart that have been devised, many of which are still being extensively used, have proved so unsatisfactory. Most of these tests utilize the effect of some effort on the heart rate, the blood pressure, or on the production of dyspnea, in order to determine the health of the heart. The fallacy of using such procedures to test the health of an organ which has so many different ways of expressing its abnormalities is apparent. It would be just as illogical to decide that the brain is normal because the hearing or vision is not disturbed. As a further illustration of this difficulty, a patient may have a history of serious syncopal attacks with complete heart block (Adams-Stokes disease) and yet when put to a test of effort will show no dyspnea or pain whatever. The reason for this apparent anomaly is that the main disturbance in function in this particular instance is one of conduction of impulses, and the other functions of the heart are essentially normal. Functional tests in current use are for the most part tests of physical fitness and not of cardiac disease. Many individuals with normal hearts may manifest a poor response to effort and, contrariwise, those with definite well-compensated heart disease may show a normal or excellent response. The differences are due to the degree of physical training or to variations of nervous stability in different individuals and do not measure the current or future status of the heart itself. The above statements will suffice to throw some light on the present status of functional tests of the heart and to indicate that the proper appraisal of problems in heart disease necessitates a complete survey of all factors that may have any possible bearing on the situation.

CHAPTER 2

Rheumatic Fever

The term "acute rheumatic fever," long used in clinical medicine, is an extremely unsatisfactory one. The disease is often subacute or chronic rather than acute. There may be no "rheumatism" or pains, and fever may be very slight or absent. The term "rheumatic state" has come into use and has the advantage that it focuses attention on a "state" or peculiarity of the host, and yet a case of smoldering chorea need show no rheumatism. There is not even a constant pathologic finding, for the Aschoff nodule in the myocardium or elsewhere which is so characteristic is not always present. This is one instance in which it might have been advantageous to have a disease bear the name of some famous physician until its exact etiology were discovered, a custom in medicine that is often perplexing to students and practitioners. In this chapter rheumatic infection is meant not to include rheumatoid arthritis, although in some cases the former seems closely allied to the latter.

Rheumatic fever is the most important infection that is directly related etiologically to the development of heart disease, particularly in younger people. With this is included chorea, or St. Vitus' dance. The exact etiology of this disease is not known, although the streptococcus is thought by many to be the cause. It is very likely that certain hemolytic streptococci play a role in this connection, as the disease so frequently follows in the wake of sore throat, tonsillitis, or other streptococcic infections. The occurrence of epidemics of rheumatic fever in camps or institutions, where large groups are crowded together, following beta hemolytic streptococcus infection of the throat affords strong evidence in favor of the view that there is some causal relationship between the streptococcus organism and rheumatic fever. The exact relationship, however, is not well understood.

Much has been written about the allergic nature of rheumatism, comparing it to asthma, hay fever, and urticaria, only that the sensitivity in the cases of the latter is to proteins and in the former it is to bacteria and their products, particularly streptococci. This conception has aided in the understanding of some of the manifestations of the disease. It can explain why joints may swell in response to a sore throat without the presence of bacteria in the joints. Under such circumstances certain tissues (e.g., the skin or joints) may respond to infection or streptococci in distant parts of the body (e.g., the tonsils, teeth, or sinuses) because

7

of local alterations in sensitivity. This point of view gives a different aspect to the idea of "focus of infection" in its relation to rheumatism.

At the outset it becomes very important to have a clear understanding of this particular infection and its various manifestations. The rheumatic infection often appears seven to fourteen days after some primary illness or upset. This primary cause generally is a streptococcus infection, like a sore throat, but it may be an ordinary surgical operation, the injection of some foreign protein, a chilling or exposure. Some maintain that in all such instances streptococci are still the primary cause and can be isolated from the throat in these cases. Scarlet fever is one of the trigger mechanisms that may start this series of events, but it cannot be regarded as a cause of rheumatic fever or rheumatic heart disease. On careful analysis it will be found that in only 2 to 5 per cent of cases of scarlet fever are there cardiac complications. This percentage corresponds to the number of individuals in the general population who are vulnerable to rheumatic infection. It is generally true that the cardiac murmurs which follow scarlet fever occur in that small number of patients who showed mild arthralgic symptoms about ten days after onset of the disease. In other words, the scarlet fever infections uncover those individuals who are constitutionally rheumatic or vulnerable. It is possible that if the scarlatinal infection had occurred at some other time when the particular host was not vulnerable it would not have resulted in a rheumatic bout.

We are all familiar with the typical attack of acute rheumatic fever in a child or a young adult who is suddenly afflicted with painful joints which are tender, warm, swollen, and red, the symptoms jumping from one joint to another in rapid succession. During such a condition there is a moderate fever and slight leukocytosis. This may last a few days, a few weeks, or even months. We are also familiar with the typical attack of chorea in which the child insidiously develops involuntary nervous muscular movements or twitchings of a peculiar character. Both these conditions may properly be regarded as different manifestations of the same rheumatic infection, for they frequently occur together; they attack the same type of individual and in a sense produce the same disabilities in the heart. When either of these two conditions occurs in a typical form, it is very easily recognized. However, when the symptoms are slight, they are frequently overlooked both by the patient's family and by the physician, remain unrecognized, and lay the same foundation for the subsequent development of rheumatic heart disease. I have often seen children who have appeared somewhat nervous or fidgety, in whom it was extremely difficult to tell from the symptoms that chorea existed, and yet in whom there was sufficient evidence of a subsidiary nature to make it certain that a true Sydenham's chorea was present. The same has frequently been true of mild cases of rheumatic fever. Here the patient may only have vague aches and pains in the limbs, often called "growing pains," and yet, because of these same secondary manifestations of the rheumatic infection, the true character of the underlying disease became evident. We must, therefore, be ready to make the diagnosis of rheumatic infection in many atypical cases.

ATYPICAL CASES

The failure to recognize atypical cases of rheumatic infection accounts for the fact that in many instances outspoken valvular disease of the heart is seen in adults when no past history of rheumatic fever or chorea can be uncovered. In fact, if we take a condition like mitral stenosis, which I believe is due to only one disease, namely, rheumatic infection, in only about 50 per cent of the cases will there be a definite history of rheumatic fever or chorea. In the other 50 per cent, I believe that rheumatic infection occurred years previously, but presented itself in an atypical form, although with sufficiently characteristic features to be recognized if these unusual aspects of the rheumatic infection had been appreciated.

We must look upon the rheumatic infection as a very protean disease, in many respects similar to syphilis. Apart from the more commonly known organs that are involved, attention has been drawn to rheumatic lesions in the lungs and kidneys, and in the blood vessels of other structures. It affects almost the entire body. A child has an attack of rheumatic fever at the age of 9, recovers satisfactorily, and then presents himself twenty years later with mitral stenosis. A young adult has a chancre at the age of 20, and presents himself with aortic insufficiency twenty years later. Chorea may be regarded as the nervous manifestation of rheumatism, as meningitis is of syphilis. Both diseases have cutaneous symptoms, i.e., the nodules and erythema multiforme of rheumatism as compared to the secondary rash or later tertiary syphilid. In both, the heart is frequently involved. The analogy may be carried further, for the joints and other organs are affected in both conditions. It is also true that the predominance of one type of symptom or another varies considerably from patient to patient in both diseases. In some syphilitics, the cutaneous features are very prominent; in others they are almost absent, and the central nervous system involvement is the outspoken lesion. Likewise, in some rheumatics, the element of arthritis may be entirely absent, and the nervous manifestation in the form of choreic movements may be the sole feature of the disease. In others, there may be neither joint nor nervous symptoms, and the disease will be confined entirely to an affection of the heart or of the skin. There are numerous instances in childhood in which the illness is characterized by gradual fatigue, lassitude, slight pallor, mild sweats, loss of appetite and weight, and a slight fever without any limb pains or chorea. Sometimes such a child will be considered as suffering from tuberculosis, possibly involving the hilar glands. The rheumatic nature of the disease is often overlooked and in fact could be suspected only by the most careful consideration of the secondary factors of rheumatism. In these cases it will frequently be found that the heart sounds are hyperactive or that a murmur over the precordium will be present, either of which should direct attention to the possibility of rheumatism. One may be left in doubt as to the diagnosis only to see the child at some subsequent time go through a similar illness, this time associated with typical poly-arthritis or chorea. We must, therefore, not confine the diagnosis of rheumatic infection to those patients suffering from typical polyarticular rheumatism or St. Vitus' dance.

The various manifestations of rheumatism are best looked upon as resulting from differences in the type of response on the part of the host rather than from differences in strains or virulence of the infection. We do not all respond to the same insults in the same way. This applies to psychic, bacterial, or mechanical trauma. One patient loses his entire fortune and then commits suicide, another after suffering a great financial loss takes to drink, and a third grits his teeth and starts all over again. Similarly one patient has a primary chancre and despite good treatment develops a stubborn skin syphilid. A second with little or no treatment has few or no skin lesions and only becomes aware of his plight when, twenty years later, he has involvement of the central nervous system. A third has no involvement of the nervous system but develops an aortic aneurysm. Likewise two individuals cut their hands and blood flows. One faints at the sight of the blood, and the other has enough presence of mind to put his handkerchief over the wound. These are differences in the response of the host, and such differences are of extreme importance in rheumatic fever, for they explain the multiplicity of the symptoms. It must also be remembered that the host changes during different periods of life, so that the response in childhood may differ from the response in adult life or old age.

DETECTING ATYPICAL FORMS

Appreciating the fact that the rheumatic infection need not appear in its typical form as polyarthritis or chorea, what means have we of detecting the atypical forms of this disease? Numerous clues which have frequently been invaluable in diagnosis may be called subsidiary or secondary features of the disease. None of them is characteristic enough to be pathognomonic, for they are vague and may occur in many other diseases; but it is surprising how often, when considered in toto, they make up a distinct clinical picture. In the first place I have reference to *epistaxis*. It is well known that nosebleeds occur in many normal individuals and in a variety of diseases, but I know of no group of individuals who have repeated epistaxis as frequently as rheumatic children. I do not refer to the nosebleed that comes from trauma. The epistaxis here is spontaneous and may occur for some years before the outspoken attack of rheumatic fever takes place; it may occur during the active rheumatic infection while the child is sick in bed with fever and polyarthritis, or after recovery while the child is feeling well and attending school. Whether this is due to a peculiar vulnerability of the small blood vessels of the body in these individuals, or whether the actual cause of rheumatic fever which lurks in the body for many years produces specific pathologic changes in the mucous membrane of the nose, is not clear. It must be appreciated, however, that the rheumatic infection has a predilection for synovial membranes. It affects the endocardium, the pericardium, the pleura, the peritoneum, the synovial membranes of the joints, and the mucous membrane of the eye and possibly of the nose. At any rate, a history of repeated nosebleeds, together with other features, which may be of doubtful significance in themselves, should make one strongly suspect that the patient is rheumatic.

Another symptom, although not quite so frequent as epistaxis, but one which may be similarly valuable in indicating a diagnosis of rheumatic infection, is *repeated vomiting spells.* The child may be ambulatory, attending school, and suddenly have an attack of vomiting. This is generally painless and accompanied by only slight nausea or none at all. To be sure, vomiting is a frequent occurrence in many nonrheumatic children, but it has impressed me that recurrent attacks of vomiting are more common in this disease than can be accounted for as an accidental phenomenon. Sometimes, with or without this vomiting, there is pain in the abdomen and tenderness. One can readily see from this brief description how a child might erroneously be operated on for acute appendicitis because of the symptoms of nausea, vomiting, pain in the abdomen, slight tenderness, fever, and leukocytosis. I have personally seen several instances in which this mistaken operation had been performed. It is in these unusual cases that one may be entirely dependent on other features of rheumatism, such as hyperactive heart sounds, murmurs, family history, and nosebleeds, to arrive at a proper diagnosis.

FAMILIAL FACTOR

Further peculiarities of rheumatism pertain to the family history and the constitutional type of the individual. There is now no doubt whatever that there is a strong familial factor in rheumatism. What is not clear is whether the high incidence of rheumatic infection in members of the same family is due to a particular hereditary element or whether it is due to the fact that members of the same family are exposed to the same environmental influences. If the disease has a contagious or infectious element in it (and well-established epidemics of rheumatic fever have been reported), it would not be surprising that two or more children in the same household should have the same disease. Even if it is not contagious, but dependent upon factors like dampness, unhygienic surroundings, overcrowding, and diet, one would also expect to find an apparent familial incidence of the disease. I am inclined to the opinion that apart from the infectiousness of the disease, there is a distinct hereditary predisposition. In one family I know of two sisters and a brother who lived in different parts of New England, yet one or more of the children of each sibling has had rheumatic fever or chorea. In this same family the children have had one or another form of rheumatic infection and their parents and grandparents have shown marked evidence of degenerative vascular disease, namely, hypertension and angina pectoris. Here we have a striking example of familial vascular vulnerability, the children developing the infectious type of circulatory disease and the parents the degenerative form. I have seen this combination of rheumatism in children and angina pectoris in the parents too frequently for the relationship to be entirely coincidental. The inference to be drawn at this point is, I believe, that there are families with vulnerable vascular systems and that this vulnerability is both to the infectious and to the degenerative form of heart diseases.

Apart from the familial predisposition to rheumatic infections there are rare instances of intrauterine rheumatic involvement of the fetus. It would be difficult otherwise to explain the finding of well-marked mitral stenosis in an eight-month-old child who showed this finding at autopsy. This can be called an instance of fetal endocarditis.

CONSTITUTIONAL FACTOR

Much attention has been given to constitutional or anthropologic features of the individual in relation to disease. I have been interested in this problem in so far as it bears upon three distinct clinical conditions, namely, pernicious anemia, angina pectoris, and rheumatism. There seems to be no doubt now that there is a type of individual with fair skin, blue, gray, or light brown eyes, and fair hair (prone to early grayness) that more readily develops pernicious anemia. Highly pigmented individuals are only rarely affected by this disease. In a similar manner, there seems to be a certain type that frequently develops angina pectoris. I refer here to the well-set, stocky, strong man (mesomorph), who has always enjoyed good health. In this type the muscles seem to be hard, the skin tight, and the forearms well rounded rather than of flat configuration. There are also some striking characteristics in the rheumatic cases. It is surprising how many freckled and red-haired children, frequently with hyperextensive fingers, are seen in our heart clinics. This is the type characterized in England as having the rheumatic diathesis. Although I have not any statistical control studies, I am quite certain that the incidence of such individuals among patients with heart disease exceeds that in the population at large. Another finding of possibly less importance is the appearance of the sclerae. Many of the rheumatic children show pinkish coloration of the sclerae, which is due to an increase in the number of capillaries that come in from the periphery toward the iris. This peculiarity, however, may not be constitutional, but rather the result of infection. The foregoing constitutional considerations, although not as yet established on a firm scientific basis, cannot be lightly brushed aside. They seem to be important enough to deserve further study and have actually proved distinctly useful in diagnosis.

REGIONAL AND SEASONAL DISTRIBUTION

Other peculiarities of rheumatism pertain to its regional and seasonal distribution. There is no longer any doubt that rheumatism, meaning by this term rheumatic fever and its allied conditions, is distinctly more common in certain parts of the world than in others. It is much more prevalent in New England, for example, than in the southern states. For some time this was not believed to be true, and the apparent difference was explained by the fact that in any statistical study the terminology was confusing. In the North the disease might be catalogued under the term "rheumatic fever," and in the South under some other name such as "infectious arthritis" or "polyarthritis." When it was found that the incidence of mitral stenosis at autopsy in a general hospital of a large southern city was about one-tenth as great as in a similar hospital in Boston, one could not avoid the conclusion that rheumatism must vary a great deal in its frequency in different parts of the country. No matter what the original infection was called in the two cities, if the disease were equally frequent, mitral stenosis, the common result of this disease, and a condition which is eventually fatal, would necessarily have been found with the same frequency in any large series of autopsies performed in the two places. This regional difference in the incidence of the disease is important entirely apart from its possible bearing on the nature of the malady, for, where the disease is prevalent, the physician must suspect its presence even on slight or doubtful evidence.

The seasonal variations are also of some importance. Until the specific etiology is known, we shall have no explanation of many of the features and peculiarities of rheumatism. Among these are the variations in the prevalence of the disease during the different months of the year. The early spring is a particularly precarious time, both for the development of new cases and for recurrent attacks in old cases. There is a practical inference in this observation, for, if we have any measures of protection or prophylaxis which may be beneficial, it is during the months of February, March, and April that these measures should be carried out most energetically.

CARDIAC DAMAGE

Rheumatic disease is primarily important in so far as it affects the heart. The acute problem, whether in polyarthritis or chorea, is the disabling condition, but this is a state from which recovery is almost always complete. It may last, however, a very long time. The painful joints or the active chorea may come and go over a period of years. This aspect of the disease is trying on the patient, on his family, and on the doctor, but they may all find comfort in the knowledge that eventually all this disappears. The most distressing feature of the condition is the great frequency of cardiac damage, even when the original infection is apparently mild. It is difficult to estimate how frequently the heart is involved, because one would have to define what is meant by heart damage. If all the means now available to detect abnormality of the heart are utilized in studying this question, it will appear that close to 100 per cent of the patients show some evidence of heart damage. To be sure, many of these changes are slight and transient; others, although permanent, may produce no bodily discomfort to the patient nor diminish his future usefulness. However, it is fair to say that more than half the patients subsequently suffer a more or less serious organic cardiac condition.

It must be clear from the foregoing remarks that, whereas the rheumatic infection may show manifold symptoms, it may also appear in a singularly pure form. In one case there may be a great deal of polyarthritis; in a second case there may be rheumatic nodules, and vomiting and nosebleeds may occur; in another none of these symptoms will be present and only active chorea will be noted. The disease is the same in all instances, but the response of the body is different. What is much more important is that in a fourth case none of these symptoms may be manifest, but there may be an acute affection of the heart. Here again the cause is the same rheumatic infection.

It is quite conceivable and logical that rheumatic infection is a great deal more prevalent than has been recognized. It can be compared to the situation that exists in relation to infantile paralysis. In this disease there is reason to believe that, for every case in which paralysis occurs, there are many others in which the same infection took place but no paralysis developed. Likewise, may there not be numerous instances of rheumatic fever in which the rheumatism is either absent or very slight? There are probably frequent instances in which the child has a slight fever and sore throat, shows no appreciable arthritis, but develops a heart murmur. Such patients would be considered as developing valvular disease of the heart not due to rheumatic fever, but rather as a result of a simple sore throat or without any discoverable cause. In other words, there are probably many patients with mild infections, rheumatic in nature, which affect the heart but which go unrecognized, who later constitute that large group of patients with organic valvular disease in whom no past history of rheumatic fever can be obtained.

CLINICAL FEATURES

Let us now consider briefly some of the clinical features presented by the patient who comes down with a rheumatic attack. The onset of the disease may be abrupt or insidious. It often follows a sore throat or acute tonsillitis. The patient may, within a short time, complain of rather severe pains in one joint or another, show a moderate fever, and begin to perspire. It is characteristic of this disease for the condition in one joint to clear up rather quickly, and for another to become troublesome. In the fulminating case, the joints are extremely tender to the least motion, and there is swelling, redness, and increased warmth of the affected parts. Sometimes these symptoms recede spontaneously, or as the result of salicylate therapy. In other cases, the arthritis remains refractory to treatment for a considerable period of time. There are great variations in the severity, duration, and stubbornness of the joint manifestations. Occasionally, the entire illness seems to subside within a few days or a week, and the patient recovers. More frequently there is an amelioration of symptoms, but the infection keeps smoldering for weeks, months, or even years. During the acute stage of the disease, the patient is apt to develop some secondary anemia, and looks pale. In almost all cases, the heart is accelerated out of proportion to the degree of fever. This is an important feature of the disease. There is hardly any other condition in which the heart rate continues as rapid with a temperature of 100 to 101° F. for as long a time as in rheumatic fever. It is a common experience to see the heart rate continue around 120 for months with a fever of only one degree. Even if practically all the symptoms have disappeared and the patient feels fairly well, a slight fever and a rapid heart may persist. I have seen instances in which a temperature of about 100° F. and a heart rate of about 110 lasted for several years. During all this time the patients were feeling quite well, attending school, and undertaking ordinary activities. Finally, without any particular treatment, the temperature and heart rate gradually returned to normal. There is no better proof of the chronicity of this disease than such experiences. This also throws light on how the rheumatic infection may lurk within the body, smolder in a comparatively inactive way, and suddenly, without any evidence of a reinfection, flare up and new symptoms appear. Reactivation is a term that well describes this peculiarity.

At different times during the period of activity of the disease there is frequently pain in the precordium. This sometimes is fairly severe and troublesome, and may occur without any clinical evidence of either pericarditis or pleuritis. The heart sounds have a hyperactive quality. This pounding of the heart troubles the patient, and he complains of palpitation. The quality of the sounds resembles very much that heard in hyperthyroidism. It is always a matter of great importance to determine, if possible, whether any part of the heart is being involved during the acute infection and, if so, to what extent. Similarly one should try to foretell whether certain suspicious evidences of damage are likely to indicate a permanent structural injury or not. In many cases this is rather difficult, and at times may be impossible. A more detailed discussion of this question will be taken up in the following chapter.

DIAGNOSIS

The typical case of acute polyarthritis with involvement of one joint after another and complete subsidence of the condition in the previously affected part is easily recognized. The response of the fever and the pain to salicylate therapy is fairly characteristic but by no means conclusive evidence. In some cases salicylates are not very effective and at times other types of fever or pains respond to this drug. In the atypical cases a complete knowledge of the subject will be necessary to identify the condition as rheumatic fever. The family and past history, the season of the year, the occurrence of epistaxis or vomiting, the feeling of listlessness and fatigue, the presence of sweating or anemia, the peculiar acceleration of the heart and the increased intensity of the sounds, the development of cardiac murmurs, the detection of a skin rash like erythema multiforme or erythema marginatum, and the presence of small rheumatic nodules in the scalp, elbows, feet, and spine, or over ligaments are all important aids in diagnosis. The sedimentation rate of erythrocytes is increased, but so it is in almost any infection and therefore this finding is not particularly helpful. It does aid in estimating whether or not the process once identified is still in the active stage, and with the presence of fever and leukocytosis may serve as a guide as to the length of bed rest to be carried out. Furthermore, there are peculiar immunologic reactions that occur with rheumatic fever. During the week or two following the initial streptococcus infection those persons who are rheumatic or who are prone to develop symptoms of rheumatic fever are likely to show a high titer of antistreptolysin in the blood. In fact, when such bodies do not appear, rheumatic symptoms are not likely to develop. However, this is by no means infallible, and the antistreptolysin titer cannot be used as absolute evidence that rheumatic fever will or will not develop. However, if the antistreptolysin titer is normal it is extremely unlikely that the patient is suffering from rheumatic fever at that time. It seems that some change or response in the host is necessary before the manifestations of rheumatic infection can take place.

Finally, there are changes in the electrocardiogram that are of considerable diagnostic importance. Many patients with rheumatic fever show an increased conduction time or P-R interval (see Chapter 21). Inasmuch as this is quite rare in other infections, its presence is presumptive evidence of rheumatism. Likewise alterations in the R-T complex of the electrocardiogram somewhat resembling those seen in coronary thrombosis are not infrequent in rheumatic fever. The duration of the Q-T interval is also lengthened during the active stage of the infection and this has been used by some as a guide to the continuation of rest treatment. These changes, especially in the P-R interval, at times are the main or sole evidence upon which a proper diagnosis can be made.

Infectious arthritis may at times be confused with rheumatic fever. Very rarely the same patient may have both diseases at different times. Arthritis rarely involves the heart, and rheumatic fever does not permanently cripple the joints. Disseminated lupus erythematosus may closely simulate rheumatic fever. The former is practically always fatal; it usually occurs in females during the years of menstruation, and there are apt to be characteristic skin lesions on the face. Both diseases are alike in that they may involve the endocardium, pericardium, lung, pleura, kidneys, and other organs. At times tuberculosis, periarteritis nodosa, undulant fever, subacute bacterial endocarditis, and other infectious diseases need to be considered in the differential diagnosis.

TREATMENT

The Treatment of Acute Rheumatic Fever.   In the past, treatment has been entirely symptomatic. Various vaccines proved useless. Artificial fever was employed without real beneficial results. The only medication that appeared to be helpful was some form of salicylate therapy, either sodium salicylate or acetylsalicylic acid (aspirin). At least salicylates had a specific effect on the joint pains. It was and still is thought that they had little if any effect on the extent of cardiac damage. Therapy is now much more promising. It may be divided into three aspects, namely the treatment of acute rheumatic fever once it has developed, the prevention of rheumatic fever at the time that the threatening streptococcal sore throat occurs, and finally the over-all prevention of its occurrence in one who has already had a first bout or in one who has never had an attack but is vulnerable to rheumatic fever.

The introduction of sulfonamide compounds and the later discovery of penicillin and other antibiotics have changed the entire problem of treatment, especially that of prevention. Once acute rheumatic fever has developed chemotherapy may not accomplish much. There is still some question whether a particular attack is controlled any more effectively by giving penicillin or aspirin or adrenal steroids. Certainly, it is reasonable to suppose that penicillin, by eliminating the offending streptococci, will make it less likely for the illness to remain protracted. How favorably it will affect the cardiac damage following that attack is not so certain. One wonders whether the barn door has been closed too late. In any event it would seem wise to administer penicillin rather vigorously in the hope of ameliorating the immediate as well as the ultimate course of the illness. One may give 500,000 to 1,000,000 units parenterally daily in two to four divided doses, depending on the size of the individual. This should be continued for ten to fourteen days, the dose then being gradually diminished, depending on the state of fever, leukocytosis, and other evidence of active infection. It would be desirable to take repeated throat cultures with the aim of attaining and maintaining a streptococcus-free state.

During this time salicylates are given, preferably in the form of aspirin, using enteric-coated tablets if necessary. Four to eight grams daily in divided doses may be given. The salicylates may be administered rectally (one dose daily in 50–100 cc. of water) if there is much nausea or vomiting. As the acute phase subsides, the dose can be decreased. Some clinicians continue a maintenance daily dose of aspirin of 0.3 to 2.0 gm. for a considerable period.

If there has been severe cardiac involvement with congestive symptoms during the acute rheumatic infection measures to counteract heart failure should be instituted. Digitalis may or may not be helpful but should be tried. Diuretics such as aminophylline and particularly mercurial preparations are of considerable value, and sodium intake should be restricted. The value of adrenal steroids is debatable. It has seemed that in some desperately ill patients with acute pericarditis and pancarditis dramatic improvement has followed cortisone administration. At present Meticorten would be preferable because of the lack of sodium retention that follows its use. The dose of about 50 to 75 mg. of cortisone every six hours orally or its equivalent would be appropriate, the amount being gradually decreased or continued as seems necessary. Small doses of 25 mg. two or three times a day may be continued for several weeks.

Although some of the acute phases of rheumatic fever and acute carditis appear to be better controlled by the adrenal steroids than without them, it is not certain that the degree of later permanent cardiac damage differs any from that following use of aspirin and penicillin alone.

The Prevention of Rheumatic Fever.   Specific means are now available for preventing the development of rheumatic fever. The close relationship between a streptococcal infection and the subsequent appearance of the rheumatic state makes it imperative to treat all acute infections, especially those that are definitely or likely to be streptococcal in nature, with antibiotics as promptly and as effectively as possible. Bacteriological studies will better fortify the physician in carrying out his program. In any event, a sore throat or an upper respiratory infection should be assumed to be due to a hemolytic streptococcus unless proved otherwise, especially in children and even more so in those who have rheumatic stigmata, such as a family history of rheumatic fever or other evidence of vulnerability to this condition.

Treatment consists of the administration of penicillin, in one of several ways. The choice will depend on various circumstances, especially the size of the patient and the urgency and progress of the disease. It may be given intramuscularly as a single injection of benzathine penicillin G, in children in a dose of 600,000 to 900,000 units and in the adult in a dose of 900,000 to 1,200,000 units. An alternate intramuscular method is to administer procaine penicillin with aluminum monostearate in oil every three days for three injections, in a dose of 300,000 units in children and 600,000 units in adults. The oral route may also be employed; the dose required is 200,000 to 250,000 units three times daily for a full ten days.

The Prevention of Recurrences of Rheumatic Fever.   Rheumatic fever shows a strong tendency to recur. It is thought that recurrences are due to repeated hemolytic streptococcus infections. In fact, the opinion prevails that if the patient can be kept free of streptococcal infections reactivation of rheumatic fever will be prevented. For this reason it is wise to institute prophylactic chemotherapy in any patient who has once had a rheumatic infection. Some physicians go so far as to advise prolonged preventive therapy in all siblings of a rheumatic individual. It is given throughout the year despite the fact that recurrences are most common in the early spring and fall, although some advise omission of the medication during the summer months. This should be continued for some years, at least until the child has attained full growth, and possibly indefinitely. Only future experience will guide us in some of these decisions. There are two possible courses to follow. The first is an oral dose of 100,000 units of penicillin one half hour before each meal or possibly a 200,000 unit tablet morning and night. The second plan is to give 1.2 million units of long-acting benzathine penicillin (Bicillin) intramuscularly every four weeks indefinitely. Alteration of the exact schedule of doses and the manner of administration may be necessary under various circumstances or be dictated by broadening experience during the coming years, but it is already fairly well established that recurrences of rheumatic fever can be minimized or abolished by this type of prophylactic treatment. If for some reason penicillin cannot safely be taken, sulfadiazine or Gantrisin therapy should be instituted but is less satisfactory. These drugs are given in doses of 0.5 to 1.0 gm. once daily.

Other Therapeutic Considerations.   During the active stage of acute rheumatic fever, the painful joints should be protected by proper support in the form of pillows, and frequently it is necessary to place a hood around the feet and legs as even the weight of the bed covers may be distressing. Bandaging the tender joints after applying oil of wintergreen may give added comfort. Occasionally, the pains will be so distressing that sedatives such as codeine or even morphine may be advisable for short periods of time. These details in the care of the patient are of considerable importance, as they are supportive and help to spare his vitality which is needed to combat an illness that frequently is chronic.

There is no particular problem in the care of the bowels except that it is advisable that the patient have one movement a day, with or without the aid of any cathartic. Inasmuch as rheumatic fever is frequently accompanied by a great deal of sweating, it may be necessary to change the patient's clothing frequently and to watch the condition of the skin. The heart itself, in the vast majority of cases, needs no specific medication, although in patients who have precordial pain an ice bag may be helpful. Although digitalis is often given because the heart is rapid, I have seen no evidence of any beneficial effects except in rare instances when simultaneously with the acute infection there is congestive heart failure as well. The matter of food is of considerable importance. The diet should be liberal and nutritious. One should welcome an actual gain in weight, for, in most cases, the patient is already undernourished. I know of no reason for limiting the diet in any way. Every attempt should be made to encourage extra nourishment. The diet should be adequate in vitamins, especially in fruit juices, all the more so because it is thought by some that deficiency in vitamin C is an important factor in the development of rheumatic fever. In fact, it has been suggested by Massell that very large doses of ascorbic acid (1 to 4 gm. daily) produce dramatic effects on active rheumatic fever.

It is always a matter of considerable moment to decide how long to keep the patient in bed. This, of course, will depend a good deal upon the severity of the illness and upon the extent to which the heart is involved. One would prefer to continue bed care until there are no symptoms and the temperature, pulse, white count, and sedimentation rate have been normal for at least one month. In many cases, to accomplish this, the patient would have to be bedridden for many months, particularly if one waited for the normal heart rate to be resumed, for, as has been mentioned above, tachycardia may continue even for years. When the disease persists and smolders, showing only slight evidence of activity, the practical problem becomes extremely difficult. To obtain the desired result, one might have to confine the patient to bed for one or more years. At some point in the course of the illness, the question of diminishing returns comes in. In the average public clinic patient, if such a drastic procedure is carried out in the attempt to obtain a slight and somewhat questionable advantage by means of a time-consuming and troublesome plan of treatment, the child frequently loses years of schooling. When recovery takes place, which might possibly have been accomplished without the loss of so much schooling, the child finds himself handicapped economically in later years of life. There is also to be considered the additional cost to the family of this prolonged medical care. When the advantages from prolonged bed rest are obvious, the decision is simple. Almost any sacrifice should be made if permanent and severe injury to the heart can be obviated. It is only when this advantage is either very slight or doubtful that these economic features enter directly into the decision. I often permit a child of humble means to continue at school after a previous trial of bed care, although there are slight fever and a few joint pains, whereas if the economic status of the family permitted private nursing and tutoring I should advise the child to remain in bed. The importance of these considerations would be evident to any one who has charge of large numbers of clinic patients.

In making these decisions the general appearance of the patient, the sense of well-being, the state of nutrition, and particularly a gain of weight may prove to be more reliable guides than the presence or absence of a slight fever or leukocytosis.

Realizing that a sore throat or acute tonsillitis may initiate rheumatic fever, and recalling the problem of "focus of infection," the question arises as to the advisability of tonsillectomy. There has been a great deal of discussion *pro* and *con* concerning this matter. At first it was hoped that tonsillectomy after the initial attack of rheumatism would actually diminish the number of recurrences that would take place and the degree of subsequent damage to the heart. If this is true, it certainly is so only to a slight extent, for we often see the disease persist unabated after the most careful tonsillectomy. After this disappointing experience, it was thought that, once the disease had started, removing the tonsils was like closing the barn door after the horse had escaped. It was then argued that the infection had spread from the tonsils and was lurking elsewhere in the body. It would follow, therefore, if this premise were true, that by removing the tonsils in healthy children, before the first infection took place, rheumatism would either be prevented or at least diminished in its incidence. This, of course, would require very elaborate and extensive statistical study. Such a study was carried out in Rochester, New York, where many thousands of normal children with tonsils and without tonsils were followed over many years. The results were only slightly indicative of beneficial effects so far as diminution in the occurrence of rheumatism and rheumatic heart disease was concerned. Certainly, large numbers of children have their first attack years after tonsillectomy. At present it would be fair to state, however, that children who have had their tonsils removed are slightly less liable to have rheumatism in the future than those who have not had their tonsils removed.

There are other practical aspects to the whole question of tonsillectomy that merit our consideration. If this operation is to be done it is safer during childhood than in later years. Although post-tonsillectomy lung abscess is a rare complication, it occurs much more commonly in adults than in children. The same is true of subacute bacterial endocarditis which occasionally develops after tonsillectomy in adults with valvular disease, and almost never in children. Finally, the operation is a much simpler procedure in children, requiring only a day or so of hospitalization. These are additional reasons for early tonsillectomy in rheumatic children. When a tonsillectomy of election is being contemplated it is better to have it performed in the month of May or June than in August, September, or October, because during the latter months poliomyelitis is more prevalent and there is a possibility of development of a severe post-tonsillectomy bulbar type of poliomyelitis that might otherwise have been avoided.

A factor that interests me a great deal from the point of view of prophylaxis is the question of weight. It seems to me that the obese child is rarely stricken with an initial attack of rheumatic infection. This has been particularly true with regard to chorea, although many such children become obese after the disease has started if they progress favorably. One may contend that the apparent relationship between the rheumatic infection and the lowered state of nutrition is that the latter is the result of the former rather than the cause of it. It is difficult to offer scientific proof in this regard one way or another, and one would, therefore, have to depend for the present on general impressions. However, as a result of observation of a great many rheumatic patients, I cannot avoid the conclusion that undernutrition is conducive to the development and the prolongation of this disease and that a diet particularly rich in proteins should be given to vulnerable children.

This discussion brings up the relation between normal or average weights and optimum weights. Doctors and parents often refer to standard weight tables when they consider the weight of children. We must appreciate that the normal figures given in these tables are average ones, derived from thousands of so-called "normal" individuals. These figures are, therefore, averages of good, bad, and indifferent weights. One should strive, not for average figures, but for optimum ones. The best weight at any part of life may be quite different from the average. I feel that the best weight for children and young adults is distinctly above the average, and, as we shall see later in discussing degenerative heart disease, the best weight for the second half of life is distinctly below the average. If this view is true, the practical inference follows that a deliberate attempt to keep infants and children overweight might actually diminish the ravages of rheumatic fever. Such attempts might be more particularly applicable when other features like a positive family history or peculiar constitutional characteristics indicate that the child is more than ordinarily susceptible to rheumatism. The same efforts in the dietary care should be carried out even after the first attack has occurred. Recurrences, I feel, are less likely to develop, or are less likely to be damaging, if those who once had rheumatism gain weight or actually become somewhat obese.

There are other measures of a preventive nature that deserve some attention. It is a frequent experience that an attack of rheumatism quickly follows exposure to wetness and chilliness. I have seen instances in which the first attack came immediately after the patient was soaked through to the skin in the rain or was chilled from lying down on cold, damp ground. This should make us caution our patients to avoid getting their feet wet or their body chilled, and we should call these matters to the attention of the parents of these children so that they may take appropriate prophylactic measures. It is a simple matter for the physician to tell the patient or his parents that he ought to avoid sore throats or catching cold. This is easier said than done. No doubt upper respiratory infections have an intimate bearing on or are often responsible for initial or subsequent attacks of rheumatism, but we have, as far as I know, no certain or specific measures for avoiding these infections, except the general ones that pertain to bodily hygiene. Mouth cleanliness and appropriate dental care should be carried out. Much is being said about the importance of the teeth in their relation to systemic disease, especially rheumatism and rheumatic heart disease. I cannot convince myself that I have ever seen an instance in which this causative relation existed as far as rheumatic heart disease is concerned. Teeth have a more important bearing on the development of subacute bacterial endocarditis than they have on rheumatic fever. Notwithstanding this doubt and skepticism as to the role of infected teeth, I do urge all these patients to keep their teeth in a satisfactory condition.

Two other procedures, the value of which has not yet been demonstrated but which deserve attention, are vaccination against colds and x-ray treatment of the throat. The former, in the opinion of some authorities, will diminish the incidence of upper respiratory infections. I am very skeptical about this and at present do not recommend it. The latter has some theoretical justification for its use. We know that radiation can destroy adenoid tissue in the throat. It has been used as a substitute for tonsillectomy by some physicians. There are numerous miliary tonsils on the posterior pharyngeal wall that cannot be enucleated surgically, each one of which might be regarded as a possible focus of infection. I have, therefore, advised radiation of the throat in some cases in which sore throats have persisted after tonsillectomy.

What good has been accomplished thereby in these cases is still uncertain. There is a further use of the x-ray that deserves consideration. In a small number of cases a series of six daily "spray" x-ray treatments given to the entire body has been of help for troublesome aches and pains of smoldering rheumatic fever. The dose used is 25 r. The beneficial results in such cases probably come from an effect upon the immune or reactive state of the host rather than from any antibacterial action of the x-ray.

An upper respiratory infection with fever deserves more than usual consideration in a rheumatic individual. During an ordinary "cold" many of us continue our daily work with the hope that it will pass by without any further ado; the risk is so great in an individual with a possible rheumatic infection that it is imperative that he start penicillin therapy promptly, as discussed above, and remain at rest until the illness is well over.

A final consideration in the matter of prevention concerns the question of climate. As mentioned earlier in this chapter, there are parts of the United States in which rheumatism is comparatively rare. The question arises whether we can utilize this factor in a prophylactic way. Will an individual who might come down with rheumatic fever while living in Boston, for example, avoid the disease if he spends his life in Florida, Southern California, or in a city like New Orleans, where the disease is less common? There are no statistical studies to give the answer to this question. It is logical to think that the disease might be avoided in this way, but this has reference to patients who have not as yet suffered from the first attack. The matter is quite different when we consider what might happen to a patient who has already had a rheumatic attack and then goes to a region where the disease is less prevalent. In other words, will recurrences be less frequent in one place than in another, or does the fact that the disease has once obtained a foothold make its occurrence independent of external surroundings? I have on occasion advised parents to move their families out of New England to warmer climates when one of the children persisted in having recurrences of rheumatism despite all therapeutic measures that we carried out. Although such instances have been too few in my experience to draw any definite conclusions therefrom, it seemed that good was accomplished when a change to a warmer climate was made. However, uprooting the whole household is extremely costly and drastic, and naturally can be undertaken only by a few families. Furthermore, the present prophylactic means available by the use of penicillin are so promising that such migrations are now entirely unnecessary.

From a sociologic and public health point of view progress is being made and much more is to be hoped for. There is already statistical evidence that rheumatic fever and rheumatic heart disease are on the decline in the United States. Rheumatic fever is mainly a disease of urban populations, and its incidence is directly related to factors such as crowding, dampness, and poverty. As these conditions are ameliorated rheumatic fever will be more satisfactorily controlled. In this regard, there is reason to suspect that improved ventilation will help matters considerably, as droplet infection appears to play some role in the spread of streptococcal infection.

Finally, it is to be hoped that with the improved control of streptococcal infections by the use of antibiotics the total incidence of rheumatic fever and rheumatic valvular disease may show the same decline in the coming decades that we have witnessed in syphilitic heart disease in the past few decades.

PROGNOSIS

The ultimate prognosis in any single attack of rheumatism is most variable. Recurrences are numerous. In only a small number of instances (1 to 2 per cent) does death occur with the acute stage of rheumatism, and then it is as a result of a pancarditis, frequently associated with nephritis. In half the cases, at least, permanent heart damage results. It has been thought that, the more frequent the attacks, the more likely there is to be a cardiac complication. This may need some qualification for in many cases there are repeated bouts without any further cardiac involvement. Some patients, in fact, suffer no permanent heart damage after several attacks. Thus, in some instances, we might be led to believe that the "all or none" law applies; i.e., if the heart is to be attacked the damage will be done in the first attack and the degree of cardiac involvement will be as great in those who have one as in those having multiple attacks. The younger the individual at the time of the first attack, the more likely it is that the heart will be involved. There are certain peculiarities in the outcome, depending on the original type of rheumatic infection, which at present remain unexplained. Although we rightly regard chorea and rheumatic fever as merely different manifestations of the same disease, yet there are qualitative differences in the type of heart damage that results from them.

When a child has chorea and no other manifestations of rheumatic infection (pure chorea), the heart is more rarely involved than when rheumatic fever occurs with or without chorea. This applies to the events during the immediate few years after the infection. I do not believe, however, that chorea will prove to be as benign as it seems, if these same patients are seen years later. I feel that many will still show valvular disease, in some because recurrent rheumatic infection will have taken place and in others even though there has been no subsequent infection. In other words, the child who had chorea at the age of 11 may show no evidence of heart disease at the age of 15 and yet appear at the age of 30 or 40 with mitral stenosis, never having suffered from any relevant illness in the meantime. I have not infrequently seen women over 50 with mitral stenosis who only then began to have symptoms of heart disease, who had had chorea in childhood and no subsequent illness. It is baffling to conceive of what was taking place in the mitral valve all those forty or fifty years between the original illness and the development of significant valvular disease. If chorea were as benign a disease as an early follow-up study would lead one to believe, there ought to be a considerable number of adults who give a past history of chorea in childhood but who show no evidence of heart disease. This has not been my experience.

In fact, a later follow-up study of patients who had had chorea, made at the Good Samaritan Hospital, Boston, showed that whereas there was only a very rare instance of mitral stenosis during the first five years, 30 per cent of the subjects showed this lesion 20 years after the initial infection.

A further peculiarity of chorea is the predilection for involvement of the mitral valve when there is a cardiac complication. Although the mitral valve is the one most commonly affected, no matter what type of rheumatic infection may have been the cause, this is particularly true when the antecedent illness is chorea, for aortic involvement and pericarditis are rarely seen in those who have had only chorea.

These qualitative differences in the cardiac complications are rather difficult to explain if we accept the prevailing view that rheumatic fever and chorea are due to the same underlying cause, for one would then expect similar types of complications as far as the heart is concerned. Two possible explanations may have a bearing on this. In the first place, there may be different strains of organisms that cause rheumatism, one having a predilection for the nervous system and the other for the joints. The organism with a predilection for the nervous system may more easily affect the mitral valve than the pericardium or the aortic valve. One may draw an analogy between this state of affairs and syphilis. It used to be thought that there were strains of spirochetes with a predilection for the central nervous system and others with a predilection for the cutaneous system. The other possible explanation is that the cause is the same, but that the hosts differ. Certain other factors lend emphasis to this latter view. Chorea, for example, is more prevalent in the female than in the male, whereas the reverse is true with regard to rheumatic fever. Here one might say that sex alters the type of response to the same virus, the nervous system of the female being more vulnerable than that of the male. May there not be certain anatomic differences in the valves of the heart between those who develop mitral stenosis and those who do not or who develop aortic disease? Investigation has shown that in some individuals the heart valves contain blood vessels and in others they do not, whereas previously heart valves were thought to be entirely devoid of blood vessels. May it not be true that whether mitral stenosis develops will depend upon the presence or the extent of the blood vessels in the mitral valve, and that those which are entirely or comparatively avascular escape? Such anatomic considerations may account for the discrepancies in the kind of cardiac complications that follow rheumatic infections.

Chorea

The general considerations relating to the treatment of rheumatic fever apply with equal force to chorea. Just as the presenting complaint in the one, i.e., painful limbs, may vary in degree from practically no pain whatever to extreme, exquisite pain, likewise the nervousness may be manifest in all gradations from merely that shown by a "fidgety child" to the extreme "chorea insaniens." Occasionally there is marked weakness and paresis of an affected limb. I once saw a patient in whom poliomyelitis was mistakenly diagnosed. During active chorea there is apt to be no fever or only a very slight rise in temperature, and the heart rate is generally slow or at least not so accelerated as during active rheumatism. The treatment for active chorea is a prolonged period of rest in bed and general nursing care. Although various medicines are used and each physician may have his preference, there is little evidence of a specific value that can be attached to any of them. Some prefer bromides or barbiturates, others use arsenic in the form of Fowler's solution, while a third group believe that sodium cacodylate intramuscularly is of value. At times the nervousness seems to be helped by daily warm tub baths. As I have watched the various methods used I have thought that isolation in a hospital with good nursing, bed care, and forced feeding were the main factors in recovery. When the chorea is of the extreme or maniacal type morphia may be indicated or even Avertin by rectum (70 mg. per kg. body weight) may be given. Fever therapy has been advocated and found beneficial in shortening the duration of active chorea. The temperature of the body is raised to about 105–106° F. by means of a "hot box" and kept at that level for several hours. Such treatments are repeated once or twice at intervals of three to five days. In all but rare instances recovery takes place, for the cardiac complications during active chorea are hardly ever of any great immediate concern. The nervous twitchings may continue in a mild form with irregular exacerbations for several years.

There is one type of chorea that deserves special mention, i.e., the chorea of pregnancy. Both rheumatic fever and chorea occur most frequently in the second decade of life, particularly during the ages of 10 to 13. When either form of the disease has once appeared there is a marked tendency for subsequent attacks. In some patients the same manifestations return year after year, while others who first had chorea will later develop rheumatism, or vice versa. After full growth has been achieved and the patient has reached the age of about 18 years, recurrences become much less frequent. From then on, more purely cardiac complications become manifest with repeated bouts of fever. Rheumatic pains and even outspoken rheumatism, however, are not at all rare in the third and later decades. Occasionally even the first attack of rheumatic fever may take place during these later decades. Curiously, this is hardly ever true of chorea. I have not seen a single instance of chorea occurring for the first time in a patient past the second decade, except in the rare instances when it is associated with pregnancy. Even then there probably will be found a history of some manifestation of previous rheumatic infection. The great prevalence of chorea (and, for that matter, rheumatic fever) during the period of active growth of the child, and the fact that chorea is never seen again except in association with pregnancy, bring to one's mind the possibility that the endocrine balance or the calcium metabolism is in some way related to the susceptibility to rheumatic infection. During both of these periods there is a great disturbance of the glands of internal secretion and an unusual demand on the calcium metabolism in the production of the long bones of the individual during growth and in the laying down of new bones in the fetus during pregnancy.

A final sidelight on the nature of the rheumatic infections is the peculiar seasonal incidence mentioned above. Both first attacks and recrudescences of the disease seem to be most prevalent during the early spring. This has interested me a great deal and particularly so in the light of work on animals at the Rockefeller Institute that showed seasonal variations in the susceptibility to experimental syphilis. It was found in this research that the weight of the various parenchymatous organs, particularly the glands of internal secretion, varied a great deal during different months of the year. February and March were found to be months during which animals were particularly susceptible to experimental syphilis. During these months, moreover, the relative weight of certain glands was especially low. It was also found that the calcium content of the blood varied in different months. May not similar factors be playing important roles in human susceptibility to rheumatic infections? In this connection the following experience is of interest. I once saw a young boy, 11 years old, who had just come down for the first time with an attack of chorea. It began during the month of February. I learned from the boy's mother that her brother (the patient's uncle) had had chorea when he was 11 years old and that he was first taken ill with it during the month of February. Thus, the same disease occurred in two members of the same family at the same age and during the same month. It makes one think that perhaps there is some inherent hereditary defect in metabolism associated with growth or with the glands of internal secretion that renders some individuals particularly susceptible to some noxious agent that is fairly generally prevalent. This concept that changes in the internal environment, especially the endocrine system of the host, may have a bearing on whether or not an individual will develop a rheumatic infection deserves more investigation than it has received, for it may suggest methods of prevention. It at least gives added meaning to some vague phenomena, such as "growing pains" and "spring fever," that characterize this mysterious disease.

It is not unlikely that much valuable information will come to light in the future concerning the relation of the endocrine glands to many other diseases. Excision of the testes has already been found to have a favorable influence on cancer of the prostate. The fact that disseminated lupus erythematosus is so overwhelmingly confined to women during their years of menstruation leads one to think that the ovaries play some role in this disease. The disappearance of a stubborn acne of the face directly after radiation of the ovaries is another example. The very low mortality of patients with untreated lobar pneumonia at the age of 10 in contrast to the high mortality of those at the age of 70 may be related to differences in the endocrine system. Patients with thyrotoxicosis appear to have a much greater incidence of concomitant rheumatic heart disease and hypertension than other persons in the same environment. Women have very much less arteriosclerosis than do men and live several years longer on the average. Does this depend upon some function of the endocrine system? One might cite other illustrations, all of which lend support to the view that the endocrine glands may have an important influence on vulnerability to infections as well as to the development of some noninfectious or metabolic diseases.

The above discussion concerning the possible relation between the endocrine system and rheumatic fever and other diseases is similar to that in the first edition of this book in 1936. It is interesting to see that developments have borne out this speculative prediction. Since the discovery of the dramatic effects of Compound E on rheumatoid arthritis by Hench and Kendall this endocrine product has been administered for many other conditions with profound results. It is much too early to draw any final conclusions, but already favorable improvement has been observed in acute rheumatic fever, lupus erythematosus, and gout, apart from the original observations on rheumatoid arthritis. The implications from this discovery are great and remain to be unraveled by future study. It is obvious that adrenal steroids are not bactericidal agents. In some way they must alter inflammatory tissue response. It seems that these endocrine products change the internal environment of the host so that more normal metabolic activity is restored, at least temporarily. There is reason to hope that fundamental advances in our knowledge of many metabolic processes and new approaches in the treatment of hitherto incurable conditions will result from this work.

CHAPTER 3

The Development of Rheumatic
Heart Disease · Mitral Valve Disease

Acute Rheumatic Carditis

The development of rheumatic heart disease may best be studied by considering two aspects of the disease: first, what is taking place during the acute rheumatic infection, and, second, the progressive changes occurring later which go to make up the whole picture of chronic rheumatic valvular disease. During the acute rheumatic infection it is frequently difficult to tell whether or not the heart is being affected at all and whether certain changes that are noted indicate transitory or permanent cardiac damage. Often one has to leave the question open, and delay a final decision for some months or years. During this time the condition may possibly be called "potential heart disease." Certain criteria, as we shall see, afford quite conclusive evidence that the heart is involved. There are other changes that are common accompaniments of many febrile reactions and, therefore, have not the same significance. The distinction between these two types of changes is a most important one to appreciate in following a case of rheumatism.

During the active infection, there is naturally some fever and acceleration in the heart rate. The tachycardia is frequently out of proportion to the degree of fever. This is quite typical of a rheumatic infection, but need not indicate that the heart is seriously damaged or that it will show structural changes after the infection is over. If the patient develops signs of circulatory insufficiency, such as marked dyspnea, congestion of the lungs and liver, or peripheral edema, which are not common during the acute stage of the disease, we must assume that some serious injury is taking place in the heart. Even under these circumstances it is surprising how much improvement may eventually occur and how little evidence may remain, after a long convalescence, to indicate any permanent organic heart lesion. When these symptoms are severe and a satisfactory recovery occurs, we cannot avoid the conclusion that there must have been an acute rheumatic myocarditis in which healing took place without impairment of cardiac function.

29

SYSTOLIC HEART MURMUR

The most difficult feature to appraise properly during the acute infection is the development of a systolic heart murmur. We all are familiar with the fact that a very slight systolic murmur may be present during fever, whatever its origin, especially when the heart is rapid and hyperactive. The significance of a systolic murmur is discussed in more detail in Chapter 17. However, the louder the systolic murmur that one hears during acute rheumatic fever, the more likely it is to be permanent and to indicate some organic lesion. This is more particularly true if a murmur of moderate intensity is present while the heart action is comparatively slow. As the heart slows, what might be regarded as a benign or functional murmur ought to diminish in intensity, for with the slowing the hyperdynamic element becomes less prominent. Loud systolic murmurs rarely disappear. Faint systolic murmurs may disappear, but if they persist they may be practically disregarded. The murmur of moderate intensity needs to be carefully followed. If it persists as the infection disappears, I believe that some injury, possibly minor in nature, has occurred although it need not incapacitate the patient in any way. It is clear from this discussion that we must pay some attention to the loudness of the murmur and to its persistence. When it is interpreted as indicating a structural damage, it generally points to involvement of the mitral valve, especially if its intensity is loudest in the apex region of the heart. This may be true even when the point of maximum intensity is at the base, although this is not so certain. We now know that the rheumatic infection may affect the wall of the aorta and this may add to the confusion of interpreting the causation of the basal systolic murmur.

DISTURBANCES IN CONDUCTION

A more certain indication that the heart is being affected during the acute disease is the finding of disturbances in conduction in the mechanism of the heart beat. Not infrequently during ordinary bedside examination one detects an actual heart block, an occasional omission of an entire heart cycle, or a dropping of the beat. This indicates an acute myocarditis, for the conduction apparatus of the heart lies within the musculature, and there must be some toxic process or some structural lesion, such as an Aschoff nodule, affecting the auriculoventricular node or the bundle of His. Although it has recently been shown that this delayed conduction may disappear on full doses of atropine, indicating that it is vagal in origin, it is difficult to believe that such observations mean that the heart muscle has not been involved. Minor evidence of this disturbance in conduction which does not produce an actual blocking of beats may be detected by the use of the electrocardiograph. Here it is found that the time it takes an impulse to go from auricle to ventricle is merely prolonged, although the beats all reach the ventricle. The normal conduction time for impulses to go from auricles to ventricles is less than one-fifth of a second. It is considered delayed if this upper limit is exceeded. The heart will then be perfectly regular and it might be impossible by bedside examination to discover this disorder. One may suspect it on detecting a gallop rhythm on auscultation, or on observing that the first heart sound is weak or fainter than it was formerly. If careful studies are made of the heart during the acute infection, changes in conduction are found to be quite common, and they are one of the best proofs that the heart muscle is being involved, at least temporarily. Fortunately, recovery from such damage is very likely to be complete since, when the infection has passed, the conduction disturbances tend to disappear. Even in the rare instances, when some permanent defect remains as evidenced by the continued presence of a delay in the conduction time (P-R interval), the efficiency of the circulation may be perfectly normal.

ELECTROCARDIOGRAPHIC CHANGES

There are other changes of a qualitative nature, as shown by the electrocardiogram made during the acute process, that are fairly characteristic and that also indicate that the heart is being affected by the disease. The changes to be sought for are evidence of auriculoventricular heart block or abnormalities in the configuration of or lengthening of the QRST complex. This means of diagnosis is a more specialized one and can only be utilized by those clinicians who are carrying on electrocardiographic work. Suffice it for the present to bear this possibility in mind, for occasionally such changes in the form of the ventricular complex (see Chap. 21, Figs. 185, 186) may be helpful from a diagnostic point of view, and may aid in determining whether or not a certain vague infection is rheumatic in origin. In fact, there will be instances in which the electrocardiographic changes will be the only evidence that the illness is of rheumatic origin. A girl of 13 who complained of listlessness, nausea, and vomiting was seen by her physician. He found a slight fever (100° F.), slight tenderness in the right lower quadrant, and a leukocytosis of 14,000. The child was sent to the surgical service to be operated on for acute appendicitis. A few hours after admission the temperature was only 99° F., and the white blood count was 12,000. The surgeon noted a faint abnormal sound over the precordium. There was very little evidence of any abnormal condition in the abdomen, but the electrocardiogram showed a P-R interval of 0.30 second. It seemed to me that the child had an atypical form of rheumatic fever of the abdominal type with a mild acute myocarditis, without any rheumatic pains. On rest in bed and salicylate therapy the patient recovered and the P-R interval returned to normal (see Chap. 21, Fig. 123). When the abdominal pain and tenderness are more marked than in this case, an unnecessary appendectomy is likely to be performed.

ENLARGEMENT OF THE HEART

In the attempt to determine whether or not the heart has become affected during an acute rheumatic infection, the question of hypertrophy or dilatation of the heart is a matter of considerable importance. Although during the acute stages it cannot be said that a heart which is normal in size is not diseased, it may be safely accepted that, if the size of the heart increases or is greater than normal, it is diseased. In fact, we may make the generalization that enlargement of the heart is always a definite sign of disease of that organ. There are important exceptions to this general rule. Appreciable dilatation without hypertrophy occurs with severe anemia, especially in children. This will naturally increase the percussion outlines and the x-ray silhouette of the heart. Such dilatation of the heart disappears completely when the blood returns to normal. Dilatation without increase in weight of the heart is also found occasionally in acute toxic states, particularly when the heart muscle is affected. It is, therefore, important to try to estimate the presence or absence of hypertrophy or dilatation. Ordinarily this is done by percussion and palpation. When it is possible to feel the apex impulse quite distinctly beyond the nipple line, it is fair to assume that the heart is enlarged. Frequently one is in doubt as a result of bedside examination whether the heart is enlarged or not, and further information in this regard may be obtained with the aid of the x-ray and the electrocardiogram. The electrocardiograms may give indirect evidence of preponderant hypertrophy of one ventricle over another and occasionally may throw light on whether the auricles are dilated or hypertrophied. Precordial electrocardiography is often more helpful in detecting hypertrophy of one or the other ventricle than is roentgenography. This type of data needs to be weighed most carefully, for there are numerous difficulties in interpretation. If it is decided by one means or another that the heart has become enlarged during the acute process, we must conclude that the heart has been affected.

OTHER EVIDENCES OF ACUTE RHEUMATIC CARDITIS

While following any particular patient during an acute rheumatic attack, if enlargement of the heart has not been noted, if a systolic murmur is either absent or only slight, and there are no obvious evidences of circulatory insufficiency, what other features are to be watched for? The development of a *pericardial friction rub*, which may appear any time during the acute illness, will, of course, be definite evidence of cardiac involvement. Not only will the detection of a typical to-and-fro pericardial friction sound be proof of an acute pericarditis, but it may be assumed that in most such cases the heart muscle is also affected. Another condition that can develop during the acute process of the disease is an *aortic diastolic murmur*, heard in the aortic area and better still in the third left interspace near the sternum. This aortic diastolic murmur may be entirely absent on one day, appear as a faint blow a few days later, and then be quite definite within a week or so. When it appears, it persists and is definitely indicative of an aortic regurgitation for it only rarely disappears. A diastolic murmur of mitral origin is not to be expected to develop at this time, if we assume that the patient is now suffering from the first attack of rheumatism. It takes months or years for contraction and constriction of a valve to occur, for this is a chronic scar tissue process, whereas an insufficiency or regurgitation of a valve may take place within a few days. To produce the latter, it is only necessary for the valves to become slightly retracted or distorted by inflammatory reaction resulting in a slight incompetency. That same incompetent valve years later may contract as a result of scar tissue formation and then be stenosed. The important point is that in the acute infection we may look for insufficiency of valves, but if evidence of stenosis is detected, it is likely that the valve was previously injured and that we are not witnessing the first rheumatic infection but a recurrence.

Occasionally in children, during acute rheumatic carditis, a faint, short *diastolic murmur* may be heard at the apex resembling the murmur heard in mitral stenosis. Such murmurs must be interpreted cautiously for they may be due to dilatation of the heart or to some other mechanism and not to mitral stenosis, and they may disappear entirely. They are not likely to have the same rumbling quality that is found in older patients with mitral stenosis. In fact, errors of this type in the interpretation of the apical diastolic murmur as a sign of mitral stenosis are very rare in adults although not uncommon in children.

The main pathologic evidence of acute or active rheumatic carditis is the finding of Aschoff nodules in the myocardium. Such lesions are common in fatal cases of rheumatic fever in children. However, they are by no means rare in patients over 40 years of age who die of valvular disease. They are occasionally found in older cardiac patients without valvular disease, and even in patients who gave no clinical evidence of rheumatic fever or heart disability and died of some noncardiac cause.

The entire question of assessing the evidence of rheumatic activity is confusing. All seem to agree that joint pains, fever, leukocytosis, increased sedimentation rate, skin nodules and rashes, and certain cardiac findings are all clinical evidences of activity. Sometimes one or another of these features may persist for months or years when other findings are so benign that from a practical point of view the condition may be regarded as quiescent or inactive. On the other hand, the extremely common detection of Aschoff nodules in biopsies of the left auricle during surgical operations when there had been none of these so-called clinical features of rheumatic activities has impelled a revision in our thinking. We really do not know what the Aschoff nodule signifies or how to interpret its clinical significance. These pathological changes evidently may be present for years or possibly they come and go while the patient is otherwise well. We know they may be very abundant at autopsy in patients who die while the disease is in a very acute ravaging state, but we also know they may be silent. It is often easier to decide that the rheumatic state is active than to know that it is quiescent. When the patient feels and looks obviously sick there is little doubt that the condition is active, even if some of the expected evidence is lacking. In doubtful instances, for many years, I have taken the view that if the patient looks well, is not sweating, has a sense of well-being, has a good appetite, is gaining weight (not due to edema), and does not display outspoken evidence of rheumatic activity the condition is quiescent. This view appears to have been sound when questions of surgical operations have come up or when the problem of allowing the patient to get out of bed or to increase his physical activities has to be met. At times a slight fever or increased sedimentation rate and the possible presence of Aschoff nodes in the heart may need to be disregarded in making these decisions.

Mitral Insufficiency

Let us assume that the patient did not develop any of the definite signs of heart involvement during the acute stage of the illness and that if there were minor changes, such as a delayed conduction time or a slight change in the form of the electrocardiographic tracing, they were transitory. We assume that the patient had been in bed for some months with a smoldering fever, a rapid heart rate, and vague fleeting pains in the limbs, and finally all these symptoms subsided. Let us also assume that he was left with a systolic murmur of moderate intensity heard best at the apex and that when he recovered he was symptom free. In the course of time he returned to his ordinary activities either at school or at work and felt quite well. As we observe this patient during the following years, let us trace what possible changes may take place. He may remain well, never have a return of rheumatic fever, and always show a systolic murmur on examination. Such a patient would either be denied life insurance in his later years, or be considered an increased risk and receive a high rating in his insurance examination. Occasionally the systolic murmur may gradually diminish in intensity. Rarely, it may disappear entirely. He may, therefore, live out his life as a normal individual and never be embarrassed by his heart. This, I think, is the exception, unless with recovery no murmurs whatever remained.

In a fair number of patients in whom all the findings on examination, including the systolic murmur, were considered benign, some years later, usually a decade or two, subacute bacterial endocarditis will develop. The remainder, either as a result of recurrent bouts of rheumatism and reinfections of the heart, or possibly because of the inherent nature of the original infection with its subsequent chronic progression and contraction without any recognized reinfection, will develop signs of mitral stenosis or aortic stenosis at some future time.

When this same patient whose progress we are following does not develop mitral stenosis but persists in manifesting a moderately loud systolic murmur while well and ambulatory, he may be considered as having organic mitral insufficiency. This is especially true if there is pulsation or dilatation of the left auricle or general cardiac hypertrophy.

It formerly was maintained by certain authors that organic mitral insufficiency does not exist or is extremely rare, and that in cases in which such diagnoses are made there is either no disease of the mitral valve or there is mitral stenosis. This point of view was a reaction against the previously prevailing belief that every patient with a systolic murmur had mitral insufficiency. We now know that in many such cases there is no structural disease of the mitral valve. They were often instances of nervous or hyperdynamic hearts with a benign systolic murmur or cases of myocardial failure of the degenerative type with a relative mitral insufficiency but with no endocarditis. Another group of patients at postmortem examination showed mitral stenosis. The conclusion was drawn, especially from postmortem data, that organic mitral insufficiency did not exist without stenosis. The difficulty with this point of view is that we cannot deny the presence of a disease which is generally nonfatal by the use of autopsy data. It would be just as fallacious to maintain that acute tonsillitis and chickenpox are extremely rare because one almost never finds cases at autopsy. So it is with organic mitral insufficiency. This condition may develop into mitral stenosis, which eventually is fatal, although for many years only an incompetency of the valve is present. As long as it is only a regurgitation, the patient is likely to be in good health. Even this is not invariably so for some patients die from heart failure showing a markedly dilated heart and mitral insufficiency without stenosis. Only occasionally have we an opportunity of examining the valve before stenosis develops, e.g., if subacute bacterial endocarditis becomes superimposed on mitral insufficiency. Then we see that the past history of rheumatism and the moderately loud systolic murmur indicated a true rheumatic mitral endocarditis, producing a regurgitation but no stenosis of the valve, for the pathologic examination will show both the old rheumatic and the recent bacterial lesions. Furthermore, during life many patients who have mitral insufficiency without stenosis show a definite systolic expansile pulsation of the left auricle on fluoroscopic examination, which finding affords further evidence of regurgitation through the mitral valve. The conclusion from the foregoing is that, although the diagnosis of organic mitral insufficiency should be made with caution, it is a condition that actually exists, especially in young and middle-aged rheumatic individuals.

During the past several years, since cardiac surgery for valvular disease has been revived, many more cases of rheumatic mitral insufficiency have been recognized. The patients present themselves with evidence of moderate or advanced congestive failure, often complaining more of weakness, and with markedly enlarged heart with striking enlargement of the left auricle and hypertrophy of the left ventricle, and generally are fibrillating. They always show an apical systolic murmur and frequently have a slight, moderate, or loud diastolic murmur, fairly typical of mitral stenosis as well. Some have a third heart sound in early diastole which can be mistaken for the opening snap. It comes later than the opening snap and its presence suggests that the primary lesion is mitral insufficiency and that there is left ventricular failure. Some actually have a certain degree of stenosis of the valve, and others have pure regurgitation. The valve may be very patulous, somewhat like an open diaphragm, resulting in little if any obstruction to the diastolic flow from left auricle to left ventricle but in considerable reflux in the opposite direction with systole. This condition is now frequently observed during surgical operations on the mitral valve. At times it is quite difficult to determine clinically what degree of stenosis and what degree of insufficiency are present in a given case of rheumatic mitral valve disease. This problem will be discussed later.

From the foregoing it would seem that there are two kinds of cases of rheumatic mitral insufficiency. There is one with little or no evidence of cardiac disability. The patients have a moderate or loud apical systolic murmur, a regular rhythm, and no or very slight cardiac hypertrophy, and carry on very well. They are subject to bacterial endocarditis. The other type presents the picture of advanced heart failure with features described above. What the relation between these two types may be is obscure. Does the one gradually develop into the other? If so, does this progression depend on repeated reactivation of the rheumatic process? Or is the original injury in the more severe type so great that marked incompetency of the valve quickly develops with its inevitable disastrous results? These are questions that at present remain unanswered. More careful data will be necessary, noting the changes that take place over the course of many years in those who are left with an apical systolic murmur following a rheumatic infection.

Mitral Stenosis

Let us now discuss the development of the signs of mitral stenosis. How soon the changes to be described will occur is variable. Upon rare occasions they begin within one year, although generally many years elapse between the original infection and the development of definite evidence of mitral stenosis. During these years, the symptoms may be none or few, such as slight dyspnea and palpitation. If we examine the patient from year to year, little change may be noted, until finally, as the first indication that the mitral valve is becoming stenosed, we commence to detect a snapping quality or accentuation of the first heart sound as heard at the apex. During these same years the pulmonary second sound may have become somewhat accentuated and reduplicated. As an aid in diagnosis, I have found the quality of the pulmonary second sound of distinctly less value than the quality of the first sound. In other words, an accentuation of the first sound is frequently the first suspicious evidence of early mitral stenosis. This, however, is not sufficient to enable one to make a definite diagnosis, for there are other conditions in which it occurs, such as hyperthyroidism, a short P-R interval, anemia, cardiac neurosis, and some cases of hypertension.

When this snapping quality of the first heart sound is heard, it is well to listen carefully to the heart in order to hear the early development of presystolic or mid-diastolic murmurs. At this time no murmur whatever may be heard during diastole on ordinary examination, but if one listens directly after a brief effort or with the patient in the left lateral position, in some cases a presystolic murmur may thereby become audible which otherwise might be entirely overlooked. I have frequently brought out this very important physical sign which made a definite diagnosis of mitral stenosis possible when, under ordinary examination, it was entirely inaudible. This typical rumble which is quite pathognomonic of mitral stenosis may also be uncovered by the use of the *amyl nitrite* test. Here the patient inhales amyl nitrite for a few seconds and one auscults carefully during the acceleration of the heart that follows the inhalation. It is better to use the bell rather than the diaphragm attachment of the stethoscope. Only light pressure should be applied, otherwise the bell is transformed into a diaphragm. In practice, it is sufficient to listen at the apex with the patient in the left lateral position or directly after a brief period of exercise, e.g., twenty-five hops. Whether a diastolic or presystolic murmur is heard or not, frequently a short sharp sound may be audible in early diastole at the apex. This is called the "opening snap" and is strongly suggestive of mitral stenosis. In many cases it is also followed by a rumbling murmur, but at times the latter only becomes clear months or years later. When the presystolic or mid-diastolic murmur is heard, no matter how it is brought out, and the first sound is snapping in quality, the patient may be considered to have mitral stenosis. Just as is true of most useful rules in medicine there are always exceptions. I recall examining, in 1939, a 12-year-old boy who showed a definite mid-diastolic murmur. When he was placed in the left lateral position a clear presystolic murmur became audible. In addition there was an apical grade II systolic murmur. I believed he had definite mitral stenosis. Seven years later when I examined this boy quite carefully I could hear no murmurs whatever, even in the left lateral position, and was of the impression that he had no valvular lesion.

At some later time it will be found that the same mid-diastolic or presystolic murmur will be audible even with the patient at rest or lying recumbent. It will be much better heard with the patient in the recumbent than in the upright position. Furthermore, the murmur may be quite sharply localized over a very small area in the region of the apex. As years go on and the degree of stenosis of the mitral valve increases, the presystolic or late diastolic murmur lengthens so that the time is reached when almost the entire diastolic pause is filled with the murmur. The early portion of this long rumbling murmur may have a diminuendo quality and the latter part a crescendo element, terminating in the accentuated first sound.

At this time we are not considering the development of generalized circulatory failure, which may come at any time during the patient's progress, but which generally does not occur until the mitral stenosis is well advanced. In the meantime the heart has been essentially regular in its rhythm, although there may have occurred occasional extrasystoles either of ventricular or auricular origin. The dominant rhythm, however, is likely to have been regular. Some time during the life of this patient who has already developed mitral stenosis, auricular fibrillation is apt to develop. This complication is very rare during the first decade, becomes more frequent the next decade, and is most common about the ages of 35 or 40. Whereas the heart during all these previous years was regular, the beat now becomes tumultuous and grossly irregular. This change is sudden when it occurs, so that on one day a normal slow heart rhythm may have been present and on the following day it may be found to be very rapid and absolutely irregular. Not infrequently this auricular fibrillation is transient and recurs in the form of attacks. Each attack may last several hours and then disappear, the heart returning to its slow regular rate. Some weeks, months, or years later the same phenomenon may be repeated. During the attack, the patient may suffer with a good deal of palpitation, dyspnea, and general nervous agitation. If the state of the reserve strength of the circulation is not great before the attack, the clinical condition of the patient may become quite serious. Edema of the lungs, cyanosis, and orthopnea may develop. When an attack of auricular fibrillation with a rapid ventricular rate produces no evidence of cardiac failure, it denotes a satisfactory state of myocardial reserve. After a variable number of transitory attacks of auricular fibrillation, the condition is apt to become permanent. In fact, in most cases, once the heart becomes grossly irregular, it remains so indefinitely.

It is most important to be able to recognize this type of irregularity, first because it is extremely common, and second because much in the way of treatment can be done for it. Furthermore, a proper understanding of this phenomenon aids greatly in comprehending the changes that take place when it occurs as evidenced in the physical examination of the heart. When auricular fibrillation develops, the auricles cease contracting, remain distended in diastole, and show fine fibrillary twitchings throughout the musculature. The ventricles, on the other hand, begin to contract rapidly and very irregularly. In auricular fibrillation, there is an extremely large number of impulses traversing the auricles. The number is in the vicinity of four hundred or more. Only a small proportion of these impulses succeed in reaching the ventricles, the remainder being blocked at the junctional tissue. In other words, the conduction apparatus between the auricles and ventricles (the auriculo-ventricular node and bundle of His) is unable to transmit such a large number of irregular impulses from the auricles and only a third or so get through. The result is that the ventricles contract irregularly at the rate of about 120 to 150. These contractions are grossly irregular. The pulse is also irregular, both in time and in force, and there is very apt to be an appreciable pulse deficit; i.e., the pulse rate as counted at the wrist will be distinctly less than the heart rate at the apex.

It is not difficult to recognize this condition on bedside examination, using only the apparatus that the physician carries in general practice at all times. A rather simple and fairly satisfactory rule of thumb may be described as follows: Given a patient who obviously has heart disease, who shows a heart rate as counted at the apex of over 100 and has a pulse rate that is distinctly less (a pulse deficit of 10 or more), if the rhythm appears to be grossly irregular the condition is auricular fibrillation nine times out of ten. There are rare exceptions in which this rule would not apply. One would feel even more certain of the diagnosis of this arrhythmia under the above circumstances if it were known that the patient had mitral stenosis and a history of rheumatic fever. The triad of rheumatic fever, mitral stenosis, and auricular fibrillation is so frequently found in the same individual that as a practical matter, knowing that two exist, the physician should suspect and seek for the third.

One final point may be helpful in detecting auricular fibrillation at bedside examination when there still remains some doubt as to the diagnosis. Occasionally numerous extrasystoles coming quite irregularly or from different foci of the heart may produce such a tumultuous rhythm, even with an appreciable pulse deficit, that it would be difficult to distinguish it from auricular fibrillation. One important distinction between the two conditions, however, will be noted on auscultation. In both conditions, quick beats and long pauses seem to be coming irregularly, resulting in sudden acceleration and sudden retardation of the heart beat. When the condition is due to extrasystoles, every time there is a long pause it is a compensatory mechanism and therefore follows a previous quick beat. The same succession of long pauses after quick beats also obtains in auricular fibrillation. The phenomenon that distinguishes the two, however, is the appearance of a long pause that is *not* preceded by a quick beat, for this occurs only in auricular fibrillation and not with extrasystoles. In other words, it is important to auscult carefully over the apex of the heart for a sufficient time to detect a sudden lengthening of the heart cycle and to recall whether the previous cycle was short or long. If a cycle of average length or one of longer duration is followed by a long pause, the condition is due to auricular fibrillation. Furthermore, the quality and intensity of the first heart sound vary much less with cycles of different length than is the case when the irregularity is due to extrasystoles. In addition to the foregoing observations, whenever it is possible to do so, an exercise test may help in diagnosis. When the rate accelerates in this manner, extrasystoles generally disappear and the irregularity of auricular fibrillation becomes more prominent.

Apart from the bedside method of diagnosis, auricular fibrillation is easily diagnosed by the use of graphic measures, such as the polygraph or the electrocardiograph. After a mechanical registration of the venous pulse is made, one obtains certain waves, two of which are primarily the result of the contraction of the right auricle and the left ventricle, respectively. The contraction of the right auricle sends an impulse upward through the vena cava and produces a slight wave in the jugular vein. The contraction of the left ventricle sends an impulse upward through the aorta and produces a wave in the carotid artery. The first is called the *a* wave, and the second, the *c* wave. When auricular fibrillation is present, the auricles are no longer contracting, and, therefore, the *a* wave disappears. Likewise, in the electrocardiograms, the representative of auricular contraction (the P wave) disappears. In its place there may be found numerous fibrillary waves (*f* waves) running more or less throughout the heart cycle. These small waves represent the numerous fibrillary twitchings that are going on in the auricles in patients with this condition. In Chapter 21 these matters are taken up in greater detail. At this point, it may be stated that, whereas electrocardiography gives the final proof of the diagnosis of auricular fibrillation, it is possible in the vast majority of cases to make accurate diagnoses by the use of simple bedside methods.

Let us now consider the effect of auricular fibrillation on the physical signs in a patient who has mitral stenosis. Before doing so it is necessary to review briefly the process involving the flow of blood from auricles to ventricles. As the ventricle begins to relax and dilate in diastole after the previous systole, blood flows from the left auricle into the left ventricle merely as a result of differences in pressure and of gravity. The pressure in the ventricle starts from zero at a time when the left auricle has already received considerable blood from the lungs and has developed some pressure. In fact, normally about seven-eighths of the blood flows from the left auricle to the left ventricle through the mitral valve by this mechanism. Only the last bit of blood is propelled by the contraction of the auricle, which gives the ventricle its final stretching just before it contracts. It follows that the early and middle portions of the diastolic murmur of mitral stenosis are produced independently of auricular contraction, and it has been proved convincingly that only the presystolic portion is produced by auricular systole. Now, if auricular fibrillation develops in the patient we are considering, who had a murmur practically filling diastole, that portion of the murmur due to auricular systole will disappear because in auricular fibrillation the auricles cease contracting. In actual practice this is just what happens.

If, therefore, we examine the patient on one day when the heart is regular and find a murmur completely filling diastole, we should observe on the following day, if auricular fibrillation is present, that the presystolic interval is now clear and that the murmur extends only through the first portion of the diastole. It may be difficult or impossible during the early days after this change has occurred to appreciate the actual disappearance of the presystolic murmur. This is so because the heart rate is still rapid. When the rate is rapid, the diastolic pauses are short and they do not permit the silent portion of the diastolic interval to appear. Each first heart sound comes so soon after the previous second sound that, although the early portion of the diastolic murmur alone is present, it actually extends throughout the short diastole and gives one the impression that the presystolic murmur is still present. If, however, one listens carefully when the heart rate is slower, one finds that the diastolic murmur has remained unchanged. When the pauses are long enough and the following first heart sounds are sufficiently removed from the previous cycle, nothing whatever will be heard in presystole; i.e., the presystolic murmur has disappeared with the development of auricular fibrillation. This discussion may seem complicated, but it is of some importance and deserves emphasis. The presystolic murmur by definition has its constant relationship with the following *first* heart sound, no matter how long the diastolic pause may be. If mitral stenosis exists and there is a normal mechanism, toward the end of the diastolic pause a rumble will often be heard. The earlier and mid-diastolic portion of the murmur of mitral stenosis is not due to auricular systole and has its constant relationship with the previous *second* heart sound. It is that portion alone that persists when auricular fibrillation is present.

It is possible for auricular fibrillation to develop in a patient with mitral stenosis at any time, even when only the presystolic murmur had previously been present. The degree of stenosis may not be sufficient, or the dynamics may be such that the velocity of the flow of blood from left auricle to left ventricle is too slow to produce a rumble. One can readily see that if this occurred we might lose the only murmur in diastole that existed. The presystolic murmur would disappear entirely because the auricles were no longer contracting and there was no other murmur in diastole. I have seen such cases in which the diagnoses were properly made and proved to be correct at postmortem examination. These, of course, are rare experiences. In one case, the patient was still thought to have mitral stenosis despite the absence of any murmur in diastole because on x-ray examination the left auricle was unusually prominent and the electrocardiograms showed right ventricular preponderance. These additional aids in the diagnosis of mitral stenosis will be taken up in greater detail below. In general, there are two types of cases of mitral stenosis when a murmur in diastole may be very faint or entirely inaudible. In the first type the stenosis is very slight and the state of the circulation very efficient. In the second type the stenosis is moderate or marked, but the degree of heart failure is considerable. The preceding discussion and particularly the experience just cited sufficiently emphasize the importance of the relation between auricular fibrillation and the murmurs of mitral stenosis.

I have paid considerable attention to auscultatory findings in mitral stenosis because I regard them to be of primary importance. One may gain the impression that the value of the stethoscope is being greatly overemphasized in this whole matter. To be sure, one obtains the most satisfactory appraisal of the degree of cardiac embarrassment from a brief inspection of the patient. The history of the symptoms of circulatory insufficiency, the degree of dyspnea, the distention of the cervical veins, and the amount of passive congestion in the body give one much more important information concerning the state of the circulation than the determination of the presence or absence of a diastolic murmur. However, in the vast majority of cases the final decision as to whether the patient has or has not mitral stenosis will depend upon auscultation. Symptoms and peripheral signs of congestion tell us whether or not a patient has *heart failure*, but auscultation tells us whether or not there is *valvular disease*. Patients have valvular disease for many years before and for a longer time than they have heart failure. In fact, during the early years before cardiac insufficiency develops, without most careful auscultation it will frequently be impossible to tell whether the patient has organic heart disease or no heart disease.

There are other criteria that are useful in the diagnosis of mitral stenosis. The finding of a definite thrill in the apex region that is diastolic in time is quite reliable evidence of the diagnosis of mitral stenosis. When the heart rate is not rapid, the proper timing of this thrill is not difficult. When the rate is 100 or more, it is almost impossible to distinguish the thrill that occurs in diastole from the vibration that is produced in a hyperactive heart. Such vibrations which are really systolic in time may be felt in patients with hyperthyroidism, in those who are in the acute stages of rheumatic infection, and in those with certain nervous states. I have frequently observed instances in which such vibrations were misinterpreted and considered to be diastolic thrills with the result that mistaken diagnoses of mitral stenosis were made. It has been my general experience that when the diastolic thrill could be detected with certainty, auscultation would easily confirm the diagnosis, whereas in many cases in which the diagnosis of mitral stenosis was quite certain, thrills were entirely absent. The finding of the diastolic thrill, however, may have greater importance when there is a combined lesion of the mitral and aortic valves.

When hypertension is absent the volume of the pulse in mitral stenosis is customarily small (pulsus parvus). Cyanosis of the lips, cheeks, and other portions of the face is common in mitral stenosis. Even when actual cyanosis is not present such patients are apt to have a rather florid countenance. This is in contrast to the pallor that typifies aortic disease. Mitral stenosis is also more common in the female than in the male. Another feature that characterizes mitral stenosis in contrast to disease of the aortic valve is its chronicity. Patients with mitral stenosis may continue to show cardiac failure over a great many years, with repeated intervals of improvement. It is possible for such a patient to have congestive heart failure and be alive and in fair comfort five to ten years later. This does not occur with anything like the same frequency in aortic valvular disease, for here the life expectancy is very short once decompensation develops. Hoarseness from pressure on the left main bronchus and dysphagia from pressure on the esophagus may result from enlargement of the left auricle. Rarely aphonia and paralysis of the left vocal cord occur from pressure of the dilated pulmonary artery on the recurrent laryngeal nerve. Pulmonary infarctions occur in mitral stenosis because of a tendency for the formation of mural thrombi within the cavities of the auricles, particularly in the auricular appendages when auricular fibrillation is present. From these thrombi, which may remain silent for many years, emboli may be dislodged. If they come from the right auricle they produce infarction of the lung; if they come from the left auricle they produce peripheral emboli in the greater circulation with resultant hemiplegia, or other embolic complications. Pulmonary infarction is by no means always due to cardiac emboli, for it is a common finding in chronic congestion of the lungs, no matter what the cause may be, and can result from local thrombosis of the pulmonary vessels or much more frequently from thrombosis of the veins of the pelvis or leg. *Hemoptysis* is also common in mitral stenosis apart from its occurrence as a result of pulmonary infarction. Such hemoptysis may be quite brisk, the patient raising a mouthful or more than a cupful of bright red blood. This may bring to one's mind the possibility of pulmonary tuberculosis or bronchogenic carcinoma, both of which conditions need to be searched for in doubtful cases. It is striking how clear the lungs may be shortly after an attack of hemoptysis in mitral stenosis, as if the bleeding resulted from a rupture of a small dilated vessel and did not reflect a high degree of generalized passive congestion. In some ways the hemoptysis resembles nosebleeds that occur in rheumatic individuals.

Considerable light has been thrown on this type of hemoptysis by Dock. It has been found by injection experiments that the bronchial veins can be enormously dilated in cases of mitral stenosis, whereas normally they are very small and difficult to visualize. They resemble miniature varices similar to those found in the esophagus in cases of cirrhosis of the liver. This mechanism does not apply to the cases in which bloody sputum is raised as a result of pulmonary infarction or in those in which there is acute pulmonary edema. In the former the sputum is blood stained or contains blood clots and in the latter pink, forthy sputum appears, while in the condition now being considered there is considerable pure blood in the absence of much obvious pulmonary congestion.

X-RAY AND ELECTROCARDIOGRAPHY

There are times when the diagnosis of mitral stenosis is doubtful, even after the most careful bedside examination. There remain at our disposal two means which may further aid in this regard, i.e., x-ray and electrocardiography. As a result of stenosis of the mitral valve, the pressure in the left auricle increases and this chamber dilates. This dilatation may be apparent on an x-ray film of the heart exposed in the ordinary manner. A bulge may be seen in the left upper border just below the pulmonary artery. Sometimes it is quite prominent. Occasionally it is difficult to distinguish this, except by fluoroscopic examination, from the dilatation of the pulmonary artery that occurs with patent ductus arteriosus or other conditions. Furthermore, the left auricle may extend with undue prominence posteriorly and bulge into the posterior mediastinal space. On occasions the left auricle will be so dilated that it will actually extend across the midline and form the right upper border of the heart. The large left auricle may produce a definite angulation of the esophagus and push it to the right. This can be observed on fluoroscopic examination or on a roentgenogram taken while barium is being swallowed. Even the left primary bronchus may be seen on x-ray examination to be raised upward or constricted by a dilated left auricle. These observations may sometimes be extremely helpful in distinguishing mitral stenosis from congenital heart disease. Finally, with improved x-ray technique, it has been possible to see calcification of the mitral valve on fluoroscopic examination and less frequently on the flat x-ray film. When this is disclosed by proper examination it always means mitral stenosis and it can be distinguished from calcification of the annulus fibrosus which usually causes no disturbance in the function of the heart and is an unimportant finding. Rytand has called attention to an auscultatory sign that might lead one to suspect the presence of a calcified mitral annulus. It consists of detecting a short apical diastolic murmur in elderly patients with or without a systolic murmur who also have heart block. The sound is due to auricular activity. The detection of calcification of valves has proved of great aid in diagnosis, especially when combined lesions are present.

The electrocardiogram occasionally gives helpful indirect evidence of mitral stenosis. As a result of hypertrophy and dilatation of the auricles in this condition, the auricular complex (P wave) may develop a peculiar form, become unduly large, prominent, and notched, and have a flat top (see Chap. 21, Figs. 140, 141). When these changes are marked they are almost invariably indicative of mitral stenosis. A further change that results from mitral stenosis is hypertrophy of the right ventricle. The pulmonary pressure is increased, and with it a compensatory hypertrophy and dilatation of the right ventricle take place. Inasmuch as the electrocardiograms give some measure of preponderant hypertrophy of one ventricle over another, in mitral stenosis they may show certain alterations from the normal. These changes consist of prominent downward deflection of the initial ventricular complex in Lead I and a prominent upward deflection in Lead III. In addition there are changes in the precordial leads that are even more valuable in detecting hypertrophy of either ventricle. Such curves, however, must be interpreted with great caution, for not infrequently they may be obtained in subjects with emphysema or in patients with certain forms of congenital heart disease. Simultaneous recordings of the electrocardiogram and phonocardiogram may also throw light on the diagnosis. In mitral stenosis the interval between the Q wave and the first apical heart sound (M_1) is prolonged. The normal Q-M_1, interval is about 0.04 second, whereas in mitral stenosis it averages 0.06 second with a range from 0.04 to 0.09 second. When the interval is 0.07 second or greater, the diagnosis of mitral stenosis is very likely. The interval between the second sound and the opening snap is shorter as the stenosis is more advanced. It is also thought that these changes become less pronounced after a successful valvuloplasty.

Electrocardiography in general has not been very valuable as an aid in diagnosis of valvular disease, but occasionally this evidence, coupled with other data which of themselves might not have been sufficient, enables one to make a proper diagnosis.

Now that accurate anatomical diagnosis of valvular disease is so important when operative therapy is being considered, other diagnostic methods are being employed in doubtful cases. Ballistocardiography is thought to show changes that are helpful in the diagnosis of mitral stenosis. These findings need further study and confirmation. Catheterization studies of the heart may show increased pulmonary wedge pressure (pulmonary capillary pressure). This is common in cases of mitral stenosis but is also present in other conditions accompanied by left ventricular failure. Another diagnostic procedure consists of injecting dye and visualizing the left auricle and even the constriction of the mitral valve. This method is unsatisfactory with ordinary technique, or the chambers of the left side of the heart are poorly visualized by the x-ray. When the dye is injected directly into the left auricle either through the back or by bronchoscopy, as is done by some, much more satisfactory results can be obtained. Finally, pressure determinations in the left auricle and left ventricle, determined by inserting a catheter into the left auricle and through the mitral valve, may afford convincing evidence of mitral stenosis. The finding of a distinctly greater diastolic pressure in the auricle than in the ventricle is fairly diagnostic. One can see that extreme measures may be necessary to establish a preoperative diagnosis in some doubtful cases.

CLINICAL CRITERIA FOR DIAGNOSIS

One can recapitulate the clinical criteria for the diagnosis of mitral stenosis. In order of importance they are (1) a diastolic or presystolic apical murmur, (2) calcification of mitral valve on fluoroscopy, (3) broad prominent notched "P" waves with evidence of right ventricular hypertrophy in the electrocardiograms, (4) an accentuated apical first heart sound, (5) an opening snap, and (6) x-ray evidence of left auricular and right ventricular enlargement. The evidence of an accompanying or predominant mitral insufficiency will be (1) a loud apical systolic murmur, (2) *marked* cardiac enlargement especially of the *left auricle*, (3) left ventricular enlargement on x-ray or electrocardiographic examination, and (4) systolic expansion of the left auricle. Although there are various combinations of the findings typical of mitral stenosis or of mitral insufficiency in the same case, the greater the evidence for one or the other the more prominent the respective lesion will be. It must be borne in mind that exceptions do occur, for even tight mitral stenosis may exist with no audible diastolic murmur, and no significant mitral insufficiency may be present with a very loud apical systolic murmur. In this connection the past history of rheumatic fever or the presence of unexplained auricular fibrillation may point to valvular disease but will not differentiate mitral insufficiency from mitral stenosis.

COMMON SIGNS OF HEART FAILURE

Throughout this discussion nothing has been said about the common signs of heart failure that may be found in a patient with mitral stenosis, such as engorged liver and cervical veins, generalized edema, or enlargement of the heart. These are not particularly characteristic of mitral stenosis, although it must be stated that enlargement of the heart is more apt to be transverse, especially to the right, in mitral stenosis, than it is in other forms of heart disease. The signs of heart failure associated with mitral stenosis will be taken up in detail when discussing the problem of general cardiac failure.

Little has been said about the presence of a systolic murmur at the apex in mitral stenosis. This, of course, is a very common finding but does not indicate that the mitral valve is stenosed. It means that there is a concomitant mitral insufficiency or it has the questionable significance that accompanies systolic murmurs in general. It has been generally taught that mitral stenosis is almost always associated with mitral insufficiency. Whether or not regurgitation of blood actually takes place in many of these cases is difficult to ascertain. The only physical evidence of this would be the presence of an apical systolic murmur. It is not sufficiently appreciated that, in a large number of cases of clearcut mitral stenosis, no systolic murmur whatever can be heard. The same may be said of stenosis of the aortic valve. I am of the opinion that mitral stenosis without any insufficiency is very common, and that it often develops in patients who previously never had a systolic murmur.

It also must be understood that mitral stenosis is not always the sole valvular lesion of the heart. There may be additional involvement of the aortic or more rarely of the tricuspid valve. The diagnosis of combined lesions is no simple matter, but, in so far as it can be determined, it will depend upon the proper utilization of the criteria for each individual lesion with some regard for the effect of one upon the other.

MITRAL STENOSIS AND BLOOD PRESSURE

This discussion would not be complete without some mention of the relation between mitral stenosis and the blood pressure. The old term "pulsus parvus" reflects the general impression that the pulse is small and the blood pressure is low in this condition. In a study of almost 800 cases of mitral stenosis, it was found that when the disease was present in young people the blood pressure tended to be lower than that for the average population of that age group. However, in patients with mitral stenosis who were in the higher decades of life the average blood pressure increased decidedly until it reached 180 systolic and 95 diastolic for patients 60 to 69 years of age. This I feel cannot be an accidental finding, for certainly no group of patients suffering from some unrelated condition, such as cancer of the breast or ulcer of the stomach, has hypertension as a general rule. It is hard to believe that mitral stenosis itself accounts for the hypertension, for when mitral stenosis is present in young persons the pressure is even lower than normal. Yet how is the frequent association of mitral stenosis and hypertension to be explained?

One may at the outset maintain that the mitral stenosis in these older hypertensive patients is not rheumatic in origin and that it is due to sclerotic changes in the mitral ring, similar to the peripheral arterial sclerosis with which the hypertension is associated. One might object to the accuracy of the diagnosis of mitral stenosis in these elderly hypertensive persons on the ground that the presystolic gallop rhythm which is common in hypertension might be mistaken for the presystolic murmur of mitral stenosis. In answer to the latter it may be said that the diagnosis in a sufficient number of these elderly patients has been confirmed at autopsy. As far as the former criticism is concerned, apart from the general view that I have expressed before, that mitral stenosis is probably due to no other cause than rheumatism, a past history of rheumatic fever or chorea was found in 50 per cent of these hypertensive patients, a percentage which corresponds fairly closely to that of a rheumatic history in any group of patients having mitral stenosis. Inasmuch as mitral stenosis per se does not produce hypertension, it is possible that the underlying chronic rheumatic infection insidiously produces arterial changes that terminate in hypertension. Another possibility is that a long-standing disease process in the heart by some reflex mechanism can initiate hypertension. Furthermore, the great frequency of hypertension in the older patients with mitral stenosis may be due to the fact that the elevation of the blood pressure enabled them to survive and reach the later decades of life. A more likely explanation, it seems, is that mitral stenosis and hypertension are commonly associated because the underlying rheumatic infection has a predilection for patients who have a vascular vulnerability. The disease has a tendency to select certain types of people and this so-called "vascular" type is vulnerable both to the infectious and to the degenerative form of heart disease. The frequent association of rheumatic heart disease and angina pectoris in the same family is additional evidence in favor of this concept.

There is also some clinical and statistical evidence to indicate that the hypertension developing in patients with mitral stenosis need not produce any deleterious effect but on the contrary may be actually helpful. Although it may add certain symptoms as a result of the hypertension itself, when these are not severe there is reason to believe that it delays the progress of mitral stenosis. It is very curious that so many patients with mitral stenosis over 50 years of age have hypertension in addition. I believe that the hypertension prolongs their lives and enables them to reach the later decades, for the great majority of patients with mitral stenosis without hypertension die before they reach the age of

50. One may explain the beneficial effect of hypertension by supposing that as a result the cavity of the left ventricle tends to remain large and somewhat dilated and that this dilatation tends to counteract or delay the antagonistic, progressive contraction that is going on in the mitral ring as a result of the rheumatic mitral stenosis. Another possible factor is that mitral stenosis is a burden on the right side of the heart and hypertension embarrasses the left side of the heart. In this way the two burdens are equalized, and if congestive failure is due to an imbalance of the two ventricles, as is believed by many authorities, the effect may be beneficial. I have frequently seen elderly patients with mitral stenosis and hypertension continue to do fairly well many years after it was expected that they would die. It therefore appears to be a somewhat favorable sign to find an increasing blood pressure in cases of mitral stenosis. A final possible explanation is that cases with slight or moderate constriction of the mitral valve are more likely to reach the later decades of life when hypertension is more common. In any event, one might look upon the combination of mitral stenosis and hypertension with some degree of optimism.

CHAPTER 4

Diseases of the Aortic and Tricuspid Valves

There are certain striking differences between diseases of the aortic and the mitral valve. Aortic valve disease is more common in males than in females, and the reverse is true for mitral disease. Pain in the chest of the type that is characteristic of angina pectoris is frequent in aortic disease and is rare in mitral disease. Pallor and sweating are more typical in the former, whereas plethora or at least a florid countenance is more typical in the latter. Patients with aortic valve disease, although frequently complaining of chest pain and palpitation, have much less dyspnea compared with those having mitral disease. They generally also have better bodily strength and remain ambulatory and able to do work for a longer time with outspoken evidence of valve disease; however, when general circulatory insufficiency does develop, with dyspnea, congestion of the lungs and liver, or peripheral edema, they have not the recuperative power that is commonly seen in patients with mitral stenosis. In other words, when decompensation is once developed in a patient with aortic valve disease, the outlook is rather grave. The average length of life after such an occurrence is not apt to be more than two or three years. In mitral valve disease, on the other hand, frequently several attacks of decompensation occur, each followed by a partial restoration of circulatory efficiency. The patients are thereby enabled to continue for many years on restricted activities. Pulmonary infarctions are less common in aortic than in mitral cases. This may be partly but not entirely accounted for by the fact that auricular fibrillation is rare in disease of the aortic valve and very common in mitral stenosis. Disturbances in conduction, such as heart block and bundle branch block, are more common in aortic than in mitral disease. The same is true of attacks of syncope and sudden death. A final difference that has impressed me is that subacute bacterial endocarditis is more common in aortic disease than in mitral stenosis. This does not mean that the mitral valve is less frequently involved in subacute bacterial endocarditis, for in most cases when the mitral valve is involved there is only an insufficiency of the valve but no stenosis.

There are three general causes of disease of the aortic valve; namely, rheumatism, syphilis, and arteriosclerosis. The young are apt to be rheumatic, the middle-aged, syphilitic, and the aged, hypertensive or sclerotic. This division is quite arbitrary, as many cases overlap from one

49

age period into another. Aortic valvular disease may also be an occasional complication of chronic arthritis, especially when the spine is involved. In certain sections of the country almost all cases of aortic insufficiency will be syphilitic in origin. This discrepancy has made some authors state that aortic insufficiency is invariably due to syphilis. In a locality like New England, more individual cases of rheumatic aortic insufficiency are seen than any other type, although frequently this is associated with other valvular disease. On rare occasions aortic insufficiency may be functional or transient. This may occur during the very asthenic stages of marked anemia of the pernicious type and in hypertension.

Aortic Insufficiency

The two types of lesions of the aortic valve to be considered are aortic insufficiency and aortic stenosis. Let us first take up aortic insufficiency. The heart in this condition will become hypertrophied in the course of time and in some cases this enlargement becomes extreme. The left ventricle is the chamber that bears the main brunt of the leak and therefore it becomes not only thickened but eventually considerably dilated. This enlargement extends downward more than outward, so that the apex impulse may be felt in the sixth interspace outside the nipple line or even lower. The apex impulse is apt to be heaving and forceful, denoting a thickened musculature of the left ventricle. It is well to become familiar with this type of impulse no matter under what circumstances it is felt, for it gives a fairly satisfactory indication that the wall of the left ventricle is thickened and sometimes enables one to decide that the heart is hypertrophied, even when percussion outlines are doubtful. One gains the impression that with systole the apex impulse lifts the palpating finger and keeps it elevated for an appreciable time before it recedes. It does not merely tap the finger. Only on rare occasions can a diastolic thrill be felt at the base of the heart in aortic insufficiency. Percussion merely aids in estimating whether the heart outline is enlarged or not, and in no way helps in identifying aortic valvular disease. Auscultation reveals the decisive evidence of the diagnosis. In uncomplicated conditions, the heart rhythm will generally be found regular. Almost invariably a systolic murmur will be heard at the base of the heart and often there is a systolic murmur at the apex as well. The apical systolic murmur is due either to a relative mitral insufficiency or to a concomitant mitral endocarditis. When the aortic insufficiency is due to syphilis or sclerosis the apical systolic murmur should be regarded as due to relative mitral insufficiency and not to a true endocarditis, because a true organic mitral insufficiency practically never results from syphilis or arteriosclerosis. Here the left ventricle becomes markedly dilated and the mitral ring, although essentially normal, is large and the leaflets do not completely close the opening during systole. When the condition is rheumatic in origin, it will always be difficult to decide whether or not the mitral valve is structurally diseased unless additional evidence is obtained pointing to mitral stenosis as well. If aortic stenosis is also present an apical systolic murmur may actually be coming from the aortic valve.

There are three possible explanations of the basal systolic murmur in aortic insufficiency. First, it may be due to an actual structural or relative stenosis of the aortic valve. This I think is more common than is recognized. Secondly, it has been thought that a roughening of the aortic wall such as is found in syphilis and arteriosclerosis may produce a systolic murmur. This I think is fallacious, for I have frequently heard no murmur when later at autopsy the aorta showed extreme degeneration. Finally, the murmur may be due to the hyperdynamics of the circulation at that moment. There may be a momentary increase in the rate of flow of the blood during systole that accompanies aortic insufficiency. I believe that the latter factor is more important than is generally assumed.

The apical and basal systolic murmurs discussed in the foregoing paragraphs, although generally present in aortic insufficiency, are in no way diagnostic, for they occur when the aortic valves are competent. The most important and characteristic finding is the presence of a diastolic murmur heard at the aortic area, and even with louder intensity at the third left interspace near the sternum and propagated downward. This murmur has a blowing quality, starts directly with or replaces the second heart sound, and is diminuendo in character. At times it is quite faint and requires most careful auscultation for its detection. In some cases it will be audible only if searched for with the patient sitting up and examined during deep expiration. In general it is unwise to make the diagnosis of aortic insufficiency without this finding.

Although the detection of an aortic diastolic murmur is valid evidence of aortic incompetency, especially if there are peripheral signs as well, postmortem examination may occasionally fail to confirm the finding of valvular disease. This does not mean that the diagnosis was incorrect, for the valve may have been incompetent in life and still show no structural disease at autopsy. When the heart is examined post mortem we do not see the structures as they existed with their normal tone and under blood pressure relations that prevailed during life. The valves may have been relatively insufficient because of dilatation of the aortic ring. Such relative aortic insufficiency is not uncommon in hypertension and in marked anemia when the valves are structurally sound. Similar dynamic dilatation has been repeatedly observed in the aorta itself. I have seen instances in which the x-ray showed very marked dilatation of the aorta, pointing strongly to the diagnosis of aneurysm, when at autopsy a perfectly normal small elastic aorta was found.

There are instances in which a presystolic murmur will be heard at the apex in cases of aortic insufficiency. This is the so-called "Austin Flint" murmur. It may be difficult to interpret the significance of an Austin Flint murmur, for it has the same time and quality and is heard in the same place as the murmur of mitral stenosis. It must be admitted, however, that this murmur can be present when mitral stenosis is absent. The practical point of view I have taken in this regard is that if the so-called Austin Flint murmur is heard in syphilitic aortic insufficiency I would accept it as real, but that when it is present in a rheumatic case I would be apt to regard it as due to concomitant mitral stenosis. This is based on the empirical pathological experience that syphilis never produces mitral stenosis and that rheumatism frequently does, even when aortic disease is also present. However, I have seen instances of rheumatic aortic insufficiency in which not only a presystolic murmur was present at the apex, but also a presystolic thrill and x-ray evidence of a prominent left auricle were noted in cases in which at postmortem examination mitral stenosis was not demonstrated.

PERIPHERAL SIGNS

There are, in addition, very important peripheral signs of aortic insufficiency which are more or less dependent upon the increased pulse pressure that accompanies this condition. The most striking one of these is the hyperactive agitated pulsations of the arteries, especially the carotid arteries. They beat violently so that the entire lateral portions of the neck seem to pulsate. The radial pulse has a water-hammer quality, the so-called "Corrigan" pulse. In general, the lower the diastolic pressure the greater the degree of aortic insufficiency. There is a capillary pulse that may be made out on observing the fingernails while exerting mild pressure. This may also be detected in watching a flush come and go after rubbing the forehead or while pressing on the inside of the lower lip or the lower lobe of the ear with a glass slide. In addition, there is the so-called "pistol shot" in the femoral artery that one may detect with the stethoscope. Here, if pressure is applied during auscultation, a systolic murmur may be heard. This murmur is really a normal phenomenon, but what is more significant is that in many cases of aortic insufficiency with appropriate pressure over the femoral artery, one may hear a distinct diastolic murmur (Duroziez's sign). These various peripheral evidences of aortic insufficiency are by no means pathognomonic. They occur to a less marked degree in a variety of conditions. In many states in which there is a lax atonic peripheral vascular tree the patient may present these signs. They are commonly seen in association with hyperthyroidism, certain types of anemia, especially pernicious anemia, fevers, nervous hearts, and in some cases of hypertension. In most of these conditions the pulse pressure will also be found greater than normal. I have frequently observed the capillary pulse and a Corrigan pulse in conjunction with the above conditions, sometimes even noting pulsation of the retinal arteries.

The peripheral signs of aortic insufficiency, although in general not so helpful in diagnosis as the diastolic murmur, nevertheless are valuable when there are combined valvular lesions. This is especially true in rheumatic aortic insufficiency. Here, it may be difficult to interpret the origin of a diastolic murmur heard along the left sternal border. Such a murmur may have various causes. At times the diastolic murmur of mitral stenosis may be so prominent and loud that it is actually well heard even toward the base of the heart. The diastolic murmur, on the other hand, may be due to an aortic insufficiency, which is combined with the mitral stenosis. It may be a so-called "Graham Steell" murmur. This latter murmur is supposed to be due to a relative pulmonary insufficiency occurring in mitral stenosis, and is heard in the pulmonary area (second left interspace) and along the left sternal border. Moreover, the presence of a diastolic murmur in this area, together with the systolic murmur that is also present, may be attributed to congenital heart disease. Finally it can be the result of organic tricuspid stenosis. Frequently it is impossible to make an accurate differentiation. In such instances the peripheral signs may decide the question as to whether aortic insufficiency is present or not. One may have to utilize all available means of diagnosis to arrive at a proper decision. The presence of auricular fibrillation will point definitely to mitral stenosis and the snapping quality of the first heart sound should make one suspect its presence. The x-ray finding of a dilated pulmonary artery will suggest the diagnosis of a patent ductus arteriosus or some other congenital lesion. When the patient has obvious aortic insufficiency and the question of an additional mitral stenosis comes up, if auricular fibrillation exists both valves are probably involved. Also, if there is evidence of right ventricular hypertrophy in the electrocardiograms or a prominent left auricle on x-ray examination, it is likely that the lesion is not confined to the aortic valve, but that mitral stenosis is also present, for if aortic insufficiency were the sole lesion we would expect marked left ventricular preponderance in the electrocardiograms. Although this evidence is not indisputable, it is helpful. In order to make the diagnosis of a Graham Steell murmur, it would be necessary to find this diastolic murmur present in the absence of peripheral signs of aortic insufficiency. One would also expect that the patient would be decompensated and that the murmur should either disappear entirely or at least diminish in intensity as improvement in the circulation occurred. Although in most cases the interpretation of the basal diastolic murmur is not difficult, when it is doubtful it is likely to be of only academic interest, unless cardiac surgery is contemplated.

Aortic Stenosis

Stenosis of the aortic valve is frequently due to rheumatic infection, is occasionally the result of arteriosclerosis, is rarely congenital, but is never syphilitic in origin. There was a time when the diagnosis of aortic stenosis was made much too frequently, as many patients who merely had a basal systolic murmur were regarded as suffering from this condition. This was followed by a period of undue caution when it was regarded as a very rare disease. At present we must take a middle course, for there is ample experience to teach us that it is fairly common, and that it is frequently overlooked.

The younger individuals with aortic stenosis are generally regarded as suffering from rheumatic valvular disease, whether the aortic lesion is found to be an isolated one or is combined with mitral or tricuspid involvement. Individuals with aortic stenosis who are over 50 or 60 years of age, who frequently show no significant involvement of the other valves, have been regarded as arteriosclerotic. It has been my impression that many, if not most, of such patients are also rheumatic. It is curious that even in this older group a positive history of previous rheumatic infection will be elicited in almost 30 per cent of the cases. This is true notwithstanding the fact that the interval between the possible early infection and the present illness might have been forty to fifty years, that a history of rheumatism may easily have been forgotten, and that many years ago atypical rheumatic infections were doubtless overlooked. Furthermore, as a result of a better understanding of the pathologic findings in rheumatism, pathologists are now willing to admit that cases which they formerly had called arteriosclerotic they are now ready to call rheumatic. Another argument against the arteriosclerotic origin of many of these cases is that as a rule the ascending aorta, where sclerotic processes in general are so extensive, is apt to show comparatively few atheromatous changes in aortic stenosis. This may, however, be due to a protective effect that the stenosed valve exercises in buffering the systolic impact of the aorta. It is also conceivable that some cases of aortic stenosis are the result of a previous nonrheumatic infection of the aortic valve, or may even represent the healed stage of a previous subacute bacterial endocarditis. Furthermore, some of the cases very likely are congenital in origin. If it is known that a systolic murmur or some cardiac abnormality was detected shortly after birth or during the first few years of life the diagnosis of congenital aortic or subaortic stenosis is more tenable. Finally, the likelihood that arteriosclerosis alone can be responsible for a portion of the older cases cannot be entirely dismissed.

The general clinical features of aortic stenosis resemble those of aortic insufficiency in that it is more common in males, it is found in hearts with a regular rather than an absolutely irregular rhythm, and it is rarely associated with emboli or pulmonary infarction. The left ventricle is often enormously hypertrophied, with only very little dilatation. The heaviest hearts are those with aortic stenosis, although the largest silhouettes on x-ray examination are those of mitral disease. This is so because of the marked dilatation that occurs with the latter condition. Dyspnea comes late, the patients maintaining rather good health for long periods of time until congestive failure finally intervenes. When this occurs, the prognosis is grave, for death is likely to intervene within two or three years. The foregoing generalizations do not hold, however, when there is combined mitral and aortic valvular disease.

One frequent complication of aortic stenosis is angina pectoris. This,

I believe, is often overlooked. It has currently been taught that angina is a common accompaniment of aortic insufficiency and little mention is made of its association with other valvular lesions. The explanation given is that the heart is nourished in diastole, for during the actual systolic contraction blood flows out through the aorta while the coronary arteries are practically occluded. In aortic insufficiency blood is regurgitating back to the left ventricle from the aorta during diastole and with the diminished diastolic pressure there is inadequate nourishment of the heart muscle. Although this seems to be a logical explanation, there are certain conflicting clinical facts. In patients with aortic insufficiency the occurrence or severity of angina by no means follows the level of the diastolic pressure. Furthermore, in cases of syphilitic aortic insufficiency in which the mouths of the coronary arteries are not occluded the degree of regurgitation is very often of an extreme degree and yet angina is rare. On the other hand, it has seemed to me that in patients with aortic valvular disease and angina pectoris the element of stenosis has been more prominent than that of regurgitation. In fact, I have frequently seen angina with aortic stenosis when there was no evidence of aortic regurgitation.

The explanation of the frequency of angina in aortic stenosis is obscure. Possibly several factors are involved. It is now believed that there is coronary flow during systole as well as diastole. The ventricular wall is generally thicker in aortic stenosis than in pure aortic insufficiency or in other types of heart disease. This may result in a greater degree of relative myocardial anoxia because the coronary blood supply may not keep pace with the hypertrophy, and oxygen diffusion into thick muscle fibers is more difficult. Furthermore, the work of the heart must be enormously increased to expel blood through such narrow valves. Also the velocity of the blood ejected through the stenosed valve must be terrific to maintain a normal output per minute. This rapid stream may possibly exercise a suction action on the mouths of the coronary arteries which lie just beyond the valve. If this happens, blood actually is extracted from, rather than fed to, the heart during systole. Finally, numerous cases have additional significant coronary sclerosis to account for the angina. However, I have seen young patients with aortic stenosis and angina in whom sudden death occurred, and postmortem examination showed normal coronary arteries. Here some of the above mechanisms may have been involved.

Angina is frequently overlooked in aortic stenosis because insufficient attention is paid to minor complaints such as mild sternal distress on hurrying. Often the patient will not even mention it to his physician and it will have to be brought out by direct questioning. This accounts for the frequent occurrence of sudden and unexpected death that is so common in aortic valvular disease. Granted that an integral part of the symptom complex called "angina pectoris" is a likelihood of sudden death, eliciting a proper history will often forewarn the physician of possible sudden fatalities in aortic cases that otherwise would remain unexplained. Furthermore, when no such previous history of angina can be obtained it is not inconceivable that a first attack of angina may end fatally. I once saw a man of 55 who was suffering from congestive heart failure. After his condition had improved it was planned that a complete thyroidectomy would be performed. Many other physicians and I had seen him over a period of a year and we all were in accord in the diagnosis of aortic stenosis. Finally, on direct questioning, I found that he had a definite history of anginal distress of about two years' duration, a fact that he never mentioned before because his primary complaint was breathlessness. The day before the time set for the operation, while he was apparently in good condition, he suddenly expired. If the diagnosis of angina had not been made this patient's demise would have been regarded as one of those unexplained sudden deaths in aortic disease. Experiences similar to this one are not uncommon.

Another peculiarity of aortic stenosis is that it is frequently accompanied by a tendency to faintness or to actual syncope. The exact explanation of this is obscure but it may be linked up with peculiarities in the carotid sinus reflex. It is now well known that if this reflex is hyperactive, giddiness, weakness, and fainting attacks can occur. It is, therefore, necessary to study the condition of this reflex in cases of aortic stenosis in the hope of throwing further light on this otherwise obscure phenomenon. So far, however, in most cases a normal sensitivity of the carotid sinus has been found. Syncope occurs particularly on effort and in the last analysis is probably due to cerebral anoxemia. It is unlikely that it is due to temporary heart block, despite the fact that conduction defects are common in aortic stenosis. May it be due to a temporary increase in heart rate with a decrease in cardiac output? The problem is still unsolved.

In this connection it is of interest that in aortic stenosis the heart rate is often slow. This may be so even when gross evidence of congestive heart failure is present. In fact there are few conditions apart from aortic stenosis in which advanced congestive heart failure will be found with a heart rate under 70 or 60, in which the slow rate cannot be accounted for by heart block or by the administration of digitalis. This point has been useful in first directing suspicion to the diagnosis of aortic stenosis and then detecting the direct clinical evidence of the lesion by careful examination. This slow heart rate may possibly be due to the same factor that makes the patient subject to syncope or may in some way be related to the vagus apparatus.

For some unknown reason, the basal metabolism may be elevated in some cases of aortic stenosis. This may occasionally occur when there is little or no evidence of congestive failure. The increase in metabolism may be as great as 20 to 40 per cent. I have seen several proved instances of aortic stenosis in which repeated examinations showed such readings and yet on gross and microscopic study of the thyroid gland nothing abnormal was found. The explanation that the increase is due to the marked cardiac hypertrophy hardly seems valid as many other cardiac patients with great enlargement of the heart have shown a normal metabolism. This problem needs serious consideration when the question of latent thyrocardiac disease comes up.

The clinical diagnosis of aortic stenosis in the past has generally depended on finding a systolic thrill at the base of the heart. If one waits for this finding to be present the diagnosis is likely to be correct but many other cases will have been overlooked. It is now necessary and possible to make accurate diagnoses of aortic stenosis without detecting the systolic thrill. When it is marked it can readily be felt in the second right interspace or over the upper or middle portion of the sternum. It is often missed because careful palpation is not practiced or because it is not searched for properly. A fainter thrill may only become apparent if palpation is performed during a held expiration with the patient sitting upright or leaning forward. The thrill can be confused with systolic thrills that accompany congenital heart disease, but the differential diagnosis is generally established without difficulty by the presence or absence of other findings such as cyanosis, clubbing of the fingers, electrocardiographic changes (right ventricular hypertrophy with pulmonary stenosis and left ventricular hypertrophy with aortic stenosis), and x-ray examination. One must be careful to interpret as a thrill only that condition in which a real purr of significant duration is felt. In this way it will not be mistaken for systolic or other impacts of the chest that are common in hyperactive hearts or in thin-chested individuals. This differentiation is important, for true basal systolic thrills in the absence of congenital heart disease generally mean aortic stenosis.

A second indisputable sign of aortic stenosis is the finding of calcification of the aortic valve on x-ray examination. This is best detected by fluoroscopic examination but may even appear on the flat heart film. It needs to be distinguished from calcification in the mitral valve or in the myocardium. This can be easily done by a trained observer, the main differential points being its location and the fact that at the very beginning of systole calcification in the mitral valve will be seen to move upward whereas the aortic valve moves downward. It is obvious that calcification of a valve must be a late process, and when it is sufficiently advanced to become visible the valve must have been diseased for years. In fact, in many cases in which calcification is not very extensive it will not be detected. It is surprising, however, how frequently this diagnosis was made on x-ray examination and in all such patients that were examined post mortem the x-ray diagnosis was confirmed. Although calcified aortic stenosis is generally seen in older people it is not at all rare in younger persons. In the younger group the disease is obviously rheumatic in origin and I suspect that in many of the older group it is also of rheumatic source, although the older patients have been generally regarded as arteriosclerotic. It must be borne in mind that calcium deposits are often found in any long-standing chronic inflammatory process and if a patient survives an aortic lesion long enough calcification may result.

The other clinical signs of aortic stenosis are less important because they are more difficult to interpret. The second aortic sound is diminished in intensity or absent in many cases. The difficulty is that the pulmonary second sound may be audible in the aortic area making it impossible to distinguish the origin of these sounds. A systolic murmur will be present in practically every case of aortic stenosis. This murmur is best heard in second right intercostal space (the aortic area) or not infrequently over the upper precordium and midsternal region. It is generally a fairly loud murmur and coarse in quality. The difficulty is that basal systolic murmurs are common in such a variety of circumstances that this alone cannot constitute reliable evidence for the diagnosis of aortic stenosis. When it is appreciated, however, that the constricting process, which eventually becomes sufficient to produce a palpable systolic thrill or calcification of the valve detectable by x-ray, is a very slow one extending over many years, it is evident that the diagnosis can only be suspected in many instances during these intervening years. When phonocardiograms are taken the classic systolic murmur has a peculiar diamond-shaped appearance (Fig. 212). Although this is not pathognomonic it is sufficiently characteristic to distinguish it occasionally from the murmur of mitral insufficiency. It is obvious that a very loud murmur must have been fainter or even very slight years before or at its onset. I am convinced that many patients who merely show systolic murmurs of moderate or faint intensity without much other evidence of heart disease have aortic stenosis, even when the systolic murmur is louder at the apex than at the base of the heart. I have followed such cases long enough to see the true nature of the lesion develop. At first a systolic murmur would be heard when there were no symptoms. Such a patient may have been refused insurance because of it. At this time a thrill, a diastolic murmur, or appreciable hypertrophy would be absent. The murmurs might have been called functional systolic murmurs. I might have made the diagnosis of mitral insufficiency, because in some of these cases the murmur was quite prominent near the nipple as well as toward the base of the heart, or the murmurs may have been designated as instances of "systolic murmurs, cause unknown." Then as years went on a definite basal thrill would become palpable or calcification of the valve would be found on x-ray examination. Dyspnea or anginal pain were frequent eventual developments in such patients.

Although most cases of aortic stenosis in which the diagnosis can be made will have moderate or very loud murmurs (grade III to VI), there will be some with only faint basal murmurs. I recall a man I followed for twenty years who always showed a grade I (rarely grade II) aortic systolic and diastolic murmur. He had had an early history of rheumatic fever and remained quite well all these years. He had a fairly large chest with an increased anteroposterior diameter. Although the murmurs were very faint, calcified aortic stenosis could be seen fluoroscopically, which was confirmed eventually post mortem. In such cases the systolic murmur is faintly heard because of the thickness of the intervening space between the heart and the outside of the chest.

The lesson to be drawn from these experiences is that we should be more ready to make the diagnosis of aortic stenosis before all the classical signs are present.

Insufficiency so frequently accompanies stenosis of the aortic valve that one should make a careful search for a basal diastolic murmur. When it is found it will lend support to the diagnosis that the aortic valve is at least diseased and that the systolic murmur, which can be due to so many other causes, is in fact the result of aortic valvular disease. Even the presence of a systolic and a diastolic murmur at the aortic area does not necessarily indicate stenosis of the valve. Both murmurs are present in most instances of free aortic regurgitation without stenosis, such as occurs in syphilitic aortic insufficiency, a condition which never results in stenosis of the valve. It is sometimes taught that when there is stenosis of a valve there must be insufficiency; i.e., if a valve is so deformed and scarred that it cannot open it would similarly be impossible for it to close completely. Although this view sounds logical and one is further impressed by its validity on seeing the rigid calcified valves post mortem, the fact remains that in many instances of aortic stenosis no diastolic murmur will be audible nor will there be any peripheral signs of aortic insufficiency. The same holds true for mitral stenosis, for here in many instances, although there may be a long diastolic rumble indicating a fair degree of stenosis, no systolic murmurs will be heard after the snapping first heart sound.

There are other auscultatory signs in aortic stenosis. Murmurs may be present at the apex of the heart indicating an additional organic involvement of the mitral valve or a relative insufficiency of that valve. The basal systolic murmur and thrill may be transmitted upward into the vessels of the neck. The finding of a systolic murmur and thrill over the vessels of the neck, without similar signs over the chest, cannot be relied upon as certain evidence of aortic stenosis, because they may be present in other conditions, such as hyperthyroidism, anemia, and nervous states. Furthermore the apical systolic murmur may merely be transmitted from the aortic valve and may not signify any additional lesion.

The plateau form of radial pulse is fairly characteristic of aortic stenosis. It is often overlooked because the examiner does not think about it. When it is present the pulse will be found to rise and remain sustained longer than in other conditions. It will obviously be absent if there is also sufficient aortic insufficiency, for this will counteract the plateau character with a collapsing quality.

The blood pressure in aortic stenosis is variable. In the classic case the systolic level is apt to be low and the diastolic level comparatively high, producing a small pulse pressure. One frequently finds readings such as 110 mm. systolic and 90 mm. diastolic. Two other factors, however, affect the blood pressure so that almost any reading might be found in different cases, i.e., an accompanying aortic insufficiency and an independent essential hypertension. The result is that both the systolic and the diastolic pressure may vary from extremely low to extremely high levels.

The x-ray in typical aortic stenosis will show a prominent, rounded left ventricle producing a boot-shaped heart. The electrocardiogram will reflect the degree of left ventricular preponderant hypertrophy that is present and occasionally disturbances in conduction.

Just as occurs in mitral stenosis, there are times when the diagnosis of aortic stenosis is in dispute or the degree of stenosis is uncertain, and contemplation of cardiac surgery makes this information necessary. There are then other diagnostic procedures that are available. A tracing of the brachial pulse may show the slow upstroke that is characteristic of aortic stenosis. Determination of the pressure in the left ventricle may establish even the degree of obstruction, because when the gradient between the left ventricle and the aorta is great the stenosis must be severe.

Disease of the Tricuspid Valve

Although functional insufficiency of the tricuspid valve is common, organic disease of this valve is rare. It is easy to understand the frequency with which this valve becomes relatively incompetent. When there is congestive failure, the heart is generally dilated. If the right ventricle dilates, the tricuspid ring is thereby stretched and the valve, although normal in structure, will no longer be able to close the enlarged opening. This will necessarily result in a regurgitation of blood from the right ventricle into the right auricle. This condition is common in all types of heart disease, but particularly in mitral stenosis, when the burden on the right side of the heart eventually becomes great. Under such circumstances, the patient is apt to have not only marked evidence of cardiac failure with cyanosis, edema, and engorged liver, but regurgitation of blood through the tricuspid valve may show itself in other ways. There may be an actual systolic pulsation of the veins of the neck and limbs, and a pulsating liver. It is no simple matter to detect these changes, for normally there are pulsations in the jugular veins which are difficult to time. Likewise it is difficult to distinguish systolic pulsations of the liver from pulsations of the right side of the heart and abdominal aorta. By placing both hands around the lower right axilla and right upper quadrant of the abdomen, one may at times be able to sense an actual systolic expansion in the liver region with each heart beat as one hand moves forward while the other moves backward. In many cases the significance of a systolic pulsation is misinterpreted because it can be due to an impact from the neighboring abdominal aorta or the overlying heart. More reliable clinical evidence of tricuspid regurgitation is the detection of faint pulsations in the veins of the forearms or forehead. As a result of tricuspid insufficiency, there is also a systolic murmur heard in the tricuspid area over the lower sternum. It is very difficult to identify this murmur or to distinguish it from the systolic murmur of mitral origin heard at the apex that is invariably present and has the same quality. It is thought that having the patient hold a deep breath may accentuate the systolic murmur if tricuspid insufficiency is present. It probably is true that many patients with advanced cardiac failure have a functional tricuspid insufficiency even when no such diagnosis is made, for frequently at postmortem examination the tricuspid ring is found dilated.

True tricuspid endocarditis is practically never a pure lesion. It has the same etiologic background as disease of the mitral valve, and in my experience it has invariably been associated with mitral stenosis with or without aortic stenosis. The diagnosis of organic tricuspid insufficiency or tricuspid stenosis is extremely difficult. Many authorities have considered it impossible to make this diagnosis. However, with the recent increased interest in this condition, more and more cases are being recognized. There are certain features which, although not pathognomonic, should arouse suspicion of the presence of tricuspid stenosis.

Patients with tricuspid stenosis have in general the same symptoms as those with mitral stenosis. Cyanosis in this condition is apt to be more intense, infarctions of the lung are very common, and the liver is invariably enlarged. A striking feature in some of the cases is the fact that the liver may remain enlarged for a long time, even years, while the patient is comparatively comfortable and ambulatory. One common and fairly characteristic observation is the rapid change in the appearance of the face when the patient changes from an upright to a recumbent position. Within a minute or so the face, which appeared normal or merely showed a very slight tinge of cyanosis, becomes markedly suffused and intensely cyanotic. The veins of the neck and head will also become very distended. This change probably results from the fact that on assuming the horizontal position the increased venous return to the right side of the heart cannot be delivered quickly through the constricted tricuspid valve and backs up in the veins. For similar reasons this sign ought to be present in cases of constrictive pericarditis.

Ascites may also be very prominent and require frequent abdominal tappings. The same thing may be true of hydrothorax, especially on the right side. Patients with tricuspid stenosis seem to tolerate these evidences of advanced heart failure with less dyspnea and general distress than do patients with other cardiac conditions. It is thought by some observers that in the course of time these patients are apt to develop a peculiar appearance of the skin, consisting of a slight olive discoloration. I have seen this in several instances and it has seemed to be the discoloration of a mild chronic jaundice with a slight greenish tint to it. It probably is the result of prolonged enlargement of the liver and no doubt may develop in other cardiac patients when the same long-continued stasis takes place. Polycythemia is also an occasional finding in tricuspid stenosis. Abdominal symptoms are common, particularly pain and tenderness in the liver. What is more impressive, however, is the degree of comfort and the comparative absence of dyspnea and peripheral edema in the presence of a persistently enlarged liver and recurrent ascites. To this extent it resembles constrictive pericarditis which is distinguished from tricuspid disease by the absence of significant enlargement of the heart and murmurs.

On physical examination the cervical veins are almost always found to be distended and prominent. These characteristics may occur in all types of right heart failure. The distinguishing feature in tricuspid cases is that the condition is not only very marked but it persists for long periods of time, even when the patient is in a fairly good state of compensation. The same will be true of the venous pressure. It not only will be elevated, but with improvement it will not return so closely to the normal level as in other cardiac diseases, with the exception of constrictive pericarditis. The blood pressure is practically never significantly elevated in tricuspid stenosis (over 150 mm. systolic). Hypoproteinemia is common, probably the result of prolonged hepatic insufficiency.

Enlargement of the right side of the heart is very striking. The right auricle dilates tremendously and may even extend beyond the right midclavicular line. There is almost invariably a right ventricular preponderance in the electrocardiograms. Auricular fibrillation, although often associated with tricuspid stenosis, is not so frequent with the same degree of heart failure as in cases of mitral stenosis alone. This means that a fair number of these patients will show gross heart failure with a regular rhythm. The murmurs are similar to those that occur in mitral stenosis, but they are well heard over the lower sternum or to the right of the midline. When it is appreciated that in a series of 32 cases of tricuspid stenosis every case also showed well-marked mitral stenosis, difficulties in the interpretation of murmurs become apparent. When the systolic murmur and particularly the diastolic murmur are better heard near the midline than at the apex of the heart, it would lead one to suspect that the tricuspid valve is diseased. If these murmurs near the lower left sternum become accentuated with a deep inspiration they are more likely to be tricuspid in origin; if they become diminished they are more likely to be mitral in origin. Also auricular sounds may be audible over the right clavicle in cases of tricuspid stenosis and in other conditions in which there is increased pressure in the right auricle. The frequent association of tricuspid stenosis with mitral stenosis, aortic stenosis and even adhesive pericarditis makes accurate diagnosis extremely difficult.

It is of considerable interest that, among patients with chronic rheumatic valvular disease, those with tricuspid stenosis die at the earliest age. The age at death in these cases (34 years) is about twelve years less than in those with mitral stenosis alone (46 years) and nineteen years less than in those with aortic stenosis alone (53 years). However, the duration of symptoms or evidence of congestive failure is much greater in patients with tricuspid disease than in those in whom the other valves are involved. One study has shown comparative figures to be seven and five-tenths years for tricuspid stenosis, four and six-tenths years for mitral stenosis, and three and one-tenth years for aortic stenosis. In other words, although death occurs at the youngest age in the tricuspid cases, the patients with this disorder live longest once failure develops. This is because they have a mechanical embarrassment of the heart comparable to constrictive pericarditis, but the constriction is inside the heart at the tricuspid valve, and not outside in the pericardium. This process is more static and does not necessarily imply heart muscle failure. We, therefore, are witnessing in such cases evidence of right-sided failure, such as venous distention, enlarged liver, and ascites, which has essentially a mechanical cause. Such congestion would obviously be much less serious or progressive than if it resulted from pure heart muscle failure.

It follows that if a patient with known mitral stenosis carries on fairly well for years with evidence of right heart failure and shows persistently engorged cervical veins and enlarged liver, especially if this is out of proportion to the degree of dyspnea, and there is no hypertension, the diagnosis of tricuspid stenosis must be considered.

With the introduction of cardiac catheterization more accurate diagnoses of tricuspid disease can now be made. The form of the pressure curves may be typical of tricuspid regurgitation. An appreciable gradient between the level of diastolic pressure in the right auricle and that in the right ventricle (the former being greater) is reliable evidence of tricuspid stenosis. This kind of study may be necessary in certain cases when cardiac surgery is being contemplated.

CHAPTER 5

Diseases of the Pericardium

Disease of the pericardium is almost always secondary to some other primary condition, whether it be an infection or some other morbid process. The pericardial abnormality may impair health or threaten life in one of several ways. As part of an inflammatory process, pus may form and give rise to the hazards attendant on a closed empyema. Sterile fluid, an exudate, a transudate, or a hemorrhage may be so abundant that it produces cardiac tamponade, i.e., interference with the normal movements of the heart. Finally, as a result of a previous infection or some other pathologic condition, scars, adhesions, or bands may form in the pericardium impeding the free contraction or expansion of the heart. This latter process can conveniently be divided into two clinical types: *chronic constrictive pericarditis* and *chronic nonconstrictive pericarditis,* the latter embracing the condition generally called *chronic mediastinopericarditis.*

The various common types of acute pericarditis will first be discussed, then pericardial effusion, and, finally, chronic constrictive and chronic nonconstrictive pericarditis will be considered.

Rheumatic Pericarditis

Acute rheumatic pericarditis generally develops about two weeks after the onset of the rheumatic infection. Its occurrence, however, is variable. At times it ushers in the rheumatic infection, actually preceding any other manifestation of rheumatism. In fact, it may be the only evidence of the rheumatic infection, there being no joint pains whatever. On the other hand, it can develop after the original attack of rheumatism has subsided, just as one is ready to allow the patient to get out of bed. It is more commonly associated with aortic disease than with mitral stenosis. This may be explained when we consider the anatomic relation between the pericardium and the valves of the heart. At the base of the heart there is only the thickness of the aortic wall between the visceral pericardium and the aortic valves, while the entire musculature of the ventricles intervenes between the visceral pericardium and the mitral valve. If the process of infection is one of extension, no matter in which direction, it is easily conceived how pericarditis would be more often associated with disease of the aortic than with disease of the mitral valve.

SYMPTOMS

The symptoms of acute rheumatic pericarditis consist essentially of an accentuation of those symptoms that already exist as a result of the underlying rheumatic process. The heart, already rapid, becomes further accelerated so that a rate of 130 or more is not at all unusual. The respiratory rate becomes unduly rapid. Although this need not be associated with actual dyspnea, in some instances the rate of respiration may be 50 and the patient may be able to lie flat in bed. In most cases, however, there is actually some respiratory distress. The marked increase in the heart and respiratory rates is out of proportion to the degree of fever, which often is no more than 101 or 102° F. Very frequently there is a rather peculiar and characteristic cough. This is short, hacking, irritative, and unproductive. Often there is pain in the chest. It was formerly thought that this chest pain was due to the inflammation of the pericardium, but there is now considerable doubt about this explanation. There are frequent painless instances of acute rheumatic pericarditis. Certain studies on human beings indicate that the pericardium for the most part is insensitive to pain. It may be, therefore, that the pain in pericarditis is due to an associated pleuritis. Notwithstanding the different possible explanations, pain in the heart region is fairly common in pericarditis. Occasionally the early pain is in the abdomen rather than over the heart, and, with the fever and leukocytosis that accompany it, an acute surgical condition of the abdomen may be simulated.

DIAGNOSIS

The diagnosis may be suspected from the evidence described in the preceding paragraph, but will finally rest upon detecting the to-and-fro pericardial friction rub. This is generally a harsh, grating sound, best heard in the third or fourth left interspace. It can remain localized or spread over a larger area. On auscultation, the sounds seem to be close to the ear and the intensity may be augmented by firm pressure with the stethoscope or by having the patient bend forward. This to-and-fro friction on rare occasions is quite transient, lasting only some hours, but generally it persists for days. When it is loud, it seems to envelop the heart sounds rather than to follow them. When it is typical, it has two portions to it, one with systole and one with diastole, but I have seen instances in which for about twenty-four hours there was only a systolic element and later the diastolic portion was heard. At times, the continuity of the sounds is interrupted so that it may give one the impression that there are three or four portions to the entire friction rub. Because of the frequent association with aortic insufficiency, which has a to-and-fro systolic and diastolic murmur, it is sometimes quite difficult to distinguish a to-and-fro pericardial friction rub from the signs of aortic insufficiency. In fact, both conditions may be present. In some cases, it is necessary to delay judgment. If the to-and-fro murmur disappears, it must obviously have been due to a pericarditis. If it persists indefinitely, it is due to aortic insufficiency. The detection and proper interpretation of a pericardial friction rub is most important because it may be the only distinctive evidence that there has been an acute pericarditis.

There is another frequent development in acute rheumatic pericarditis that is helpful in diagnosis, particularly if by chance the pericardial friction was either missed or indistinct. This is the so-called "Ewart's sign." It consists of dullness and bronchial breathing heard below the angle of the left scapula. These findings are supposed to be due to atelectasis and compression of the left lower lobe of the lung from fluid accumulating in the posterior pericardial sac. It is not certain whether this explanation is true, but it is clear that the above signs which resemble pure lobar pneumonia frequently occur in acute rheumatic pericarditis. The bronchial breathing in this condition is apt to be quite loud, and generally is unassociated with any rales. The resemblance to pneumonia accounts for the frequent history obtained from rheumatic patients that they had pneumonia in childhood. I have seen numerous such instances in which the physician thought the child was suffering from pneumonia. Had not the proper diagnosis been made, such patients would have presented themselves later with aortic insufficiency and the valve disease could have been attributed to no other infection than the pneumonia. The development of Ewart's sign generally follows by some days the appearance of the pericardial friction rub. It may, however, actually precede it. I recall an experience with a patient thought to have pure lobar pneumonia, in a ward given up solely to the care of pneumonia patients. Because the patient had some of the secondary features of rheumatism discussed in Chapter 2, namely, repeated nosebleeds and a family history of rheumatic heart disease, and because he already had some aches in his joints, it was predicted that a pericardial friction would appear and other features pointing to rheumatic infection would develop. This occurred during the following days. I cite this case to illustrate the importance of accurate diagnosis and the indirect means by which proper diagnoses are sometimes made.

The third characteristic of rheumatic pericarditis is the frequent development of disturbances in conduction. Heart block is very common in this condition. When actual blocking of beats occurs, it is easily detected by auscultation. The rhythm, which is rapid and regular, will suddenly be interrupted by pauses. These pauses will not be preceded by a premature beat, which distinguishes it from extrasystoles. A complete heart cycle every now and then actually drops out. When the disturbance in conduction is less marked, no actual blocking of beats occurs. The heart remains perfectly regular. It is almost impossible to detect this change without graphic methods, although the presence of a gallop rhythm or a decrease in intensity of the first heart sound arouses one's suspicion. If an electrocardiogram is taken, the conduction time indicated in these curves will be found above the upper limits of normal, which is 0.2 sec. These slight changes are earlier evidence of what becomes heart block when the process is more marked. Disturbances in conduction indicate a simultaneous myocarditis which frequently accompanies pericarditis. Except for occasional cases of coronary thrombosis, this is the only form of pericarditis in which conduction disturbances are apt to occur. Apart from the friction sound, Ewart's sign, and the conduction disturbances, there is little that is distinctive on physical examination in cases of rheumatic pericarditis.

It is likely that in most cases of rheumatic pericarditis an effusion of a greater or lesser extent develops. When it is slight, it is impossible to detect it. The inflammation gradually subsides and the fluid is absorbed. The pericardial friction disappears after lasting a few days, but the signs of compression of the left lower lobe of the lung and the conduction disturbance may persist for two weeks or more. Gradually both of these signs also disappear, although on rare occasions the electrocardiograms may continue indefinitely to show a delayed conduction time. Changes in the ventricular complexes of the electrocardiograms may also be present (Chap. 21, Figs. 185, 186).

PROGNOSIS

After a prolonged illness, generally lasting months, the patient recovers. The prognosis in rheumatic pericarditis in general is good. The immediate mortality is about 15 per cent. The physician should always keep before him the possibility and even the likelihood of a favorable outcome in the face of what seems to be a very stormy disease. One must appreciate that we are dealing primarily with an infection which at this time is in an acute fulminating stage and that the acute process can subside. Patients may be desperately sick and make an excellent recovery even if signs of congestive heart failure develop. Acute rheumatic pericarditis practically never leads to constrictive pericarditis.

The ultimate outcome, if immediate recovery takes place, will depend in a great measure upon whether the valves have been affected during the acute process. If during the attack of pericarditis no diastolic murmur develops, recovery may be complete from a symptomatic point of view. The presence of a systolic murmur will have the same significance as systolic murmurs in general. This matter is discussed in detail in other chapters. I have seen numerous instances in which, after a most violent and desperate attack of rheumatic pericarditis, recovery was complete and the patient was subsequently able to carry on even strenuous physical work. In such cases there may even be no evidence of heart disease whatever in later years. The subsequent health of the patient and ability to work are quite different when evidence of valve disease develops. Such experiences have impressed upon me most forcefully the importance of the valves in heart disease. Recovery from injury to the myocardium after acute infections seems to take place most satisfactorily, but when the valves are structurally involved, in many cases there appears to start a progressive vicious cycle, with subsequent development of circulatory insufficiency.

Great emphasis has rightly been placed on the importance of the myocardium in heart failure. This applies primarily to nonvalvular heart disease. In chronic rheumatic heart disease a fairly healthy ventricular musculature is noted on postmortem examination. If the myocardium rather than the valves were of primary importance in rheumatism, it is surprising that we do not see patients in later life, who have had rheumatic fever in childhood, dying of heart muscle failure without valvular disease. Apart from the fatalities that occur during acute rheumatic carditis when the state of the myocardium is all important, death due to heart damage in subsequent years is limited to those patients who develop valvular lesions, while those who recover from the acute infection without murmurs or without valvular injury may never have any further trouble from the heart. The degree of valve deformity is not the sole final cause of failure of the circulation, although it is a most important factor in the disability; the so-called "accidents" of heart disease intervene, such as bacterial endocarditis, infarctions, emboli, and infections. When these accidents do not occur, then the valvular damage present at the time of heart failure will be found to be adequate to explain the situation in most cases without recourse to any significant role played by the heart muscle.

TREATMENT

The treatment for a patient with rheumatic pericarditis comprises little more than that employed for the underlying rheumatic fever. It is customary to give salicylates either by mouth or by rectum, as described in Chapter 2. Some believe that large doses of salicylates actually produce absorption of the pericardial effusion. Digitalis will have no beneficial effect unless there is evidence of congestive heart failure. The patient, of course, should be made as comfortable in bed as possible and requires careful nursing to spare him any unnecessary effort. He generally will find it more comfortable to be in the semirecumbent or at times in the upright position. Codeine in doses of $\frac{1}{4}$ to $\frac{1}{2}$ grain may be given every four hours, even to children, for precordial pain or cough. The only additional therapeutic measure that may be helpful is the use of an icebag over the precordium. This sometimes alleviates the heart pain and diminishes the sensation of palpitation. In only a very rare case will it be necessary to tap the pericardium. The fluid then will generally be serous but occasionally may be hemorrhagic. Tapping the pericardium may be a life-saving measure and will be taken up under the general discussion of pericardial effusion.

In addition to the above symptomatic care penicillin should be administered as has been outlined in a previous discussion. Occasionally in fulminating cases adrenal steroids may produce dramatic and prompt improvement.

Pericarditis in Pneumonia

Pericarditis due to pneumonia is now extremely rare. There are certain distinctive features in this condition. It occurs almost exclusively in those cases of pneumonia in which there is empyema of the pleura. Furthermore, it is more commonly associated with empyema in the left pleural cavity than in the right. In fact, if a diagnosis of pericarditis is made in a patient with pneumonia, empyema of the pleura, especially on the left side, should also be sought for. Pericarditis, when it does occur, is apt to develop in the later days or after the crisis or lysis would be expected. A most important difference between the pericarditis in pneumonia and in rheumatic fever is that the pneumococcus is likely to produce pus and rheumatic fever never produces pus. For this reason the diagnosis of the former is important.

The diagnosis of pericarditis with pneumonia will rest almost entirely upon detecting the pericardial friction rub. When pericardial friction rub occurs and is heard, its interpretation is a good deal more simple than in rheumatic fever, for there are no endocardial murmurs to confuse the picture. If it is not heard, pericarditis may yet be suspected in occasional cases of pneumonia if during the second week of the disease there develops a left pleural empyema which is satisfactorily treated and yet a septic course continues. One must remember that a patient suffering from pneumonia may have an empyema cavity in the pleura, well cared for, and yet die of an empyema of the pericardium. If there is any suspicion of this, an exploratory puncture of the pericardium is indicated because the effusion under such circumstances is purulent and not likely to heal spontaneously. If pus is found in the pericardium, surgical drainage should be instituted. This complication of pneumonia is a most serious one.

Since the introduction of sulfonamide and penicillin therapy pneumococcus pericarditis, which formerly was uncommon, has become extremely rare. However, it is not unlikely that unrecognized subclinical cases are occurring and the patients are recovering without surgical drainage. May not some of these cases form the background upon which subsequent constrictive pericarditis will develop?

Acute Pericarditis (Benign, virus, non-specific, idiopathic)

During the past few decades the incidence of pericarditis due to tuberculosis, pneumonia, pyogenic infections, and even rheumatic fever has decreased sharply. The reason for this change is fairly obvious. However, the relative frequency of acute pericarditis of unknown origin has increased. It is called by various names such as benign, virus, non-specific, and idiopathic. This merely indicates the lack of precise knowledge as to its etiology.

It occurs in all ages from youth to old age, but most frequently in young adults and predominantly in males. In its typical form it runs an acute course with predictable clinical features. The most common and almost invariable complaint is pain over the heart. This pain is often accentuated by cough or respiration or movements of the trunk. It may extend upward toward the left clavicle and left side of the neck and shoulder. The pain is not very severe and it lasts days rather than hours. With this illness there is moderate fever, leukocytosis, and increased sedimentation rate. One might reasonably assume that a pericardial friction is present in all cases at one time or another and is generally detected without difficulty. It lasts for days so that careful auscultation daily should not miss it. In many instances there is an accompanying left pleuritis with some pleural effusion. The heart rhythm is likely to remain regular throughout. Cardiac dullness to percussion and the cardiac silhouette on x-ray examination are generally increased and at times considerably so, not because of hypertrophy or dilatation but as a result of pericardial effusion. This increase and decrease in the size of the heart shadow may recur through two or more cycles over the course of a few months.

Electrocardiographic changes may occur with this form of pericarditis and they may be confused with those of coronary artery disease or myocardial infarction (Chap. 21, Fig. 186). However, significant Q waves do not occur, and the elevation of the ST segment, when present, is likely to be found in both Leads I and III of the conventional leads, rather than to have reciprocal relationship in these two leads as is found in myocardial infarction. Somewhat inverted and deformed T waves are frequent and may persist for some weeks before complete return to normal.

This disease generally runs a benign course as fatalities are very rare. The average case lasts a few weeks, although some run through two, three, or more cycles, lasting several months and possibly longer. The chest pain, fever, pericardial friction, and actual pericardial effusion may keep recurring until final recovery takes place.

There is no special treatment for this condition. Broad-spectrum antibiotics are often given, but there is no adequate proof of their value. Symptomatic care and rest, such as one plans for any infection, are all that is available at present. It must be an extremely rare occasion that pericardial tap for tamponade would be necessary. One expects a complete recovery. How often constrictive pericarditis develops in these cases is at present in doubt. I have not seen a single convincing instance in which this complication took place, although such cases have been reported.

The main difficulty that confronts the physician is in diagnosis. When an adult male has precordial pain and develops a pericardial friction rub, fever, leukocytosis, and increased sedimentation rate, one generally thinks about the diagnosis of myocardial infarction. Only the most careful analysis of the type of pain, the exact details of the electrocardiographic changes, the persistence of the friction rub, and the appraisal of other features, such as the presence or absence of shock or cardiac arrhythmias, will prevent serious error. The determination of the serum transaminase or lactic dehydrogenase may be of great help in the diagnosis. The differentiation between acute benign pericarditis and myocardial infarction is extremely important because of the differences in therapy one would outline and, what is more important, the differences in prognostic implications in the two conditions.

Tuberculous Pericarditis

Tuberculous pericarditis is very rare in general practice. Its mechanism and development are quite similar to those of tuberculous pleurisy. In both conditions the process may be dry or fibrinous, or a serous or serosanguineous effusion may be poured out and adhesions may develop. Tuberculous pericarditis, however, is a much more serious complication of tuberculosis. It is always secondary to tuberculosis of the pleurae, lungs, or mediastinal glands. The diagnosis of this condition in the early stages will depend almost entirely on the detection of a to-and-fro pericardial friction rub as in other types of acute pericarditis. There will be no evidence of either heart muscle disease or of valvular disease, for the heart proper is very refractory to the tuberculous infection. The striking characteristic of tuberculous pericarditis is a tendency to large pericardial effusions and it is the one condition that may require repeated tappings. The exudate will be found to be sterile on ordinary bacteriologic examination, just as occurs in rheumatic effusions. Here, on the other hand, inoculating some of the fluid into a guinea pig may prove that it is tuberculous or occasionally the tubercle bacilli may be found on staining part of the fluid or on culture. Whenever a large effusion is found (800 to 1200 cc.), especially if there is a tendency for reaccumulation, tuberculosis should be suspected. Effusions are apt to be larger than in rheumatism because they are poured out slowly, allowing the heart and pericardial sac gradually to accommodate themselves to the increased pressure, and because the heart itself is not diseased. In rheumatic pericarditis, the reverse is true. The accumulation of the fluid is more rapid and either the heart muscle or the valves are generally affected. The heart then would have failed before such extensive effusions as occur in tuberculosis could have been poured out.

It is quite likely that many cases of tuberculous pericarditis are unrecognized, run a mild course and heal, thereby forming the basis of chronic constrictive pericarditis in later years. In some instances evidence of constrictive pericarditis may develop within a few months after the first detection of acute pericarditis. There may not be a large pericardial effusion, and what fluid there is may be pocketed and not free.

Although in the past there was no specific treatment for this condition except for the occasional pericardial tap, now streptomycin, para-aminosalicylic acid, and isoniazid would be indicated. In fact, successful use of instillations of streptomycin into the pericardial cavity has been reported.

Pericarditis with Chronic Nephritis

Pericarditis is a very common complication of chronic nephritis. Its exact nature is not altogether clear. Although it may be due to a terminal infection, in some cases bacteriologic examination of the pericardium and pericardial fluid at autopsy shows no evidence of any infectious organisms. In other cases, streptococci are found. More likely the condition is purely vascular in origin and similar in its mechanism to the ulcerations in the bowel that are frequently found in cases of uremia. It develops insidiously in those who have advanced chronic nephritis with marked nitrogen retention. There frequently is a slight fever and leukocytosis with the pericarditis. These need not be present. The disease may be entirely painless. Uremic pericarditis may rarely result in massive effusion. As large an amount as two liters has been found, which may give rise to cardiac tamponade as a terminal event in the course of this disease. The diagnosis will rest on the finding of the pericardial friction rub. It is only important from the point of view of prognosis for it denotes quite definitely that the end is near. Out of twenty-four cases of pericarditis and nephritis that I once studied, in twenty-three instances death occurred within three weeks. The other patient was practically moribund when he was last seen. More recently one patient survived four months after the friction was first detected. Pericarditis sometimes develops in an ambulatory patient who has advanced chronic nephritis and even here it indicates that a fatality is to be expected within one month. There is no therapy whatever that can be offered for this condition, for it is the underlying nephritis with its uremic manifestation that is the real problem. With the use of the artificial kidney life may be prolonged a few months in some of these cases. While following a patient with advanced chronic nephritis, it is important to watch for acute pericarditis purely as an aid in estimating the prognosis, for sometimes such information is needed in giving certain advice to the family and patient.

Pericarditis with Coronary Thrombosis

A more detailed discussion of coronary thrombosis will be taken up later (Chap. 6). At this point the single feature of pericarditis which frequently develops in coronary thrombosis needs to be considered. Following an attack of partial or complete occlusion of a coronary artery, the part of the ventricles supplied by this vessel becomes infarcted. When the process of infarction is sufficient to extend from within the ventricle to its surface, the pericardium is necessarily involved. At this point, a localized fibrinous exudate develops and therefore a true serofibrinous pericarditis will result. It is obvious that if the infarction does not extend to the visceral pericardium, no pericarditis occurs, or if the site of the lesion is in the posterior part of the heart or over the dome of the diaphragm, even if the pericardium is involved, a friction rub

means necessarily true, for frequently large effusions will be seen with the persistence of a loud to-and-fro rub. It has been quite definitely shown that, in some cases of pericardial effusion, there is a true pulsus paradoxus. Here the pulse, which is already small, may diminish markedly or actually disappear with inspiration. Pulsus paradoxus has been observed in cases of pericardial effusion and found to disappear with the removal of the fluid, only to return when the fluid reaccumulated. An interesting observation in this regard was made some years ago showing that most normal individuals may make the pulse disappear in the radial artery by throwing the clavicle backward entirely independently of the respiratory cycle. By this manipulation, the subclavian artery is compressed, obliterating the pulse wave to the arm. With normal inspiration, the clavicle is thrown backward to some extent. This mechanism is probably in a measure responsible for the production of pulsus paradoxus. The other clinical findings that a patient with pericardial effusion may present are those that are more intimately associated with the underlying disease, such as rheumatism, pneumonia, leukemia, and the like.

X-ray examination serves as a most valuable aid in this diagnosis. In general, it confirms more accurately the heart outlines, and gives a better picture of the peculiar globular shape taken on by the heart shadow. A further point that is obtained in this way is the lack of demarcation between the left auricle and left ventricle which ordinarily is made out either fluoroscopically or by flat x-ray films. On fluoroscopic examination, the individual contractions of the various chambers of the heart are difficult to distinguish, and, instead, indistinct wavelike movements are seen at the outer portions of the heart. The configuration of the heart will also change materially if two films are taken, one with the patient recumbent and one upright. The shadow at the base of the heart will be found broader in the former than in the latter. Angiocardiography, involving the injection of opaque medium to visualize the cavities of the heart and the great vessels, can elicit very definite evidence of pericardial fluid. There will be a large area between the opaque medium within the ventricles and the outside border of the pericardial sac. Although x-ray examination is extremely helpful, it is by no means infallible. The differential diagnosis generally consists in distinguishing a pericardial effusion from a grossly enlarged or dilated heart. This is occasionally quite difficult and at times the only proof will come by making an exploratory puncture of the sac.

PERICARDIAL TAPPING

The question now comes up, when and where should pericardial tapping be performed? It should not be performed in the vast majority of patients with rheumatic pericardial effusions since they so frequently do well if left alone. If there were no risk in tapping the pericardium and it were as simple a procedure as a puncture of the pleura, it probably would be helpful in shortening the illness of many patients with rheumatic pericardial effusion, but there is danger of an immediate fatality. The danger does not consist merely of piercing the heart. In the experimental animal, heart's blood may be obtained repeatedly by puncture without any deleterious effects. Another danger lies in piercing one of the coronary vessels. These lie very superficially just below the visceral pericardium and have no supporting tissue covering them. If one of these vessels is punctured there may be a continuous gradual ooze with a fatal hemorrhage into the pericardial sac. I have seen two instances in which fatalities occurred. There are times, however, when tapping a rheumatic patient is indicated and may possibly be life saving. If the general condition grows worse, the stage may be reached when tapping seems safer than allowing the fluid to remain. Exactly how to estimate this point is difficult to describe; it will depend more upon judgment and general experience than upon any single indication. If the systolic blood pressure is still maintained satisfactorily it is generally safe to delay. It is surprising how extremely sick such a patient may be and recover satisfactorily without tapping.

There are various sites for performing a pericardial puncture. Different physicians prefer different procedures and I judge that it is a matter of custom rather than that one method has any advantage over another. The method I prefer is to go in at the fifth left interspace, just inside the border of dullness and outside the apex impulse. It is well to inject Novocain into the skin at this point. The needle is inserted inward, backward, and slightly upward. One should select a trocar with a dull point to avoid unnecessary scratching and piercing of blood vessels. It should be pushed in slowly, and it is better to have it attached fairly intimately to a syringe rather than to a suction bottle, for it is then more easily manipulated, and by frequent trials with the plunger of the syringe one can more quickly and instantaneously tell when fluid is obtained. If the needle is pushed in very gradually, applying frequent suction, fluid may be obtained even without ever feeling the pulsations of the heart. If these are felt with the tip of the needle, it should immediately be slightly withdrawn and suction continued. When fluid is obtained, it should be removed slowly and as much should be taken out as comes freely. It is not wise to spend time looking for fluid if none is obtained at the outset, because it is this aimless exploration which may prove disastrous. The danger in the puncture is greater if it turns out that there is no pericardial effusion than if a large amount of fluid is present.

Another method for pericardial puncture is the so-called "Marfan's procedure." This consists of inserting the needle just below the lower border of the ensiform cartilage, going upward, backward, and inward. This avoids the peritoneal cavity and enters the pericardium from above the diaphragm. Another method is to reach the pericardial sac from the right of the sternum, inserting the needle in the fourth interspace about 1 inch from the right sternal border. Finally, some clinicians prefer to puncture the pericardium from behind, and insert the exploratory trocar below the angle of the left scapula. On one occasion I removed 500 cc. of fluid from the pericardium by this last method after no fluid had been obtained by exploring through the fifth left interspace. In general, it may be said that tapping the pericardium should be regarded as a major procedure and should not be undertaken except after the most careful consideration.

In cases of rheumatic effusion, it is practically never necessary to tap the pericardium more than once. On occasions, however, within a day or two after the tapping, extensive effusions will develop in the left pleural cavity. It is not unlikely that when this occurs the fluid actually continues to be poured out from the pericardium through the hole made by the trocar into the pleural space. I have seen two instances when this occurred, and during this time the patient seemed temporarily a good deal worse than before the pericardium was tapped. In each instance, marked improvement resulted after tapping the pleural cavity and removing about 2 liters of fluid.

Tuberculous pericarditis with effusion frequently requires repeated tappings, in contradistinction to rheumatic pericarditis. Favorable results have been reported from the reinjection of air after the removal of the fluid. It has been recommended that, when this is done, the volume of air injected should be about half the volume of fluid removed. A more promising method of treatment would be the use of streptomycin, previously discussed. In hydropericardium occurring in cachectic conditions or with advanced cardiac failure, there is little to be gained by tapping the pericardium. It is conceivable that, under certain circumstances, the patient's life may be slightly prolonged by releasing the pressure on the heart produced by a tense pericardial sac, but unless there is hope that the underlying condition may be improved subsequently, the relief will be only very brief. The finding of bloody fluid in the pericardium, not produced by trauma, should make one think of a neoplasm of the pericardium.

Chronic Constrictive Pericarditis

The type of chronic pericarditis now to be discussed, i.e., constrictive pericarditis, is of particular importance because it is amenable to surgical treatment. Because of some previous infection or inflammatory reaction in the pericardium a slow progressive fibrosis results, often with considerable calcification, that produces a constricting influence on the movements of the heart. In the course of months or years the heart may become greatly embarrassed so that it is unable to expand or dilate properly. It is obvious that if the right side of the heart is prevented from performing an adequate diastole or dilatation, it cannot receive the normal amount of blood. It follows, therefore, that the heart cannot expel an adequate amount of blood in any given period of time, for it cannot propel more than it receives. The result is a decreased cardiac minute output. Because of the impediment to a free inflow into the right heart the venous pressure or back pressure increases. This affects the superior and inferior venae cavae as they both empty into the right auricle. The pressure in the pulmonary arteries is also increased because of additional constrictions around the left ventricle or as a result of accompanying myocardial involvement. Only in recent years has it been appreciated that the left ventricular musculature itself is often involved and fibrotic in this condition. For that reason both sides of the heart need to be explored by the surgeon, and one may not obtain complete recovery even if all mechanical constriction of the pericardium is removed, because of the inherent involvement of the myocardium.

The disturbances in the dynamics of the circulation just mentioned take place irrespective of whether the ventricles are capable of normal systolic contractions or not. Even if there were no other abnormalities, such as myocardial, valvular, or hypertensive disease, and the heart were otherwise perfectly normal, pericardial constriction would necessarily produce some of these changes. There often is another disability resulting from these pericardial scars that makes it more difficult for the heart to contract after it has dilated. The pericardium may be bound down to neighboring firm structures, such as the ribs, and the work of the heart thereby increased. This handicap in contraction is much less important in cases of constrictive pericarditis than is the difficulty in expansion.

The etiologic factor in this condition is not always discernible. A large number of cases are due to tuberculosis, some to a staphylococcus, and others to a pneumococcus infection. Other undetermined infections, originally minor in nature, may prove to be the cause of some of the cases that at present have not been classified. It is quite evident that in many cases no definite past history of acute pericarditis can be elicited. If the pneumococcus and streptococcus have been playing a frequent etiologic role in the past, realizing that such types of acute pericarditis formerly were often fatal, we may predict that, with current antibiotic therapy, in many more acute cases recovery will take place and possibly form the background for a larger number of chronic cases of pericarditis in future years. A most impressive fact in considering etiology is that rheumatic fever, such a common cause of acute pericarditis, is practically never the cause of chronic constrictive pericarditis. However, I have seen one patient with constrictive pericarditis who was considerably improved by surgery for about ten years, who showed definite rheumatic mitral stenosis at autopsy.

Pericardial constriction now also results from another cause. As a result of the great number of patients subjected to cardiac surgery, it is not surprising that occasionally the operative insult to the pericardium might result in chronic constriction. It is well known that encapsulated blood may end up with calcification. Thus a few cases of constrictive pericarditis have followed accidental trauma to the chest. One such case that I saw showed calcification of the pericardium and of the pleura. The patient had had an automobile accident in which several ribs were fractured and left hemothorax developed. Very likely hemopericardium was present at that time but was overlooked, and this formed the background for the subsequent calcific pericardial constriction. Some years later cardiac symptoms appeared. Pericardial resection improved the circulatory difficulty, although constrictive pleuritis persisted.

The same sequence of events can now occur after cardiac surgery, if blood is retained in the pericardial sac in any considerable quantity. I have seen a patient on whom six months previously an operation for aortic stenosis had been performed. Not long after the operation definite and progressive evidence of right-sided failure developed, with enlarged liver, ascites, markedly increased venous pressure, and edema of the legs, with very little dyspnea. A second operation confirmed the diagnosis of pericardial constriction, whereas at the first operation it had been clearly noted that the pericardium was normal. I have heard of two other cases of pericardial constriction which followed operations on the valves of the heart. Although such postoperative complications following cardiac surgery must be extremely rare, they no doubt occur and indicate the desirability of preventing persistent hemopericardium after operations on the heart.

SYMPTOMS

Let us now consider the symptoms and clinical findings in constrictive pericarditis. Such patients may complain of weakness, shortness of breath, abdominal distress, and, later, swelling of abdomen and legs. The amount of embarrassment that will be present and the severity of symptoms will obviously depend on the degree of constriction around the heart and the stage at which the patient is being observed. In general there are two types of conditions that it might imitate and with which it is often confused. Because of breathlessness, fatigue, and cardiac findings, it may resemble the other more common forms of heart disease and, because of the enlarged liver and possibly ascites, it may erroneously be regarded as cirrhosis of the liver.

DIAGNOSIS

Physical examination of the heart often reveals nothing abnormal. The rhythm is generally regular, although in a small number of patients auricular fibrillation may be detected. Gallop rhythm is not uncommon. No murmurs are present or only a slight systolic murmur may be heard. Frequently a faint and sometimes a loud third heart sound is heard at the apex during diastole. This may even be the loudest sound heard during the cardiac cycle. The first sound is likely to be decreased or at least not accentuated. Although this may resemble the opening snap or the short mid-diastolic rumble of mitral stenosis, the absence of a snapping first sound, a dilated left auricle, and other features should enable one to distinguish the two conditions. The heart is quiet and inactive. The customary apex impulse is absent or feeble, and in its stead there may be a prominent diastolic thrust most marked with inspiration. One of the most significant findings is the absence of any marked cardiac enlargement. In almost all other forms of congestive heart failure (with which this is confused) the heart is enlarged. This is best determined by x-ray examination, which is discussed below. The blood pressure is almost always within normal limits or lower than normal and the pulse pressure tends to be decreased. The pulse is small, somewhat rapid, and frequently shows a pulsus paradoxus. The latter finding consists of a marked diminution or disappearance of the pulse with inspiration, and can be elicited by palpation of the radial artery, or, better still, by auscultation during blood pressure determination.

The liver is always enlarged and generally palpable, and in later stages ascites may develop. In cases of long standing, repeated abdominal taps may have been performed. For a considerable time peripheral edema is likely to be absent, but eventually swelling of the legs will appear. Probably, as a result of the prolonged hepatic congestion, hypoproteinemia may be present and this in turn helps to produce a stubborn form of edema. Unlike other types of heart disease, constrictive pericarditis is characterized by breathlessness only late in the course of the disease and paroxysmal dyspnea or orthopnea does not occur. The pulmonary findings may, therefore, be inconspicuous, unless evidence of pulmonary tuberculosis is present. Eventually, however, true congestion of the lungs and even hydrothorax may appear. The electrocardiograms may be of low amplitude and often show flattening or inversion of the T waves in Lead I or II.

The venous pressure is increased. This is detected by noting the distention of the cervical veins while the patient is sitting upright or in the semirecumbent position, when normally the veins ought to be collapsed, or in finding distended veins on the dorsum of the hand or forehead. Venous pressure in the arms should be determined and will always be found elevated, generally over 200 mm. This increase in venous pressure will also be found in any case of right-sided heart failure, no matter what the cause may be, and especially in tricuspid insufficiency or stenosis. The striking point in constrictive pericarditis is that the venous pressure is elevated when the other evidences of heart failure are not very impressive; it remains elevated even after the employment of vigorous therapeutic methods that are ordinarily helpful in cases of heart disease. The pressure in the veins of both the arms and the legs is elevated, whereas in cases of cirrhosis of the liver with ascites or in some other abdominal conditions the increase in pressure will be confined to the veins of the legs.

An interesting alteration in the dynamics of the circulation is decrease in the minute output of blood. What is even more significant is that whereas a normal heart can increase its output per minute five- or tenfold with physical effort, here the mechanical handicap prevents any such response. This explains the fact that these patients may be comfortable at rest but become markedly fatigued on effort or actually find it impossible to do very much physically.

Quite recently it has been observed in some cases by electrokymographic technique that the interval between the inward movement of the left ventricle and the systolic expansion of the aorta and the onset of the first heart sound was decidedly delayed. One would suspect that the same phenomenon might also result in other conditions, such as severe myocarditis, in which ventricular contractions were markedly weakened. Studies of the movements of the ventricular border by kymography have shown a distinctive "flat top and V" pattern. This parallels the changes in the ventricular volume curve. The ventricular filling is more rapid than ventricular ejection and stops abruptly early in diastole and is unchanged throughout the remainder of diastole. The protodiastolic sound occurs toward the end of the rapid filling phase at the point when the ventricle can no longer accept any more blood. The sound may be produced by this abrupt halt in filling. It occurs closer to the second sound than a third sound gallop. Lateral ballistocardiograms show marked diastolic excursions which relate to the palpable apical thrust.

The x-ray findings are often of primary importance in the diagnosis of constrictive pericarditis. On fluoroscopic examination the heart beat is found to be quiet. The movements of the cardiac borders are diminished. This decrease in contraction of the cardiac chambers, although visible to some extent throughout the heart, is often more marked over certain areas. Careful search should be made particularly in the region of the right auricle and ventricle, for this is the favorite site for fibrotic plaques to produce constriction. Kymograms may furnish permanent records of the actual amplitude of contraction of the cardiac chambers and serve for comparison in judging postoperative results. Furthermore, in many instances, calcification of the pericardium even to an amazing degree may be detected. In some cases, especially those due to tuberculosis, calcification of the pleura may also be found. It was previously stated that the heart is not enlarged. That is certainly the general rule, but occasionally because the pericardium is so thick, or because of pockets of fluid, the cardiac silhouette may be increased. Although the x-ray findings are very valuable in detecting disease of the pericardium, whether or not the condition causes constriction of the heart must depend on other observations, especially the increased venous pressure, for there are instances of marked pericardial calcification in which the dynamics of the heart are not disturbed.

Once the possibility of constrictive pericarditis has been considered, the foregoing features and examination findings enable the physician to make the diagnosis. These cases are often not detected because the condition is not thought of and will be confused with two general groups of other cases. It is among patients who are regarded as having heart failure, in whom the ordinary causes are lacking, i.e., hypertension, coronary sclerosis, valvular disease, hyperthyroidism, etc., or who are thought to have cirrhosis of the liver, that constrictive pericarditis will be found.

Another aid in diagnosis is the response to medical treatment. Whereas most cardiac patients with congestive failure improve on rest, digitalis, and diuretics, patients with constrictive pericarditis only occasionally show any appreciable response. The venous pressure may fall slightly but will remain distinctly above normal despite all efforts. In this respect the condition resembles tricuspid stenosis, from which it can be distinguished by the absence of any valvular disease or marked cardiac dilatation. There are very rare instances in which the venous pressure may actually return to normal temporarily with satisfactory clinical improvement on medical management, only to have the symptoms return later.

One may repeat that constrictive pericarditis needs to be sought for among patients who, generally 20 to 45 years of age, appear to have some form of heart disease or cirrhosis of the liver, who have a small, slightly rapid, often paradoxical pulse, generally regular in rhythm although occasionally grossly irregular, who have no hypertension, significant murmurs, or cardiac enlargement, and who always show an increased venous pressure and an enlarged liver.

The foregoing describes the more usual features of constrictive pericarditis. With increased experience more and more "exceptional" cases are seen. During the past few years I had two men over 60 years of age under observation. They both had been regarded as having coronary artery disease. They had vague atypical distress in the chest and shortness of breath. They showed no significant murmurs or hypertension. The liver was enlarged and there was marked distention of the cervical veins in both instances. One had a considerable and the other a slight amount of fluid in the right pleural cavity. The electrocardiograms showed some nonspecific abnormalities of the ventricular complexes which were interpreted by their physicians as "consistent with coronary disease." This expression is commonly used and may be a necessary one, but it can be misleading. Even a normal electrocardiogram is "consistent" with the presence of coronary sclerosis. In these two cases the tracings helped to fortify the mistaken diagnosis of coronary disease. In one the suspected diagnosis of constrictive pericarditis was readily confirmed on finding marked calcification of the pericardium and left pleura on x-ray examination. In the other case the clinical diagnosis was made because the venous pressure persisted at about 260 mm. despite medical therapy, there was striking suffusion of the face on recumbency, and there was a definite mid-diastolic sound and diastolic apical thrust. In both cases striking improvement followed surgery.

The inference from these experiences is that even elderly patients may have this condition and one should not accept the diagnosis of coronary disease without adequate evidence. These patients had neither a clear-cut story of angina nor acute myocardial infarction. Mere age, sex, and atypical abnormalities of the electrocardiogram are not sufficient for the diagnosis of coronary disease. Simple clinical clues were important guides to the correct diagnosis.

Very recently another exceptional case was seen. This man, 40 years old, had been sick for five years. He puzzled many physicians and consultants. Auricular fibrillation was present. He carried on fairly well for four years with increasing disability, but finally became invalided because of breathlessness. The unusual features here were marked left ventricular enlargement and a forceful apex impulse. Those who had examined him before either never considered the possibility of pericardial constriction or dismissed it because of the marked left ventricular hypertrophy and other features. The two points that were odd were the continued marked elevation of the venous pressure and the unusual history that the first and main complaint for a year or two was abdominal discomfort and fullness. He had had an enlarged liver at the onset and for a long time had no dyspnea whatever. These two clinical features could be best explained on the basis of pericardial constriction. Despite the absence of calcification on x-ray examination exploratory surgery was performed and the diagnosis was confirmed.

When catheterization of the heart was introduced it seemed for a while that this technique might afford definite evidence of constrictive pericarditis. Pulmonary capillary pressure, pulmonary arterial diastolic pressure, right ventricular end-diastolic pressure, and mean right atrial pressure are moderately elevated and tend to be at the same level. There was what one might call a plateau in the elevated pressures. At first this was thought to be characteristic of pericardial constriction. Later, after more extensive experience, it was learned that similar pressure readings were found in cases of diffuse myocarditis and even in a rare case of endocardial fibroelastosis. It is evident that the diagnosis will be difficult and at times impossible to make. There will be instances in which it will be advisable to explore the pericardium surgically, as is practiced in the abdomen or chest, even if exploration proves to be negative. In fact I have had two instances in which exploration revealed nothing. In neither was the patient any worse for the operation.

TREATMENT

The treatment for patients with this condition is surgical. Some temporary improvement may result from medical management, mainly from use of diuretics, and restriction of salt and fluid intake. Digitalis is occasionally of value but may aggravate the condition. When the protein content of the blood is low a high-protein diet should be given and infusions of plasma may be helpful. Inasmuch as the fundamental problem is mechanical, surgical resection of the pericardium (Delorme's operation) is the only satisfactory means of relief. The surgeon should be one especially expert in cardiac surgery for the operation is difficult and not without risk. Owing to the work of White and Churchill, Burwell and Blalock, Cutler and Beck, and others, sufficient progress has been made so that operative results are now very satisfactory. Some patients are actually cured and many others are considerably relieved. A few are no better because the lesion is too extensive and the surgeon is unable to free enough of the heart to permit adequate expansion, or the heart muscle is also extensively involved. Rarely the lung is similarly bound down to the thorax, so that respiratory failure continues despite a satisfactory restoration of cardiac mobility. Occasionally secondary operations are necessary because sufficient relief does not result following the first attempt. Age need not be a contraindication for surgery. I had a woman 75 years old who obtained a satisfactory result after operation. Finally, the physician should be patient in appraising the operative result. Although some subjects may make a dramatic recovery in a few weeks, others show little gain for many weeks or even months and yet finally make satisfactory recovery.

In performing the operation due regard must be paid to the eventual dynamic relations of the circulation. If the right side of the heart is freed of constrictions and enabled to fill normally and the left ventricle remains bound down, the situation may be no better or even become worse than it was before. Now, added pulmonary congestion may develop because of the inability of the left ventricle to receive or expel its quota of blood. In other words, the dissection must be carried out so that a balanced state of the circulation results. In fact, it would seem wise to free the left side before the right so that even during the operation acute pulmonary edema might be prevented. One need have no fear of the ability of the heart to take care of the increase in work. Finally, it is of interest to know that when improvement or cure is obtained it is maintained. Follow-up studies so far have shown that constriction does not redevelop, at least for the years that these patients have been observed.

Chronic Nonconstrictive Pericarditis
(Adhesive Pericarditis, Mediastinopericarditis)

The details of the development of chronic nonconstrictive pericarditis are meagerly understood. It is fair to assume that the condition is the result of a single or of repeated infection of the pericardium. What is not known is whether recovery in any individual case of acute pericarditis takes place with or without subsequent adhesions. One physician may see a patient with acute pericarditis and twenty-five years later another physician sees the same patient with heart failure. At this time, if chronic pericarditis is present, it rarely is discovered, or if it is correctly diagnosed the past history of acute pericarditis is not known. We have very little reliable data from which to ascertain the frequency with which any one of the primary causes of acute pericarditis produces chronic pericarditis. The complexity of the problem is increased by difficulties in diagnosis. There is reason to suspect that while infection with the tubercle bacillus, the pneumococcus, staphylococcus, and possibly the streptococcus are responsible for chronic constrictive pericarditis (discussed in the preceding pages) these same infections may account for other cases of chronic pericarditis that are nonconstricting. However, when there is also chronic valvular disease with chronic pericarditis it would appear that rheumatic fever is the main etiologic agent. Furthermore, it is of considerable interest that such rheumatic cases rarely produce the picture of constrictive pericarditis.

From a clinical point of view cases of chronic nonconstrictive pericarditis may be divided into two groups; in one the subjects are symptomless and in the other there is significant heart disease and eventually heart failure. In the former group are persons in whom the condition is found at postmortem examination who had shown no symptoms referable to the heart during life. Small bands or synechiae may be found extending between the visceral and parietal pericardium, or at times the entire pericardial cavity may be obliterated and yet there will be no embarrassment to the circulation. Such changes in the pericardium can be seen in patients dying of entirely unrelated conditions, such as brain tumor or abdominal cancer.

The second group concerns us here. The affliction in these patients is generally designated as *chronic adhesive pericarditis* or *chronic mediastinopericarditis*. The adhesions in the pericardium are so extensive and firm as to bind the heart to neighboring structures such as the ribs, pleura, and diaphragm. Thus the free contractions of the heart are impeded and its work is increased. The condition is found associated with marked cardiac hypertrophy. The adhesions were at one time thought to be the cause of the great hypertrophy. This is probably untrue, for very large hearts with chronic pericarditis also have valvular disease, which alone produces considerable cardiac enlargement. The fact that the pericardial adhesions do account in part, but only in part, for the hypertrophy was shown in a comparative study of the weights of hearts with and without pericardial involvement. The average weight of forty-three hearts with various forms of valvular disease with adhesive pericarditis was 125 gm. greater than that of sixty-two hearts with similar valvular involvement but without pericardial disease.

DIAGNOSIS

The diagnosis of chronic nonconstricting pericarditis is difficult, but from a practical point of view is not important. Inasmuch as this type of pericarditis is associated in the main with advanced valvular disease, the physical signs and the symptoms can for the most part result from the cardiac condition irrespective of the pericardial changes. Such patients will have the customary symptoms of valvular disease and, eventually, of heart failure. They will show the signs of some form of rheumatic valvular disease, often aortic, and with it considerable cardiac enlargement. In addition there may be signs (to be discussed in the succeeding paragraphs) that have often been ascribed to the pericardial adhesions. The liver is frequently enlarged and the spleen is occasionally so. In the type called "Pick's disease" there may be perisplenitis, peri-hepatitis, chronic peritonitis, and pleuritis. In fact, the affection that used to be called Pick's disease was rather ill-defined, and this designation might have been used to include constricting and nonconstricting types of pericarditis.

Signs. The so-called "signs" of adhesive pericarditis are very numerous and bear the names of many prominent physicians, but for the most part they are unreliable diagnostically. Studies throughout the entire world tell the same tale, i.e., that this condition is generally first recognized at the autopsy table. The main difficulty is that most of the "signs" may be present when the heart is markedly enlarged and the pericardium is normal. Nevertheless, it is well to enumerate some of the signs and to comment upon them briefly.

Systolic retraction of the apex region is a common finding. With systole the heart actually pulls the interspaces inward rather than out-ward. The heart is also immobile. The apex impulse and left border normally shift an inch or so when the patient is moved from the left lateral to the right lateral position. In chronic adhesive pericarditis the heart is comparatively fixed. On deep inspiration the left border of cardiac dullness may be unaltered because the left lung is prevented from extending over the heart by adhesions between the heart and the anterior chest wall. As a corollary to this phenomenon, on watching both nipples during deep inspiration the left may be seen to lag behind or even to remain stationary while the right moves forward (Wencke-bach's sign). On examining the interspaces below the angle of the left scapula, a systolic retraction may be seen on careful inspection (Broad-bent's sign). A diastolic shock may be felt in the apex region and a sudden diastolic collapse of the jugular veins may be present. A diminu-tion or disappearance of the radial pulse with inspiration (pulsus para-doxus) has also been described as a sign of adhesive pericarditis. An electrocardiographic sign has been proposed by Dieuaide. This may be detected by taking electrocardiograms with the patient in the dorsal and in the left and right lateral positions. Normally the heart shifts under these circumstances, thereby altering the electrical axis. If the pericardial adhesions are sufficient to render the heart immobile, one would expect to find no appreciable change in the electrocardiograms. This test seems to have a sound theoretical basis, but the validity of its practical application is not so certain. I have seen a case in which no shift in the electrical axis occurred by this technique and yet the peri-cardium was found to be normal.

Finally, the x-ray may throw light on the diagnosis. Irregularities in the contour of the heart as a result of adhesions may be seen. With inspiration the heart may fail to descend, as it normally should, if it is adherent to the anterior chest wall, or tugging of the diaphragm or pleura may be detected with each systole on fluoroscopic examination. Other x-ray findings, such as diminution of movements of the cardiac borders or marked calcification (concretio cordis), are generally indicative of constrictive pericarditis and have been discussed.

The foregoing long list of signs of adhesive pericarditis is an indication in itself of the difficulty of diagnosis and would lead one to suspect that the signs are not very reliable. In fact, except for the roentgenologic evidence, I have seen practically all these findings in patients with enlarged hearts who showed no pericardial disease whatever. I recall a case that seemed quite typical of Pick's disease. The patient was a woman 45 years old who showed evidence of advanced cardiac failure. The liver was enlarged, the abdomen was full of fluid, and there was a hydrothorax. There were signs that seemed typical of mitral stenosis. In addition there was marked systolic retraction of the apex and immobility of the heart. There was a prominent Broadbent's sign, which was demonstrated to several undergraduate classes in physical diagnosis. The abdomen and chest were tapped many times. The patient was observed very carefully over a period of four years and was always thought to have mitral stenosis, adhesive pericarditis, and polyserositis. On postmortem examination the pericardium was found to be perfectly normal, the heart was enormously enlarged and dilated, and there was stenosis of the mitral, aortic, and tricuspid valves. This well illustrates the difficulties in diagnosis.

TREATMENT

As has been indicated, the importance of accurate diagnosis of chronic pericarditis of the constricting type is great because surgery offers the only effective treatment. This is not true of chronic nonconstrictive pericarditis or chronic adhesive pericarditis. For the most part, this condition occurs in patients having rheumatic valvular disease and enlarged hearts. They suffer from cardiac disabilities that are not particularly the result of the adhesions. Such patients would be receiving treatment for heart failure anyway, and in most cases the treatment would be no different even if it were known that adhesive pericarditis was present.

Many years ago Brauer devised an operation for the relief of chronic pericarditis which he called "cardiolysis." At that time the essential differences between the constricting and nonconstricting aspects of pericarditis were not so well distinguished as they are today. The procedure consisted of removing several ribs and a portion of the sternum over the precordium, thus permitting the heart to tug away at flexible soft tissue rather than at an unyielding bony chest. This operation did not necessitate the exploration of the pericardium and heart. Although carrying much less risk than the Delorme operation, in which the heart itself needs to be explored, it is performed very little nowadays. It can do no good for constrictions that may be present. Its only effect would be to diminish the work of the heart in its contraction or to give an enlarged heart a little more room, serving as a decompression of the chest. Inasmuch as the pericardium is not explored, the presence of pericardial adhesions is not confirmed by the operation. Some patients appear to have been improved by this operation and in a few of these who were subsequently examined post mortem no pericardial adhesions were found. Improvement could then only be ascribed to a decompression effect on an enlarged heart.

CHAPTER 6

Angina Pectoris and Coronary Thrombosis

Angina Pectoris

Angina pectoris is a distinct clinical entity in the sense that, when it is properly understood, it can be diagnosed accurately, the subsequent course of the disease can in a great measure be predicted, and the type of pathologic changes in the heart at autopsy can be foretold. The likelihood of sudden death is a necessary corollary of the term "angina pectoris." In addition, one may expect certain measures that are helpful in some heart conditions to be comparatively useless in angina pectoris, and other means not ordinarily employed to be of benefit. For example, nitroglycerin may relieve an attack of angina and have no influence on the precordial pain of cardiac neurosis or mitral stenosis. It therefore becomes imperative to isolate from among those patients who suffer chest distress the ones who have true angina pectoris.

A patient either has or has not angina pectoris. There is no room in this discussion for terms such as pseudo-angina, false angina, juvenile angina, and anginoid. The use of such terms has served to spread confusion and to distort the truth. It may be proper to call a condition pseudo-angina if the symptomatology is quite characteristic of angina and yet one infers that there is no true anginal element whatever in the problem. Furthermore, the term "mild angina" is often equivocal. If the term means that the complaint is not very troublesome its use is proper, but it must not be inferred necessarily that the disease is mild or trivial. An anginal patient with only mild complaints may be dead of heart disease in a few days, for the underlying process may be out of proportion to the symptoms.

Much of the confusion concerning angina has resulted because of the lack of uniformity in the explanations of the mechanism of the attacks that characterize the disease and in the underlying etiology. So divergent have the hypotheses been that one authority has insisted that angina has nothing to do with the heart and is only the result of disease of the aorta, another has maintained that it is due to spasm of the coronary arteries, a third that it is due to heart fatigue, and a fourth that it is a neurosis. Although it is not proposed here to discuss the various theories concerning angina pectoris, one thesis propounded seems to be worthy of mention. It has been suggested that the invariable

89

mechanism which causes an attack of angina is anoxia of the myocardium no matter how brought about. This can explain the overwhelming frequency of angina pectoris in disease of the coronary arteries. It accounts for its occurrence in some cases of anemia with comparatively normal coronary arteries, for here anoxia of the heart might well result from lack of hemoglobin. It also accounts for the disappearance of angina in some cases of thyrotoxicosis when the demands on the heart are decreased by diminishing the body metabolism. This hypothesis satisfactorily explains many other features of angina which other theories do not, and I feel that at present it is the one most worthy of our consideration.

GENERAL CONSIDERATIONS AND ETIOLOGIC FACTORS

Despite the extensive studies of coronary artery disease from a clinical, pathological, physiological, and epidemiological point of view there remain many features that are puzzling and unanswered. Although atherosclerosis is generally a widespread process, often involving many structures of the body, there are numerous instances, especially among younger men, when fatal coronary disease occurs and the sclerosis is essentially limited to the coronary vessels. The arterial disease may even be confined to one portion of one coronary vessel, the other arteries of the heart and those of the rest of the body being practically normal. It would be difficult to explain such cases on the basis of a general or constitutional cause. If some disturbance in cholesterol or lipid metabolism is an underlying cause of coronary sclerosis, why would one vessel (the left descending coronary artery for example) be chosen to manifest this abnormality? One might go farther and inquire why only one small portion of one artery becomes thrombosed so frequently, sparing the rest of the arterial tree. If a patient had jaundice with hyperbilirubinemia and the jaundice were limited to a finger or to an eye, one would naturally look for some local cause in the finger or eye to explain the localization of discoloration. This would be necessary even if there were an additional condition, like a common duct stone, which caused the jaundice.

These experiences force one to the inference that there is some reason in the heart itself for localization of the sclerotic process in a particular vessel in some cases. May there not be some peculiarity or defect in the anatomical architecture of the arteries in some individuals? We inherit similar structures from our ancestors—the color of the eyes, the shape and size of the ears, etc. When we speak of hereditary disease or a familial tendency to a certain condition, we often lose sight of the fact that in last analysis we inherit certain definite structures. When the final valid explanation is discovered, an inherited disease will be found to be due to the inheritance of an excess or deficiency or peculiarity of certain cells or granules or some other chemical or anatomical structure of the body. May we not inherit a certain size or bend of a branch of the coronary tree that lends itself to greater mechanical trauma with each contraction of the heart? With forty years of torsion a particular vessel, which originally was a little different in its anatomical structure, might develop sclerosis more quickly than another vessel with a more normal original structure. This would explain the familial factor in coronary disease, one of the few features of the disease that is well established.

There is already some work of a suggestive nature that lends support to the local anatomical factor in coronary artery disease. Dock has presented some evidence that the male heart, even at birth, contains more localized thickened areas in the intima of the coronary arteries than does the female heart. If this work is substantiated, it would help to explain the great predominance of angina in the male sex. Another anatomical difference among hearts was observed by Schlesinger. He found that there were three general types of distribution of the two main coronary vessels. In one the left coronary artery extends to nourish a fair portion of the right as well as the left ventricle. In a second group the right coronary extends over to supply a portion of the left ventricle. The third type is the one in which the two main vessels mainly supply their respective ventricles. He also inferred that an occlusion of the left coronary artery in an individual belonging to the first group is more serious, because a larger part of the heart is thereby impaired. The point to emphasize is that there may be other important differences in the architecture of the coronary arteries which have a bearing on the problem of coronary sclerosis, entirely apart from more general or constitutional or dietary factors.

Another intriguing and puzzling question is the actual mechanism of the pain in angina. Where does the pain originate? Is it made in that part of the heart muscle that is temporarily anoxic? Is it produced by pressure of a spasmodic vessel impinging on nerve endings in the arterial wall itself? Or does the pain come from distention of the vessels proximal to the point of spasm? We all readily accept the premise that anginal pain results from the *lack* of sufficient oxygen to a certain part of the heart muscle. It does not seem intellectually satisfying to propose that the *lack* of something causes pain; it is more logical to assume that the *presence* of some chemical is the cause. Is the irritant lactic acid or some other catabolite that produces the pain (the so-called "P" principle of Lewis)? There are numerous instances when there must be profound anoxia of the entire heart and yet pain does not occur. Patients may bleed to death and remain conscious until a short time before death and yet have no chest pain. One has a general feeling that anginal pain is more likely to occur if a local portion of the heart is anoxic, while the rest of the heart is better supplied with blood and contracting vigorously. It also would appear that, under certain conditions, whatever makes the heart contract less vigorously decreases the pain and, contrariwise, whatever increases the force of contraction aggravates the pain; e.g., angina at rest may disappear when marked congestive failure with a low output develops. Similarly, angina at rest may be present during the thyrotoxic state and vanish when hyperthyroidism is cured. During the former state the heart can be seen on fluoroscopic examination to be beating very actively, whereas during the latter the beat is quiet and calm. The accepted explanation is that angina lessens in such cases because the demand on the heart decreases as the basal metabolism is restored to normal. The difficulty with this reasoning is that the output is also decreased. If it were a question of improvement in the ratio of demand and supply to the heart the disappearance of anginal pain could only result if the decrease in demand was greater than the decrease of coronary flow. If both decreased equally the heart would be in no better state. One wonders whether we have accepted too readily the general premise that lack of oxygen is the cause of many of the features of heart disease.

I strongly suspect that, when a local part of the heart is anoxic and pain develops, if the vessel could be supplied with a greater amount of fluid which did not contain an abundant amount of oxygen the pain would let up. In a word, it may not be an actual increased amount of oxygen that is needed but rather an increased amount of blood flow to wash out the noxious catabolite that causes the pain. In that sense the difficulty may be *ischemia* rather than anoxia. Might not the pain disappear if the involved part were better irrigated, even with salt solution, provided the ventricular contractions did not produce an excessive amount of the substance causing the irritation? Or the pain might possibly disappear if the rest of the heart were made to contract more feebly.

Another puzzling event is the occurrence of sudden ventricular fibrillation. This can readily be produced in animals by ligation of one main coronary artery and is regarded as a common mechanism to explain sudden death in patients with coronary disease. It has been shown in animals that if both coronary arteries are simultaneously ligated near their origins the heart gradually dies, but ventricular fibrillation is not so likely to occur. Certainly there is more myocardial anoxia if both vessels are ligated than if only one is. Furthermore, if one coronary artery is ligated but the proximal portion of the vessel is allowed to bleed and expel its blood freely, ventricular fibrillation may be prevented. Here there must be more anoxia than if the vessel were not allowed to bleed, and yet the arrhythmia is inhibited. It would appear that tension in one vessel proximal to its occlusion may be important as a trigger mechanism to initiate ventricular fibrillation. In general, discrepancy in blood supply to neighboring parts of the heart may set up potential differences which are responsible for increased irritability of the myocardium.

In all considerations concerning anginal episodes it must be realized that the basic anatomical condition of the heart is essentially the same all day long, and yet an episode of pain may occur and last a few minutes. What goes on during those few minutes? The structure of the coronary artery, the hyperthyroid state, or the degree of aortic stenosis is the same during the twenty-four hours, and yet the pain is only fleeting. When the pain results from increased physical effort, like hurrying, or from excitement, we look upon the spell as a result of a discrepancy between demand on the heart and supply to the heart. When an attack comes at night during sleep we think it may be due to a dream with its acceleration of heart rate. If the patient denies that he had a dream, we may say that he forgot the dream or that it was a subconscious dream. Does the vessel go into a temporary spasm? There are other possible explanations of attacks of angina in bed or during sleep, such as slowing of the circulation or an increase in the return flow of blood to the right side of the heart. The point to bear in mind is that there must be trigger mechanisms, not well understood, that have a bearing on the production of anginal spells. These may possibly be related to the nervous system and possibly to the production of excessive epinephrine.

Another peculiarity that has puzzled physicians is the effect of posture on anginal pain. When an attack occurs while the patient is lying down he will almost always want to sit or stand up. He has learned that the pain will continue longer or grow more intense if he remains recumbent and will disappear promptly if he stands up. This experience refers to pain that comes early at night shortly after going to bed, not several hours after having been asleep. An observation published recently by Vugrincic of Yugoslavia helps to explain this phenomenon. If we regard the aorta as an elastic tube, shaped like a cane, the arch resembling the handle of the cane, one can readily see that it takes less effort on the part of the left ventricle to expel 70 cc. of blood with each beat if the system or cane were upright (standing) than if it were flat (lying). In the former state the ventricle merely has to propel the blood over the top of the arch of the aorta, after which point gravity and the weight of the column of blood in the thoracic and abdominal aorta aid in the process. This help obtained from the effect of gravity is lacking with the body flat or recumbent. It would appear that in a few seconds, apart from the decreased return flow to the heart in the upright position, the ventricle would have rested sufficiently (even if it put out the same amount of blood during these contractions) to rid itself of the pain. The painful chemical might easily have been washed out during this short interval, while a lessened amount would have been produced, because the heart was contracting less vigorously. In any event, it is a common experience that the upright position promptly lessens anginal pain.

Others have trouble walking to the train in the morning and yet can walk a great deal more later on during the rest of the day. It does not seem that the amount of foot pounds of work is the whole story. To be sure in some of these instances, especially during a golf game, the individual may unconsciously slacken the pace of his walking after having experienced discomfort with the first hole. This I believe is only part of the story and there must be other unknown factors that come into play to account for these apparent discrepancies. What are these secondary adjustments? Why does one patient repeatedly have his distress on shaving every morning, or another on undressing at night, and yet be able to perform much more physical effort at other times without distress? On the other hand, why is an orchestra conductor able to swing his arms violently for two hours without difficulty and yet experience an attack of anginal pain following a short annoying conversation? Why is a man able to do very strenuous physical work all day without distress and yet have anginal pain walking one or two blocks to the street car?

Some of these experiences in which spells occur repeatedly under the same circumstances over the course of years make one think of a conditioned reflex, especially when there does not appear to be sufficient physical effort involved. Dock compares it to tic douloureux. In a word, there is much about this problem that is poorly understood at the present stage of our knowledge.

Although there is no single specific organic cause of angina pectoris there are numerous etiologic factors which are definitely related to its development. It has generally been known that it occurs in males more frequently than in females, the proportion being about three or four to one. This sex discrepancy varies greatly in different decades of life. Under the age of forty the male predominance is very great, about 20 or 25 to 1. The proportion rapidly decreases with advancing years so that over the age of seventy the male predominance hardly prevails. The earlier disproportion becomes all the more impressive when it is appreciated that hypertension is more frequent in females than in males. It at least throws some doubt on the significance of hypertension per se as an etiologic factor. Probably the most important etiologic factor is heredity. There is a strong familial factor in angina pectoris. All practitioners who have treated members of the same family over long periods of years have noted that there are families with a tendency to sick headaches, others which are neurotic, some with a tendency to asthma, and still others with a liability to early death from one or another form of cardiovascular disease. I have seen three brothers all of whom died of acute coronary thrombosis during the sixth decade of their lives. It cannot be mere chance that three members of the same family should die of the same disease at approximately the same time of life. It seems as if the original tissue or structure that such individuals have at birth must be peculiar, so that ordinary wear and tear does more harm to certain vessels than is the case in other people. Another possible explanation of this familial factor of angina pectoris and its predominance in the male sex is that the peculiarities in the structure and function of the endocrine system which we inherit may be the basis of premature arteriosclerosis. There is already some experimental work in animals to show that estrogens may prevent or lessen the degree of atherosclerosis and even reverse the process once it has been produced. In fact, attempts are being made to apply this treatment in human cases. The feminizing effect of this therapy at present will obviously limit its usefulness.

As a corollary of the hereditary influence there is a distinct constitutional type of individual who is particularly susceptible to angina pectoris. I refer to the well-set, strong man who is slightly overweight and who has been especially healthy all of his life. So often these patients boast of their previous good health and remark that they "never had a sick day in thirty years," and that they "could do the work of two men." They have been physically stronger than the average, even when their daily activities did not require them to use that strength. The forearms of these individuals are muscular and round, and the skin fits snugly over their muscles in contrast to the flat-armed type. It is very striking that angina is quite rare in the undernourished and in those who have been sickly for years. It selects the vigorous rather than the weak. From an anthropologic point of view it is most common in the mesomorph (muscular), less common in the endomorph (fat), and least common in the ectomorph (thin).

The average age of patients with angina pectoris when the disease first manifests itself is about 56 for males and about 58 for females. In addition to a small number of young people who have classic coronary artery disease, angina may be seen even in the second and third decades in a few individuals who suffer from aortic valvular disease. This relation will be discussed in great detail later. Even apart from these exceptional instances, angina is not extremely rare in the fourth decade, and I have even seen an instance of typical angina pectoris followed by acute coronary thrombosis in a 24-year-old man, and one in a 22-year-old woman who subsequently went through pregnancy successfully. It seems to be occurring at an earlier age than was observed a few decades ago.

When conditions such as Buerger's disease, hyperthyroidism, and aortic valvular disease, to be discussed below, are not present, young anginal patients between the ages of 20 and 40 will generally be found to have other etiologic stigmata, such as a marked family history of vascular vulnerability, diabetes, or hypercholesteremia.

Most observers believe that angina is increasing in prevalence, both relatively and absolutely. It is obvious that with the marked increase in the span of life that has taken place during the past century and with the improvement in the methods of diagnosis, there should be a greater number of cases of those diseases that mature in persons in the second half of life. However, there is indirect evidence to show that angina is actually more common among a given number of adults than formerly. I am of the opinion that its relative and total incidence has been on the increase and that this increase is real rather than apparent. The reason for this is very obscure. It is generally explained on the basis of the "stress and strain of modern life." This still leaves us in a quandary as to the actual mechanism involved. Has there been some specific deleterious influence at work during these past decades, such as the telephone with its terrorizing clang, or the motor car with its noxious fumes, or the physical inactivity of so many of our people, or a dietary defect with an overabundance or lack of some element, or the prevalent habit of smoking? Is it even due to a process of natural selection, those with angina being the more fit and dynamic and propagating their kind, or is it merely the hustle and bustle of the twentieth century? These are important but unanswered questions.

In one study it was found that Jewish patients with coronary artery disease died on the average at a considerably younger age than non-Jewish patients. A similar though less striking difference was found in the age at death of smokers in contrast to nonsmokers, the former dying about three years earlier. If this can be confirmed and it can be shown that the over-all age of the groups studied were the same as the average age of all patients with angina, it would follow that these two factors are somehow related to the development of coronary disease.

These statistical references may sound confusing but they are important. The average age at death from coronary disease in the United States Army during the Second World War may have been 27 years, although army life may have had nothing to do with coronary disease. This is so because the average age of the entire army population was probably 27 years. The average age at death in the army from measles, mumps, or pneumonia might well have been 27 years, the same as with coronary disease. In other words the average age of the entire population in the army, from which the particular smaller group (coronary patients) was studied, is so much lower than the average age of the general civilian population that no comparisons can be made. Similarly, smoking and being of Jewish heritage could only be significant if the average age of all nonsmokers and all non-Jews were the same as that of smokers and Jews, respectively, and the average age at death from all causes other than coronary disease were the same in the two comparable groups. Because of more recent immigration of Jews and the more recent acquisition of the cigarette habit, it may well be that the general average age of all Jews or smokers is actually lower than that of non-Jews and nonsmokers and therefore the age at death from coronary disease will necessarily be less than in the control groups.

Another difficulty in appraising statistics concerning the prognosis of coronary artery disease is the matter of "sampling." One physician's study may be predominantly based on hospital cases. Here the more seriously ill patients are likely to be taken. Different diagnostic criteria may be employed in different series of cases. A consultant who answers emergency calls immediately may have a greater mortality incidence for the acute attack of myocardial infarction than one who, for one reason or another, says that he cannot see the patient for several days. The latter consultant will obviously not see some of the patients who succumbed the first day or two. Furthermore, in estimating the average duration of life in those who recover from the acute phase of the first attack of myocardial infarction, it is necessary to include only those consecutive cases that were seen by the reporting physician at the time of the first acute attack. If cases are included, even if they are consecutive, who are first seen months or years after the first acute attack, falsely optimistic figures are obtained. If the average interval between the first attack and the time the patient is first seen is two or three years, it is obvious that the coronary patients who may have died within two or three years following their first attack never could have reached the consultant. Figures obtained in this fashion would add an unwarranted bonus to the true expected life expectancy following acute myocardial infarction. This particular oversight accounts for some of the more optimistic reports in the current medical literature than my own experience could have led me to expect. There are other pitfalls in statistical studies, all of which point to the difficulties involved.

It is of some interest that females are not only less frequently afflicted with angina but that the disease occurs on the average two to three years later than it does in the males. The reason for this is obscure but the facts are beyond dispute. This may be one of the important reasons that the average age of women at death in the latter decades of life as shown by all insurance statistics is consistently three years or more greater than that of men. If the smoking of tobacco has had something to do with this difference in the sexes, as has been thought by some, it can be expected that in the next few decades, as a result of the greater prevalence of smoking among women, the discrepancy between the sexes may diminish in extent or disappear. Arteriosclerosis is much less extensive in the female than in the male sex. This merely puts the problem in different words, as the reason for this lessened susceptibility to arteriosclerosis remains obscure.

At present there is great interest in the role that diet may be playing in the development of atherosclerosis and especially of coronary sclerosis. It has been known for a long time that there is very little coronary disease among the Chinese in China. There is also much less hypertension. It is suspected that the low incidence of coronary disease is due to the low fat content of their diet. Furthermore, cardiovascular disease appeared to decrease very markedly in some European countries during the Second World War when the population had to subsist not only on a low caloric intake but on a diet that was particularly low in fat. It is also of interest that in these same localities, when the war was over and a more normal diet became available, the incidence of coronary artery disease returned to its former high level. It appears that within the same country coronary disease is more common in those cities where the consumption of fats is great than where it is less. These global statistical studies are also supported by the extensive experimental studies of Katz and his co-workers. They have abundantly confirmed earlier work that extensive atherosclerosis can be produced by high cholesterol feedings and that this process can be inhibited to a greater or lesser degree by the administration of thyroid gland or estrogen products.

The problem of diet and its fatty content is by no means very simple. It is true that the blood cholesterol level can be reduced in many, but not in all, individuals by a diet low in fats, especially animal fat. However, there are many other individuals who eat a diet high in fat or remain quite obese all their lives or who constantly show a high level of cholesterol in the blood who do not develop early coronary sclerosis. No doubt there are other factors at play. For a while it was thought that the animal rather than the vegetable fats were to blame. Another theory proposed by Gofman was that the more mischievous components were cholesterol molecules of large size rather than of small size. Quite recently it has been shown that certain oils (corn oil) may actually decrease the blood cholesterol level. It also has been demonstrated that a loss of considerable weight (about 15 per cent) will produce a considerable reduction of blood cholesterol even while the individual is eating a liberal amount of animal fat. Another point of view in this connection is that the critical factor may be the cholesterol/phospholipid ratio rather than the actual cholesterol level. It is known that phospholipids tend to maintain cholesterol in solution. Finally, we now learn that physical exercise itself lowers the blood cholesterol. An interesting study has been published in this regard by Morris and his colleagues in England. As a result of a very extensive statistical review they found that bus conductors (an active occupation) had less coronary artery disease than bus drivers (a sedentary occupation), and that the condition, when it occurred in the former, was less severe, with a lower mortality, and started more frequently with angina rather than with an acute coronary thrombosis. The same relationships also were found to be true when postmen were compared with postal clerks who were doing more sedentary work. It would appear from this that physical work in some way had a favorable influence in the development of coronary symptoms.

There remains many other important unanswered questions. What role does this high blood level of cholesterol have on the vascular lesions? Although, in general, cases of coronary sclerosis have a higher blood level of cholesterol than normal controls there are many instances in which the level is quite normal. Furthermore, individuals who have no evidence of coronary sclerosis and show an elevation in blood cholesterol are more likely to develop coronary disease than are normal controls. What are the relative roles of the exogenous and endogenous factors in cholesterol metabolism? A cow eats no cholesterol-containing food and yet makes it in large quantities which appear in its milk. Is it a factor lacking in the diet rather than something in it that is important? The intense investigations going on at present promise to throw light on these vital problems.

Another possible etiological factor that has received very little attention is the physical quality of the blood. In the days before liver therapy, when pernicious anemia was invariably fatal, it was striking that at postmortem examination these patients had unusually smooth blood vessels. The average age at death was not much less than that of patients dying of coronary disease, and yet angina or coronary sclerosis was extremely rare. Now that the anemia can be cured, coronary disease develops in patients who had pernicious anemia. To be sure such patients live longer and reach ages when degenerative processes are more likely to occur. On the other hand the association of atherosclerosis and especially of coronary sclerosis with polycythemia vera is unusually common. Furthermore, it was found that coronary disease was much less common in the same decades of life in one part of Peru where there was a great deal of anemia than it was in the cities where there was little anemia. It seems reasonable to suspect that the turgid blood, with its increased viscosity, may be conducive to sclerosis of blood vessels. In fact some patients who have polycythemia vera or who are merely full blooded and suffer from angina appear to be helped by an occasional phlebotomy.

Among the specific diseases that are etiologically related to the development of angina pectoris *syphilis* once was regarded as most important. It was particularly looked upon as a frequent cause of angina in young people. Since the introduction of the Wassermann reaction it has become evident that syphilis is an uncommon finding in angina. Years ago I once found it present in only 4 to 5 per cent of the cases, and even in these it cannot always be regarded as directly related to the angina. At the present time this figure will not be more than 1 per cent. There has been considerable confusion between syphilitic aortitis and angina pectoris. The two conditions are quite different. One need but realize that the former is extremely common in the colored race, whereas the latter is rare, to question any important bearing that syphilis could have in the development of angina. In occasional instances the syphilitic process extends down the ascending aorta and partially or completely occludes the openings of the coronary arteries. In this way anginal distress may result. Furthermore, the development of aortic insufficiency itself with its accompanying low diastolic pressure has been regarded as a cause of angina. I have considerable doubt as to this relationship. However, when there is involvement of neither the coronary orifices nor the aortic valves, it is very unlikely that syphilis is responsible for angina, even when both syphilis and angina are present. In a similar way a small number of tuberculous individuals may incidentally have syphilis without any relationship between the two conditions. It is important to bear in mind that syphilis very rarely produces changes in the main course of the coronary arteries where the customary atheromata are so common, and that when a person with syphilis has such changes it does not follow that the coronary changes are syphilitic or in any way different from those seen in nonsyphilitic patients.

A much more important disease related to angina is *diabetes*. A large number of diabetics, especially the elderly mild ones, often eventually develop coronary artery disease. This relationship probably will grow more common as time goes on, for insulin should prevent early death in diabetes and permit such individuals to live long enough to develop the vascular changes that are so prevalent in this disease. It is not altogether certain that diabetes is the main cause of such angina pectoris as develops, for the age at death of patients with angina pectoris and diabetes is essentially the same as those without diabetes. It may be that diabetes merely indicates the type of individual who has a vascular vulnerability just as the family history and constitutional type reflect those prone to this disease. For the most part it is the mild diabetic 50 or 60 years old, who may not have required the use of insulin and in whom the diabetes may be looked upon as one of the evidences of generalized arteriosclerosis, who develops anginal symptoms.

A high cholesterol content in the blood (*hypercholesteremia*) is common in patients with coronary artery disease. This is particularly true of those who have xanthomatosis or even when only isolated xanthelasma lesions are present around the eyelids. It has been maintained by many that diets high in cholesterol content produce marked sclerosis of the arteries, especially the coronary arteries. This topic has already been discussed. Suffice it to say that cholesterol metabolism probably is related to coronary sclerosis, but its mechanism is still unknown.

Similarly there are other less common diseases that are particularly associated with generalized arterial changes which are etiologically related to angina pectoris. I have reference to *gout, chronic lead poisoning, Buerger's disease, myxedema, Paget's disease,* and *polycythemia.* In these conditions the development of angina pectoris can readily be visualized as the result of alterations in the coronary arteries similar to changes going on in other vessels of the body. The development of angina in association with Buerger's disease is of special interest because it accounts for some of the cases of angina occurring in younger individuals in the thirties and early forties.

The presence of aortic insufficiency or stenosis is attended in some cases by typical attacks of angina. This relationship has been explained, but not altogether satisfactorily, by the following mechanism. The coronary arteries are thought by some investigators to be nourished during the diastolic pause of the heart beat, for when the heart is in systole the contracted muscle forcefully occludes the vessels and prevents any flow of blood. During the diastolic relaxation, however, the coronary arteries are open and it is then that the heart muscle is nourished. Aortic insufficiency is frequently accompanied by a low diastolic pressure which results in a diminished nutrition of the heart muscle. It is this relative anoxia of the heart that is supposed to make it more susceptible to attacks of angina. This mechanism does not explain the exact precipitating causes of the attack for the defect of the aortic valve is permanent and constant, present when the patient is free from attacks. Some other factor is required that sets off the spark to produce a spell of anginal pain. Other possible explanations that bear on the relationship between angina and aortic valvular disease were taken up under the discussion of aortic stenosis (Chap. 4). The relationship of aortic valvular disease and angina explains the occurrence of the latter in a small number of young individuals. There are persons of both sexes, in the second and third decades of life, who have rheumatic aortic valvular disease and typical attacks of angina. It is important to understand this clearly because, although such individuals are liable to sudden death, a characteristic of all cases of angina, they may live many years. The prognosis for duration of life after symptoms develop is about the same as that in ordinary cases of angina. These younger individuals do not as a rule develop coronary thrombosis but rather continue the course of valvular disease and eventually die of congestive heart failure or bacterial endocarditis.

There remain a few other conditions that need consideration. I refer to *severe anemia, hyperthyroidism,* and *paroxysmal rapid heart action.* If a heart that is otherwise competent and structurally sound is nourished by blood which contains 20 per cent hemoglobin or less as may occur in pernicious anemia, one can readily see that a state of relative anoxia may exist in the heart muscle. The same ischemia could result with normal vessels and impoverished blood as occurs with normal blood and narrowed vessels. To be sure, anginal attacks are not common in anemia, probably because there are other compensatory mechanisms that come into play to help nourish the heart and other tissues, such as an increase in the velocity of blood flow and in the minute output of the heart, an increase in the utilization of oxygen, and arteriolar and capillary dilation. However, such attacks do take place although it is to be expected that they will occur more frequently when the anemia is marked and when it develops in an individual whose coronary arteries are already showing degenerative changes. It is obvious in these cases that the successful treatment of the anemia may prove helpful for the attacks of angina and may even make them disappear entirely. Most patients with angina associated with anemia really have a significant degree of coronary sclerosis. I have seen one instance, however, in which classic angina was associated with severe refractory aplastic anemia in a 32-year-old woman who showed normal coronary arteries post mortem. Anginal pain may be only a very rare result of anemia when the heart is otherwise normal, because all parts of the heart are equally affected by the anoxia. If only part of the coronary tree were narrowed or sclerotic, anemia might more readily evoke angina.

This aspect of anemia and angina has been generally emphasized, but an opposite clinical relationship has received very little attention. I have seen several instances of pernicious anemia in which cardiovascular accidents developed directly after the red blood cell count returned to normal. In one such case, as the red blood count went from two to five million in three months, the systolic blood pressure rose from 140 to 240 with the development of hypertensive headaches and a terminal fatal cerebral hemorrhage. Retrospectively, it would have been wiser to diminish the liver therapy and to rest content with a blood count of four million, notwithstanding the slight risk of neurologic complications. Similarly, several cases of coronary thrombosis have occurred shortly after the restoration of the red cell count to normal in primary anemia. One, therefore, needs to be on guard for such exceptional complications. Other relationships between anemia and angina have already been taken up.

For quite a different physiologic reason angina pectoris may result from active hyperthyroidism. Here the mechanism is fairly clear, for a heart that is competent when the bodily demands are normal may find itself embarrassed if the basal demands are increased 50 to 60 per cent. Such an individual may be compared to one who is forced to walk all day long. The heart again is suffering from relative anoxia because of excessive demands. It is unlikely that a normal heart will be so affected by an elevated metabolism. What is more probable is that the thyro-cardiac patients who have angina pectoris have some disease of the coronary arteries and the increased demand on the heart produces embarrassing symptoms. Here also the cure of the hyperthyroidism may eliminate or greatly improve the anginal attacks.

Finally there is a form of angina pectoris that can occur in an otherwise healthy heart as a direct result of a sudden increase in its rate. Any of the forms of paroxysmal rapid heart action discussed in Chapter 13 may be the direct cause of such attacks. Although this relationship is not common, when it does occur it may offer considerable difficulties in interpretation. These transient irregularities may result from an attack of true coronary thrombosis and yet they can occur in an otherwise healthy heart and resemble acute coronary thrombosis. I once saw a man who had severe anginal attacks during bouts of paroxysmal auricular tachycardia when his heart rate would reach 250 and be maintained there for hours and days. He never showed any evidence of organic heart disease, remained in normal health for over twenty years, and only in later years was there angina on effort not associated with tachy-cardia. The probable explanation of the anginal pain under these circumstances is that while the heart rate is extremely rapid the pulse pressure becomes so low that there is very little effective head of pressure to drive the blood around. In the case cited above, the blood pressure for hours and days during attacks was about 96 systolic and 88 diastolic. The coronary artery flow must have been greatly impeded with a resulting anoxia of the heart. It is evident that such paroxysms of rapid heart action can occur in diseased hearts as well, but that when they occur in normal hearts the prognosis can be excellent, for the arrhythmia is generally within control or at any rate self-limited in its duration.

The above peculiar forms of angina pectoris, including those with aortic valvular disease, form only a small portion of the entire group, possibly 5 to 10 per cent. All the others have no associated anemia, hyperthyroidism, or valvular disease, and represent the type that is commonly met with in general practice. One may ask, what is the basic cause of the attacks in these individuals? There have been endless discussions and numerous theories as to the cause of angina and the final solution has not yet been reached. The evidence points more and more to the view that anoxia of cardiac muscle is the most important factor. An observation which supports this theory is the reproduction of anginal attacks in patients suffering from this disease by the inhalation of air containing decreased amounts of oxygen. The theory of aortic origin of anginal pain is losing ground and now most authorities look to the coronary arteries for the underlying defect. I have rarely failed to find some disease of the coronary arteries in any of my own patients with angina who have come to postmortem examination, with the exception of the few who had some other condition, such as valvular disease or anemia. It is conceivable that under most unusual circumstances even fatal angina might occur with a structurally normal heart. Men working with nitroglycerin have been known to drop dead instantly on slight effort after being away from their work for a few days. These observations have been made by Cecil K. Drinker and lend support to the theory that the mechanism of coronary spasm is a cause of angina.

To be sure, there are patients who pathologically show sclerosis of the coronary arteries in whom angina was not detected in life. This, I believe, does not invalidate the coronary hypothesis as the origin of angina. Even if the coronary view is accepted it is not clear whether the pain is the result of spasm of the coronary vessels, whether it is due to the dilation of the vessel proximal to the spasm, or whether the pain sensation comes from metabolites that are not adequately removed from the area of relative ischemia of the heart. Finally, a most important unsolved question is the precipitating cause of an attack which occurs while the patient is at rest. Organic changes in the heart do not come and go. The coronary artery is no less sclerosed a few minutes before than during a typical attack of angina. What trigger mechanism lies behind the temporary explosion? May it not be the endocrine system, particularly the adrenals or thyroid gland? Some experiments I performed several years ago suggest this hypothesis, for it was found that Adrenalin almost invariably brought on typical attacks in patients suffering from angina and had no such effects on control individuals. The whole problem of anginal pain, although nearing a solution, still has many mysteries to be cleared.

DIAGNOSIS

The diagnosis of angina pectoris depends on the proper interpretation of symptoms. For this reason the history is all important. The patient will complain of a peculiar distress in the chest. It is frequently described not as a pain but rather as a disagreeable feeling, like "indigestion." It is so frequently associated with the belching of gas that both the patient and the physician are only too prone to regard the condition as abdominal in origin. It is well for the physician to elicit carefully the character and location of this distress complained of. Too often he regards it as a pain in the precordium when it is neither a pain nor located over the heart. Most commonly the location is in the center of the chest, in the sternum or just to the left of the sternum. Much less frequently it is located over the precordium and very rarely at the apex of the heart. It may arise anywhere from the epigastrium up to the root of the neck and characteristically radiates down the arms, through to the back, the neck, the jaw, the teeth, the face, or to the shoulder. The radiation is more common to the left than to the right, but not infrequently both sides are involved. Occasionally the pain starts peripherally and radiates to the chest, and rarely it is only in the throat, arms, or back, and not in the chest. The discomfort is generally described as a constriction, a feeling of tightness, a burning sensation, a feeling of fulness, a choking, a distress, or just an uncomfortable pain. Some will say that their clothes suddenly feel tight and others will state that they want to lift or loosen their shirt. The peculiar terms used by different patients to describe the symptoms are very illuminating and it is well to write down the history in the very terms used by the patient. In this way the physician quickly learns the character of the pain and becomes more proficient in recognizing this peculiar type of distress. Sometimes the patient cannot put his feeling into words; he may merely say "I have a funny feeling in my chest that I cannot describe." Often the complaint is so mild that the patient refuses to call it a pain and resents taking it very seriously. The mild complaint may nevertheless be very ominous.

The manner of development of the distress is also peculiar. It comes on fairly suddenly and especially on effort. The activity that is most likely to bring on a spell is walking. Patients often are able to do a great deal of hard physical work indoors and yet not be able to walk a block or two in the street. The effort of walking up a slight grade is particularly difficult. Two other factors accentuate this distress. These are a full meal and cold weather. Frequently a patient may be able to walk to his luncheon but have difficulty in returning; or he may have attacks when the air is cold or the wind blowing and none when the weather is warm. Chilling only a part of the body by placing ice cubes in the hands can diminish the exercise tolerance of patients with angina so that attacks come more readily. Another peculiarity is that the pain may come at one time after a brief walk and then at other times it may not occur after a much longer and more difficult walk. Some will complain that they may have an attack during the first or second hole of golf and then no more during the rest of the game, or have a spell going to the train after breakfast and be free the rest of the day. Furthermore, there are peculiar efforts in individual cases that bring on attacks, such as shaving in the morning, taking a bath, undressing at night, or getting into bed between cold sheets. Only careful history-taking will uncover these variations in symptomatology.

Next in importance to physical effort is mental excitement or agitation. Many patients will have an attack on coming into a consultant's office. In this way I have frequently been able to witness in my office the entire development of the anginal spell. Sexual intercourse is another precipitating factor that is not uncommon. A heated argument, suddenly being informed of pleasant or unpleasant news, or any form of nervous excitation may be the precipitating cause of attacks. Finally anginal attacks may come without any apparent precipitating cause while the subject is at rest. They may even awake patients from sleep; in such instances we try with only partial success to blame the attacks on dreams. A division has been made by some observers between "angina of effort" and "angina of rest," but I see no useful purpose that can be attained by this distinction. The latter frequently follows the former, although occasionally the first attack may be of the form described as angina at rest. There are no important practical differences between the two types except that it has seemed to me that those who have angina and hyperthyroidism are very prone to have attacks at rest.

When the attack comes, the patient is generally brought to a sudden halt. When it occurs in the street he is apt to walk slowly to a shop window, not to attract attention, and wait for the distress to relax. He quickly learns that if he remains stationary for a few minutes the pain disappears and he is able to continue. He also learns that if he does not stop the pain persists and may grow more uncomfortable. In rare instances the attack does not prevent continuation of the effort. During the period of pain in most instances there is no shortness of breath, but some will complain that they have difficulty in breathing. It is hard to distinguish true dyspnea from a certain immobility of the chest that may accompany the attack. The patient may not want to move his chest even by the act of breathing for fear of aggravating the pain. Occasionally a patient will find that taking one or two deep breaths will relieve the pain. When this occurs I suspect the relief comes because of some slowing of the heart rate that follows deep breathing. When true breathlessness occurs with the attack it generally signifies that there is an additional factor of heart muscle insufficiency which for the most part is absent in angina. The occurrence of fear of death is variable. It is often, but by no means always, present. It will depend on the severity of the pain and the psyche of the individual. There is something fearful and ominous about the sensation, however, even though it is not severe. The same patient who dreads an attack of angina may suffer a very violent attack of renal colic requiring repeated hypodermic injections of morphia yet experience no fear.

There are rare instances in which attacks of angina are related to hypoglycemia. Patients may observe that spells are most likely to occur when they are hungry, or may be prevented by eating something sweet. One should particularly suspect this relationship if attacks occur late at night. In these cases blood sugar studies are useful.

Much more commonly meals are aggravating influences. Patients often state that food brings on attacks and therefore are convinced that they have stomach trouble. On close questioning it will be found that if they remain at rest after meals the spell will not come, but that it occurs only if they exert themselves directly after eating. One often hears the story that the patient has no trouble walking to lunch but has pain returning to his office. There are rarer instances in which true anginal attacks come during or directly after eating without physical effort.

There are other cases in which attacks have developed directly after severe trauma to the chest or after a very violent sudden effort. There is now reason to believe that under such circumstances the coronary arteries may actually be traumatized with resultant symptoms of coronary insufficiency. The relationship between trauma and coronary artery disease is a very difficult one to disentangle, because so much depends on subjective complaints which may not be reliable when matters of litigation arise. However, when it is known that an individual was well before such an accident and begins to suffer from definite anginal pain hours or a few days afterward, it is reasonable to assume that there is a relationship of cause and effect. The same is true when one suffering from simple angina becomes markedly worse or develops evidence of a coronary thrombosis directly after significant trauma.

When a patient is seen during an attack he will appear slightly pale and introspective and there may be slight perspiration. He will not want to converse but will prefer to remain quiet until the attack is over. The pulse rate during this time may be unchanged but more generally it is somewhat accelerated. The rhythm remains regular in the vast majority of cases but occasionally extrasystoles may suddenly appear during the attack. Such patients may be helped by quinidine. The blood pressure, if taken during the pain, will rise almost invariably. It is not the pain that produces the rise in pressure in these patients, for I have found no rise in these same persons during the pain of severe renal or biliary colic. Occasionally there is an increased flow of urine or of saliva during attacks. After a few minutes, either spontaneously or as a result of a nitroglycerin pill, the distress disappears and the patient feels quite well again.

The preceding details have been repeated because upon their proper evaluation will depend the diagnosis of angina pectoris in the vast majority of cases. The physical examination and all our laboratory tests are so often of no help that it is only from a true understanding of the nature and character of the symptoms that these cases will be recognized. It is the failure on the part of the doctor to appreciate the importance of complaints of mild distress in the chest that leads many patients with angina pectoris to be overlooked entirely or to be treated for indigestion or gas. It is imperative that we deliberately inquire into the history of all our patients over 40 years of age, asking whether they have chest distress on effort no matter what their primary complaints may be, for they may not volunteer this information. The lesson that needs to be emphasized repeatedly is that this common and serious malady is generally associated with no significant abnormal findings on physical examination.

PHYSICAL EXAMINATION AND LABORATORY TESTS

Although examination reveals very little that is characteristic of angina one frequently detects some abnormalities in the cardiovascular apparatus. Generally there is evidence of arteriosclerosis in the peripheral vessels or on ophthalmoscopic examination. Often, however, there is no more than would be expected at the patient's age, and at times there is even complete absence of any detectable vascular disease. The blood pressure is variable and may be anywhere from subnormal to markedly elevated.

There is a curious and most important difference in the blood pressure findings in the two sexes. Whereas the average readings for males were found to be 149 mm. systolic and 89 mm. diastolic, the corresponding figures for females were 190 mm. and 102 mm.

Whenever the problem of angina or coronary thrombosis arises in a woman less than 55 years old who is known to have had a normal blood pressure, one should look for other noncardiac causes of the symptoms or for particular stigmata of vascular vulnerability. In this way overlooked instances of diaphragmatic hernia, gallstones, etc. may be found. When these conditions are not present one often may find hypercholesteremia, a marked family history of coronary disease, or evidence of diabetes mellitus. There still will remain a small number of women with classic angina without hypertension who have none of the above conditions. The inference is that although normal or low blood pressure is common among males with angina, the absence of hypertension in females, except following a coronary thrombosis, makes one strongly doubt the diagnosis.

The heart in most instances is enlarged, although frequently the enlargement cannot be detected without x-ray examination. Occasionally calcification of the coronary arteries can be seen fluoroscopically or on the x-ray film. Although such calcification always means coronary sclerosis, is distinctly pathologic, and generally establishes the diagnosis of angina, it occasionally may be found in the absence of angina. It must be remembered that the term "angina pectoris" denotes a physiologic state, and sclerosis of coronary arteries is a structural condition. Although such sclerosis is by far the most important cause of angina pectoris, each on occasion may exist without the other.

There is a dominantly regular rhythm in practically all cases. Occasional extrasystoles may be present, but auricular fibrillation is rare. There seems to be some antagonism between auricular fibrillation and angina. If the former exists it is unlikely that the latter will subsequently develop. The presence of both does occur but is rare. Auricular fibrillation can develop in a patient with angina pectoris following an attack of coronary thrombosis or after angina has been present for some time.

The heart shows no murmur whatever in about one half of the cases and in the other a systolic murmur is heard at the apex or base of the heart. A small number, possibly 5 to 10 per cent, show a diastolic murmur. This includes the very rare patient (1 per cent) with mitral stenosis who has angina, the young group of rheumatics with aortic valvular disease, and a few older patients with aortic insufficiency due to syphilis or hypertension. On the whole the quality of the heart sounds is of no aid in diagnosis. In most instances the sounds are normal in character, but in some the intensity of the first heart sound is distinctly diminished. A diminution of the intensity of both heart sounds can be due to a thick chest wall or to overlying emphysematous lungs and the like, but if the first sound is muffled and the second sound is distinct, it at least makes one suspect that the P-R interval is prolonged. In some a gallop rhythm may be heard. There is no evidence of congestion in the liver, lungs, or extremities unless there is an added element of congestive heart failure, which will be found in a comparatively small number.

Two other examinations are commonly carried out in studying patients with heart disease, i.e., determination of the vital capacity of the lungs and electrocardiography. The *vital capacity* is the greatest amount of air one can expire after inspiring as much as possible. This varies mainly with the height of the body. Normal standards have been established, and although formerly they were calculated with reference to given heights, this was later changed and comparisons were made with reference to the surface area of the body. In this latter calculation the surface area is determined from the height and weight of the body. This change in calculation seemed more scientific and accurate when it was first introduced, but I have always felt that the reverse is true. One can obtain a closer reading of the expected or normal vital capacity from the height than from the surface area of an individual. The following example will make this clear. A young man 25 years old, in good health, weighs 135 pounds and is 67 inches tall. His vital capacity is 4000 cc., which is perfectly normal. In ten years he gains 40 pounds, is still in perfect health, the vital capacity is still 4000 cc., and his height is the same. The surface area has increased, and the "expected or normal" vital capacity has increased. Calculating on the basis of height his vital capacity is 100 per cent of normal, whereas in terms of surface area it has fallen to about 80 per cent. This gives one a false impression, for his circulation has been normal throughout. There is no reason why one should expect a greater vital capacity because the subject has become obese. In fact, the reverse occurs when obesity is marked. A patient may have no disease of the cardiovascular system and yet have a distinct diminution in the vital capacity of the lungs from obesity alone. When the added weight is sufficient, it may inhibit the expansion of the chest and the descent of the diaphragm. This often results in dyspnea on effort. This type of diminished vital capacity and shortness of breath does not indicate heart disease, is not of itself progressive, and must be carefully distinguished from the other more serious types of breathlessness. This may entirely disappear with appropriate dieting and a consequent loss of weight. A corollary of the foregoing is that a thin cardiac who is short of breath is apt to be in a worse state than an obese cardiac, for, in the case of the latter, part of the dyspnea at least is due to the benign obesity. Similarly, a low vital capacity reading is more ominous in a thin than in a stout individual. It is apparent that the readings must be interpreted in the light of the constitutional type of physique of the individual.

Age likewise influences the vital capacity to some extent. Practically all the normal standards with which readings are compared have been obtained from young men and women, generally college students or young hospital interns and nurses. The result is that the vital capacity of patients with angina pectoris is being compared with that of normal young people. The readings thus obtained would indicate that in angina the vital capacity is diminished about 20 to 25 per cent. If suitable comparisons could be made this difference would be much less and probably would show that when unassociated with myocardial insufficiency the vital capacity in angina is essentially normal. What has just been stated about the vital capacity in relation to age and weight needs to be borne in mind in interpreting readings. It is difficult to compare the reading in one patient with that in another unless the differences are marked, and yet smaller changes occurring in the same individual from time to time may have more definite significance. This is particularly true in study of the same patient over the course of years.

In the interpretation of the relation of the vital capacity of the lungs to breathlessness, two other factors need consideration. The first is the general muscular strength or tone of the body, especially the muscles of respiration. With marked anemia or with general asthenia, although the total breathing space is normal, the effort of taking deep breaths rapidly is exhausting and cannot be kept up for any length of time, and breathlessness results. The second is the speed with which the respiratory cycle can be completed. In marked emphysema, expiration is so difficult and prolonged that the number of respiratory cycles per minute is considerably reduced. In the last analysis it is not only the actual vital capacity of the lungs but the facility with which a given amount of air can be inspired per minute that determines the development of dyspnea.

The *electrocardiographic findings* in angina pectoris are variable. Frequently they are perfectly normal or they show preponderant hypertrophy of the left ventricle, which has no diagnostic significance. On the other hand, in a good many cases there will be distinct abnormalities of the ventricular complex. Not all of these changes are particularly indicative of angina. In fact, some of these are also found in association with heart disease other than angina, but in so far as they direct attention to a pathologic condition of the heart they aid in avoiding the error of diagnosing a normal heart. Although a Q wave in Lead III is found not infrequently in a person with a normal heart it has appeared to be much more common in those suffering from coronary artery disease. There are other changes that point more clearly to angina pectoris, inasmuch as they are so commonly associated with disease of the coronary arteries. Among these are spread and delay in the QRS complex, bundle branch block, and initial ventricular complexes of low amplitude. All such alterations occur in heart disease other than angina but for the most part are not found in normal hearts. Other abnormalities that more clearly point to coronary artery disease are certain changes in the QT complex or in the T wave. These changes will be discussed in greater detail under coronary thrombosis, but in so far as some of them are observed in cases of angina they often are diagnostic. Occasionally opportunities have been afforded for obtaining electrocardiograms of patients during an attack of angina, and some have shown slight but distinct alterations of the RT complex resembling those seen in coronary thrombosis. The R-T segment is somewhat depressed or elevated in one or another lead as compared with the form that is seen in the tracings before or after the attack. This has been regarded as additional evidence to support the theory that anginal attacks are due to myocardial ischemia. The importance of the electrocardiograph is that, although often it is of no help, in some doubtful cases of angina the tracings may be the only evidence of the grave condition that exists, and that without such evidence the patient would be regarded as having a normal heart.

When the diagnosis of angina is still in doubt there are some tests that may prove helpful. The first is to have the patient exercise with the purpose of bringing on the distress of which he complains, or significant electrocardiographic changes. This can be done by making him walk upstairs until pain is produced, or by using a so-called Master "two-step" test. If the type of pain of which the patient complained is reproduced by the exercise test it would tend to support the diagnosis of angina. In the majority of cases no such pain results, but the decision will rest on the electrocardiographic changes. The most reliable evidence is a depression of the S-T segment of more than 1 mm. (especially if it is as great as 2 mm.). This is most commonly observed in Lead V_3 or V_4.

Another test is to have the patient breathe an atmosphere poor in oxygen content (10 per cent). If this is continued for ten to twenty minutes, anginal attacks may be reproduced in those suffering from this disease. Furthermore, breathing low concentrations of oxygen may produce in the R-T segment and T wave abnormalities which do not occur in normal hearts. Somewhat similar electrocardiographic changes may be produced by a brief effort. When these are marked, as shown in Figure 172, the diagnosis of coronary sclerosis is quite clear. However, an appreciable number of cases of angina (approximately 30 per cent) may have a negative anoxia test. Finally, I have employed an Adrenalin test for angina that merits a word of explanation. It was found that the subcutaneous injection of 0.5–1 cc. of 1:1000 solution of Adrenalin reproduced attacks of angina pectoris in most cases and failed to do so in control cases. In some patients even smaller doses were effective. Unfortunately Adrenalin injections are dangerous when given to patients who have heart disease and especially angina. This test, therefore, should never be employed when the diagnosis is quite definite, and the amount employed in performing the test should be small at first (e.g., 0.3 cc.), the amount being increased if necessary on subsequent examinations. When the results are positive, the patient will start complaining of the same sort of pain in the chest five to fifteen minutes after the injection is given. The pain will generally be accompained by a rise in pulse rate and in blood pressure. Just as soon as the pain is reproduced, nitroglycerin, amyl nitrite, or, if necessary, morphine is given to bring the attack to an end. I believe that the test can be helpful in some doubtful cases, particularly when it is thought that the condition is functional rather than organic. It must be borne in mind that performing any functional test for angina is dangerous, for instant fatalities have occurred.

There are several conditions that particularly must not be confused with angina. First, there is the large group of patients suffering from some form of organic heart disease, valvular or hypertensive, who complain of pain in the chest. For the most part the pain is at the apex, not in the sternum, and is often associated with hyperesthesia of the left breast. Then there is the group who have functional heart disease. Here the pain is also apical and generally comes while at rest. Furthermore, arthritis of the spine, subdeltoid bursitis, and muscular pains from trauma and similar conditions may simulate angina. The confusion becomes increased because many patients with coronary disease develop a troublesome pain in the left shoulder, arm, and hand that resembles causalgia and is not due to the heart. They may, therefore, have two different types of pain in the left arm, one of an anginal type brought on by effort and another related to motion of the left arm or shoulder. The two need to be carefully distinguished, because of differences in treatment. For the shoulder pain local heat and aspirin may be all that is required; occasionally stellate ganglion block will be helpful. Disabilities in the hands have been reported as associated with coronary artery disease, especially following myocardial infarction. Dupuytren's contraction and stiffness of the fingers resembling sclerodactylia presumably due to vascular constriction have been observed. These various features are distinct enough to be called the "shoulder-arm syndrome" and constitute a frequent complication in patients suffering from coronary artery disease. It is much more common on the left side but may involve the right. In some stubborn or severe cases of shoulder-arm syndrome adrenal steroids have been helpful; as an extreme measure a few patients have required and have been cured by manipulation of the arm and shoulder under Pentothal anesthesia.

A most important and common differential diagnosis is that between angina and gallstones. The difficulty is increased because so many patients have both conditions. X-ray of the gallbladder is of great value in this connection. Other conditions such as diaphragmatic hernia, herpes zoster, cervical rib, thoracic tumor, or aneurysm may also cause confusion. However, a complete review of those features that characterize angina pectoris will generally lead to the correct diagnosis.

A new test has interested me a great deal in recent years, i.e., the carotid sinus test. It has been found that if a patient is having anginal pain, slowing of the heart by carotid pressure will make the pain disappear or lessen almost instantly. I have employed this test hundreds of times without any mishap and frequently found it helpful to prove or to rule out the diagnosis of angina. It is a common experience for my presence or my examination or my eliciting the medical history to evoke an anginal spell in the patient. This has afforded abundant opportunity to make these observations. When the patient has his customary pain or distress the physician should stop everything and auscult the heart. The patient is not told what to expect. A nurse or another physician, if present, is asked to hold the stethoscope in place so that auscultation is clear. If not, the patient holds the stethoscope. Then he is asked whether he is still having distress. If so the right carotid sinus is massaged for a few seconds. If this does not produce appreciable cardiac slowing, the left side is massaged. Just as soon as the heart slows for several beats pressure is released and the patient is asked whether the pain is worse. The purpose is not to ask a leading question but, on the contrary, to try to misdirect him. If the heart has been slowed, almost invariably the patient will pause for a second or two, seem to be looking into himself, and reply, "the pain is gone" or "it is letting up." The disappearance or lightening of the pain occurs in seconds, not in minutes. In fact, I observed one instance in which the pain actually disappeared while the heart was not beating. In this case a long asystole of seven seconds was produced. That patient was instructed to say "now" when the pain let up, and it was during that pause that it ceased. When no slowing occurs from carotid stimulation the pain is unaltered and no conclusion can be made. In some the distress lessens and as the heart resumes the more rapid rate the pain returns to its original severity. That particular attack often is completely controlled or after a few minutes it may return and again respond as in the first instance.

When I first made these observations, which were similar to those made cursorily by others, I thought the effect was due to a nervous reflex, a release of coronary spasm, as it occurred so instantaneously. But when it was noted that relief came only when slowing occurred and pain in the *left* arm would disappear following pressure on the *right* carotid sinus, a purely nervous mechanism did not seem to be the explanation. It is more likely that with slowing of the heart some irritating substance, a catabolite such as the Lewis "P" factor, possibly lactic acid, is washed out of the heart. Inasmuch as most of the coronary flow occurs during diastole, with the longer pauses of the heart more of the noxious factor may be removed than is made and the pain therefore disappears.

As a practical matter this test has been of considerable value in some puzzling cases. Whenever a definitive positive test was obtained, except for very rare functional cases, other evidence or the subsequent course of events proved that the diagnosis of angina was correct. When no slowing occurred no conclusion could be drawn. With other types of pain, such as those due to gallstones, arthritis, or carcinoma, no such prompt relief can be obtained. Contrariwise, if good slowing is produced and the pain is neither relieved nor lessened, it is not likely to be anginal. It may yet be due to a coronary thrombosis. Here the pain is either not altered at all or is only slightly and very temporarily lessened.

The value of the carotid sinus test is illustrated by the following experience. A 50-year-old man was being observed by an expert gastro-enterologist. A careful study of the case revealed definite gallstones on x-ray examination. All other objective evidence was negative, including electrocardiograms. His complaints were not easy to analyze. Besides recurrent upper abdominal pain and gas there was an odd distress in the region of the lower sternum, not typically related to effort. As I began to question the patient he developed this particular symptom. Within a few seconds after applying right carotid sinus pressure the distress was gone. I felt quite certain this patient had not only gallstones but angina as well, a combination frequently met with. This was a new observation to the gastroenterologist and appeared to him to be too feeble evidence to make such an important diagnosis. The patient left the hospital only with the diagnosis of gallstones. Four months later he was found dead in bed. It so happened that some time later I had an exactly similar experience with the same physician. This time at least the patient was discharged with the diagnosis of gallstones and question of angina. Subsequent events again confirmed the latter diagnosis. It must be borne in mind that the test is only valid if an actual episode of pain can be observed and does not rule out the diagnosis of angina if no slowing is produced. Although the main value of carotid sinus manipulation is diagnostic, some patients have been taught to abort these attacks in this fashion.

Another procedure has now come into use that may throw light on myocardial function and indirectly may aid in the diagnosis of coronary artery disease. The ballistocardiogram affords some information concerning the efficiency and quality of myocardial contraction. It is supposed to afford some measure of cardiac output; but what is more important it is claimed that even when the output is normal it tells us whether the heart is performing its function easily or with difficulty. A weight of 25 pounds may be lifted 1 foot from the ground quite easily by one person and by another only with difficulty and awkwardly. In both instances the same amount of work is done, but the expenditure of energy may be different in the two. Similarly, the normal 60 to 70 cc. of blood may be expelled by the ventricles with each contraction. The ballistocardiogram, which reflects the efficiency of contraction, may be quite normal in one case and very abnormal in another. Already a great deal of data has been accumulated on this subject, but there is dispute concerning the significance of the findings and even about the proper instruments to use.

It is true that the great majority (but not all) of the patients with coronary artery disease have abnormal ballistocardiographic curves. In fact, many have abnormal tracings before they have symptoms. When abnormal ballistocardiograms are found in the absence of other evidence of heart disease, follow-up studies in subsequent years have shown a much greater incidence of coronary artery disease than where the tracings were normal. How soon such early changes may actually mature and do material harm to the heart may not be predictable in any individual case.

This method of study may prove to have value for insurance companies in aiding them to appraise risks, but at the present state of our knowledge it is not likely to help greatly in individual diagnostic work. It must be realized that various kinds of heart disease are associated with abnormal ballistocardiograms. In some the changes are specific and even diagnostic. This method of study has already proved of some use. Where the differential diagnosis is angina or no heart disease at all the finding of a grossly abnormal tracing would weigh heavily in favor of the diagnosis of angina. Furthermore, when a patient has recovered from an acute myocardial infarction the return of the ballistocardiogram to a good normal pattern, as occurs in some instances, would indicate an excellent recovery of myocardial function. Although this subject is still being explored some value has already been derived and much more is to be expected in the future from this technique.

Despite all our routine methods of study many patients with angina will show either nothing abnormal or only those minor alterations that are common in otherwise well people in the later years of life. Even when abnormalities are found they do not always characterize the anginal state. The description of the type of distress is by far the most important feature from a diagnostic point of view. Despite the great dependence on the subjective symptoms and notwithstanding the fact that they may be atypical and simulated by diseases other than angina, the diagnosis of angina pectoris by and large can be made with a high degree of accuracy.

PROGNOSIS

The prognosis in any case of angina pectoris is most uncertain. Sudden and unexpected death which characterizes this disease may occur at any time. It probably is just as well for all concerned that accurate predictions of this fatal outcome cannot be made. There is no other condition in which sudden and instant fatalities take place with the same degree of frequency. In fact, when the diagnosis of angina pectoris is properly made the possibility and likelihood of this eventuality is always inferred. A word about instant death may be appropriate at this point. There are very few conditions that cause instant death. Physicians are too prone to make the diagnosis of cerebral hemorrhage, stroke, or apoplexy when a patient dies suddenly. In my experience, rupture of a cerebral vessel from hypertension or from a cerebral aneurysm, or cerebral embolism never kills instantly. Such patients may suddenly become paralyzed or comatose, but death, when it occurs, follows after several hours or more commonly in a few days. Rarely a massive cerebral hemorrhage may kill in some minutes or in an hour. I have seen death occur in eighty minutes in an apparently well woman, 48 years old, who post mortem showed a ruptured cerebral arteriovenous aneurysm with massive intracerebral, subarachnoid, and intraventricular hemorrhage. Major peripheral emboli do not kill instantly. Even a large pulmonary embolus presents a picture of sudden respiratory distress and suffocation, and, when it is fatal, death is apt to be delayed for a period of ten minutes or more. Occasionally rupture of an aortic aneurysm may produce death instantly. In fact, most of the cases in which death occurs instantly, i.e., within seconds or one or two minutes, are directly due to the heart and moreover are the result of a limited number of causes.

Instant death may result from rupture of the ventricle. This is by no means an uncommon event in those suffering from coronary heart disease, and is also an occasional end-result in subacute bacterial endocarditis. Another cause is complete heart block. Here the circulation may be quite adequate and compatible with a considerable degree of physical activity as long as the ventricles contract at a rate of 30 or more. When there is an attack in which the ventricle fails to respond (Adams-Stokes seizure) unconsciousness results, and if the asystole lasts more than a few minutes consciousness does not return and the attack is fatal. There is a very rare condition in which inhibition of the heart occurs. It is not a matter of blocking of heart beats but rather that the beats do not arise; the pacemaker stops functioning. This can be due to an oversensitive carotid sinus. It is known that the heart may be completely arrested for as long as ten seconds by this mechanism and it is conceivable that rarely a fatality may occur. The constant use of ephedrine in patients who present this peculiarity is of considerable value in preventing attacks. Sudden fatalities occasionally occur during the administration of quinidine. Some light has been thrown on this by a few observations in which it was found that occasionally quinidine causes inhibition or paralysis of the auricles. Such cases have shown a temporary disappearance of the auricular complexes (Fig. 56). If this same inhibition which has been shown to affect the auricles should affect the ventricles, the heart beat would suddenly stop. In this way sudden death during quinidine administration, not the result of other causes, may be explained. A similar mechanism rarely follows excessive digitalis (Chap. 21, Fig. 55). It is also conceivable that quinidine in very rare instances may also cause ventricular fibrillation with sudden death.

The last type of disorder that causes instant arrest of the circulation is ventricular fibrillation. This must not be confused with fibrillation of the auricles. In the latter condition the ventricles are contracting irregularly but actually expelling blood from the heart. In the former the ventricles are essentially immobile, producing no effective systole whatever and no flow of blood. There are many reasons to believe that this mechanism is probably an important cause of sudden death. In animal experimentation the heart is frequently seen to stop as a result of the onset of ventricular fibrillation after ligation of one of the coronary arteries. This has generally been considered as the cause of the sudden type of death that characterizes angina pectoris. Besides the above indirect experimental evidence in support of this explanation, there has been more direct proof of this point of view. During some routine work it so happened that a patient suffering from angina pectoris was having an electrocardiogram taken. He died in the attack while the third lead was being taken, and postmortem examination showed disease of the coronary arteries but no acute occlusion. The electrocardiograms were typical of ventricular fibrillation. This was direct proof that instant and unexpected death in angina pectoris could be brought on by ventricular fibrillation. This mechanism is very likely a common cause of sudden death accompanying coronary artery disease. When a patient with angina drops dead instantly one should not assume that he suffered from a fresh attack of coronary thrombosis. Postmortem examination is likely to show coronary sclerosis and narrowing but no new fresh lesion. When an acute thrombosis occurs he is more likely to survive for minutes, hours, or longer, and live long enough to be seen by a physician.

On occasions a surgeon is confronted with the problem of sudden arrest of the heart during an operation. This may occur without the presence of organic heart disease. In a few such instances electrocardiograms have shown that ventricular fibrillation was present. Under these circumstances it is best to massage the heart manually and rhythmically and to spray the heart with 0.5 to 1.0 per cent procaine hydrochloride. Five or 10 cc. of the solution can also be injected intravenously. Satisfactory recoveries have occurred with this technique.

Electrical methods are also employed in the operating room to defibrillate the ventricles, but the results are uncertain. When sudden arrest of the heart is not due to ventricular fibrillation, external electrical stimulation with the Zoll pacemaker may be very helpful and at times life saving. This apparatus is particularly applicable to medical cases with Adams-Stokes syncope.

Because of the unpredictable occurrence of sudden death in cases of angina pectoris the prognosis in any given instance is very uncertain. Patients may die in the first attack or shortly after the onset of the first symptoms or may live in comparatively good health for over twenty years. There is very little in the clinical features that enables the physician to distinguish one type from the other. In the past the average length of life after the first symptoms developed was about five years for both sexes and the average age at death was 61 years for the males and 63 years for the females. A more recent review by White indicated more than seven years as the average length of life after the first symptom. This increase, to a large extent, may be explained by more careful history-taking. If, on accurate questioning, an earlier date of onset of symptoms is elicited, the duration of angina will obviously be lengthened. It was found that whether the tonsils had previously been removed or not made no difference in the course of the disease. I believe that foci of infection have no important relation to this problem. Slight differences in average life expectancy may be predicted on the basis of certain factors, but on the whole such considerations do not help materially in estimating prognosis. When angina develops before the age of 50 years the duration of the disease is about two years longer than when it first begins in later years. Those who have a low blood pressure develop the disease a few years earlier and live a little longer after the onset of the disease than those who have hypertension.

There is one significant factor that aids in prognosis, i.e., the hereditary one. Those patients with angina pectoris whose parents died at an older age lived distinctly longer than those whose parents died at a younger age. In this study of heredity it was also found that although males suffered from angina about four times as frequently as females, the inherited defect of vascular vulnerability was transmitted more prominently through the mothers of these patients than through their fathers. In other words, the females transmit this tendency more than do the males but are themselves less affected. This, I believe, helps to explain the fact that, in the latter decades of life, all vital statistics show that females outlive males by more than three years.

The relation between angina pectoris and cardiac decompensation is of some interest. Although it is generally stated that the former disappears when the latter develops, this frequently is not the case. In fact there are instances in which both conditions are present simultaneously and the disappearance of the evidences of decompensation is accompanied by the disappearance of anginal attacks. In addition, it is obvious that with congestive failure patients cannot walk briskly and may not experience anginal pain because of their inability to exert themselves sufficiently to evoke this symptom. This applies to other cases in which individuals, as a result of intermittent claudication, of old age, or of incapacitating conditions, are unable to perform that degree of physical effort which would have been necessary to bring on heart pain. This I believe explains many instances of sudden death or coronary thrombosis that occur in people who were regarded as having no previous heart disease. The presence of hypertension makes it more likely that congestive heart failure will develop sometime during the course of the angina. The duration of life, however, after the onset of angina is one year longer in those who decompensate than in those who do not. The great frequency of hypertension in women, therefore, explains the more common occurrence of cardiac decompensation in this sex when angina has been present.

Obesity was not found to affect either the age of onset or the duration of angina pectoris. I believe that if obesity per se acted deleteriously as a causative or aggravating factor the obese patients should have developed the disease earlier in life and died at a younger age than those with normal or subnormal weights. The fact that this was not found to be true suggests that obesity has no important direct relationship to angina pectoris but merely reflects the constitutional type that is more prone to the disease.

Although electrocardiography is often of considerable value in the diagnosis of coronary artery disease, its aid in prognosis is very slight. In a study of over 100 cases in which electrocardiograms were taken it was found that the duration of the disease was one year longer in those with normal curves than the average, but inasmuch as angina developed earlier in life in the former than in the latter, these patients died at an earlier age than those with abnormal electrocardiograms. The duration of life after the onset of angina was one year less in those with inverted T waves in Lead I or II than in those without such changes. In a small number of instances showing other electrocardiographic changes, such as prolongation of the P-R interval or the QRS complex or QRS waves of low amplitude, the prognosis was slightly better than for the entire series. It must be recalled that, in many of the cases with these latter electrocardiographic abnormalities, the anginal features had become less prominent and the element of myocardial insufficiency with dyspnea and limitation in physical activities had become more important.

It is of some interest to know what type of exitus is to be expected in patients with angina. Approximately 50 per cent were found to die suddenly. In addition about 30 per cent died of coronary thrombosis. In these latter cases the patients were seen and lived long enough for the physician to make this diagnosis. Many of the "instant deaths" in the former group no doubt were also due to coronary thrombosis. That this is not invariably true is attested by the fact that in some cases of sudden death from angina pectoris there was no evidence of an acute thrombosis although atheromatous changes were noted in the coronary arteries. Somewhat less than 10 per cent of the subjects died of congestive heart failure and the remainder died of miscellaneous causes such as cerebral hemorrhage, bronchopneumonia, cancer, and other conditions. The fact that there was such a high incidence of that type of death which one would expect in cases of angina pectoris is valid proof of the great accuracy of the clinical diagnosis.

TREATMENT

The treatment of angina pectoris may be divided into two problems, the treatment of the specific attack and the general care of the patient with the hope of diminishing the severity or frequency of recurring attacks. Patients with angina should be instructed concerning the use of nitroglycerin. This is the simplest and on the whole the most useful medication for the attack. They should always carry some pills with them. The dose should be $\frac{1}{100}$ grain or $\frac{1}{200}$ grain (0.6 or 0.3 mg.). Although most patients find $\frac{1}{100}$ grain to be the suitable dose some will find either $\frac{1}{200}$ grain or even $\frac{1}{400}$ grain to be sufficient. When nitroglycerin is first given it is wise to start with the smaller dose, as occasionally the ill effects from the full dose so alarm the patient that he refuses to use it any more. The pill should be placed under the tongue and should be dissolved in ten to twenty seconds. This should occur either spontaneously or as the result of sucking the tablet or crushing it between the teeth. Tablets that are hard and dry and require minutes for complete dissolution should not be used. The occurrence of a sensation of warmth or pounding in the head serves as a guide to the potency of the pill. The patient should be told to use it whenever he has the anginal distress unless it is so mild and of such short duration that it would be hard to know whether nitroglycerin really did much good. Those suffering from angina generally learn before long whether the pill is helpful or not. If its use appreciably diminishes either the duration or the severity of the attack it should be used. The physician should further advise that nitroglycerin is to be used to ward off attacks. During the daily routine patients often learn that a particular act or set of circumstances frequently precipitates attacks. Shaving in the morning, undressing at night, walking to the train, attending a business conference, and the act of sexual intercourse are common precipitating factors and nitroglycerin can serve as a preventive in anticipation of such attacks. Occasionally patients may find that taking a pill every two hours during the day may be helpful. I have seen no ill effects resulting from the liberal use of nitroglycerin when it seemed indicated. One woman consumed 1000 $\frac{1}{100}$ grain pills in one week without ill effects, and many patients have used 100 pills a week continuously for many years.

It is very rare that amyl nitrite is needed or will accomplish what nitroglycerin will not. The inhalation of amyl nitrite acts somewhat more quickly and more violently, but is not so simple for daily routine use. On the whole, amyl nitrite is used very little. Alcohol in the form of suitable drinks is often of considerable help either during a spell or, better still, as a preventive. Some individuals find $\frac{1}{2}$ to 1 ounce of whisky taken before bedtime will prevent attacks from coming at night. Finally, the patient should either stop the activity that brings on the spell or should at least slacken his pace. Although it is well to give this advice, it is generally unnecessary as sufferers from angina quickly learn that if they carry on and do not heed the distress it will continue or grow worse, and if they stop still the pain lets up. Some attacks are severe and protracted enough to require morphine.

The second aspect of the treatment is much more difficult and less effective. In most cases the transient attacks are readily controlled by the measures just mentioned, but how is the recurrence of these attacks to be diminished so that they will not prevent the patients from walking or working or conversing? There is no simple specific procedure that has proved very valuable for this purpose. At the outset the question arises whether or not to enforce a period of strict rest in bed. There have been two diametrically opposite views in relation to this method of treatment. In one the importance of a period of bed rest for as long as several weeks or even months has been propounded. In the other it has been maintained that this is not desirable, but it has been recommended that the patient remain ambulatory and walk or exercise to the limit of his tolerance; i.e., he should avoid the effort that brings on the distress if possible. The very fact that such different views have been expressed and carried into practice by equally learned clinicians must mean that neither one can be universally applied and that there can be no great difference in the results obtained. Many considerations must be taken into account, especially economic ones. One hesitates to put a man to bed for four weeks when the resulting loss of income would work great hardship on the family. Particularly would this be true if such a procedure would jeopardize the patient's job or subsequent work. Working men and women over 50 years of age are readily discharged by their employers, only to have their places filled by younger employees, and find it extremely difficult to replace themselves in industry. These are matters that the physician must constantly keep in mind, for too often the social and economic status of patients is ruined without any significant gain in their health to compensate for this preventable loss. On the other hand, when the person in question has no occupation, is retired from business, or has sufficient means to enjoy the luxuries of life one would be more ready to try a period of prolonged rest.

When attacks are recurring very frequently and are quite severe, or when they actually prevent a person from attending to his work, it is wise to try a period of rest for several weeks. He need not be confined to bed and, in fact, is more likely to obtain the maximal mental and physical rest if he is allowed to relax in a comfortable chair with his feet down for most of the day. In some cases this alone improves the condition or at least renders the patient free from attacks or diminishes their frequency for a considerable period of time. In some patients who suffer primarily from nocturnal attacks, placing 9-inch shock blocks under the head posts of the bed may eliminate attacks in bed. The explanation of this beneficial effect of posture may be that return flow to the heart and therefore heart work may be decreased by this simple procedure. Although the rigidity of the rest treatment will vary with different circumstances, in so far as possible it should provide complete mental and physical relaxation. When kept at bed rest such patients should be permitted to leave their beds for movements of the bowels. They should avoid all annoying experiences such as disturbing visitors and business conversations. If pressing personal or business matters which could be straightened out by a visit of a few hours at the office or by a conference are preying on the patient's mind, it is better to have it over with before instituting the rest treatment. In other words, all reasonable measures should be employed to procure the rest that is desired. It is generally better to do this in the patient's home or better still in a hospital than to send him off for a vacation, a procedure that is often ill-timed, expensive, and ineffective.

Another consideration in this treatment is the diet. Five small meals a day are preferable to three larger meals. It is well to advise a period of rest directly after meals whenever possible or at least to urge against any avoidable physical or mental effort on a full stomach, as attacks are very common under these circumstances. A high carbohydrate diet has been recommended by many and even the intravenous injection of concentrated glucose solution is practiced by some. I have seen too little good come from the latter to advise its use, although I frequently suggest the taking of sweets in the absence of diabetes. It is important that the diet contain the necessary vitamins.

There is a great interest at present in the role of cholesterol in the causation of atherosclerosis. It has become clear that the serum cholesterol level is determined not only by the dietary cholesterol intake but also by the quality and quantity of consumed lipids. It therefore seems reasonable, even in the present uncertain state of our knowledge, to advise a low-fat, low-calorie diet in all cases of coronary disease and possibly in all individuals vulnerable to coronary disease. It is of interest, furthermore, that certain oils with unsaturated fatty acids, like corn oil (Mazola oil) can actually lower the blood cholesterol concentration. I now advise its use for general household purposes. It also can be taken as a medication, i.e., 8–12 cc. in orange juice, two or three times daily.

Rarely when other measures have been without avail and the patient continues to experience frequent angina even at rest, a strict semistarvation diet for several days to a week may quiet down the stormy state. This may account for the beneficial effects, recorded by our predecessors, that were obtained from the Karell diet (200 cc. of milk four times daily and no other food).

Whether the patient has started the rest treatment or remains ambulatory, a loss of weight is desirable in most cases. When the amount of overweight was considerable I have seen marked improvement result from a gradual loss of 30 to 40 pounds in instances where nothing else was done, the patient remaining at work and taking no medication. When the weight is normal at the start, a slight loss of weight might be advised.

The relation of "gas in stomach" and anginal attacks has always been puzzling. A great many patients are certain of the association so that they think they have stomach trouble or "indigestion" and are never convinced that they have anything wrong with the heart. They feel that gas brings on the attack and if they raise the gas the attack stops. It is possible that gas is swallowed before or during the attack and later expelled. On close examination it generally becomes clear that gas may be an accompaniment or result of the attack but that some physical or mental effort is the real precipitating cause and that gas with the patient at rest produces no distress. Notwithstanding this, some patients would be a good deal more comfortable if the condition of the gastrointestinal tract were improved. This is no simple matter and taxes our ingenuity to the utmost. Proper bowel habits and whatever measures that will prevent constipation and straining at stool are indicated.

One should not forget that peptic ulcer is by no means rare and that disease of the gallbladder, with or without stones, is very common in patients suffering from angina. When these additional diseases are present their symptoms must and can be distinguished in most instances from those resulting from the heart disease, and the conditions merit appropriate treatment. It must not be expected that removing the gallstones will cure the patient of angina. When this is supposed to have occurred I feel certain that the diagnosis of angina was incorrect. I have had a great many patients with both conditions and found that, when the gallbladder and stones had been removed surgically, those symptoms due to biliary disease disappeared but those due to the coronary artery disease persisted although they may have been ameliorated.

When the question of smoking came up in former years I used to tell patients to smoke moderately, i.e., not more than eight cigarettes or two cigars daily. Now I am more inclined to urge omitting tobacco entirely. It is generally believed that tobacco has vasoconstricting effects on the peripheral arteries. It should always be avoided in a condition like Buerger's disease. We now know that tobacco produces temporary depression of the T waves in the electrocardiograms in some individuals. In fact, marked electrocardiographic changes characteristic of extensive myocardial infarction have been observed to appear shortly after smoking and entirely disappear within fifteen minutes. This makes one think that a major coronary artery was temporarily in spasm, producing local ischemia. Furthermore, the ballistocardiogram is generally temporarily worsened by smoking. Although I have never seen tobacco per se produce angina in the sense that the disease would disappear on omitting its use, one does find patients who have fewer attacks if they do not smoke. It therefore seems wise to greatly curtail or eliminate its use in cases of angina. One should individualize in this matter. One might wisely urge a man 40 years old who has been smoking 40 cigarettes a day to give up smoking entirely and yet permit a man 70 years old to smoke a pipe or a cigar after each meal. In the first instance there is good possibility that the patient may live many years, whereas with the older individual the number of pleasurable experiences may already have become quite limited.

A variety of drugs have been used for the purpose of diminishing the frequency and severity of attacks and of enabling the patient to do more work without discomfort. The great diversification of these drugs is ample evidence of their inefficiency. Potassium iodide (10 drops three times daily) has long been used in all forms of vascular disease, including angina pectoris. The frequent reference to the value of this drug that is so prevalent in the older medical literature no doubt is due to the striking results that were obtained in some cases of masked hyperthyroidism and in syphilis when their etiologic significance was not understood. Whether it is of any value in other cases is problematical and at least doubtful. Digitalis has been used a good deal and it has been found that when angina is unassociated with dyspnea, general myocardial insufficiency, or congestive failure it has been of no use. There are some who believe it can aggravate angina pectoris. It should be tried only when there is dyspnea apart from the anginal pain or when there is definite or suspicious evidence of congestive failure.

The use of atropine was once advised by Sir Clifford Allbutt on the basis that the sudden fatal outcome in angina is due to "vagal inhibition of the heart." There has been no proof either of this mechanism of death in angina or that atropine acts beneficially. Inasmuch as some believe that an increase in heart rate is an important factor in the development of attacks and atropine can increase the heart rate by diminishing vagal tone, the therapeutic indications for this drug are at least open to question.

The common experience that all physicians have had in finding that emotional factors seem to precipitate attacks of angina has led to the use of sedatives. Sir James Mackenzie believed that more good was to be obtained from bromides than from any other medication. The purpose is to diminish the nervous receptivity or instability of the patient so that those reflexes that are involved in the production of the attack or in the sensation of the discomfort will be dampened. For this purpose 1 gm. (15 grains) of sodium or potassium bromide or 0.015 to 0.03 gm. ($\frac{1}{4}$ to $\frac{1}{2}$ grain) of phenobarbital may be used three times a day. I have witnessed occasional instances in which patients who were having frequent short attacks at rest have promptly become entirely free from attacks following such medication. Unfortunately this is not the usual result. At times it is distinctly valuable to use a preparation such as sodium amytal, 0.2 gm. (3 grains), every few hours, to render the patient seminarcotized for a day or two to break up a storm of recurrent attacks of angina. In general I believe that the use of some form of sedatives, especially bromides, has a distinct place in the treatment of those patients who have frequent attacks of angina.

Because of the importance of the psychic and nervous factor it is best, whenever possible, for the physician to avoid the term "angina pectoris" in talking to his patients. It carries too great a dread in the mind of the average lay person today. When it is necessary to give explanations it is less shocking to state that the arteries within the heart are not so flexible or patent as normal, or that the heart is simply tired.

A sojourn to a warm climate is often advisable when circumstances permit this luxury. It is a common experience that patients who cannot walk a block during the winter in New England without pain are able to walk long distances in Florida. Not only is it warmer, but the weight of the clothes worn is less and the individuals are more relaxed.

During recent years there has come into vogue a series of new preparations that are supposed to dilate the coronary arteries and increase the blood flow through the heart. There is considerable experimental evidence in animals to show that these drugs do increase coronary flow. Whether similar effects are produced in human beings and especially in those who already have atheromatous changes in the coronary arteries is another matter and more difficult to prove. There is clinical evidence, however, although not all are agreed on this point, that some patients are more comfortable and can do more while taking these drugs. Of this group the common ones employed are Diuretin (0.3 to 0.5 gm. three times daily), aminophylline (0.1 to 0.2 gm. three times daily), Phyllicin (0.25 gm. three times daily), quinidine sulfate (0.2 to 0.3 gm. three times daily), Theocalcin (0.3 gm. three times daily), Theominal (0.3 gm. three times daily), Theobrominal (0.3 gm. three times daily), Erythrol tetranitrate (0.03 to 0.06 gm. three times daily), theobromine and sodium acetate (Thesodate) (0.5 gm. three times daily), choline theophyllinate (Choledyl) tablets (0.2 gm. three times daily), papaverine (60 to 120 mg. three times daily), and others. When attacks occur frequently during the day, or keep recurring regularly at night, Nitrol ointment is worth trying. About one inch of the ointment is smeared (not rubbed) over any portion of the skin. This can be repeated in several hours. There are instances in which this has a beneficial effect and decreases the need for nitroglycerin. Occasionally a rectal suppository of 0.5 gm. aminophylline once or twice daily is helpful. Physicians should employ those preparations that are least expensive and should omit them entirely if their observations indicate that no clinical improvement takes place. It is well to try patients on such a preparation for one month, then omit it for a month, alternating in such fashion and then deciding whether attacks are more or less troublesome on one regimen or another.

As has been mentioned before, if congestive failure is present digitalis and diuretics may also help angina if that is a concomitant symptom. For this reason it is wise to try an intramuscular injection of mercury in stubborn cases of angina, even when there is little or no peripheral pitting edema. At times such patients have latent edema and a successful diuresis may result, with improvement in the anginal pain.

Intramuscular injections of various tissue extracts have also been tried, but there is little valid evidence of their value. Cobra venom injections have been employed, with some success, in stubborn cases when attacks were recurring frequently. Although numerous other drugs have been used at one time or another they have generally proved disappointing. These few which have just been discussed, however, are worth a trial, but great expectations should not be based on their administration. Of these, aminophylline and theobromine, and their allied preparations, and quinidine are the most promising.

A drug, proposed by Anrep and his colleagues for the treatment of angina, called khellin, is derived from a plant (*Ammi visnaga*) that grows wild in Egypt. Experimentally this has been found to increase coronary flow. Only a few clinical reports have appeared which seem to be favorable. It is thought to act beneficially in angina and also in bronchial asthma, according to some observers. I have had some experience with it and feel that occasionally it is helpful. It is given orally in doses (tablets) of 50 mg. three times daily. It can be given intramuscularly, but experience with this method is very limited. The difficulty is that in about one third of the cases the drug causes ill effects such as nausea and dizziness, and has to be discontinued, although in none are there any serious complications. In some a smaller dose, i.e., 50 mg. once or twice daily, could be tolerated and proved helpful. Further observation will be necessary before final judgment can be made, but at present it would appear that khellin (Eskell) has possible value, especially if the toxic effects can be eliminated. The same may be said of Peritrate, a new preparation that has recently come into use. The dose is 10 to 20 mg. orally three to four times daily before meals. Although it is too early to be certain, this is thought by some to be more valuable than any of the ordinary oral preparations for prolonged use as a method of diminishing the incidence of anginal attacks.

There are several observations that point to the sex glands as possibly related to coronary sclerosis. Males in general far outnumber females among those suffering from coronary disease. This is strikingly true below the age of 40 or 50 years. In the latter decades, after the age of 70 years, the incidence is almost the same in the two sexes. It is also thought that hysterectomy or the normal menopause makes the female more susceptible to coronary disease. Finally, the administration of estrogens experimentally in animals tends to inhibit the development of atherosclerosis otherwise produced by high cholesterol diet. For these reasons attempts are being made in human males to prevent further progress of the disease in cases of angina or previous coronary thrombosis by long range estrogen therapy. This work is in its infancy. The feminizing effects of such treatment with the development of gynecomastia are obvious undesirable effects. It is hoped that, with further research, compounds might be found that eliminate the undesirable action of such hormones and yet retain its beneficial effect on the arteries.

The value of many of the drugs commonly employed in the treatment of angina pectoris have been appraised by various investigators. This has always been a difficult problem because of spontaneous variation in the course of the disease and particularly because the main index of favorable or unfavorable progress is the subjective complaint of chest distress. The effect of suggestion and emotional factors increase the difficulty. Using the double blind method of administering drugs, in which neither the observer nor the patient knows whether a placebo or the tested drug is used, patients who have been observed to be in a stationary condition have been studied. An individual is tested repeatedly and found to be able to take about 25 steps at a certain pace before developing pain. Then a given medication is administered and the test is repeated under similar circumstances. In this way many drugs have been found to have no value and others have been found to increase exercise tolerance. In such experiments digitalis was generally observed to have a deleterious effect. At times it is stated that certain preparations cause a 50 per cent improvement, when the patient can take 30 steps whereas during a control period he can take only 20 steps without pain. The reader may derive a false impression as to the value of such a drug, because 50 per cent improvement sounds like a great deal—one half a cure. In point of fact, all this gain really signifies is that the patient may be able to walk one block and a half instead of one block. He normally should have been able to walk a hundred blocks or more without chest pain. One can readily see that even if we accept the observations as valid the effect from these drugs cannot be very great.

As happens in any chronic disease for which no specific effective treatment is available, many bizarre therapeutic methods are suggested and often supported enthusiastically by their respective sponsors. X-ray treatment over the adrenals has been recommended on the basis that epinephrine acts as the trigger mechanism responsible for attacks of angina. Testosterone propionate given intramuscularly has been heralded as a valuable cure. I have tried all these medications and have failed to be convinced that they have any real specific value. The same may be said of vitamin E. It has been claimed by some that this produces striking benefit in cardiac disease, especially angina pectoris. Most critical observers have failed to confirm this view. The same is true for the intramuscular use of heparin. A critical study has indicated that it has no value in the treatment of angina. Finally it is thought by some that a snug abdominal belt applied so that pressure is exerted upward, elevating the diaphragm, can prevent attacks of angina on effort. This type of belt does help breathing in cases of emphysema and possibly in cardiac patients with congestive failure, and also makes patients with enlarged liver more comfortable. It therefore may indirectly be of some value in selected cases of angina. In fact, more recent observations seem to confirm the original view of Kerr that a definite minority of patients with angina are helped by use of an appropriate abdominal belt. Even an abnormal ballistocardiogram may become less abnormal in some patients with angina as a direct result of such a belt.

SURGICAL PROCEDURES

The recognition of the limitations of ordinary medical treatment for many diseases, the lack of specific therapy, and the rapid development of surgical technique and newer surgical procedures have brought the general surgeon into contact with problems that not so long ago were entirely confined to the attention of the physician. This has been true of practically all the organs of the body. The most recent spheres of surgical interest have been the lungs, the brain, and, last of all, the heart. We are now seeking surgical aid in the treatment of cardiac disease because of the failure to give our patients relief by use of the older methods. The problem of heart disease in this respect is difficult for many reasons. The morbid processes are for the most part progressive. The fundamental cause that is responsible for these changes is generally poorly understood, so that further progress of the processes can be altered but very little. Finally, the obvious technical difficulty of surgical manipulation of the interior of the heart has impeded the kind of therapeutic progress that has taken place in the treatment of disease of the kidneys, lungs, and other organs. Despite all this, attempts which at first might have appeared to be desperate have been made. Early in this development simple accidental wounds of the heart were repaired. Some 50 years ago Brauer introduced the operation of cardiolysis for adherent pericardium. This formed the stepping stone for further surgical work that has proved of real value in some otherwise hopeless cases of pericardial disease. Some years ago Cutler and Levine reported the first case of valvulotomy for mitral stenosis. Although the first patient survived the operation and seemed to be somewhat improved, the great operative mortality of the procedure rendered it impracticable. The surgeons likewise have been playing their role in attempts to relieve anginal pain.

The first surgical attempts to relieve attacks of angina pectoris consisted in removing the cervical sympathetic ganglia. This was first performed by Jonnesco, following the suggestion made many years ago by the physiologist François Franck. At first the entire chain, consisting of the superior, middle, and inferior ganglia, including the stellate ganglia, generally on the left side, was removed. Later a simpler operation in which only the superior ganglion was removed was proposed by Coffey and Brown. The results obtained by these operations were variable. It seemed that in about one half of the cases some relief was obtained, but it was impossible to predict who would and who would not be improved. I have had some patients who were greatly helped by this simple operation, including one who was enabled to walk miles without distress, and yet others who seemed equally promising subjects were hardly relieved at all. There was much controversial discussion concerning the rationale of these operations as the sensory and motor pathways to and from the human heart were not well understood. The most recent point of view is that the logical method of interrupting the painful impulses is through the upper four or five dorsal ganglia and not through the cervical ganglia. This has led to procedures consisting of alcohol injections of the upper dorsal nerves or extirpation of these nerve roots. The former type of operation carries with it almost no surgical mortality but often results in uncomfortable pains due to alcohol neuritis, whereas the latter is an elaborate surgical procedure which, when carried out on patients with angina, will entail an appreciable immediate operative risk. At present alcohol injections are very rarely performed, but interest in upper dorsal sympathectomy continues. This latter operation can afford satisfactory relief in a large majority of patients who survive the operation. Smithwick has performed a total dorsolumbar sympathectomy in a small number of hypertensive patients who also had angina, with no operative mortality and with very satisfactory clinical relief of the anginal pain. It would seem that operation on the sympathetic nervous system still has its place in a limited, well-selected group of patients suffering from intractable angina with or without hypertension.

I recall an instance in which a 16-year-old boy was suffering from intolerable attacks of angina as part of marked rheumatic aortic valvular disease. The heart was markedly enlarged, but there was no congestive heart failure. The boy's condition was pitiful, for he had terrific attacks of anginal pain accompanied by palpitation. During these spells the blood pressure would rise markedly. The pain was very severe and would spread across the upper chest, making the boy cry and beg for relief. Nitroglycerin would alleviate and shorten the distress. These attacks occurred frequently even while the patient was at rest in bed. We contemplated surgical treatment as all medical methods had failed. The possible procedures that occurred to us were a simple decompression of the chest (there was marked cardiac hypertrophy with a bulging of the precordium), a thyroidectomy, or a complete left-sided cervical sympathectomy. It was decided to try the latter. The therapeutic result was most gratifying. The painful attacks disappeared. Although the boy had spells, they consisted of palpitation and the terrible agony that previously accompanied them was gone. Instead of being a most distressing, bedridden cardiac cripple, he was able to return to school, gained weight, and was happy. Similar favorable results in cases of severe angina accompanying aortic valvular disease have been reported following alcohol injections of the dorsal ganglia. I have had other instances in which, after such operations, patients who previously had been greatly handicapped were improved and enabled to walk and carry on without pain. The puzzling feature of all this is that the same operation often proved to be a complete failure in cases that seemed promising. It appears, however, that these operations may yet be indicated in selected cases for the relief of pain, although there is no evidence that they prolong life or that they prevent the subsequent occurrence of sudden death or coronary thrombosis.

Another operation that was formerly employed is total thyroidectomy. During the several years after 1932, when it was first introduced, many patients with angina were subjected to this procedure. Relief of pain was generally obtained for a considerable period of time. The untoward effect of the induced myxedema detracted from the value of the operation so that in the course of time it was given up. The purpose was to diminish the metabolism of the body, thereby decreasing the demands on the heart. It must be recalled, however, that the output of the heart and therefore the coronary flow is likewise decreased. It would be helpful to a patient with coronary sclerosis if the decrease in total work of the heart exceeded the decrease in coronary flow as a result of lowering the body metabolism. Inasmuch as favorable effects do follow lowering of the total metabolism in cases of thyrotoxicosis with angina, it is logical to assume that similar effects might result if one started with a euthyroid state.

Since this drastic operation (total thyroidectomy) was abandoned, Blumgart re-introduced the application of the same principle by the administration of radioactive iodine. A medical complete or partial thyroidectomy could be produced by this simple means without any risk. Fairly satisfactory results have been reported from various clinics. I have employed this procedure in a good many instances. Treatment is not always successful, but some patients are helped considerably. Appreciating that this treatment is used only in stubborn refractory cases, it appears at present that radioactive iodine has a distinct place in our methods of treatment in a small selected group of patients suffering from intractable angina.

Finally, different attempts have been made to increase the coronary circulation by surgical measures. Beck sewed the left pectoral muscle to the pericardium overlying the left ventricle. O'Shaughnessy anastomosed a portion of the omentum through the diaphragm to the ventricle. In both instances elaborate experimental work was first carried out in animals which seemed to show that new blood vessels developed in the heart muscle. Later a considerable number of patients with coronary artery disease were subjected to these operations. Also the left coronary sinus has been ligated and the nerve fibers resected from the coronary arteries by Fauteux in a small group of patients with coronary artery disease. Here also the purpose was to encourage increased arterial supply to the myocardium.

Beck devised a more elaborate operation with the hope of increasing coronary blood flow. He anastomosed the subclavian artery (or some other vessel) to the coronary sinus, bringing arterial blood to the myocardium in a reversed direction through a coronary vein. (This procedure has now been abandoned.) Later Vineberg introduced the technique of inserting the mammary artery directly into the myocardium of the left ventricle. More recently Beck has been practicing and advocating a different procedure consisting of mechanical abrasion of the epicardium and parietal pericardium, partial ligation of the coronary sinus, instillation of powdered asbestos, and the application of mediastinal fat and pericardium to the heart. The objective is to stimulate intercoronary communication to bring additional blood to the myocardium.

The most recent operation that is being advised is ligation of both internal mammary arteries below the phrenic division. The claim is made that this increases the blood flow to the myocardium through the branches that reach the pericardium. This operation is very simple, it should carry very little risk, and excellent results are already being reported. More time, however, is needed for final appraisal of its merit.

Another and simpler method of increasing blood supply to the myocardium has been employed by Thompson and Raisbeck. They spray powdered talc over the visceral pericardium to induce adhesions of the two pericardial layers. The report of their experiences seems encouraging.

Certain modifications in this "talc" operation have been introduced by other surgeons. Believing that the usual pericardium may act as a barrier to the growth of new blood vessels into the myocardium, Harken denudes the pericardium by the application of phenol and also sews the lingula pulmonalis to the ventricle. This operation is called de-epicardialization–poudrage–pneumonopexy. Operative mortality is low, in contrast to that following the more elaborate operations that have been proposed. Although it is still too early to be dogmatic and certain of the value of this procedure (as anginal pain may alter its course spontaneously in a most bizarre fashion), it appears that striking relief of pain has occurred in some cases. I have advised this operation in a selected group of patients who have frequent attacks of anginal pain, especially if they occur at rest without cause, or in whom the pain on effort prevents the carrying on of essential daily duties. They should also have a sense of well-being when free from pain, for the main effect to be hoped for from surgery is amelioration of the pain.

Each author has reported satisfactory results from his own procedure. For the present these operations should be regarded as still in the experimental stage. That does not mean that they should be condemned. The heart is the last important organ for the surgeon to explore. It is an encouraging sign that such numerous and varied attempts at surgical treatment for chronic heart disease and for coronary artery disease are being made. This is especially desirable as medical management at present is far from satisfactory.

Coronary Thrombosis

The clinical recognition of acute coronary thrombosis forms one of the most interesting chapters in the history of medicine. Although there were isolated instances in which a clinical antemortem diagnosis of occlusion of a coronary vessel was made, such as that by Hammer in 1878, and although there were other reports that touched upon the question in one way or another, the first publication that discussed the clinical features which might help us in differentiating an attack of coronary thrombosis from one of angina pectoris was by Obrastzow and Straschesko in 1910. A second one by Herrick appeared in 1912. Only then did it become clear that there were certain findings obtainable ante mortem which differentiated the two conditions. In fact, Herrick first emphasized that the condition need not be fatal. Before this a great deal was known concerning the condition from a pathologic point of view, but the clinical findings in the living patient remained entirely confused and were obscured by terms like "status anginosus" and "myomalacia cordis." It is difficult to understand how the great clinicians of the past, many of whom had performed many postmortem examinations, could have overlooked this problem, especially when it is appreciated that the recognition of coronary thrombosis developed from a purely clinical study of patients without the use of any of the elaborate procedures or laboratory methods that characterize the modern era of medicine.

Despite these publications in the early part of the second decade of this century, very few physicians became familiar with this condition for some years. This important work seems to have been overlooked for a decade or more, except by a very few. In 1916 I had the opportunity of seeing two cases of acute coronary thrombosis, both presenting the picture of an acute surgical abdomen. In the first case I advised immediate exploration and the surgeon agreed to operate. This patient died on the operating table, and postmortem examination to our amazement showed an acute coronary thrombosis and infarction of the myocardium. The second case was seen several months later and, based on the previous experience, a clinical diagnosis of coronary thrombosis was made. The patient died a short time later, and postmortem examination confirmed the clinical diagnosis. These were my initial experiences with coronary thrombosis, a condition which has interested me ever since.

In considering the etiologic factors, all that has been discussed under angina pectoris applies more or less with equal force to coronary thrombosis and infarction of the myocardium. All those influences that are conducive to or associated with arterial disease naturally form the background upon which coronary thrombosis develops. Most important is the familial factor. Males overwhelmingly predominate. The majority have had hypertension previously. A large number have had diabetes. Only a few are syphilitic. Some have had conditions like gout, Buerger's disease, polycythemia, and hyperthyroidism. Some who had a rheumatic valvular lesion had in addition disease of the coronary arteries. The great majority of patients have had a previous history of angina pectoris, either of short but more often of long duration. Frequently this early history of angina is overlooked and the sudden attack of coronary thrombosis is then regarded as the first indication of any serious heart disease. I have frequently elicited such definite evidence by direct questioning when it had previously been assumed by both the patient and the physician that all was well. There are, however, many instances in which an attack occurs without warning, like a bolt from the blue, and in which it can clearly be said that no element of angina preceded it.

Conditions associated with an abrupt fall in blood pressure or marked slowing of the circulation may be conducive to the development of acute myocardial infarction with or without coronary thrombosis. Occasionally coronary thrombosis may develop as a sequence of shock that follows a brisk hemorrhage from a peptic ulcer. It also may occur during or following any surgical operation if there is a significant fall in blood pressure. This complication is particularly to be feared when spinal anesthesia (Fig. 165) is administered and a fall in blood pressure is not prevented or quickly controlled. It is fair to assume that the hazard does not exist except in those patients who already have coronary sclerosis with vulnerable blood vessels. This explains the occurrence of such accidents in elderly patients subjected to prostatectomy and in old debilitated individuals who are in a state of shock for any reason. Failure of cerebral circulation may occur as a result of the same mechanism that has just been discussed.

Coronary thrombosis is related to angina pectoris in much the same way as an occlusion of a vessel of the leg with gangrene is related to intermittent claudication. The anginal state may be regarded as a transitory one, leaving the heart in practically the same condition after an attack as before. When a partial or complete occlusion occurs, the muscle supplied by that vessel suffers to a lesser or greater degree. Sometime during the life of those suffering from angina a thrombosis of a coronary artery is apt to occur. This is the common cause of death in angina, although not a necessary one. There are a few cases of angina, even among those in which death occurs instantly, in which no acute thrombus can be seen. Such hearts in my experience have almost always shown significant atheromatous changes in the coronary arteries. In fact, I have seen but two cases of angina in which the coronary arteries were normal, except when there was one of these associated conditions discussed above, such as aortic or mitral valvular disease, that adequately explained the condition. One was a case of severe refractory anemia and in the other there was extensive amyloidosis of the myocardium.

It has always been puzzling to explain the precipitating causes of an acute thrombosis. There is both clinical and pathological evidence to make one believe that it occurs at the site of a previous sclerotic or atheromatous area in a coronary vessel. The occlusion, partial or complete, then occurs rather suddenly. It is not due to an embolus dislodged elsewhere, for coronary emboli are very rare and are likely to be associated with vegetation at or near the aortic valve. Do further platelet thrombi develop on the roughened surface of the vessel which lead to greater narrowing of the channel? This seems reasonable, but does not quite explain the extreme suddenness of some of the attacks. Or does the final occlusion result from the rupture of a miliary subendothelial atheromatous "abscess" as some experimental studies of Leary suggest? The latter hypothesis would explain the abruptness of the symptoms better than the former. Another possible mechanism that has been postulated is that minute hemorrhages first occur within the layers of the wall of the coronary arteries and these are followed by changes in the vessel wall such as narrowing and thrombosis. Possibly all mechanisms are involved in different cases.

A new method of studying the coronary arteries by a special type of injection devised by Schlesinger has thrown considerable light on this problem. It has revealed that many thromboses occur that are not recognized in life and that are not accompanied by the clinical features of an acute attack to be described shortly. It has also been found that thromboses occur without infarction and that infarction can also take place without thrombosis. Most hearts have shown two or more occlusions, even as many as ten in rare instances. This technique has revealed many new, interesting, and important clinical pathological correlations.

Another perplexing aspect of coronary thrombosis is the frequency with which a particular part of the coronary system is involved. A common site is in the descending branch of the left coronary artery, about 1 inch from its origin. Sclerotic changes and thrombosis are so common at this particular spot as to make one suspect that a mechanical factor is involved. Is it possible that as the heart contracts there is a greater bend or torsion of the artery at this point? If this were so it could throw some light on the hereditary factor that is so striking in this disease. We do inherit specific anatomic characteristics such as the color of the iris and configuration of the nose. May not those several members of a family with early coronary artery disease inherit a peculiar architecture of these vessels which puts them under greater mechanical strain as a result of the normal twisting and bending that goes on with the motion of the heart? This presents an anatomic and physical problem about which we have entirely too few data.

THE CLINICAL PICTURE

Before taking up the clinical aspects of acute coronary thrombosis it will be helpful to review briefly the pathologic process that is taking place. When a coronary vessel becomes partially or completely occluded the area of heart muscle supplied by that vessel becomes infarcted. Early in the process there is extravasation of blood, then muscle fiber necrosis and finally repair by scar tissue. If the involved area extends to the periphery a localized aseptic pericarditis may develop, and if it extends inwardly the endocardium may be involved, resulting in a large secondary ventricular mural thrombus attached to the area of infarction. The local area of necrosis may become sufficiently softened to perforate during the early days or the wall may be weakened to such an extent that a localized aneurysm of the ventricle results. When satisfactory healing takes place due to the anastomosis of collateral vessels, which occurs more frequently in the heart than was formerly thought, a healthy scar forms. This simple review enables one to picture some of the clinical events that occur.

Attacks of coronary thrombosis seem to occur more frequently at rest than during effort. Furthermore, the patient may become restless and walk around or pace the floor instead of remaining still. In this respect it differs from angina pectoris. It is a common experience to find that the patient is aroused from sleep with the attack. On close questioning many will confess that during the preceding day or two they had not felt quite so well and may have had more or less mild discomfort in the chest. Occasionally one may suspect that a coronary thrombosis is impending when a patient who previously had ordinary attacks of angina promptly relieved by rest or nitroglycerin suddenly starts having attacks without effort, lasting a half hour or so and not responding to nitroglycerin; also, if similar severe symptoms occur without preceding angina, an outspoken coronary attack not infrequently follows in a few days.

In its typical form the pain of coronary thrombosis becomes very severe, almost unbearable. The location and severity of the pain varies a great deal in different cases just as there is a striking variability of most of the clinical features of the disease. Although no single sign or symptom is found in all cases, there generally is enough evidence of one form or another to make the diagnosis fairly definite. The amount of pain may vary from none at all to the most severe agony any mortal can suffer. It takes the form of a pressure or terrible crushing or squeezing sensation. Its location most often is in the middle of the chest centering around the sternum, or between the two nipples. It can either begin in or even be limited to the upper epigastrium near the ensiform. It often radiates to the upper midback, shoulders, and arms. It must be borne in mind that in some the distress is not very marked and in fact there are a few who are not prevented from carrying on their activities throughout an attack. The duration of the pain is also variable, lasting from an hour or two to several days. In some it comes in waves, each lasting about fifteen minutes, until it becomes continuous. Generally after six or twelve hours the severity has abated although a milder soreness persists. Not uncommonly after the pain has subsided it returns in varying degrees for several days or longer.

Breathlessness may be the presenting complaint, particularly in those occasional instances in which pain is very slight or absent. Although dyspnea is not present in most cases there are a few in which the clinical picture is one of acute pulmonary edema. Even when the respiratory symptoms are not so fulminating, orthopnea or other evidence of embarrassed breathing may be apparent.

In many instances there is a peculiar and rather characteristic appearance of the patient during the height of the attack. He seems to be in shock. The skin is cold and moist, and takes on a gray ashen color. The face is anxious and one is quickly aware that something profound has happened. In the early hours and days sweating is often very marked, resulting in dehydration and a loss of salt from the body. In fact, a very moist skin may persist for weeks and gives one the impression that the underlying process of myocardial infarction is still active or insecure. In some atypical cases a moist skin may be the first clue that the illness which was painless and consisted mainly of weakness is due to an acute coronary thrombosis. Great weakness is often very striking, even when there are but few other complaints. With this there is generally a fall in the blood pressure. This fall occurs in varying relation to the onset of the attack. Sometimes the first reading that the physician obtains is extremely low or the patient may already be pulseless. Not infrequently the blood pressure is still elevated during the first few hours and falls subsequently. On very rare occasions no significant change takes place at all. In the typical case the systolic pressure that was around 170 mm. gradually falls to 110 mm., this change possibly taking place over several days. With the progress of the case it may return to its previous level or be permanently lower to a greater or lesser extent. Practically always the pressure returns approximately to the original level during the following year or two.

Gastrointestinal symptoms are often prominent and may be troublesome from a diagnostic or from a therapeutic point of view. The abdominal pain and tenderness which occur in a few cases resemble an acute surgical condition. Even slight icterus may be present. Nausea, vomiting, and distention may be distressing and at times resemble the symptoms of acute intestinal obstruction. Vomiting is very common during the first hours of the attack and may become even more prominent after the frequent injections of morphine are given which are necessary to control the pain. Occasionally annoying hiccoughs develop. Usually all these symptoms disappear after one to several days.

A slight fever and leukocytosis are very common accompaniments of coronary thrombosis. They both require some time to develop and are generally present in twenty-four to forty-eight hours, although they may be found at times as soon as six hours after the onset. The fever is often overlooked if the temperature is taken by mouth, as these patients are in shock and the periphery of the body may be actually cold in the presence of a true fever. This error will be avoided if a rectal temperature is taken. I have often found the latter to be ±101° F. when the mouth temperature was only 98° F. The slight fever lasts from three to seven days, rarely longer. The leukocytosis ranges around 15,000 to 20,000 and also lasts several days. The sedimentation rate of the erythrocytes is also increased, probably as a result of the myocardial infarction. This increase is apt to occur a few days after the onset of the attack and may persist for two weeks or more even after the fever and leukocytosis have disappeared. Occasionally the sedimentation rate may indirectly aid in differentiating an attack of coronary thrombosis from one of angina pectoris or other conditions or may help in the decision as to whether an extension or aggravation of the myocardial infarction has taken place.

Enzyme chemistry has now come into use in following cases of coronary disease. It has been found that the serum glutamic oxalacetic aminopherase (transaminase) and other enzymes such as lactic dehydrogenase increase sharply in the blood as a result of myocardial infarction. The rise may begin in several hours, reaches its maximum in one or two days, and then gradually returns to normal in several days or longer. The maximum increase may be two- to twenty-fold. This rise does not occur in angina or simple acute coronary insufficiency. There may be a slight rise in congestive heart failure, pulmonary infarction, and certain diseases of the liver. The test for such enzymes promises to be of considerable diagnostic value in doubtful cases of myocardial infarction.

The findings on examination of the heart are variable. The sounds generally diminish strikingly in intensity so that at times they are almost inaudible. However, in some the first heart sound may be normal or occasionally increased in intensity if the P-R interval is short. The rate becomes accelerated to about 100 to 120 and in many instances a definite gallop rhythm can be heard. Just as is true of all these individual features, there are numerous exceptions. Occasionally there is no acceleration of the heart rate. A small number of patients will show a transient pericardial friction rub. When this occurs it is extremely helpful in diagnosis but its development will depend upon the location and extent of the myocardial infarction. Almost any of the disturbances in rhythm with which we are familiar may develop during the early days following an acute coronary thrombosis. When they do occur most of them are transient and the normal rhythm returns. Of the important arrhythmias, transient auricular fibrillation is most common. Auricular flutter is rare but ventricular tachycardia is not uncommon. Extrasystoles are also common. Some patients will show partial and a few will develop complete heart block even with Adams-Stokes attacks of syncope. Conduction defects are more apt to develop with posterior lesions. The apex impulse disappears as a result of the feeble contraction. Although one might think that with such a profound injury to the cardiac mechanism dilatation would occur, x-ray studies have shown no such change.

The examination of the lungs will frequently show some rales at the bases, especially on the right side. Occasionally typical evidence of acute pulmonary edema will be found with moist or bubbling rales all over the chest. In fact, an attack of coronary thrombosis may be ushered in by this type of onset even without chest pain. Sudden dyspnea may, therefore, replace sudden pain as the presenting complaint. Cheyne-Stokes breathing is very common even when there is no subjective respiratory distress. The abdominal examination is generally not remarkable, although in a few cases the findings resemble an acute surgical condition, for there may be tenderness and muscular spasm in the epigastrium or right upper quadrant. In some cases at least these findings are due to an acute passive congestion and enlargement of the liver with the accompanying tension on the liver capsule. In one case in which the abdomen was explored as a result of a mistaken diagnosis this was observed.

The urinary findings deserve some mention. Many patients will show marked oliguria and some will void practically no urine for twelve to twenty-four hours. This is the result of the low blood pressure and the state of shock. It is unwise to catheterize the bladder during these early hours merely because little urine has been voided. Generally only a few cubic centimeters will be obtained and often a local infection requiring antibiotics and other troublesome procedures will result unnecessarily. The urine that is voided is concentrated and may show an appreciable amount of albumin and numerous cells and casts. Glycosuria is very common, first because so many diabetics develop coronary thrombosis and because others who never had glycosuria before may temporarily show sugar in the urine as part of the coronary attack. Some of the latter are possibly mild or potential diabetics but it seems that in others, who temporarily show glycosuria, it is entirely precipitated by the heart attack. What is important to bear in mind is that the urinary findings indicative of renal disease need give us no great concern as they always clear up if the circulation improves. The same may be said of the glycosuria. It rarely if ever requires insulin during the acute stages. In general it is better to disregard the diabetes unless, as very rarely occurs, there is a significant acidosis as shown by a lowering of the carbon dioxide–combining power of the blood.

Electrocardiography has been a most important aid in the diagnosis of coronary thrombosis. Although Herrick very early in his work suspected that certain electrocardiographic changes might possibly be the result of coronary thrombosis, it was Pardee who first established the fact that, during the early hours or days after an attack, the ventricular complex may take on a peculiar form. This consisted of a high take-off of the T wave from the QRS complex before the latter reaches the isoelectric line in one or another of the customary three leads. This does away with the normal short flat interval between the initial and final phases of the ventricular complex. It has also been found that rapid alterations in the complexes occur during the succeeding days or weeks following an attack. The T waves become rounded and dipped (coveshaped) and finally peculiarly inverted (Chap. 21). At any one particular time these tracings may appear essentially normal, but if a series of several electrocardiograms is taken during the first two weeks most if not all will show definite or at least suspicious alterations. The introduction of precordial leads by Wilson, Wolferth, and Wood has further increased the usefulness of electrocardiography, for there are some instances in which the area of infarction is so located that the customary limb leads fail to show any significant aberrations while the chest lead will bring forth definite evidence of heart muscle injury.

Electrocardiography has not only been valuable in diagnosis, but has enabled us to predict in many instances the exact location of the area of infarction. Injuries to the anterior part of the heart generally occurring in the lower lateral portion of the left ventricle near the apex and resulting from a thrombosis of the descending branch of the left coronary artery are associated with one type of electrocardiogram. Similar injuries to the posterior part of the ventricle, either resulting from a thrombosis of the circumflex branch of the left coronary artery or of the right coronary artery, produce a different set of changes. In the former the high take-off of the T wave with subsequent inversion of the T wave and the appearance of a Q wave occur in Lead I. In the latter type these similar changes occur in Lead III. Wilson has indeed shown that while the changes in the T wave are often transient with even complete restoration of the normal appearing upright T wave, the changes in the initial ventricular complexes, notably the Q wave, are apt to be permanent. In this way one may be enabled to suspect months or years after an attack that one previously had taken place. Further electrocardiographic details will be presented in Chapter 21. All forms of conduction disturbance are found, such as partial or complete heart block and bundle branch block. Also in some the ventricular complexes are of unusually low amplitude. Unless the changes are quite characteristic, caution must be exercised in accepting alterations in the complexes as unequivocal evidence of myocardial infarction, as they may occur in a variety of other conditions such as pulmonary embolism, acute dissecting aneurysm, acute nephritis, uremia, and rheumatic carditis.

In an uncomplicated case of coronary thrombosis of moderate severity the patient is apt to become free from pain after the first day and thereafter to remain quite comfortable. In other patients pain returns irregularly over a much longer time. Those whose respiratory function becomes embarrassed may have marked dyspnea and orthopnea. The various irregularities of the heart previously mentioned may suddenly change the clinical status and require special attention. At any time during this illness sudden death can occur either as a result of ventricular fibrillation or rupture of the softened infarcted area of the ventricle or possibly from complete heart block. Ruptures do not usually occur until about the fourth to seventh day.

When the infarction involves the ventricular septum and is extensive it may rupture. The main evidence of this is a sudden appearance of a loud systolic murmur over the midprecordium and near the apex. With this complication there is likely to occur a sudden change for the worse with collapse. Bernheim's syndrome may develop, i.e., right-sided heart failure with increased venous pressure resulting from bulging of the interventricular septum into the right ventricular cavity.

Another type of complication is embolism. In many of these cases a fresh mural thrombus develops in one of the ventricles, generally the left, contiguous to the area of infarction. Portions of this thrombus may become dislodged and occlude other vessels, producing secondary embolic lesions. If they come from the left ventricle, hemiplegia, renal, splenic, or mesenteric infarcts may result, or gangrene of one of the extremities. If they arise in the right ventricle, pulmonary embolism or infarction occurs. These are most likely to take place after the first few days. The pericarditis that occasionally is found requires no particular concern as it almost never results in empyema or pericardial effusion. It is evident, therefore, that the exact course which any individual case may take can vary greatly.

Death may occur with great suddenness even when everything seems to be going most favorably. In other patients there is a gradual weakening of the pulse with a low blood pressure, marked weakness, and a quiet, peaceful end. In some there is a great deal of dyspnea and air hunger.

There are three possible causes of sudden death during these early days. The first two types could only be identified if a chance electrocardiogram happened to be taken the moment the catastrophe occurred, i.e., a sudden complete heart block with ventricular asystole or ventricular fibrillation. The third is rupture of the ventricle. This latter complication is the cause of about 10 per cent of fatalities from acute myocardial infarction and most commonly takes place between the third and the tenth day. It is much more likely to occur in those cases which maintain an elevated blood pressure, where the infarction is transmural and the area of necrosis is comparatively free of fibrosis, showing poor collateral vessels and little evidence of old infarction or previous angina. Unusual physical effort during the acute stage of the disease is thought to predispose to ventricular rupture. Rupture is less likely to occur in the presence of congestive heart failure even when the patient is receiving digitalis.

When recovery takes place we must also anticipate different sequelae. There are some who, having suffered from angina pectoris, either have no symptoms at all after an attack of coronary thrombosis or have much less trouble than they had prior to the attack. These patients are apt to be the ones who previously had hypertension in whom the pressure becomes permanently lowered after an occlusion of one of the coronary arteries. In others anginal attacks return with the same frequency, and in some angina pectoris may appear for the first time after a coronary attack. There is a large group of patients who, never having shown any dyspnea or congestive heart failure, first begin to manifest these symptoms after an attack of coronary thrombosis. Occasionally this occurs during the first week following the attack, but more commonly the patient becomes ambulatory and only months or years later begins to have general circulatory failure.

A localized aneurysm of the left ventricle with thinning and weakening of the wall occasionally results from a previous infarction. Curiously enough, rupture of the ventricle, which is by no means rare during the early days of an acute attack, rarely if ever occurs at the site of such chronic fibrosed ventricular aneurysms. They are present after recovery has taken place and the patient is ambulatory, and the condition is compatible with a fairly satisfactory state of the circulation. The diagnosis of ventricular aneurysm will rest on a previous history of myocardial infarction, the finding of a visible and palpable apex impulse well inside the outer border of dullness, a diminished first heart sound, certain suggestive electrocardiographic changes (Fig. 171), and roentgenographic findings. X-ray will show a localized bulge, and on fluoroscopic or kymographic examination this bulge will be observed to expand outwardly with systole as the neighboring musculature contracts inwardly. At times an apical systolic murmur, even with a presystolic murmur, may be heard in cases of ventricular aneurysm.

PROGNOSIS

The prognosis for patients with acute coronary thrombosis with myocardial infarction is variable. When large series of these patients were first studied it seemed that about 50 per cent recovered and the other 50 per cent died during the acute attack. The true figures are now much more favorable, because in the former studies only classic, severe, easily recognized cases were included, Now, with more advanced methods of diagnosis, many milder cases can be included and the immediate mortality will vary between 10 and 25 per cent, depending on the accuracy of the diagnosis.

In an extensive review of the immediate mortality certain points of interest came to light. Anterior and posterior lesions were equally serious. The mortality was lower if significant electrocardiographic changes were slight or absent, was slightly higher for women than for men, and was definitely higher in older than in younger individuals. A previous history of angina improved the immediate prognosis, while a pre-existing hypertension made it worse. A marked fall in blood pressure, especially if the level was maintained below 80 mm. for some time, made the outlook quite grave. The severity of dyspnea was more ominous than the degree of pain. In general, the immediate mortality was greater if the customary clinical features of acute coronary thrombosis, i.e., a higher fever, more rapid pulse, greater leukocytosis, and more profound shock, were more prominent.

After recovery from an acute coronary thrombosis had taken place the duration of life was found to vary greatly, the average being about three and one-half years. There was little difference in the length of survival between subjects with anterior and those with posterior infarctions. Those with only minor alterations in the electrocardiograms lived longer. One fourth had succumbed in one year, one half in two years, three fourths in five years, and the remainder died at varying intervals up to more than twenty-five years. Two thirds had angina some time after the attack of coronary thrombosis and about one fourth developed congestive failure. The latter complication occurred more frequently with anterior than with posterior infarction. About 30 per cent of the subjects resumed essentially full duties for varying lengths of time and the remainder were more or less restricted. The survival period for women was much shorter than for men, and it was much shorter for older subjects than for younger ones.

The observations just mentioned concerning prognosis were derived from the study of hospital cases. They are weighted unfavorably, as the more severe cases are sent to a general hospital. If a larger number of milder cases that are quite common had been included, the figures would obviously have been much more optimistic. In estimating prognosis individual circumstances must be appraised. The outlook would be better the younger the patient, if the heart remains normal in size, angina or congestive symptoms are absent, the electrocardiogram is normal or nearly so, the rhythm regular, the blood pressure within normal range, and the family history favorable, than it would be if some of these clinical features were otherwise.

In appraising statistics concerning prognosis the source and type of material need careful analysis. If the figures are compiled by a physician who mainly sees ambulatory patients he obviously cannot include those who are quite sick or confined to their homes. He also cannot be including many who already have died, either during the acute attack or during the first few weeks or months after the attack. If the consultant is reluctant to see acute emergencies or because of his work cannot answer sudden calls, he may avoid seeing many severe cases and will have for study an undue number of milder cases. On the other hand, the figures compiled from cases observed in a large general hospital are likely to be weighted with severely ill patients. Finally, the criteria for the diagnosis of myocardial infarction influence statistics. Many patients with ambulatory angina who have never had a clinical episode of coronary thrombosis and who never required or were never advised to take a period of rest present electrocardiograms that some will regard as evidence of old myocardial infarction and others will not. Such differences in interpretation will greatly influence the final statistics obtained in the study. One can readily see how difficult it is to compare one study with another.

As an illustration of the difficulties in prognosis the following experience is of interest. A physician had a severe attack of coronary thrombosis at the age of 45. During the subsequent fourteen years he had several more attacks of coronary thrombosis and many attacks of paroxysmal ventricular tachycardia. On more than one occasion he was in profound shock, semiconscious and pulseless, with a heart rate of 200 or more. With the first attack and during most of these years a definite gallop rhythm was present. He never showed evidence of significant congestive failure and there was no dyspnea. He remained ambulatory but had frequent attacks of angina which were promptly relieved by nitroglycerin. Incidentally, he persisted in smoking ten cigars daily, ate two eggs every morning, and was quite happy.

The knowledge that some can recover and carry on in good health for a long time, even fifteen years or more, permits us to encourage our patients. Furthermore, satisfactory recovery from a second and even from multiple attacks occurs but with increasing rarity. In general, the prognosis should be guarded but always hopeful, for even in the face of an extremely severe and desperate attack satisfactory recovery may take place.

DIFFERENTIAL DIAGNOSIS

There are several conditions that may at times become easily confused with coronary thrombosis. Of first importance are the conditions that resemble acute surgical states of the abdomen, such as gallstone colic, perforated peptic ulcer, acute pancreatitis, acute appendicitis, and acute intestinal obstruction. All the diagnostic methods available may be required to arrive at the correct diagnosis in such cases, and despite care there will be rare instances in which errors will be made. The presence of dyspnea with the attack and the radiation of the pain to the sternum or to the arms may be helpful in differentiation. The electrocardiograms may be the turning point on which a diagnosis will rest. There is also the opposite danger of overlooking an acute surgical condition requiring immediate abdominal operation in our enthusiasm to detect instances of coronary thrombosis, for it must be borne in mind that patients with known organic heart disease, as well as those who are only suspected of having it, may also have these very surgical conditions which require an operation.

Another condition that may closely simulate acute coronary thrombosis is pulmonary embolism or pulmonary infarction (acute cor pulmonale). In both there may be sudden circulatory collapse, dyspnea, a rapid thready pulse, and cyanosis. Pain in the chest is less common with pulmonary embolism, although it does occur and is particularly disconcerting when it takes place on the left side. On the other hand, pain may be absent in both conditions. During the early hours after a pulmonary embolism, there is no hemoptysis and examination of the lungs is apt to be of no help in diagnosis. Both conditions may occur after surgical operations, but it will help to simplify matters if a cause for pulmonary embolism, such as phlebitis, can be detected. Distention of the veins of the neck, although not an absolutely distinguishing physical finding, is more likely to be present with a pulmonary than with a coronary attack. In pulmonary embolism the pulmonary second sound is often accentuated and there is a systolic murmur in this area, probably due to the dilated pulmonary artery and the increased pulmonary pressure proximal to the embolus. Finally, the electrocardiograms may prove valuable in diagnosis. Minor changes in the ventricular complexes are common to both, but outspoken alterations, like a very high take-off of the T wave or a sharp rounded inversion of the T wave, occur only with cardiac infarction. Occasionally the electrocardiograms are sufficiently distinctive to make a fairly definite diagnosis of acute pulmonary embolism (Chap. 21, Figs. 173 to 178).

Two experiences, almost identical in detail, that had important medicolegal implications are of interest in this regard. A man about 45 years old was accidentally hit in the ankle while at work. He limped around for the rest of the day having mild pain in the leg. A few days later an x-ray revealed a slight fracture. The leg was put in a cast and the man put at rest. Two weeks later he suffered an attack which was diagnosed as acute coronary thrombosis with posterior myocardial infarction. He died a few days later, and no autopsy was performed. Three months later I received the above information and was asked by the widow's attorney to help in the litigation that was going on. Not wishing to appear in court I was ready to express an opinion in writing. I stated that if the man died of a coronary thrombosis it was questionable whether there was any relation between the original accident and the death three weeks later. However, I suspected that the correct diagnosis was a sudden pulmonary embolism from a thrombophlebitis of the right leg, and if that were true death could be regarded as a direct result of the accident. In that case the trauma, the cast, and the immobility caused the thrombophlebitis and the dislodgement of a clot caused the fatal pulmonary embolism. I therefore urged that the body be disinterred and an autopsy be performed. This was done and the predicted findings were confirmed. The heart was normal; there was a large pulmonary embolism and a thrombophlebitis of the leg was found. The second experience was exactly the same as the above. In both instances the widows rightly obtained the compensation that was their due, which otherwise would have been denied them.

The lessons to be drawn from these two experiences are (1) that the physician should think first of pulmonary embolism rather than of coronary thrombosis if some thoracic catastrophe follows a trauma, and (2) that electrocardiograms of acute cor pulmonale may resemble those of posterior myocardial infarction. Furthermore, it is apparently valuable at times to perform an autopsy even months after burial.

In reviewing the differential diagnosis I need but recall errors that have occurred, some of which I have made myself. In one instance some years ago I made the diagnosis of coronary thrombosis because of sudden suffocation and collapse occurring in a man 60 years of age. The patient seemed to be in shock with a rapid thready pulse. Although there was very little pain I thought he had had a coronary accident. It was not until the next day that I realized that one side of the chest was not expanding with respiration and there were practically no breath sounds on that side. He had a complete pneumothorax from which he recovered very satisfactorily.

Another difficulty in diagnosis is the differentiation of pneumonia and coronary thrombosis. The fairly acute onset of chest pain, cough, dyspnea, cyanosis, and the development of fever, leukocytosis, rapid pulse, and rales in the lungs occur in both conditions. There are no significant alterations in the electrocardiograms in pneumonia, however. This differential diagnosis at times is very difficult and I recall erring in each direction, considering a case one of pneumonia when it was coronary thrombosis and in another making the opposite mistake. Electrocardiograms may serve to differentiate the two. No doubt many elderly patients considered as having pneumonia really have suffered an attack of coronary thrombosis.

Diabetic acidosis and coma may be simulated by acute coronary thrombosis. Inasmuch as the latter often occurs in diabetic patients glycosuria is very common. There may also be an associated acidosis with diacetic acid in the urine and a lowered carbon dioxide–combining power of the blood. When such findings accompany a state of semistupor or complete unconsciousness one is strongly tempted to regard the condition as diabetic coma. All this, however, can result from an attack of coronary thrombosis. Inasmuch as insulin may be harmful to patients with coronary artery disease great care must be exercised in differentiating the two conditions. If the blood sugar is not high, insulin should not be given, and even when it is found to be elevated only small doses should be used unless it is certain that diabetic coma is present. In general I have very rarely found it necessary to use insulin in such patients.

Hamman has called attention to a condition that may closely simulate acute coronary thrombosis. He called it "spontaneous interstitial emphysema of the lungs." Many of us must have confused these two conditions in the past. Such patients are suddenly stricken with violent pain over the precordium with radiation to the left shoulder and left arm, and there may be an acceleration of the pulse, a leukocytosis, and slight fever. All this results from the rupture of an air sac in the lung that dissects its way along the bronchi and blood vessels and infiltrates the mediastinal tissues. The air may extend in the subcutaneous tissue to the neck or may reach the pleural space, producing a pneumothorax. The most important and characteristic finding is the presence of unusual clicking, grunting, or crunching sounds synchronous with the heart beat. These sounds may be influenced by respiration and may be entirely absent with the patient flat on his back, only to be brought out in the left lateral position. In some, the x-ray will show air in the left pleural cavity or in the anterior mediastinal spaces. This condition is essentially benign, as complete recovery is apt to occur. The only treatment necessary is sedation for the pain and a brief period of rest. The importance of the condition lies in the fact that it needs to be differentiated from coronary thrombosis and it impels us to watch carefully for these unusual auscultatory findings. It also must not be confused with noises that may on rare occasions be heard in cases of diaphragmatic hernia. Such splashing "heart noises" result from the beating of the heart against the stomach or intestines, which may lie in the chest.

There is a group of patients in whom the early symptoms of the acute stage are so mild that they are disregarded and the subjects present themselves as medical problems only after an embolus has occurred, particularly when a hemiplegia results. Some cases that are diagnosed cerebral hemorrhage fall into this group. The possibility that a hemiplegia may be due to an embolus dislodged from a left ventricular mural thrombus following a coronary thrombosis should always be considered when it occurs in a patient who has a low blood pressure. Even in elderly patients cerebral hemorrhages of the ordinary type, excluding those resulting from aneurysms of the cerebral vessels, rarely if ever occur without hypertension. A consideration of all the diagnostic points may be necessary in order to arrive at the correct diagnosis.

There are atypical cases of coronary thrombosis in which extensive experience will be necessary to avoid making erroneous diagnoses. This is particularly true in the occasional instances in which pain does not occur. Here there is apt to be sudden breathlessness and a feeling of exhaustion. In such cases the dyspnea will be found to be out of proportion to other evidences of heart failure. When this is the case, a low blood pressure, if it is known to have been high before, together with other features such as changes in the electrocardiograms, will give one the proper clue.

When the coronary vessels are slowly narrowing, infarctions of the heart may occur without any acute episode. This may take place in patients who have progressive heart failure and are regarded as suffering from chronic myocarditis. Even here a proper survey of all the data, especially obtaining a history of early angina pectoris and the study of the electrocardiograms, may enable us to anticipate the true pathologic state.

Considerable interest has developed in the diagnosis of dissecting aortic aneurysm which is often confused with acute coronary thrombosis. The pain in the former comes with even greater suddenness than that in the latter. The pain in the chest is crushing, may extend through to the back and at times even to the legs. Hypertension is generally found, and it tends to persist after the attack. Fever and leukocytosis develop, but there are none of the irregularities of the heart or a friction rub that occur in coronary thrombosis. Although the electrocardiograms in most cases remain unchanged and fail to show significant alterations in the ventricular complexes, T wave changes resembling myocardial infarction may appear as a result of pressure on one of the coronary arteries by the aneurysm. In fact, some of the peculiar findings in this condition will depend on the location of the dissecting aneurysm and the direction which the dissection takes. After splitting the wall of the aorta, the aneurysm and blood clot may extend down the abdominal aorta even to the iliac vessels. In its course it may compress any of the arteries that are given off from the aorta and produce a variety of symptoms. Giddiness and blurring of vision may result from the effects on the carotid arteries, anuria or hematuria from involvement of the renal vessels, and pain and numbness in the legs from occlusion of the common iliac artery. Paralysis of the limbs may be caused by involvement of the spinal cord. The peripheral pulse in one or another of the limbs of the body may disappear. At times there is a systolic impulse or lift to be seen or felt in the region of the manubrium or at the sternoclavicular joint.

Sudden death frequently occurs from rupture of the aneurysm, especially into the pericardium or less frequently into the pleural cavity. Although the two conditions have many clinical features in common, careful consideration of the finer differential points involved, especially the direct findings in the heart, will generally suffice to distinguish coronary thrombosis from dissecting aneurysm.

Dissection and rupture of the aorta, often arteriosclerotic in type, may take place in its abdominal portion. The symptoms can then be quite baffling and resemble acute pancreatitis, perforated peptic ulcer, or an acute gallbladder attack. There may be fever, a brisk leukocytosis, and pain in the right upper quadrant and back. The dissection may rupture into the pleural cavity.

Incomplete tear or rupture of the aorta also occurs that may or may not be followed by dissection. It is extremely difficult to recognize this condition clinically. It may account for attacks of choking or suffocation or midchest pain occurring in patients with hypertension. These tears are generally horizontal, and when they are present quite close to a commissure of the aortic valve, it appears that the valve may sag and result in aortic insufficiency. This is thought to be the explanation of an aortic systolic and diastolic murmur that may develop in some patients with incomplete rupture of the aorta. Healing of these tears can take place or dissection may develop hours, days, or even months later.

With the great increase in knowledge concerning coronary thrombosis that has taken place in recent years, the diagnosis is now being made too frequently. Whenever the evidence is not entirely convincing one should search for other conditions. Apart from gallbladder disease and gastrointestinal disturbances already mentioned, bleeding peptic ulcer and diaphragmatic hernia must be considered. The shock, weakness, rapid pulse, and fall in blood pressure resulting from hemorrhage can resemble a painless coronary thrombosis. Similarly the peculiar distress in the chest that may occur with a diaphragmatic hernia, especially in women, may simulate a coronary attack. In neither case, however, will there be found reliable evidence of myocardial infarction. Herpes zoster, arthritis of the spine, carcinoma of the lung, and syphilitic aneurysm of the aorta are other conditions not to be confused with coronary thrombosis. The list of diseases that may enter into a differential diagnosis is almost endless, as is well illustrated by an experience in which coronary thrombosis was confused with the very rare condition called diaphragmatic flutter.

Finally the differentiation of simple angina pectoris and coronary thrombosis needs consideration. Generally this is not difficult. All the features discussed in the preceding pages under these two headings help to distinguish the one from the other. Although most attacks of angina last only a few minutes, some continue for fifteen minutes or more. It is not always possible to detect evidence of coronary thrombosis when attacks last longer, although some of these no doubt result in myocardial infarction. In many cases, on postmortem examination, there have been noted several isolated areas of fibrosis from old infarction, in which a corresponding number of attacks cannot be distinguished from a clinical point of view. Furthermore, I see patients with typical angina pectoris in whom I can obtain no evidence whatever of an attack resembling typical coronary thrombosis who yet show definite evidence in the electrocardiograms of a previous myocardial infarction. The term "acute coronary insufficiency" may well be applied to attacks of prolonged coronary pain in which no evidence of myocardial infarction appears. The most careful observation of patients with so-called "attacks" of severe angina pectoris, watching for a slight fever or for significant alteration in the electrocardiograms, will be necessary to arrive at the correct diagnosis. In cases that are called "acute coronary insufficiency" there may be electrocardiographic changes indicative of temporary myocardial ischemia, such as deviation of the S-T segment or inversion of the T wave. There will be no alterations in the QRS complex. The changes in the S-T segment and T waves are likely to be transient.

TREATMENT

There is hardly any other condition in the general field of heart disease in which it is more difficult to appraise the value of specific measures of therapy than in the treatment of acute coronary thrombosis. Events occur with such suddenness that one may be too ready to attribute the last procedure employed as a cause of the result, whether favorable or unfavorable. Notwithstanding this there are certain methods of treatment that for the present meet with general acceptance and others that may be regarded as still in the experimental stage or at least open to doubt.

Of first importance is the relief of pain. This is best obtained by the liberal use of morphine. The amount necessary will vary from one dose of 0.015 gm. ($\frac{1}{4}$ grain) subcutaneously to many such doses. When the pain is very severe and persistent morphine should be repeated in one-half hour or so, and at times a grain or more will be necessary. Morphine should be given subcutaneously or intravenously, as oral administration will be entirely inadequate. Demerol in doses of 100 mg. may also be tried. Papaverine (0.05 to 0.1 gm. given intravenously) has been suggested for severe coronary pain. This may be administered every four to six hours for several days. There have been isolated instances of sudden death following within one or two minutes after intravenous injection of papaverine in coronary thrombosis. In fact, the intravenous injection of many drugs in cases of coronary disease occasionally causes instant fatality. It does not appear to be a specific result of any one chemical compound, for the variety of drugs responsible for such sudden and unpre-

dictable disasters is great. In this group can be mentioned arsenic, mercurial diuretics, aminophylline, papaverine, and caffeine. The exact cause
of this is obscure. The abruptness of the action makes one suspect that
the chemical acts as a trigger in a susceptible heart in producing ventricular fibrillation or standstill of the heart.

During the early minutes after the onset, if the patient's condition
seems very critical, he should not be moved or even undressed unless it is
extremely inconvenient to treat him as he is. These changes are often
better made a few hours later. When, as occasionally happens, the patient
quickly becomes unconscious and pulseless, the hypodermic use of
Adrenalin (0.5 to 1 cc. of a 1:1000 solution) is indicated and may help to
restore consciousness.

It has been suggested that injecting a liberal amount of 0.5 per cent
Novocain subcutaneously in the precordial region, particularly over the
painful area, may control the intractable pain of coronary thrombosis.
Although I have had very little experience with this method of treatment,
it seems quite safe and may obviate the need of repeated injections of
narcotics with their nauseating effects.

Complete mental and physical rest is paramount. The patient should
be spared all possible physical movement. Frequent tiring examinations
are undesirable. After the initial pain has subsided, sleep should be assured the first few nights, even using morphine if necessary. It is just as
well to avoid the use of enemas for one to several days despite the absence
of bowel movements. Very little food is consumed during these days, and
it is not necessary that the bowels should move every day. An enema on
the third or fourth day will often be better tolerated. Nausea and vomiting are common during the first day or so. They are partly the result of
the attack and partly brought on by the morphine that is given; generally they subside after the first day, especially if narcotics become unnecessary. Thorazine, 10 to 25 mg. parenterally, may be helpful for these
symptoms, but the blood pressure level needs to be watched.

Considerable dehydration develops in some of these patients. They
often lose a great deal of water and salt with the marked perspiration that
occurs and from the vomiting and inability to retain fluids and nourishment taken by mouth. It sometimes is imperative to administer 1000 cc.
of normal salt solution or 5 per cent glucose solution intravenously or
subcutaneously. Some observers have been very favorably impressed by
the results of intravenous injection of 100 cc. of 50 per cent glucose solution. I have not witnessed any striking improvement following this procedure. Another reason for encouraging the intake of fluid is the oliguria
that may amount to a complete anuria, which is so common after an
attack. There is also some ground to believe that the administration of
sodium chloride would be desirable, for the state of shock can certainly
be aggravated by the great loss of salt that takes place from excessive
perspiration in some cases.

Oxygen may be of use. When there is marked dyspnea and pulmonary congestion the inhalation of oxygen can improve breathing and

cyanosis. In fact I have also seen instances in which severe and persistent pain seemed to disappear promptly after the patient was placed in an oxygen tent. During the first hours stimulants like caffeine and Adrenalin may be beneficial, the former for respiratory distress and the latter for shock and a low blood pressure. The latter may be used as an emergency procedure in a pulseless patient when time and circumstances do not permit the intravenous therapy to be discussed below.

Shock is a common and serious complication. When profound, it carries a very high mortality, as only a few recover. Apart from other ill effects, such as decreased renal flow and increasing nitrogen retention, prolonged shock probably increases the area and severity of the original myocardial infarct. Treatment must be prompt if irreversible changes are to be avoided. The introduction of the vasopressor drugs, the sympatho-mimetic amines, marks a significant advance. These drugs have definitely salvaged some otherwise hopeless cases. The following agents have proved most helpful: norepinephrine (Levophed), mephentermine (Wyamine), phenylephrine (Neo-Synephrine), methoxamine (Vasoxyl), and Aramine.

Levophed in continuous infusion has been found very valuable. This preparation comes in 4 cc. ampules, equivalent to 4 mg. of active principle. One ampule is dissolved in 1000 cc. of 5 per cent glucose in water. This provides a concentration of 4 micrograms of Levophed per 1 cc. of solution. It is given intravenously at the rate of 20 drops per minute initially. The level of blood pressure should be determined frequently and the speed of administration will need to be increased or decreased accordingly. It would be well to maintain a level of about 110 to 120 mm. constantly. Inasmuch as it will not be desirable to give more then 2000 cc. of fluid daily and this treatment may be necessary for several days, difficulties may arise because of the slow intravenous drip. At times one may be forced to insert a polyethylene catheter into the brachial or femoral vein. In other patients, adding one or more ampules of Levophed to the solution, thereby increasing its concentration, may produce the desired response not obtainable otherwise. Care in the technique is vital, as extravasation of the solution may produce sloughing, and local thrombosis of the veins is common. Although troublesome, the above method of treatment has proved of value.

The other drugs mentioned above may also be helpful in the treatment of shock. Mephentermine (Wyamine), 5–10 mg. intravenously or 30–70 mg. in 500 cc. of 5 per cent glucose solution given slowly over two hours, may prove effective. Similarly, Neo-Synephrine, 5 mg. every 10 to 30 minutes intravenously or less often intramuscularly, is worth trying. Vasoxyl may be given intravenously in a dose of 5 mg., or 15 mg. intramuscularly, or as a continuous infusion in a concentration of 100 mg. per liter. Another preparation recently recommended is Aramine, 0.3 gm. in 1000 cc. of 5 per cent dextrose in water given at the rate of 50 to 100 drops per minute. The blood pressure should rise in 5 to 10 minutes, and the speed or concentration of the mixture can be varied depending on the blood pressure response. It is claimed that local sloughing or thrombophlebitis does not occur with this preparation as it may with some of the other anti-shock drugs.

Apart from drug therapy, 250 to 1000 cc. of plasma or one or more units of human albumin intravenously may be helpful. From a physiological point of view it is conceivable that an increase in blood volume produced by plasma would be desirable at one time for shock and a decrease in blood volume produced by bleeding for pulmonary edema would be desirable at another time, even in the same patient. I once saw a pulseless patient to whom 250 cc. of plasma was given intravenously and repeated in four hours. This caused a prompt, dramatic improvement and seemed to save the patient's life. Although intra-arterial transfusions are thought to be more effective for shock than intravenous, the advantage has not been clearly established.

Adrenal steroids are also being used for overt shock or shocklike states in acute coronary thrombosis. For the present, experience of this sort is still very limited, although very beneficial results have been claimed in a few instances. There is some physiological and pathological background for such therapy. With such a severe acute illness one might expect the stress reaction to be considerable. It may well result in temporary adrenal insufficiency or exhaustion. I have seen instances in which postmortem examination revealed bilateral adrenal hemorrhage with thrombosis of the adrenal veins. It was suspected that these structural changes were in some way related to the anticoagulant treatment that was given. It is also conceivable that local thrombosis of the adrenal veins might take place as a result of the very low blood pressure that occurs in some cases of acute coronary thrombosis and thereby tend to perpetuate or render irreversible the shocklike state. The above considerations make it likely that adrenal steroids, like Meticorten, might on rare occasions be valuable and possibly life saving.

The remainder of the treatment is expectant and directed at complications. Of these, two are rather important from a therapeutic point of view. First is the development of complete heart block with or without Adams-Stokes syncope. This is an infrequent complication but may be controlled very satisfactorily by the hypodermic injection of 0.5 to 1 cc. of 1:1000 Adrenalin solution. In some cases it will be necessary to give such injections frequently. In several instances I have given 0.3 to 0.5 cc. of Adrenalin every two hours for forty-eight hours to patients who had this condition and thereby prevented the pauses of the heart that were otherwise occurring, finally observing that the tendency to syncope had disappeared. It has seemed to me that in rare cases such treatment has been life saving.

The other complication to be considered is paroxysmal ventricular tachycardia. This occurs in about 3 per cent of the cases. When it develops it can quickly produce a state of collapse. The heart rate becomes very rapid (180 to 200), and the blood pressure falls still further. The condition can often be recognized by three features. The rapid rate, although apparently regular, may show slight irregularities which the ear can detect. The first heart sound may change in quality and intensity in different heart cycles, and carotid sinus or ocular pressure never produces any slowing of the heart. These points can distinguish ventricular tachycardia from other forms of paroxysmal tachycardia. Quinidine, procaine amide, and magnesium sulfate are the drugs of choice in controlling this irregularity. Digitalis will not only fail to slow it but will tend to accelerate or to perpetuate it. Quinidine can stop it but the dose required varies considerably. I have seen such an attack stop promptly after one dose of 0.3 gm. (5 grains) taken by mouth. In another case it required 1.5 gm. (22 grains) to stop an attack, and such a dose five times a day for several days to prevent the return of the tachycardia. In two instances it was found that even very large doses of quinidine merely slowed the ventricular rate and failed to abolish the abnormal mechanism. The rate would gradually return to the previously high level as the effect of the drug wore off. In these two cases the hypodermic injection of 1.0 to 2.0 mg. of atropine sulfate, one hour after a large dose of quinidine had been given orally (while the temporary slowing had taken place), promptly eliminated the ventricular tachycardia. Quinidine may also be given intramuscularly or intravenously. It would appear that the parenteral method, especially the intravenous, would carry more risk. A solution of 5 per cent glucose or normal saline is made up so that 200 cc. contains 1.2 gm. of quinidine dihydrochloride or lactate. It is given intravenously at the rate of 0.1 gm. per five minutes. It is helpful to be taking electrocardiograms during the injections so that treatment can be stopped the moment the desired result is obtained. Quinidine merely restores the normal rhythm of the heart and controls this complication. It does not prevent the other complications to which the same patient is still subject. Similarly 2.0 to 4.0 gm. of magnesium sulfate, given intravenously, may stop these attacks (see Chap. 13).

Another drug that has an action similar to that of quinidine and probably is preferable in the control of paroxysmal ventricular tachycardia is procaine amide (Pronestyl). This is best given intravenously slowly and should be administered while electrocardiograms are being taken continuously. The details of this procedure are discussed in Chapter 13.

There is a final use of quinidine that bears mention. Both clinical and experimental evidence that quinidine sulfate tends to inhibit the development of ventricular fibrillation has been advanced. It is more than likely that some of the instances of sudden death in coronary thrombosis are due to ventricular fibrillation. I formerly advised giving 3 to 5 grains of quinidine three times a day during the first two or three weeks following an acute attack, except when there is any contraindication to its use. One would want to give the smallest dose that is effective because the drug can have undesirable effects. A dose of 0.3 gm. (5 grains) may be preferable for I saw one patient who was taking 0.2 gm. at four-hour intervals. About one hour after the second dose he died instantly, and the autopsy showed acute coronary thrombosis without rupture of the ventricle. This is just the type of sudden death which quinidine is meant to prevent. In fact, I had another experience identical with the above in which sudden death, not due to rupture of the ventricle, occurred while the patient was taking 0.2 gm. of quinidine three times daily. The question arises whether a larger dose would have been effective in preventing the fatality. The main contraindication is any evidence of defects in conduction, like bundle branch block, or partial or complete auriculoventricular block. Inasmuch as quinidine can further impair the conduction apparatus it should be given with caution under such circumstances. It is difficult to prove that the routine use of quinidine as has been suggested has any practical merit or that the dose is adequate to produce the effect for which it is given. A recent study by Cutts of the value of routine quinidine administration in the prevention of sudden death in a group of cases of acute myocardial infarction failed to show any difference as compared with a control group. At present, therefore, I advise administering the drug only when certain cardiac irregularities have already appeared, especially if extrasystoles are noted.

It is the custom of some physicians to give preparations like aminophylline routinely during attacks. Although there is some experimental evidence to show that such a drug increases coronary flow and that it diminishes the extent of myocardial infarction after coronary arteries are ligated, it is difficult to be certain that it is useful in clinical cases of acute thrombosis. This subject, however, deserves further study. Such a drug has been used even intravenously during the height of pain. I have had some experience with this but it both requires and deserves further controlled observation in clinical cases to establish the usefulness of such medication.

In addition to some of the things the physician is called upon to do there are certain procedures he should not do. When a syphilitic patient has an acute coronary thrombosis it is inadvisable to give any intravenous antisyphilitic treatment. In fact, it is better to disregard the syphilitic aspects of the problem entirely during the first two weeks or so. In these cases it is not at all certain that syphilis is directly related to the coronary thrombosis for it is more likely that the latter is due to the same causes that are at work in nonsyphilitics. Reference has been made previously to the use of insulin in cases of coronary thrombosis. This should be avoided as much as possible because for an hour or two after its use the work of the heart is increased about 20 per cent if the blood sugar drops too low, and this added strain may be very serious. It is well known that attacks of angina can be precipitated by insulin, and I have seen a rupture of the ventricular wall occur about one-half hour after 10 units were given. Insulin may be given cautiously if the blood sugar is high and marked fall of the blood sugar can be avoided.

The same question of insulin administration in other cardiac disorders deserves a word of comment. I have frequently seen patients with various types of heart disease (congestive failure or angina pectoris) improve strikingly on decreasing the dose of insulin or discontinuing its use entirely. It would appear that such patients were treating the diabetic state too thoroughly, having a blue urine test quite constantly. One wonders whether it would not be desirable for cardiac patients to have a slight glycosuria. The sugar in the urine may act as a diuretic. In one case attacks of recurrent acute pulmonary edema ceased on omitting insulin and permitting the urine to contain some sugar. The attacks in this case used to come some hours after the insulin injection, at a time when hypoglycemia may have been present.

If a patient has an acute coronary thrombosis and some other surgical condition, such as an obstructing prostate or an infected kidney that needs removal, it is advisable to delay operation for at least a month or two until a satisfactory recovery of the heart has taken place. There is a final precaution in the care of patients with coronary artery disease. It has been observed that an attack of coronary thrombosis can occur directly after the intravenous injection of the iodine dye that formerly was used for cholecystography. I have seen two patients with angina pectoris in whom an attack of coronary thrombosis was brought on a few minutes after the intravenous injection of the dye. It is wiser, therefore, when a patient is either known to have or suspected of having coronary artery disease and it is desired to study the condition of the gallbladder, that x-ray examination should be made only after oral administration of the dye.

Finally, the question arises whether or not digitalis should be employed in acute coronary thrombosis, There are many theoretical reasons one could give for or against its usefulness. I have felt that it is more likely to do harm than good. If persistent auricular fibrillation is present it should be given but this condition is rare, as when it occurs during an attack it is almost always transient. Furthermore, when there is peripheral pitting edema, engorged liver, or hydrothorax, digitalis should be administered as in any case of congestive heart failure. This is rare, however, except after the first few weeks. It is uncertain whether or not it is beneficial in those cases showing rales in the lungs and dyspnea. The drug should be helpful for left ventricular failure but might be harmful for the peripheral failure or shock, and both conditions exist simultaneously in the early days of acute coronary thrombosis. The lack of cardiac dilatation would make one hesitate to use the drug. Although much more statistical evidence will be required before the question can be finally settled, at present it seems best not to use digitalis routinely during the first two weeks of acute coronary thrombosis.

The general nursing care of the patient is very important. Everything should be done to make him comfortable. The diet during the early days should be confined to liquids, gradually returning to more ordinary food in small amounts. Many of these patients are overweight and to obtain a loss of weight during this illness is desirable. It has been advised that a low-calorie diet (500 to 800 calories a day) should be used in acute coronary thrombosis and in fact is being advocated in the treatment of any severe or stubborn case of congestive heart failure (Proger and

Master). It has been found that this semistarvation diet diminishes the work of the heart and produces other favorable effects on the circulatory dynamics. Patients should be kept at rest for four to eight weeks. Occasionally the period of rest or restricted activities needs to be longer, but sometimes three weeks appear to be sufficient. From a purely clinical point of view the four- to eight-week period has been found to be adequate and it is of interest that in large animals it has been observed that two to five weeks are required to establish adequate collateral circulation after experimental ligation of a major coronary artery. It is a general biologic principle that the main stimulus for the development of collateral arterial circulation is a local need for it. Inasmuch as the present evidence favors the view that there are anastomoses from one main coronary artery to another normally, even in infancy, it is not difficult to conceive of the mechanism of recovery from myocardial infarction. Economic and social factors often will determine the exact length of time of convalescence. Whether nurses will have to be employed is also often a matter of the financial status of the patient. It generally is advisable that the patient should not be permitted to go to the bathroom for either bowel movement or urination during the early days. Usually it proves to be less of a hardship to permit the use of a commode than to require use of a bedpan. These details need to be worked out by the physician in individual cases. After the period of rest the patient is allowed to increase his activities slowly and gradually, taking a few steps at a time, then longer walks all on the same floor for about two weeks, and finally beginning to climb stairs.

The above program of rest is the one generally accepted by many physicians at the present moment. However, the entire question of *rest* for cardiac patients and how it is best attained needs reconsideration. Because this question is so important it seems appropriate to discuss it in great detail.

Rest in Bed or in Chair.   The physician at the present time is in a psychological quandary. The lay public expects patients with serious cardiac conditions to be kept strictly in bed. This is particularly true of those suffering from a so-called "heart attack," which has become almost synonymous with acute coronary thrombosis. No one is blamed if a coronary patient dies in bed. But if he had been out of bed the physician is likely to be held responsible. "If cardiacs are to die they should die in bed." This has become the standard point of view in the minds of most people, medical and lay. This view sorely needs to be corrected so that cardiac patients may obtain the maximum physical and psychological advantages that are available at present.

Rest to the affected organ is a fundamental principle in treatment of various conditions. A broken bone is put into a splint or a cast, thereby immobilizing the damaged parts and obtaining optimal union. Pneumothorax or thoracoplasty has been employed to put a diseased lung at rest to encourage more rapid healing of a tuberculous lesion. For the same reason, patients with damaged hearts often are advised to rest. In this case, the affected organ cannot be immobilized, but attempts of one kind or another are made to minimize its work. With this in mind, the current teaching in the medical profession has been to urge patients with congestive heart failure or coronary thrombosis or certain other types of heart disease to remain perfectly quiet in bed for varying periods of time, often weeks on end. The thought behind this method of strict bed rest care was that the heart obtained the maximum amount of rest if the patient was recumbent and inactive. The purpose of this discussion is to present clinical, physiologic, and experimental reasons to refute this concept.

There are two important points that have generally been overlooked in this problem. One is that the heart really consists of two parts, the right and the left side. The two ventricles must work in unison. One cannot out do the other for any length of time. If the right ventricle for any reason pumped out one drop of blood more with each beat than the left, and this continued for two or three hours, the lungs would contain an excess of about 500 cc. of blood. This could readily precipitate acute pulmonary edema. Contrariwise, if the left ventricle expelled one drop more than the right ventricle, in two or three hours there would be about 500 cc. of excess blood on the venous side of the circulation, and hepatic and other visceral engorgement would result. In other words, the circulation on the two sides of the heart must be finely adjusted. The body can tolerate an imbalance of the output of the two ventricles for only a short period of time. The bearing of this concept on the question of bed rest will become clear later in the discussion.

The second and more important misconception is the belief that the heart works least with the patient in bed. It has only recently been shown by direct catheterization studies of individuals with normal or with diseased hearts that the work of the heart is 23 per cent greater with the patient in bed than in a chair with the feet hanging down. This might easily have been predicted, and in fact was thought to be so many years ago. Since time immemorial, patients with paroxysmal nocturnal dyspnea have found that they must sit up in bed with their feet hanging over the edge, or sit in a chair, or even pace the floor in order to obtain relief. It is of interest that such spells did not usually occur directly on falling asleep but rather a few hours later, two to three o'clock in the morning. It seemed as if a certain time interval was required before the recumbent posture produced its deleterious effect. It also was evident that relief came only if the individual assumed a more upright position, and, if he continued to lie flat in bed, the respiratory suffocation would persist or grow worse.

It is surprising that the medical profession was so slow in realizing the full significance of this common clinical experience. Until recent years, and it is sad to say that even at the present moment, such patients suffering from paroxysmal nocturnal dyspnea are ordered to complete bed rest. The patient may try to rebel and insist that he feels his worst in bed, and yet, because of fear of disobeying his physician's orders, he will consent to this ill-advised program of care. Fortunately, in most cases the value of other therapy, such as digitalis, low-salt diet, and mercury diuretics, will be sufficient to undo the harmful effects of the bed, and the patient may yet make a satisfactory recovery. During the early days, morphine or similar narcotics may be necessary to control the nocturnal distress. There are occasions, however, not very infrequent, in which active therapy is not effective enough to keep pace with the harm produced by recumbency. In such cases, fatalities occur that never would have taken place if the patient had not been put to bed. I recall in my early years of practice seeing many instances in which a hypertensive patient with so-called nocturnal cardiac asthma, who showed very little peripheral pitting edema and only a few rales at the bases of the lungs, would grow quickly worse after a few days of complete bed rest. He would then show frank evidence of hydrothorax (not present before), requiring thoracentesis, and in some cases quickly deteriorate to a fatal outcome. I feel quite certain that some of these deaths were solely the result of the recumbency and would not have occurred if treatment had been carried out in a manner to be described.

A few cursory observations made some years ago threw light on this phenomenon. It was found in several cases that, twenty-four hours after strict bed rest was instituted, data obtained concerning circulatory dynamics indicated that the cardiac status had deteriorated. A thorough investigation of the effect of recumbency on the circulation in hypertensive cardiacs was made by Perera and Berliner. They found that within twelve hours after the patient lay down hemodilution occurred. With this there was increased blood volume, increased venous pressure, slowing of the velocity of blood flow, and decrease in vital capacity. It was obvious that the immediate effect of having these patients go to bed was harmful to the circulation. A more direct study by cardiac catheterization was made by Coe. He estimated that the work of the heart in both normal individuals and in cardiac patients was 23 per cent greater in bed than in a chair. The evidence is, therefore, complete that the patients' own impressions were correct; i.e., under certain circumstances the bed is just the wrong place in which to obtain cardiac rest.

It might be useful to try to express the effect of these changes on circulatory dynamics in simple language. On lying down, there is a greater and easier return flow of blood to the right side of the heart. This can take place with a greater transport of extracellular fluid to the venous side of the circulation. In normal individuals or in cardiac patients, when there is no obstruction to blood flow within the heart or when the muscular efficiency is adequate, the right ventricle accepts the increase in work, expelling the blood efficiently into the lungs. Similarly, the left ventricle receives and expels to the periphery all that has been delivered to the lungs. The result is a balanced circulation with no untoward effects. However, if a patient has mitral stenosis or if the left ventricle is the more vulnerable of the two ventricles, as often is the case in hypertensive, aortic or coronary heart disease, the right ventricle is able to meet the added load of recumbency, but the left side is not. In the course of some hours of this imbalance, pulmonary engorgement may readily result, with edema and suffocation. During these hours, the right ventricle has been pumping more blood into the lungs than the left ventricle has been expelling through the aorta. This mechanism must play a vital role in the production of nocturnal dyspnea or in the development of pulmonary congestion in many cardiac patients. It must be clearly understood that such ill effects will not result under three conditions: i.e., in normal individuals, in those cardiacs who are still able to take the added load, and in the cases in which therapy is adequate to undo the harmful effects of the recumbent position. It is only when none of these three conditions prevails that disasters from keeping patients in bed may occur.

It is a simple matter to obviate or minimize the harmful effects of recumbency. For this purpose, patients should be kept in a comfortable chair with their feet down for as much of the day as possible. Some attention should be paid to details. The back of the chair should be almost upright and extend high enough so that with or without the aid of a pillow the head will find some support. Broad side arms will enable the patient to relax his elbows and forearms, and the seat of the chair should not be so soft that the buttocks sink low, causing the upper legs to tilt upward. The purpose of the latter is to avoid buckling of the abdomen which would restrict breathing, or acute flexion of the knees which may angulate the femoral and popliteal vessels. The idea is to have the upper legs maintain a position about parallel to the floor. It will also be helpful if some method can be devised, as part of the chair itself or as an independent unit, so that a table can be placed across the knees from one arm of the chair to the other. This will permit the use of a tray for meals and will also enable some patients to relax or nap, resting their head forward on their arms placed on a pillow over the table. When a suitable chair is obtained, it becomes a simple matter in one way or another to make the patient quite comfortable. When the patient goes to the chair or returns to bed, he is not lifted unless he is unconscious; he is merely aided and guided. He first is sat up in bed, the legs being simultaneously swung over the side of the bed. Then with the help of one or two people, he is supported and guided until he actually sits in the nearby chair. To minimize the effect of recumbency during the hours the patient is in bed, 9-inch shock blocks are placed under the head posts of the bed. Any other device may be employed that will keep the head of the bed 9 inches higher than the foot.

It is conceivable that a bed may be devised that can function as a chair or at least will accomplish the same purpose. The ordinary hospital bed will not do, because the hips are still at the same level as the feet, no matter how high the back of the bed is lifted. Some beds can be cranked in positions that imitate a chair. They are not comfortable, as the bend at the knees is not sufficiently sharp, and some orthopneic patients will need to sit in a more upright position than can be obtained in any bed.

Furthermore, the beneficial psychic effect of being permitted to sit up in a chair and not being confined to bed twenty-four hours a day is lost.

When the chair method of treatment is employed in acute coronary thrombosis, it is striking how often the patient will quickly exclaim that he feels so much better. It is advisable to start this form of treatment the first day or two after the onset of the attack. This will prevent the development of pulmonary congestion, for it is very rare to see pulmonary edema or increasing congestive signs develop *after* the chair treatment is instituted. Furthermore, if the patient is kept immobile in bed for two weeks or so and then put into a chair, he is likely to feel weak and giddy. When it is done during the first few days, there has not been enough time for the same degree of muscular and skeletal weakness and atony to develop. Other advantages that result from early chair treatment are that bladder and bowel functions are less troublesome. The need of enemas or of catheterization of the bladder is likely to vanish. The constant fear that so often attends the weeks of confinement to bed with this dreaded illness, popularly known as a "heart attack," is lightened.

If allowing patients with acute myocardial infarction to get out of bed seems radical, the physician needs only to realize that the process of getting in and out of bed is identical to that employed in using a bedside commode. Inasmuch as most physicians have given up the use of the bedpan in cardiac patients because of the inherent difficulties and increase of effort involved, it seems illogical to fear the transport to a chair. Furthermore, a careful study of the pulse, respiration, and blood pressure for a half hour before and a half hour after the change from bed to chair in a series of cases of acute coronary thrombosis showed no evidence of any harmful effects or increase in the work of the heart.

There is a final physiological consideration already taken up in the discussion of angina pectoris (page 93) that has a bearing on this question of posture for cardiacs. Reasons were given to support the idea that the left ventricle does less work and would require less oxygen to maintain the same volume output of blood into the aorta with the patient sitting up than lying down in bed. The psychological advantage is very striking and is particularly noticeable in those patients who were treated by strict bed rest for a previous attack. They are likely to comment how much more pleasant and less terrifying the chair treatment is than the bed.

For some years I have treated in this manner all patients with acute coronary thrombosis who were not in shock or were not too feeble to sit up. This would include those with fever, pericarditis, arrhythmias, or any of the complications that may occur. When this treatment is begun in the first days, dramatic improvement is not obvious unless marked pulmonary edema is already present. However, when the patient has been allowed to remain strictly in bed several days and has become very dyspneic and orthopneic, if he is then promptly put into a chair and allowed to stay there several hours, astounding improvement at times may be witnessed directly after getting the patient out of bed. It was experiences such as this that originally convinced me that posture was important in the care of such cardiac patients. I was also convinced that the very pulmonary edema that may at times quickly disappear in a chair would never have developed if the patient had been treated by the chair method from the onset. The only contraindication to the chair method of treatment is a state of shock with a low blood pressure. Here the reverse posture, with elevation of the legs, may be necessary to increase cerebral blood flow.

The discussion so far has centered about the use of chair treatment in acute coronary thrombosis. The same principles apply to the care of cardiac patients in general and those with congestive failure in particular. If the work of the heart is less with patients in a chair than in bed, there is no advantage in strict bed rest in their care in most cases. One can conceive of certain circumstances in which peripheral edema would disappear more readily with the patient recumbent than out of bed with the feet down. When peripheral edema is present and there is no threat of pulmonary congestion, then lying flat will lessen the edema by encouraging greater return flow from the periphery to the right side of the heart, with resultant increase in cardiac output of the left ventricle and possible increase in urinary output. All this postulates the absence of significant obstruction between the lungs and the aorta (such as occurs in mitral or aortic stenosis) and the presence of adequate left ventricular muscular function. When these factors are not favorable, then peripheral pitting may lessen as a result of recumbency, but the fluid will now accumulate in the chest where it will do much more harm than it does in the legs. One can readily see that there are, in point of fact, very few cardiac conditions in which it is wise or necessary to institute strict bed rest care.

A final consideration with regard to the question of bed versus chair treatment in cardiac disease is the matter of convalescence. During the early days of an acute coronary thrombosis with myocardial infarction, when the patient is kept in a chair the major part of the day, he is not allowed to be any more active than if he had been in bed. If the physician thinks the patient should be fed by a nurse, that can be done just as well in the chair as in bed. The same applies to other details, such as listening to the radio, watching television, reading the newspaper, etc. These are matters entirely apart from the question of posture. Furthermore, whether this kind of care should be continued for three weeks or for six weeks is an entirely different problem. The main point is that as long as it is desirable to *rest* the heart, it is best to have the patient in a chair a good part of the day. In other words, chair treatment is by no means synonymous with early ambulation.

How long to keep a patient who is recovering from an acute myocardial infarction at rest is a debatable topic. The decision, apart from other considerations, may depend on the social and economic factors involved. In some instances this period may be shortened because of great financial loss that would result from a more lengthy stay away from work or for other reasons. The period may be greater because the illness has been more severe. The season of the year, and whether the patient may be able to take a vacation in a warm climate before returning to work, are also considerations that come up. In general, it would appear that the minimum initial period of rest should be three to four weeks. This should be followed by a second month of gradual and slow increase in activities so that part-time work may be resumed in two months from the onset of the illness. It must be admitted that whenever the economic burden of the illness is not too great, it would be preferable to extend the entire period of convalescence to three months. Thereafter, adjustments in the type and amount of work may be necessary. Here again wisdom on the part of the physician is greatly needed. If too long a period of time is taken before the patient is allowed to resume part-time duty, he may never be either willing to get work or be able to find a suitable job. New employers and even some old employers are hesitant and some actually refuse to employ persons who have had heart disease. It will be a great gain to our society and an important aid to these individuals when this point of view on the part of employers is altered.

I have observed a sharp decrease in immediate mortality from acute coronary thrombosis since the arm-chair method of therapy was introduced. Although the ultimate or long-range survival period of chair-treated patients has not been investigated, there is no reason to doubt that what was helpful during the acute phase can be anything but beneficial to the eventual process. It is at least quite striking that after chair treatment general physical and mental strength is better conserved. Marked asthenia that so frequently follows and may persist months after a prolonged period of confinement in bed, with its wasting of musculature, is prevented or at least greatly mitigated by early chair treatment. It also appears that the "shoulder-arm syndrome" which is so common after a coronary attack is quite rare in those who are treated in a chair. From every angle—physical, mental, and economic—this method of cardiac care has much to recommend it.

Anticoagulant Therapy.   New methods of therapy will necessarily be proposed in the future. Attempts will be made to prevent further thrombosis of vessels. Mural thromboses of the ventricular cavities with subsequent arterial emboli are the cause of some fatalities. One not infrequently sees patients survive the first week of the attack then, while everything seems to be progressing satisfactorily, have a sudden cerebral embolus with hemiplegia that proves fatal. In such cases if the secondary mural thrombus in the left ventricle could have been prevented from forming during the first several days after the onset of the attack, death would not have occurred. These thrombi are found in about one third to one fourth of the patients dying in the acute attack and therefore account for a considerable group.

Another frequent complication is thrombophlebitis and secondary pulmonary embolism. Emboli of one type or another are a not uncommon cause of death in cases of coronary thrombosis. Primarily for these reasons anticoagulant therapy has now come into general practice. At the time of the third edition of this book (1945) I had begun a study of this problem but the work was interrupted by the Second World War before sufficient experience could be obtained. Rather extensive studies made later by Wright and Nichols showed that the mortality from acute coronary thrombosis under anticoagulant therapy, using Dicumarol, dropped from 23 per cent in the control group to 16 per cent in those treated, and the incidence of thrombo-embolic episodes dropped from 19 to 9 per cent.

From the above figures one is led to conclude that anticoagulant therapy is valuable for acute coronary thrombosis. There are several possible beneficial effects to be achieved by its use. The first is the prevention of thrombophlebitis of the legs and subsequent pulmonary emboli, a serious and frequent complication. There is very little doubt that Dicumarol, properly administered, can prevent or markedly diminish the incidence of this complication. The second is prevention of the development of a ventricular mural thrombus that is so common, with the hazard of arterial emboli, especially to the brain. It is not so certain how effective Dicumarol therapy is in this regard. Inasmuch as these thrombi are known to form the first few days (while the thromboses in the veins of the legs occur much later), therapy might have to be effective very early and promptly. The third and more doubtful purpose is to affect favorably the actual thrombus in the coronary artery or to prevent secondary and further coronary thromboses.

There are several courses of anticoagulant therapy one might undertake. One is to use heparin, the second is to use Dicumarol or similar drugs, and the third is to use a combination of drugs. For the latter purpose Dicumarol would be started and heparin would also be given only the first thirty-six to forty-eight hours (50–100 mg. intravenously or intramuscularly every six hours) until the effect of the former drug became manifest. All these measures are difficult and expensive, and can hardly be carried out unless the patient is in a hospital. Satisfactory results comparable to those obtained with Dicumarol have been obtained by giving heparin/Pitkin menstruum, 300 to 400 mg. every second day intramuscularly. With this method the coagulation time of the blood needs to be checked frequently, trying to keep it at 30 to 45 minutes or about three times normal. If the effect of heparin is excessive or bleeding occurs, the antidote is protamine, about 50 mg. intravenously. This checks the bleeding tendency in a few minutes. The method most commonly employed, however, is to administer Dicumarol orally.

At the outset it must be realized that there are certain contraindications to anticoagulant therapy. These are primarily severe renal or hepatic insufficiency, jaundice, purpura, or severe blood dyscrasias, surgery on brain or spinal cord, or any major operation, open wounds, and severe nutritional deficiency. These conditions rarely interfere in the treatment of coronary thrombosis. Before treatment is started the prothrombin time is determined. If this is in the vicinity of 100 per cent of normal, 300 mg. of Dicumarol is given. If it is definitely lower, the initial dose is appropriately diminished. The prothrombin time is then tested every morning and the subsequent dose regulated accordingly. The aim is to keep it around 15–20 per cent of normal, or about 35 seconds. The second dose frequently will be 200 mg., and the daily dose thereafter 100 or 50 mg. It may be necessary to omit the Dicumarol entirely for one or more days if the prothrombin time is excessively prolonged. It certainly should be stopped if the time is above 40 seconds. The treatment is continued for three, four, or more weeks, preferably until the patient is at least partially ambulatory or until two or three weeks have elapsed after occurrence of the last thrombo-embolic episode.

During this treatment the patient should be carefully watched for evidence of bleeding, particularly from the nose, in the urine, or in the stools. If significant bleeding does develop or if the prothrombin time is very excessive, vitamin K_1 in 50 to 100 mg. doses intravenously should be given. If that is not effective whole blood transfusions should be used. It has been found that certain commercial preparations like Hykinone are ineffective for this purpose. If this program is carried out with care, serious bleeding will be very rare. It is obvious that this treatment is difficult and expensive. It would help greatly if some quick and reliable bedside test for prothrombin activity could be devised so that Dicumarol could be given in patients' homes. On occasions I have carried out this course of treatment at home but it required a good deal of cooperation. At present it appears that anticoagulant therapy has definitely decreased the mortality of acute coronary thromboses, mainly by diminishing the incidence of thrombo-embolic complications, and should be started as soon as the diagnosis can be made if there are no contraindications. In fact, anticoagulants ought to be valuable as a preventive in those cases that present the premonitory symptoms which occasionally appear a few days before the acute dramatic episode.

Not all physicians are agreed that anticoagulants should be employed in the treatment of acute coronary thrombosis. There are a few who do not advise it in any case. There is a larger number who do not use it in mild or so-called favorable cases. The reason given for this view is that the mortality in this so-called favorable group may be no more than 2 per cent and that the risk of anticoagulant therapy is almost as great. My own practice is to give anticoagulant therapy in all cases in which the diagnosis is definite, either mild or severe, if there are no contraindications and the laboratory facilities for determining the prothrombin time are reliable. I find it difficult at times to predict whether a case will run a mild course. One that starts with only mild symptoms and signs may become very severe and prove fatal a few days later. For that reason I advise its routine use. One precaution and complication to watch for that necessitates temporary or complete withdrawal of anticoagulants is the development of so-called hemorrhagic pericarditis. If a patient shows a pericardial friction rub during the early days and it disappears only to reappear a few days later, it is well to assume that the Dicumarol is producing a hemorrhagic pericarditis and the medication should be stopped.

The same thing may be suspected if the initial pericardial friction lasted many days. Although one cannot be sure that a deleterious hemorrhagic pericarditis is going on in such cases, the danger seems to be too great.

GENERAL COMMENTS

One of the most common and harmful errors in the management of acute coronary thrombosis is to outline a lengthy period of invalidism and convalescence. Too many patients are told to stay in bed three to six months or to spend a year away from work, "taking it easy." When there is congestive failure, there may be no other choice, but in the absence of congestion, even if chest pain continues, such long invalidism is not only fruitless but often harmful. It generally will be found that the degree of pain will be no greater if the patient is ambulatory. What is more aimless is to advise restricted activities or, as is frequently done, confinement in bed, merely because of weakness. After the first two months, such weakness will not be helped by a program of inactivity. The entire illness, coupled with the alarming precautions taken by the physician and family, produces a state of fear, which often results in a profound neurasthenia and depression. Considerable weakness is necessarily a part of the illness itself. This is further accentuated by the immobility during the early weeks in bed. To this is then added a neurasthenic state that finally may condemn the individual to a permanent useless existence.

Sometimes these prolonged periods of "convalescence" are the result of insurance considerations, for "total permanent disability" does not begin to take effect until an illness has lasted over three months. At times one is led to believe that this type of insurance has done more harm than good for it has destroyed ambition and encouraged invalidism. What is needed to help this weakness is to encourage the patient to increase his activities and to assure him that his heart has recovered sufficiently to do more. If this point of view is stressed early in the illness, much unnecessary invalidism will be prevented. Many patients ought to be doing part-time work in two months and the majority in three or four months. What has been said about prolonged bed care for patients with coronary thrombosis applies to some extent to patients with other types of chronic heart disease and to those with many other noncardiac conditions. Not only is prolonged bed rest frequently unnecessary but it may be conducive to the development of further complications such as hypostatic pneumonia, prostatic obstruction, renal stone formation, and phlebitis with pulmonary embolism.

Any patient with angina pectoris or coronary thrombosis should be cautioned to avoid active diarrhea or prolonged sweating. It appears that some acute attacks of myocardial infarction at times have followed directly after these events, as if the dehydration and increased turgidity of the blood precipitated the spell.

Finally, if a patient has had two or more attacks of coronary thrombosis and has recovered, one might be tempted to administer Dicumarol constantly. This is being done by some physicians and appears to be a reasonable procedure. The daily dose is likely to be about 50 mg., and careful observation will be necessary. One might need to perform a pro-thrombin test every week or two and try to keep the prothrombin time around 25 to 30 seconds. This method of prolonged ambulatory Dicu-marol therapy might also be applied to cases of repeated arterial emboli in valvular disease.

CHAPTER 7

Hypertensive Heart Disease, Arteriosclerosis, "Chronic Myocarditis," and Rare Forms of Heart Disease

Hypertensive Heart Disease and Arteriosclerosis

Hypertension has a most important bearing on the subject of heart disease. As a concomitant factor in heart failure it probably surpasses all others, so that, in most general surveys, hypertensive heart disease heads the list of disabling forms of heart failure. The exact role played by the actual elevation of the blood pressure is by no means clear, for so often the same degree of hypertension is well tolerated for many years by one patient and results in severe cardiac insufficiency in another. Even the causes of hypertension are difficult to understand, for it seems to accompany a variety of conditions. How much can be explained on the basis of permanent structural changes within the body, especially the arteries, and how much on the basis of an altered nervous or functional state always requires consideration. The marked and even sudden changes that have been observed in the level of the blood pressure in many individuals have necessarily resulted in the firm conviction that the emotions, the nervous system, the endocrine glands, and the vasomotor apparatus are all intimately related to this problem.

At the outset it must be recalled that there are a few distinct clinical conditions which, although not really related to the general problem of essential hypertension, produce or are accompanied by some elevation in blood pressure. It is of some importance to be familiar with these conditions for, in so far as they exist, physical examination will reveal certain findings that will explain why these particular individuals are hypertensive. In coarctation of the aorta (Chap. 11), for example, there is hypertension in the arms although the pressure in the legs is low. Here the elevation in the blood pressure that is found on routine examination is directly due to a structural abnormality. Similarly one frequently finds hypertension in patients with prostatic obstruction. In some, the pressure will remain elevated until the obstruction is relieved, e.g., by an indwelling catheter, and then it will fall considerably. Such a fall of the pressure has been observed when all other factors, such as rest in bed, have been adequately controlled. At times this fall may be excessive, and it will then

164

be necessary to temporize and delay the contemplated prostatectomy until a partial recovery of the normal blood pressure has taken place. There are many instances in which the eventual prostatectomy produces a permanent lowering of the blood pressure.

Other conditions that are associated with or in some way productive of hypertension are thrombosis of a renal artery, or some unilateral lesion of the kidney, polycystic kidneys, eclampsia, tumors of the adrenals, Cushing's syndrome, occasional instances of sudden intracranial hemorrhage, acute nephritis, and polycythemia. Hyperthyroidism is also commonly associated with hypertension, but the level of the blood pressure falls little if any after the basal metabolism is brought to normal by operation. In addition, with certain cardiac disorders there is an elevation of the pressure which is the result rather than the cause of the disturbance in the heart. When complete heart block develops, the systolic pressure is apt to rise and the diastolic to fall purely as a result of the very slow heart rate. Somewhat similar changes follow the development of free aortic regurgitation. Finally, when hypertension accompanies congestive heart failure, more often than not the pressure level falls as improvement takes place on rest and digitalis. After a considerable experience I feel convinced that some of the fall in blood pressure is a direct result of cardiac therapy and disappearance of dyspnea and congestion and not to be accounted for on the basis of psychic influences or rest. In fact, if the blood pressure does not fall while a patient with hypertensive heart failure is under treatment, it generally indicates that improvement in the heart is not taking place or will not be so great as when the pressure does fall. This relationship is mentioned because there still prevails the idea that when the heart improves this improvement is manifested by an increase in blood pressure. Although this is often the case if the blood pressure is very low to begin with, it is not the general rule when congestive failure takes place with hypertension.

One more peculiarity of the blood pressure in relation to heart disease merits consideration. There is a group of patients having hypertension and angina pectoris in whom, following an attack of coronary thrombosis, the blood pressure falls with a complete or partial disappearance of the anginal attacks. When such patients become ambulatory some will thereafter have a low blood pressure, despite the fact that their general health remains even better than before the attack of coronary thrombosis, as they no longer have anginal spells. Under these circumstances a reduction in the blood pressure has taken place following an injury to the heart. This cannot be explained on the basis of structural alterations in the peripheral vascular tree. It seems more reasonable to assume that the previous elevation in the blood pressure was caused reflexly from an irritable focus in the heart and, after the coronary thrombosis, the local cause was removed. These experiences and those cited in the previous paragraph, in which it seems that digitalis may diminish the blood pressure by improving the heart, make one suspect that apart from all other causes hypertension in some cases may have its origin reflexly in the heart.

Apart from the conditions just mentioned, hypertension is regarded as an accompaniment of chronic nephritis or pyelonephritis, or as an idiopathic or essential hypertension. The latter type is most common. One suspects that to a large extent, or at least in its early stages, it is functional or neurogenic and not based on irreversible structural disease. One cannot explain on the basis of organic disease the oscillations that the blood pressure level undergoes in some individuals. I recall seeing a woman 55 years old whose pressure had been known to be over 200 mm. for some years. After three weeks' rest in bed there was a steady gradual decline to 140 mm. from the initial level of 240 mm. Thirty minutes after she read a letter containing very distressing news the level immediately jumped 100 mm., back to the original figure of 240 mm. Such changes cannot be explained except as a result of nervous or humoral influences.

The experimental work of Goldblatt has shown that the production of renal ischemia by constricting the renal artery causes maintained hypertension in animals. It has also been shown that, even after such hypertension has lasted many months, removal of the ischemic kidney restores the blood pressure to normal. Furthermore, this type of hypertension was found to be independent of the sympathetic nervous system. The inference from this work is that some product is liberated from the abnormal kidney which circulates in the blood and causes hypertension. This concept appears to be of great promise, affords a clearer understanding of the entire question of hypertension, and has led to practical therapeutic advances. In fact, already in some cases of unilateral nephrectomy for hypertension and chronic pyelonephritis the blood pressure has returned to normal.

One particular group of hypertensive cases should be constantly kept in mind. These are occasional instances of unilateral thrombosis or occlusion of a major renal artery, generally following trauma. This may, in weeks or months or possibly longer, produce hypertension with all its dire hazards. Nephrectomy may be curative under such circumstances. When this cause is suspected, proper x-ray studies following injection of an opaque dye into the aorta can establish a very definite diagnosis by revealing the obstruction of the incriminating vessel. Greater attention should be given to this procedure, as in some of the cases with local renal vascular thrombosis there was no history of trauma. This condition should be particularly suspected where the blood pressure has been noted to rise rather rapidly from a previously known normal level.

ETIOLOGIC FACTORS

Among the few known etiologic factors the most important is heredity. There are families with strong tendencies to hypertension and others which tend to hypotension. It has impressed me that marked freckling of the back of the forearms is unusually common in hypertensives and probably denotes a vascular vulnerability. The young nervous hypertensive or potential hypertensive often has a slight fever (99.6° F.). The females predominate over the males in the proportion of about three to two. The menopause seems to be a common period in life in which these changes become prominent, although earlier evidences of this tendency are generally available. The hypertensive person will often manifest certain stigmata of neurovascular vulnerability in earlier life. Nosebleeds, menstrual disturbances, flushing (especially of the neck), migraine, palpitation, and nervousness will frequently be found. Furthermore, it will be noted that there is often a tendency to slight elevation in the blood pressure on emotional provocation years before the individual becomes permanently hypertensive. An insurance examination or a visit to a consultant may raise the pressure to a higher level than the one found by the patient's family physician. In fact, the person who is not prone to hypertension is not apt to show this rise even on nervous tension. It seems, therefore, that the pressure is unusually labile in these vulnerable individuals, and that they have transient hypertension for years before they develop what one might call permanent hypertension.

Although hypertension and arteriosclerosis are frequently associated, it is unlikely that the latter is the cause of the former. One may see extensive sclerosis of the large arteries without hypertension, and very little arteriosclerosis with marked hypertension. It is more plausible that prolonged hypertension eventually leads to sclerosis of the arteries, but that during the early years spasm of vessels otherwise sound is going on. The fact that the first portion of the pulmonary artery is rarely sclerosed except in cases of mitral stenosis or other conditions in which pulmonary pressure is elevated lends support to the role hypertension may play in producing arteriosclerosis. When the blood pressure has been elevated for any considerable length of time, although the radial and brachial arteries may not show much evidence of sclerosis, changes in the retinal arteries will almost always be present. Retinal arteriosclerosis can be judged from the irregularity of the caliber of the arteries on ophthalmoscopic examination and the nicking of the veins at the points where they are crossed by the arteries. When the process is more advanced, hemorrhages, exudate, and papilledema may be found.

There are a few diseases that, in so far as they may affect blood vessels, may eventually predispose to early hypertension, e.g., typhoid fever, syphilis, chronic lead poisoning, gout, and rheumatic fever. There is some suspicion that rheumatic fever may be a more frequent precursor of hypertension than has been supposed. There is no evidence that foci of infection in teeth or tonsils are of any importance in this regard. In the great majority of cases of hypertension, however, none of these infections has been responsible and for the present at least they are best regarded as "essential" or "idiopathic."

EFFECT OF ARTERIOSCLEROSIS ON THE HEART

Before discussing hypertensive heart disease the possible effect of arteriosclerosis on the heart must be taken up. The term "arteriosclerotic heart disease" has led to much confusion. In the minds of some this term signifies heart failure resulting from peripheral sclerosis and to others it means coronary arteriosclerosis. If it merely includes those cases in which there is arteriosclerosis of the coronary arteries then it should be called by its proper name, i.e., coronary artery disease. If the former idea is held then the term is a misnomer, for there is little if any evidence to show that sclerosis of the peripheral arteries has any appreciable effect on the efficiency of the heart. A study carried out at the Peter Bent Brigham Hospital analyzing all the postmortem material in which there was a high degree of peripheral arteriosclerosis showed that when those cases were omitted in which there was hypertension, significant coronary artery disease, or other obvious causes of cardiac disability, such as valvular disease, in the remainder there was neither clinical nor pathologic evidence of heart disease. The death of these patients was due to some surgical or noncardiac cause. In a word, it was found that even an extreme degree of peripheral arteriosclerosis had no deleterious effect on the heart. It is suggested, therefore, that the term "arteriosclerotic heart disease" be given up.

BLOOD PRESSURE DETERMINATION

A word about the actual taking of the blood pressure seems worth mentioning. After the patient has relaxed, with the arm in a comfortable position, the pressure is increased above the expected systolic level. The mercury or pressure should be permitted to fall slowly while ausculting below the cuff. Many physicians do this too rapidly, and inaccuracies of 20 mm. or more may result. Furthermore, it is important that, the first time a patient is examined, the radial pulse should be palpated to check the auscultatory determination. If this is not done one may occasionally start the examination with the pressure level at the "auscultatory gap," at which point no sounds are heard, and yet the true reading may be 40 to 60 mm. higher. It is obvious that such an error can easily be avoided, for the radial pulse would be palpable even in this silent zone and the observer would have had to increase the pressure and then would have found that sounds return. Although the auscultatory method is more satisfactory than the palpatory, the latter at times will obviate mistakes. I recall a case in which the physician remarked that he could not obtain the blood pressure. It was found that the diastolic blood pressure in this young girl was 180 mm., and the physician had always started his readings at about 150 to 160 mm. If he had palpated the radial pulse he would have known that the blood pressure must have been higher, for the pulse had not been obliterated. Finally, there are instances in which a violent or hyperdynamic pulse, such as is seen in aortic regurgitation, produces a shock and noise with each beat as it strikes the cuff and this is audible in the antecubital space. It may give a falsely elevated systolic blood pressure. In such a case palpation of the radial pulse will indicate the systolic level. I have seen an instance of this type in which the systolic pressure had been read as 250 mm., when it was actually 140 mm. In this case a definite sound could be heard with the pressure over 300 mm. but it was an impact transmitted from the top of the cuff.

CLINICAL COURSE

In following the clinical course of a patient with hypertension there are several definite things for the physician to bear in mind. The exact level of the blood pressure is by no means the important criterion of the patient's progress. The pressure or the associated arterial disease will produce clinical disease in one of several ways. Of greatest importance is what is going on in the heart. This effect may become manifest in one of two ways. Angina pectoris or coronary thrombosis may result from involvement of the coronary arteries, or congestive heart failure may develop, especially left ventricular failure with paroxysmal dyspnea.

Next in importance is the possibility of cerebral hemorrhage. There is no method that enables one to predict which hypertensive patient will develop a cerebral hemorrhage or thrombosis or when it may be expected. The current opinion is that those with high diastolic pressures are most prone to cerebral accidents. I have suspected that the reverse is true. It has seemed that most patients who develop a sudden hemiplegia have had pressure levels of about 200 to 240 mm. systolic and 100 to 120 mm. diastolic. Those with diastolic readings of 140 to 160 mm. are more apt to have general encephalopathy, or cardiac or renal failure, but not an outspoken cerebral hemorrhage. May not the high pulse pressure be the more important factor in causing rupture of a large cerebral vessel?

Another group will begin to show significant disease of the kidneys and present the picture of chronic vascular nephritis, eventually developing uremia. A smaller number will have disabilities due to arterial disease of the legs, suffer intermittent claudication or even arteriosclerotic gangrene. Finally there are some in whom the arteriosclerosis of the abdominal vessels is productive of symptoms. Many ill-defined complaints, i.e., indigestion and abdominal pain, are no doubt due to arteriosclerosis of the mesenteric vessels. In this same connection the mild diabetes that is so common in elderly hypertensives may well be due to arteriosclerotic changes in the pancreatic vessels. Frequently the same patient with hypertension may show several of these evidences of arteriosclerosis. He may have a mild glycosuria, slight diminution in renal function, and definite intermittent claudication. Another may have outspoken angina pectoris, no renal impairment, and more marked sclerosis of the arteries of the legs. Finally, extensive arteriosclerosis may be present without hypertension. It is the function of the physician to try to estimate which is the major route that the vascular degeneration is taking, and in general it will be found that the cardiac complications are the most important.

Exactly when the heart will begin to fail in an individual with hypertension is an extremely variable matter. Neither the level nor the duration of the elevation in the blood pressure can entirely account for the development of cardiac insufficiency. In many instances it is clear that the main determining factor is the integrity of the coronary arteries. Atheromatous changes and narrowing of these vessels can account for the development of cardiac embarrassment in some individuals with only moderate hypertension. But there are other instances in which the gross appearance of the coronary arteries is essentially normal and yet the heart muscle fails. This unknown factor accounts for much that determines the whole question of congestive heart failure. I suspect that this factor "X" is linked up with the finer vascular bed of the coronary system. It is well known that throughout the human body there are a great many more capillaries than are being used under ordinary circumstances. A skeletal muscle or a glomerulus of a kidney contains ten times as many capillaries as are functioning at any particular time. The others are closed and are resting for the moment. Under special circumstances the number increases, the walls are opened and blood corpuscles begin to flow through. This constitutes the reserve function of the organ, and may not "cardiac reserve" depend on this very ability to open up new capillaries? When the heart muscle fails and yet shows no obstruction in the main coronary arteries, may not the cause lie in some structural or functional defect that prevented the opening of these terminal reserve channels? It is conceivable that, if these abnormalities do exist, they might yet be overlooked by the methods of pathologic study customarily employed in postmortem examination.

In the course of time an individual with hypertension may develop cardiac failure. In some this may not occur until twenty years have elapsed, in others the downhill path begins after a short time. The heart generally becomes enlarged, but the degree of hypertrophy varies considerably in different cases and is not directly proportional to the height or duration of the hypertension. What concerns us here is the development of congestive heart failure and not of angina pectoris. The latter condition can appear any time and suddenly alter the clinical course that the particular case might otherwise have taken. Most commonly, in the former, the first symptom is breathlessness. This appears at the outset on a degree of effort that formerly was well tolerated. Dyspnea on walking is, therefore, the most frequent early evidence of myocardial insufficiency. In many cases unwonted fatigue may have preceded this, but because of the numerous noncardiac causes of fatigue it does not serve so well to identify the condition as heart failure. There is a considerable group of hypertensives in which the shortness of breath appears suddenly, especially at night, and may even take the form of acute pulmonary edema. The term "cardiac asthma" is often used to classify these cases. The term is objectionable because the word asthma is too closely associated with a bronchial condition that has nothing to do with the heart and is comparatively benign. It is better to designate the condition by such terms as "paroxysmal cardiac dyspnea," "nocturnal dyspnea," or "acute pulmonary edema," as the circumstances warrant.

When dyspnea develops, either of the gradual or of the acute form, it indicates failure of the left ventricle. Examination often shows cardiac enlargement in addition to the elevation in blood pressure. The rhythm of the heart may be perfectly regular or arrhythmias due to extrasystoles or auricular fibrillation may be present. When the auricles are not fibrillating a gallop rhythm and pulsus alternans are frequently present. These two signs are so common and so important in hypertensive heart disease that they should always be looked for. The former is detected by careful auscultation over the precordium where the sounds have a peculiar quality resembling a canter due to an extra third heart sound in diastole. The latter is detected by palpation of the radial artery or, better still, on determining the blood pressure. While auscultation is carried out below the blood pressure cuff, just as the first sounds become audible, the pressure should be prevented from falling for a moment and the sounds will be heard to alternate in intensity. This method is even more helpful than palpating the radial artery. Occasionally the same mechanism of alteration of the ventricles will produce an alternating intensity of the heart sounds, murmurs, or the apex impulse over the precordium. Similarly the gallop rhythm may result in a bifid apex impulse that can be seen and felt.

GALLOP RHYTHM

It is appropriate at this point to discuss the clinical significance of gallop rhythm. This auscultatory finding is most important, can easily be detected, but is often overlooked. The extra sound is generally heard in diastole, i.e., between the second and first heart sounds at the apex (Fig. 209). When the extra sound follows the second sound it is called protodiastolic, when it just precedes the first sound it is presystolic, and when it occurs in mid-diastole it is called mesodiastolic. Such terminology is difficult and unnecessary from a clinical point of view. Gallop rhythm occurs most commonly in hypertensive heart disease and coronary artery disease and less frequently in rheumatic valvular disease. Occasionally it is present during acute infections such as diphtheria and rheumatic carditis. Because it is rarely associated with auricular fibrillation, the contraction of the auricles must have something to do with the production of the gallop. In fact, I have seen instances in which a typical diastolic gallop disappeared with the onset of auricular fibrillation and reappeared with the return of regular rhythm. In dogs, gallop rhythm has been found to be related to increased pressure in the left auricle. In the nonvalvular cases in which gallop rhythm is manifest bundle branch block is also often present. It almost always denotes a fairly serious affection of the heart muscle, carrying with it a life expectancy of one to three years, although occasionally such patients do live longer. I have seen exceptional instances in which a true diastolic gallop rhythm was detected on several different examinations (once during pregnancy) in the absence of any other evidence of heart disease and finally disappeared, the patients remaining free of any organic heart disease. The third sound of a gallop rhythm must be distinguished from a normal sound heard in early diastole in some healthy hearts. This is not generally difficult, for the rate is slow in the latter and somewhat accelerated in the former. Furthermore, patients with a normal third heart sound are apt to be young and show no other evidence of heart disease. Another confusion may arise when a patient who is developing mitral stenosis first shows a third sound in diastole (opening snap). This may resemble a gallop, and it will subsequently be found that the extra sound was in fact the early manifestation of what later proved to be the mid-diastolic or presystolic murmur of mitral stenosis. A gallop rhythm in a patient with rheumatic carditis may be indicative of delayed conduction of impulses from auricles to ventricles (increased P-R interval). This finding may enable the examiner to predict that there is a conduction defect. The prognosis of the gallop need not be grave when it is present in young rheumatic patients. Even the ordinary gallop may disappear when the clinical condition improves, especially when it occurs in conjunction with acute coronary thrombosis or when the heart rate slows, for it is rarely present when the rate is around seventy.

The mechanism of the normal third sound and the protodiastolic gallop are believed to be the same. Both occur at the same time of the cardiac cycle, during the rapid filling phase of the ventricle in early diastole, shortly after the opening of the auriculoventricular valves. The high pulmonary venous and left auricular pressure resulting from left-sided failure may cause intensification of the phase of rapid ventricular filling. It must be added that the impaired state of the contractile properties of the ventricular musculature is an additional factor in the production of the diastolic gallop.

The differentiation between a gallop, an opening snap, and a split second sound may be difficult on auscultation although it can be readily made by means of phonocardiography. The interval between the two components of the split second sound does not usually exceed 0.05 sec., while the opening snap occurs later in diastole (0.08 to 0.12 sec. after the second sound) and the gallop sound is still more delayed (0.16 to 0.20 sec. after the second sound).

Finally a word must be mentioned about another type of gallop rhythm. When the extra sound lies between the first and second heart sounds it is called a nomal midsystolic gallop (Fig. 208). It can be distinguished from the serious diastolic gallop by the following procedure. If the stethoscope is moved from the apex to the base of the heart in rhythm with the heart beat it will be found that the extra sound, which occurs in the middle of the three sounds, gradually diminishes in intensity and finally disappears, leaving the two normal first and second heart sounds. The important point is that the midsystolic gallop rhythm is benign and the diastolic is grave.

CARDIAC MURMURS

The finding of cardiac murmurs in patients with hypertensive heart disease is inconstant. In many of these patients there are no murmurs. More often a systolic murmur will be heard at the apex or base of the heart. This can be either faint or fairly loud. When there is no additional

organic valvular lesion the louder apical systolic murmurs probably result from a relative mitral or tricuspid insufficiency and the aortic systolic
murmurs from dilatation of the aorta. The dilatation of the ventricular
cavities which sometimes is very marked can readily account for stretching of the rings at the base of the valves even when the leaflets themselves
are not particularly diseased. Occasionally even the aortic valve may
thereby become incompetent in hypertension and result in the presence
of an aortic diastolic murmur. Inasmuch as valvular lesions due to other
causes, such as rheumatism or syphilis, may coexist with hypertension,
the corresponding murmurs from these valvular defects may be found.

There is one unusual development in hypertensive cases that is
called "Bernheim's syndrome." This may also occur in other instances of
left ventricular hypertrophy and strain. It consists of the clinical evidence of right-sided heart failure without pulmonary congestion, due to
displacement of the interventricular septum to the right, resulting from a
large left ventricle with increased left intraventricular pressure. This produces obstruction through the right ventricle somewhat analogous to
what occurs in tricuspid stenosis. There is increased venous pressure and
there may be a normal circulation time. The right auricle may also be
enlarged.

NVOLVEMENT OF LUNGS

The lungs often show evidence of stasis. In the milder cases a few
moist rales will be found at the bases of the lungs. When the degree of
heart failure is more marked free fluid in the pleural cavities will develop.
In the fulminating cases of acute left ventricular failure a generalized
pulmonary edema quickly appears, with moist bubbling rales throughout
the chest, cough, and frothy pink sputum. Such a dramatic storm may
come and disappear in an hour or two. With the embarrassed respiration,
Cheyne-Stokes breathing is frequently present. This may not be detected
in some cases if the patient is not carefully observed while asleep, for it
may be absent while he is awake. The rest of the examination reveals the
changes seen in any patient with heart failure. Curiously enough there
are some with considerable breathlessness and even orthopnea who show
no peripheral pitting edema, while others may have all the degrees of congestion up to massive anasarca, marked hepatic congestion, and engorgement of the cervical veins. Occasionally as one observes peripheral edema
becoming more marked orthopnea becomes less troublesome.

ELECTROCARDIOGRAPHIC FINDINGS

The electrocardiographic findings in hypertensive heart disease are
variable. For the most part these depend on the accompanying pathologic
changes in the myocardium. In most cases there is evidence of left ventricular hypertrophy. This finding has no clinical significance as it is so
frequent in other cardiac conditions and even in normal hearts during
the second half of life. Bundle branch block or a spread of the QRS complex indicating intraventricular heart block is commonly present. Inver-

sion of the T waves in Lead I or II or those alterations in the ventricular complex that follow disease of the coronary arteries or infarction of the myocardium are also frequently found. In fact, any of the arrhythmias or other abnormalities in the mechanism of the heart beat may be present. These changes merely reflect the damage that has already occurred in the function and structure of the heart.

TREATMENT AND PROGNOSIS

Inasmuch as the treatment of hypertensive heart failure is not unlike that for congestive heart failure from any other cause it will not be taken up here (see Chap. 20). One word may be mentioned about the treatment of an acute attack of paroxysmal dyspnea or acute pulmonary edema. In most cases a hypodermic injection of 0.015 gm. ($\frac{1}{4}$ grain) of morphine sulfate with 0.6 mg. of atropine ($\frac{1}{100}$ grain) will be sufficient to relieve the attack. Sometimes a phlebotomy of 500 cc. or the application of tourniquets on the extremities with or without the above medication is necessary and effective. In some cases the intravenous injection of 0.24 to 0.48 gm. of aminophylline may be of great value. This may also be used in the evening as a preventive if nocturnal attacks recur frequently. It has recently been observed that prolonged carotid sinus massage will relieve acute pulmonary edema especially in the hypertensive patient with normal sinus rhythm. This emergency treatment should be followed by adequate digitalization and use of diuretics.

The prognosis in hypertension in general is variable. As is well known, many patients live for ten to twenty years or more with a constantly elevated blood pressure. Once either angina pectoris or congestive heart failure develops the outlook changes. But even then some carry on for years. Many different factors need to be judged and even after a complete study is made it is often difficult to make accurate predictions.

There is a form of hypertension that is called "malignant nephrosclerosis" or "malignant hypertension." It is thought by some to be distinct from the ordinary essential hypertension and by others to be merely an advanced and rapidly developing form of the same process. It is associated with a very high diastolic pressure, the readings often being 250 systolic and 150 diastolic. The course is rapidly downhill, ending fatally in about a year or two. Such patients complain a great deal of headache, may have convulsions, and show marked changes on ophthalmoscopic examination, including papilledema. These cerebral features are described by the term "hypertensive encephalopathy" and may be confused with tumor of the brain. This disease is not rare in individuals under 40 and even in those in the twenties, and is often refractory to treatment. It has been of interest to me that whereas essential hypertension in general is much more common in females, "malignant hypertension" is more common in males. Do the endocrine glands determine this difference?

The hypotensive drugs of the ganglionic blocking group are the medical agents of choice for the treatment of malignant hypertension. The results have been especially promising in the absence of significant renal insufficiency. If these drugs do not afford relief, rigid salt restriction with a sodium intake of 200 mg. daily in combination with the rauwolfia or veratrum drugs should be undertaken. When all these medical measures have failed, one may resort to surgery.

The surgical treatment for hypertension is still a matter of some debate. Many hundreds of patients have already been operated upon, some type of dorsolumbar sympathectomy having been utilized. The operation devised by Smithwick appears to have certain advantages and has gained some support. It is still too early to arrive at a final judgment, but at present it appears to be successful in an appreciable number of patients and can be recommended in selected cases. It would be well, however, to perform pyelography routinely in all cases of hypertension, if a complete study is desired, for occasionally unilateral renal disease may be detected by that method only. On rare occasions a unilateral pyelonephritis or aberrant renal artery or adrenal tumor will be unexpectedly found. In search for evidence of pheochromocytoma a Regitine test and an estimation of catechol amines should be carried out. It must be appreciated that tumors of the adrenal cause not only paroxysmal hypertension but also permanent hypertension. The importance of these unilateral lesions is that, although rare, they may be curable by surgical means.

In the selection of patients for dorsolumbar sympathectomy there are various factors to be considered. The results are likely to be better in the female than in the male, when the diastolic pressure is over 100 mm. and the pulse pressure is small, in patients with pyelonephritis than in others with the same functional state of the kidneys, and in patients under 50 years of age than in older individuals. The response to the cold pressor test is more valuable than the response to sedatives.

Because the clinical course of uncomplicated essential hypertension is so variable and unpredictable and so many may live in essentially good health for two decades or more, it will be a long time before the evidence will be convincing that surgery has been worth while. However, when operation is performed on those hypertensive patients who already show grave cardiac involvement, such as angina pectoris, coronary thrombosis, congestive failure, paroxysmal dyspnea, or gallop rhythm, it will not be necessary to wait ten or more years or to accumulate thousands of cases for statistical proof that the course of the illness has been altered. Even if a smaller number of patients with these cardiac complications are operated upon and found to be well, improved, or living five years later we will be fairly certain of the beneficial effects of surgery. I have already seen a small number of such patients improve markedly and return to a useful occupation when it did not appear possible that any such recovery would have occurred on medical management. At present, therefore, I am more interested in advising sympathectomy in those hypertensive patients who already have serious cardiac complications (provided kidney function is satisfactory) than as a prophylactic measure in those who are still in fairly good general health.

Some years ago Kempner introduced the rice diet as a treatment for hypertension. This has caused considerable controversy among many physicians. This diet, which consists only of rice and fruit, is extremely low in sodium, containing less than 500 or 250 mg. daily. It is also very low in protein, fat, total calories, and vitamins. Patients therefore lose some weight and require supplementary vitamins. There is no doubt that this rigid diet lowers the blood pressure in a large number of cases. What is disputed is whether the effect is entirely due to the low sodium intake. Most investigators believe that the beneficial effects could be obtained by the use of a more general diet if the sodium content could be reduced to the same level contained in the rice diet. As a practical matter it is difficult to outline a general dietary regimen that will contain as little sodium as the Kempner diet. When the strict rice and fruit diet is followed there is also a marked fall in the cholesterol in the blood. Occasionally the chloride content also falls, and with it a rise in blood nitrogen. This then needs to be corrected by giving more salt.

This diet is a very difficult one to take. There are not many patients who will continue on it long enough for it to be of value. Physicians who are enthusiastic about it and who impart their enthusiasm to their patients often succeed and claim very satisfactory results. In my limited experience I have seen a few dramatic results, but in most cases the patients returned to what they regarded as a more palatable diet. It is unlikely that the Kempner diet will eventually prove necessary. In the meantime it has had useful results. It re-emphasized the importance of an extremely low salt intake in the treatment of hypertension and congestive failure, a point that had been well known for many years. It has also taught us that people can live comfortably for long periods of time on a very low protein intake, even if there is a nitrogen deficit, and it has focused our attention on the great importance of diet in relation to health and disease.

A host of new drugs have come into use in recent years in the treatment of hypertension. It is not the purpose of this discussion to go into this subject in detail. Much of this work can be regarded as in the uncertain or experimental stage, as it is related to accompanying heart disease or heart failure. There is no doubt that these new drugs can lower the blood pressure, but determination of their value in the treatment of chronic heart disease awaits long-range study.

Four categories of hypotensive drugs are in current use. The most recently introduced group of agents come from *Rauwolfia serpentina*, an Indian plant. The crude root and its alkaloidal extracts have similar pharmacologic properties, except that the purified derivative (Reserpine) is 100 times as potent as the parent compound. Rauwolfia acts on the central nervous system, presumably at the hypothalamic level. It is believed that it decreases blood pressure by central sympathetic inhibition and perhaps parasympathetic stimulation. The average dose of Reserpine is about 0.25 to 1.0 mg. per day. These drugs are mild hypotensive and tranquilizing agents, and the hypotensive action is additive to that of the other hypotensive drugs.

The veratrum alkaloids are also obtained from plants. Their action is mediated via the chemoreceptors of the carotid sinus and coronary sinus, resulting in increased afferent impulses via the vagus nerve to the central nervous system. Vasodilation and fall in blood pressure are due to a decrease in efferent impulses through the splanchnic nerves. These drugs exhibit a very narrow range between therapeutic effect and toxic action. The dose must be worked out carefully, and this can best be done by trial and error. They are the best currently available drugs for parenteral administration for the control of acute hypertensive emergencies.

Hydralazine, or 1-hydrazinophthalazine (Apresoline), is a synthetic agent. It acts on the central nervous system as well as counteracts certain circulating vasopressor substances. It directly stimulates the heart, resulting in tachycardia and increased cardiac output. Angina pectoris may therefore be precipitated by its use. Continued administration has resulted in the emergence of a condition resembling collagen disease in a small percentage of patients. The syndrome clears with discontinuation of the drug. Apresoline should be reserved for advanced forms of hypertension. It is most effective when used in conjunction with ganglionic blocking agents.

Of the ganglionic blocking agents the ones finding application as hypotensive drugs are the methonium derivatives, pentolinium (Ansolysen), Ecolid, and Inversine. These drugs interfere with cholinergic transmission at the ganglionic synapses. This resulting interference with sympathetic nervous activity causes orthostatic hypotension and compensatory tachycardia. Since it blocks parasympathetic activity as well, a host of side effects are encountered. The methonium compounds are also responsible for a new disease, characterized by severe and fatal pulmonary fibrosis, which has been observed in a small number of patients.

One can readily see that there are some untoward effects from these new hypotensive agents. They therefore should be used with caution. Dosage needs to be watched carefully. Only by more prolonged observation will their proper role in the treatment of hypertensive heart disease be established.

"Chronic Myocarditis"

The term "chronic myocarditis" has formerly been used to denote a nonvalvular condition associated with heart failure. There has been much discussion concerning this term, and many substitutes have been offered. Objection has been made to the term because myocarditis denotes an inflammation, and often no clinical or pathologic evidence of inflammation can be found. At present, however, as a result of the great advances in cardiac diagnosis many of the cases of so-called "chronic myocarditis" can be more accurately named and what was once a "catch-all" term for a variety of conditions may now be reserved for only a rare occasion. As one looks back at the cases so diagnosed in the past one will become aware of several clinical entities that now can be well recognized. Some were instances of masked hyperthyroidism that were overlooked. Others were instances of "cor pulmonale" or heart failure from chronic emphysema or pulmonary arterial disease. Still others were cases in which the heart failure was due to avitaminosis (the so-called "beriberi heart"), or in which edema was present because of a low protein content of the blood. A few were cases in which there was actual valvular disease, either mitral or more frequently aortic stenosis, in which the clinical signs were not elicited or were misinterpreted. I know this has frequently happened in the past because subsequent examination would uncover a systolic thrill at the base of the heart or x-ray examination later would disclose calcification of one of the valves, and finally because in some marked valvular disease was found on postmortem examination. A large group of cases that formerly were called chronic myocarditis we now can recognize clinically as due to coronary artery sclerosis or coronary thrombosis. The increased interest in angina pectoris and the great advances in electrocardiography have enabled us to make these anatomic diagnoses in many instances previously overlooked.

There remains the large group that is now called hypertensive heart disease. This does not mean that the mechanism of heart failure that develops in these cases is adequately explained on the basis of the hypertension. The unknown factor "X," mentioned previously, still has a bearing on the problem, but we are enabled to classify such cases under the heading of hypertensive heart disease merely because there is or has been hypertension and there is heart failure without any other predictable anatomic abnormality. When all these well-recognized conditions and a few others like syphilis and anemia are carefully sought for and excluded, there still remains a very small group of patients in whom heart failure takes place. There is no hyperthyroidism, emphysema, valvular disease, coronary artery disease, or hypertension, and yet the heart muscle failed. Such hearts on postmortem examination are generally enlarged and may show an apparently normal myocardium. The present methods of pathologic study fail to explain why the heart muscle was inadequate to maintain a normal circulation. In a few there are found pathologic changes in the myocardium but no satisfactory cause is discovered for such changes. These cases form the small remainder of what was formerly called "chronic myocarditis."

Some of these cases which do show inflammatory changes in the myocardium are called Fiedler's myocarditis, although the pathologic findings in this condition are not distinctive. They generally are not very responsive to treatment and run a course lasting some months to a few years, rarely longer. Occasionally the process may be essentially confined to the right ventricle and present a picture of right-sided heart failure. Some of these more discrete but rare forms of heart disease will now be discussed.

Rare Forms of Heart Disease

MYXEDEMA HEART

With prolonged advanced myxedema certain changes take place in the circulation that are designated as "myxedema heart." Such patients not only have the customary findings, such as a low metabolism, dry skin, coarse, scanty hair, a feeling of coldness, puffy appearance of the face, anemia, and a high blood cholesterol, but show more than the usual edema of the legs and marked dilatation of the heart. In most cases what is thought to be cardiac dilatation turns out to be pericardial effusion. Rarely there may be fluid in the abdominal or pleural cavities. In most cases there actually is no true congestive failure despite the cardiac dilatation. Such patients complain of weakness and dyspnea but not of orthopnea. The electrocardiograms show ventricular complexes of low amplitude (Figs. 144, 200). The diagnosis is readily made, if the above features are kept in mind.

The important point regarding treatment is that patients with this condition do not respond to digitalis but can be cured by thyroid administration. Thyroid medication should be given slowly and cautiously. Too rapid increase in the metabolic rate can bring on acute left ventricular failure or angina pectoris. Desiccated thyroid gland, 1/2- to 1-grain tablet, administered daily is often sufficient. If anginal pain develops it may be best to accept only a partial recovery in myxedema, permitting the basal metabolic rate to remain about −10 per cent. Under skillful management the heart returns to normal size, the electrocardiograms show normal tracings, and all symptoms disappear.

HEART FAILURE FROM ARTERIOVENOUS FISTULA

There is one form of heart muscle failure which may properly be discussed in this connection, although it is in no way related to either infection or degeneration, i.e., myocardial failure from a peripheral arteriovenous fistula. Here the heart dilates and dyspnea and congestion may develop purely as a result of the increased work of the heart consequent to the short circuiting of the blood. All evidence of cardiac disease may promptly disappear after surgical removal of the fistula or aneurysm. This condition is generally traumatic in origin and often follows a gunshot or stab wound of a limb. The continuous murmur over the fistula or aneurysm, the pulsating veins distal to the lesion, the high pulse pressure and the prompt slowing of the heart rate that follows compression of the fistula are diagnostic of this condition. It is one of the few types of heart failure from purely mechanical causes that is readily amenable to curative treatment.

I once learned of a case in which a nontraumatic arteriovenous fistula developed in the pelvis of a kidney. The patient had had advanced heart failure for years and was bedridden. Her physician, Dr. F. B. Camp, of Missouri, made the diagnosis by hearing a continuous murmur over the loin. Even after being refractory to all ordinary medical treatment, the patient was cured by a nephrectomy.

RUPTURED VALVES OF THE HEART

Occasionally one sees instances of rupture of the valves. In most cases this occurs in previously diseased valves. After a sudden strain a free aortic insufficiency may develop, especially in a pre-existing syphilitic lesion, with a resulting loud or musical diastolic murmur. Without any precipitating effort this complication may arise during the course of bacterial endocarditis. Likewise, in old rheumatic disease of the mitral valve, ruptures may occur, but then they are more likely to take place in the chordae tendineae. This apparently is more frequent than has generally been appreciated, even when there was no previous disease. In such cases, either after some unusual effort or quite spontaneously, a loud apical systolic murmur of mitral insufficiency and dyspnea suddenly develop. Cardiac symptoms may appear immediately or insidiously only after some years. Males are more commonly affected than females. All these patients eventually die of congestive failure, although some have survived for months or many years. The possibility of a ruptured valve must always be considered when a loud murmur and cardiac symptoms appear abruptly.

BERIBERI HEART

In the Orient it has long been known that heart failure could result from an inadequate diet. The condition was called "beriberi heart." One form of this dietary deficiency appeared as peripheral neuritis and the other as congestive heart failure. This condition is now known to be due to a deficiency of vitamin B_1. It may take the wet or the dry form, or be a combination of both. Its occurrence in this country was emphasized by the studies of Soma Weiss. It is most frequent in chronic alcoholics and in others who have abstained from necessary foods for long periods of time. There is reason to suspect that similar vitamin B_1 deficiency with cardiac complications may be present in pregnancy and hyperthyroidism. In the severe form the clinical picture is one of advanced heart failure, both of the right and left ventricular type. The heart is rapid, generally regular, but occasionally shows a transient auricular fibrillation and often has a gallop rhythm. Dilatation may be considerable and yet complete restoration to a normal size results with recovery. Systolic murmurs are frequent, but diastolic murmurs are rare. There may be a pistol shot in the peripheral pulse and an increased pulse pressure. In fact, many of the features resemble those seen in thyrotoxicosis or arteriovenous fistula. There often are considerable peripheral edema, engorged liver, and pulmonary congestion. Mural thrombosis of the cardiac chambers with resultant emboli may be present. The electrocardiogram may show a diminution or slight inversion of the T waves in any of the leads, and lengthening of the Q-T interval. The important point is that this condition does not respond to ordinary cardiac therapy or digitalis whereas dramatic and complete recovery may follow the administration of 10 to 20 mg. of crystalline B_1 intramuscularly three times a day (Fig. 199). The subsequent diet should contain meat, flour, and yeast.

HEART FAILURE WITH ACUTE NEPHRITIS

Congestive heart failure with dilatation of the heart and the picture of either left or right ventricular failure occasionally occurs during acute nephritis. These cases will show hypertension, pulmonary rales, and peripheral edema, as well as evidence of active nephritis. Electrocardiograms at this time may show changes in the ventricular complexes, especially in the T waves, that superficially resemble those seen with myocardial infarction. A similar situation may develop during the toxemia of pregnancy. The response to cardiac therapy is likely to be satisfactory, and when recovery takes place the heart may be expected to be normal or essentially so. Restriction of fluid and salt, administration of digitalis, and occasionally intramuscular injections of 1 to 2 gm. of magnesium sulfate may be helpful.

COR PULMONALE

The right ventricle may fail as a result of increased pressure in the pulmonary circuit. This may occur acutely, as following a large pulmonary embolus (acute cor pulmonale), or more slowly, as in chronic pulmonary emphysema, silicosis, or pulmonary arterial disease (chronic cor pulmonale). These conditions are discussed elsewhere (see Chaps. 6 and 16). It must be emphasized, however, that great care is needed to distinguish the breathlessness that results from the pulmonary disease per se from that which follows heart failure. The treatment and prognosis of the two states are quite different.

SCLERODERMA HEART

It is now known that pathologic changes in scleroderma are not confined to the skin and subcutaneous tissues. There may be cardiac complications, consisting of disintegration of muscle fibers and extensive replacement by fibrous tissue. This can result in cardiac enlargement and congestive failure.

Auricular fibrillation, gallop rhythm, and slight prolongation of the Q-T interval of the electrocardiogram have been noted in different cases. I have seen instances in which, because of related findings, one case resembled chronic rheumatic heart disease and another thyrocardiac disease. The treatment is the same as that for any ordinary case of heart failure. Adrenal steroids might well be helpful in this condition.

TUMORS OF THE HEART

Both malignant and benign tumors of the heart are rare. Metastatic tumors are about ten times as common as primary tumors. The diagnosis of cardiac tumors is rather difficult, and most cases are first recognized at autopsy. Peculiar x-ray silhouettes of the heart or the finding of bloody fluid in the pericardium, not otherwise explained, may lead one to a correct antemortem diagnosis. Occasionally auricular flutter or fibrillation, transient or permanent, may be present with cardiac tumors, possibly as a result of involvement of the auricles. Such arrhythmias, not otherwise explicable, may be a clue to the diagnosis. The most common primary origin of cardiac metastases is carcinoma of the bronchus or lung. However, the diagnosis of carcinomatous involvement of the heart should always be suspected in any case of cancer, Hodgkin's disease, leukemia, etc., if evidence of pericarditis or other unusual developments occur in the cardiac status.

Although metastatic neoplastic changes in the heart are much more common than primary tumors, the former have little practical interest while the latter are now of considerable importance. There is one type of cardiac tumor that is amenable to cardiac surgery, i.e., myxoma of the auricle. With the large number of cases that are presently being operated upon, especially for valvular disease, more and more instances of this form of benign cardiac tumor are being found and a few have been successfully removed with resultant cures. Myxomas of the left auricle are three or four times as common as those of the right auricle. Those involving the left auricle present features resembling mitral stenosis and those involving the right auricle resemble tricuspid stenosis or pericardial constriction. In neither case is there a history of rheumatic fever. In both spells of dyspnea, palpitation, and weakness may be related to change of position of the body from one side to the other. This feature is not common in ordinary heart disease and may help to direct one's attention to the correct diagnosis. In myxoma of the left auricle the heart sounds and murmurs may mimic in all respects those found in classic mitral stenosis, i.e., an accentuated first sound, a diastolic or presystolic murmur, and even an opening snap may be present. These findings may be constant, but not infrequently they come and go just as the symptoms may do, most likely as a result of the change in position of the tumor in relation to the valvular orifice. At different times there may be greater or lesser mechanical impediment to blood flow through the valve as a result of the movements of the tumor, which is often pedunculated. In one case of myxoma of the left auricle that I saw the first symptom resulted from an embolus to a leg. This man, 60 years old, had had no signs or symptoms of heart disease and was quite well until a bit of the tumor became dislodged and obstructed the femoral artery.

When myxoma of the auricle is suspected on the basis of some of the above features, angiocardiography might readily establish a definitive diagnosis, by showing a localized filling defect of the auricle. This can be detected much more easily when the tumor is in the right than in the left auricle. Catheterization studies may also elicit a pressure gradient between one auricle and the corresponding ventricle. This will at least indicate that there is an obstruction at the valve orifice which may be due to a stenosed valve or a tumor of the auricle.

When the myxoma is in the right auricle the features are mainly those of right-sided heart failure, with possible spells of insufficient blood flow to the lungs and therefore to the peripheral arterial system. Because pericardial constriction often produces a somewhat similar clinical picture, though without the acute changes in signs and symptoms, the two conditions may resemble each other.

At the present time cases of myxoma of the auricle are generally being found accidentally by surgeons, during operations for valvular or other forms of heart disease, especially one to accomplish mitral valvuloplasty. It would appear from current experience that if such an unexpected lesion is found it is best to retreat and postpone therapy for a time when a more deliberate operation, possibly under hypothermia or with open technique, can be performed. Attempts to excise the tumor, more or less piecemeal, have proved disastrous and fatal. Portions of the tumor mass are readily dislodged, with resultant disseminated pulmonary or peripheral emboli. On the other hand, cures have been obtained when the operation was well planned and properly carried out.

CARDIAC COMPLICATIONS IN LUPUS ERYTHEMATOSUS DISSEMINATUS (LIBMAN-SACKS DISEASE)

A group of conditions that are closely related, if not different manifestations of the same underlying process, have come to light and have been described under a variety of terms. Although there is still confusion in the terminology and complete lack of knowledge as to the etiology, the condition we now recognize as lupus erythematosus disseminatus is known to involve the heart. It is not infrequently associated with a sterile type of pericarditis, and there may be small nonbacterial vegetations on the valves of the heart (Libman-Sacks disease, or nonbacterial verrucous endocarditis). In fact there are also rare instances in which the myocardium is involved, as manifested by a prolongation of the P-R interval in the electrocardiogram. This group of diseases appear to be closely related in the pathologic findings to rheumatic fever, periarteritis nodosa, and scleroderma, from which differentiation at times may be difficult. They all can be regarded as collagen disorders. It may also be confused with subacute bacterial endocarditis, because of many features that are common to both diseases.

It must be appreciated that lupus occurs generally in females during the years of menstruation, may run a prolonged course of months or years, may show no lesions on the face at the start or for long periods during its course, and can display cycles of high fever with intervening periods of quiescence. There is generally a leukopenia or at least an absence of leukocytosis, and there may be an increase in the globulin content of the blood. The heart may be spared but often is involved, as are other serous membranes, resulting in pleuritis, peritonitis, pericarditis, or endocarditis. There generally is albuminuria and often pulmonary consolidation. The diagnosis is likely to be overlooked until the characteristic butterfly rash appears over the nose and cheeks.

At present there is no known effective treatment. Spray x-ray treatment is being tried for lupus erythematosus disseminatus, with what appears to be favorable alleviation of symptoms. Adrenal steroids have produced the best therapeutic results and have kept the condition under control for long periods of time. When the renal function is significantly involved the outlook is almost invariably poor.

THE HEART IN ADDISON'S DISEASE

With the discovery of effective methods of treatment for Addison's disease by means of synthetic desoxycorticosterone, sodium chloride, and later adrenal steroids, a new type of heart failure is now met with. The ordinary patient with Addison's disease has a small heart, often much smaller than normal. Under this new treatment, the heart returns to a more normal size. In some cases the heart is not able to make the necessary adjustment to the rapid changes in dynamics, and, with the increase in blood volume and blood pressure, the retention of salt, and undue dilation of the heart, pulmonary edema, peripheral edema, and even rapid fatality may result. Therefore, if any of the signs of heart failure appear in a patient under treatment for Addison's disease the medication should be omitted for a while and then reinstituted in smaller doses. It should be appreciated that the main offending factor in the production of the cardiac disability is the retention of sodium.

FAMILIAL CARDIOMEGALY

William Evans of London has described a small group of cases that seem to form a clinical entity. Such patients may have slight or no symptoms in their early years. Later palpitation, giddiness, and frank Adams-Stokes syncopal attacks or transient auricular fibrillation may occur. Death may take place suddenly without congestive failure. The heart will show very little except enlargement, but the electrocardiograms may reveal various arrhythmias, such as premature beats, paroxysmal tachycardia, auricular flutter, auricular fibrillation, auriculoventricular block, or intraventricular block. The condition is met with in children or young adults, and what is particularly characteristic is that more than one member of the same family are afflicted. The cause is unknown, and it is not thought to be due to glycogen deposits.

HEART FAILURE FROM DEFORMITY OF THE CHEST

Marked deformity of the chest, especially following poliomyelitis or tuberculosis of the spine, may eventually lead to heart failure. At first only slight dyspnea on exertion or with change of body position may be present. The vital capacity of the lungs becomes considerably diminished, while the residual air increases in proportion. As the condition progresses, less and less oxygenation of the blood takes place. With this there may be attacks of palpitation, weakness, cyanosis, tendency to faintness or unconsciousness, and marked dyspnea. Such patients quickly succumb to pulmonary infections. The heart is not much enlarged, although there is often right ventricular hypertrophy. The rhythm is generally regular, and the pulmonary second sound is accentuated. The velocity of blood flow, the venous pressure, and the cardiac output per minute are within normal limits. Once major symptoms develop the patient's activities become markedly restricted and the downhill progress does not seem to be influenced by treatment.

Ordinary cardiac therapy is on the whole ineffective in this type of cardiopulmonary failure. The only hope is preventive treatment. These chest deformities produce harmful results if they occur during the growing years of life. Every effort should be made to prevent or relieve these distortions of the chest when the child is young. The orthopedic surgeon should be called in to do whatever he can in order to lessen the deformity. When cardiac symptoms are already present, exercise should be greatly restricted and respiratory infections avoided as far as possible. Oxygen and ephedrine may be helpful, and morphine should be avoided.

THE HEART IN ACUTE INFECTIONS

It has become more and more evident that many acute infections are associated with some injury to the heart muscle. In most infections whatever damage to the heart may take place must be inconsequential, for very little clinical evidence becomes apparent during the acute infection and no residual cardiac defects persist afterwards. However, careful and frequent electrocardiographic studies during infections like diphtheria, typhoid fever, pneumonia, mumps, meningococcus meningitis, mononucleosis, and many other infections have shown changes in the ventricular complexes or the conduction mechanism. These are generally transient, with complete restoration to normal. Likewise in the occasional fatal case of some of these infections, pathologic evidence of inflammation of the ventricular musculature (acute myocarditis) has been detected. Inflammatory lesions in the myocardium have been found in virus diseases such as scrub typhus, poliomyelitis, encephalitis, infectious hepatitis, and others. It has long been known that with diphtheria, rheumatic fever, and Chagas' disease, the heart muscle frequently shows extensive inflammatory injury, and heart block and electrocardiographic abnormalities are quite common. It is now clear that although in most cases this type of acute myocarditis has little clinical or practical significance, occasionally it may be the direct cause of death. What is not known is whether some of the cases of subclinical acute myocarditis which are even undetected in ordinary practice form the background for subsequent damage to the heart muscle. In other words, can some cases of unexplained cardiac hypertrophy or so-called chronic myocarditis of unknown etiology be the end-result of early injury sustained during an otherwise harmless acute infection? There is more than a suspicion that this is true. I am increasingly convinced that diphtheria, which frequently is associated with heart block during the acute stage and is then generally fatal, may be the initial cause of complete heart block and Adams-Stokes disease which occur many years later. There are probably other instances in which an acute myocarditis during an infectious illness tells its tale many years later in some form of heart muscle disturbance.

As an illustration of the frequency of mild involvement of the myocardium during acute infections one can cite the experience with mumps. Ordinarily little attention is paid to the heart in this disease. No one has associated significant cardiac complications with parotitis. However, in a series of 100 cases 15 patients showed definite abnormalities in the electrocardiograms, mainly T wave changes, and two showed complete heart block. All the abnormalities disappeared with recovery from the infection. The injury to the heart muscle was apparently mild and reversible.

The following is an instance of acute myocarditis accompanying virus pneumonia. A woman 34 years old who previously was well, never having had hypertension or rheumatic infection, developed ordinary influenza. The virus was isolated in this case and found to be type A. She quickly developed alarming cardiac symptoms. She complained of substernal tightness, showed pulmonary edema and weak pulse. There was a leukocytosis of 20,000, and the x-ray of the chest was compatible with atypical pneumonia. The electrocardiograms displayed bizarre complexes resembling potassium intoxication. There were slurred broad QRS complexes and complete auriculoventricular dissociation with a ventricular rate of about 90. Within one week she died. Postmortem examination showed extensive interstitial round-cell infiltration and much degeneration of muscle fibers. The coronary arteries and valves were normal. The heart weighed 480 gm., although she was known to have had a normal sized heart on x-ray examination two months before.

Cases similar to the above must be occurring either in a fatal form or with less extensive damage so that recovery takes place. In the past the virus origin has not been identified and it is still a difficult laboratory procedure, so that absolute proof of the nature of the acute myocarditis will rarely be established. It is reasonable to suppose that milder forms of acute myocarditis frequently go unnoticed in virus and other infections.

Unfortunately therapy is likely to be of little value in this type of acute myocarditis. Obviously the early and adequate use of specific measures when available, such as antitoxin for diphtheria, penicillin for pneumonia, and antibiotics for virus infections, will either prevent or minimize the heart muscle injury. It is doubtful whether digitalis preparations will be helpful. The state of shock may be combated with transfusions of blood or plasma with due regard to the hazard of precipitating acute pulmonary edema. Stimulants like caffeine and coramine may be employed.

AMYLOID DISEASE OF THE HEART

Amyloid deposits may take place in different organs in what appears to be a haphazard fashion. Sometimes many organs are involved, and in other cases one or a few particular parts of the body are selected. Nowadays amyloidosis occurs as a primary and unexplained condition more often than it does as a result of prolonged chronic suppuration. Occasionally the heart muscle bears the main brunt of this process so that the patient's main complaints may be those of congestive heart failure or anginal pain. Whenever the cause of a chronic cardiac disability remains obscure, the possibility of amyloid disease of the heart muscle should be considered. There are no distinctive symptoms of this condition. The electrocardiograms are almost always abnormal but not specifically so. There may be prolongation of the P-R interval or QRS complex, and abnormal inversion of T waves. The Congo red test for amyloidosis may help to identify the condition. I saw a patient with classic anginal pain who showed on postmortem examination diffuse amyloid of the myocardium with no significant coronary artery disease.

SARCOID DISEASE OF THE HEART

Inasmuch as sarcoid is a generalized granulomatous disease, it is not surprising that in some instances the heart may be involved. I once saw a case in which frequent paroxysms of ventricular tachycardia had been occurring over a period of a year. Right bundle branch block was present when the rhythm was normal. Finally this man, 55 years old, developed complete heart block and died suddenly. Extensive granulomatous lesions were found on postmortem examination in the ventricular septum, in the lungs, and in the liver.

HEART DISEASE ASSOCIATED WITH CARCINOID

Very recently a new syndrome has been described. There is a small group of patients in whom carcinoid, generally involving the small intestines, is associated with disease of the right side of the heart, with pulmonary stenosis and tricuspid stenosis or insufficiency. This is particularly true if hepatic metastases are present. These patients have attacks of marked vasomotor flushing and mottling cyanosis of the skin. It is thought that serotonin may possibly be related to the skin changes and the cardiac involvement. This is an intriguing problem, as it suggests a possible chemical clue as a cause of chronic valvular disease of the heart.

THE HEART IN NEUROMUSCULAR DISORDERS

Poliomyelitis. Minor electrocardiographic abnormalities are quite common in acute poliomyelitis, and more marked changes occasionally occur. In some fatal cases examined post mortem well marked evidence of myocarditis has been observed. Hypertension is present in severe attacks, especially in the bulbospinal type, and is thought to accompany the anoxia. The blood pressure may return to normal with improvement. Pulmonary edema occurs in the severe cases. The administration of 100 per cent oxygen, even endotracheally, may be urgently needed and life saving. Intravenous fluid should be given with great caution in cases of this type, for among fatal cases of acute poliomyelitis 20 per cent were due to acute pulmonary edema. However, when recovery takes place there is little if any evidence of permanent cardiac damage.

PROGRESSIVE MUSCULAR DYSTROPHY

Heart muscle abnormalities occur mainly in the pseudohypertrophic or childhood type of progressive muscular dystrophy, when the onset of skeletal muscular symptoms occur early in life. The heart muscle will show atrophy and hypertrophy of muscle cells, loss of cross striations, fragmentation of fibers, and increase in connective and fatty tissue. Although various changes in the electrocardiograms are fairly common, real evidence of congestive failure is not frequently found.

MARFAN'S SYNDROME

Marfan's syndrome is regarded as a hereditary connective tissue disorder affecting the musculoskeletal, ocular, and cardiovascular systems. These patients are tall and thin, with long fingers and toes, deformed chest of the funnel or pigeon-breast type, winged scapula, and high palate, and often have detachment of the lens. In addition, aneurysm or dilatation of the aorta or pulmonary artery may be present. As a result of trauma or strain, or possibly even without such precipitating causes, dissection of the aorta or rupture of the aortic valve may occur.

CHAPTER 8

Thyroid Heart Disease

Hyperthyroidism, whether due to a diffuse hyperplasia or to a toxic adenoma of the thyroid gland, produces certain disturbances in the circulation. It has been the prevailing opinion that hyperthyroidism alone does not cause permanent structural changes in the heart and that when there is gross evidence of congestive heart failure, or angina pectoris, other independent conditions will be found such as hypertension, valvular heart disease, or coronary artery disease. A review of a considerable number of thyrocardiac patients, however, revealed many instances of advanced heart failure in which no cause other than thyrotoxicosis could be found and in which complete recovery occurred after appropriate treatment. Frequently arrhythmias occur that are very troublesome to the patient which are purely the result of the toxic thyroid gland, and it may be expected that these will disappear if the hyperthyroidism is cured. There are many changes that result from hyperthyroidism, independently of other conditions, which are similar to those seen in ordinary forms of heart disease. Inasmuch as thyroid and other forms of heart disease frequently occur together in the same individual and the evidence of an overactive thyroid gland may be very obscure, it becomes extremely important to be familiar with the methods of diagnosis that serve to differentiate the one from the other. This subject is one of the most important aspects of all heart disease for it comprises the one large group of cases in which the difference between accurate and inaccurate diagnosis and treatment is the difference between chronic invalidism or death, and restoration of health and life.

Symptoms

We are all familiar with the typical picture of exophthalmic goiter. It is not the purpose here to discuss in detail but rather to mention these features briefly. The main emphasis is to be directed at the group of cases called "masked thyrocardiacs." At the outset it must be appreciated, just as is true in many diseases, that no single sign or symptom is invariably present but that even in the obscure cases the composite picture is sufficiently suggestive to enable one to suspect the proper diagnosis. The cardinal diagnostic points of hyperthyroidism are exophthalmos, thyroid enlargement, nervousness, and palpitation. When exophthalmos and a palpable thyroid are absent, as is the case in this particular group of patients, the other symptoms and signs of an overactive gland become more important because only by constant search into these features will the correct diagnosis be made. It must also be borne in mind that these patients, who are nevertheless suffering from hyperthyroidism, come to the physician complaining of the same symptoms as do other patients with heart disease but without hyperthyroidism. Their primary complaints will be shortness of breath, palpitation, weakness, chest pain, coughing, swelling of the legs or abdomen. Inasmuch as they often lack the obvious evidence of thyroid disease and have evident organic heart disease of one form or another, they are treated for the latter with little if any success and the former is entirely overlooked.

It is always necessary to have the possibility of masked hyperthyroidism constantly in mind when treating cardiac cases. This is especially true if certain peculiar clues are detected. Of first importance is transient auricular fibrillation. Although this phenomenon occurs in other conditions, of none is it so characteristic and in none does it occur so commonly as in hyperthyroidism. It, therefore, should be the invariable practice to suspect a toxic thyroid gland whenever this arrhythmia is observed even when other forms of heart disease such as mitral stenosis are also present. Undue loss of weight, nervousness, tremor of the fingers, and excessive perspiration are frequently not investigated with sufficient care when present in cardiac patients. They are too often attributed to the customary forms of heart disease with which they are frequently associated, whereas in some cases a latent hyperthyroidism proves to be the more important cause. This is particularly true if the loss of weight takes place in the presence of a fair or good appetite. Other common findings in these patients are transient glycosuria and transient periods of mild diarrhea or hyperactivity of the bowels. These patients, therefore, are at times treated for diabetes or for some gastrointestinal disorder. The diabetes here is rarely of much importance, the patients often stating that they have had to pay very little attention to their diet and that it did not seem to matter very much whether they followed a diet or not. It is also of some interest that whereas the ordinary inactive cardiac patients generally need cathartics, those suffering from latent hyperthyroidism as a rule do not.

APPEARANCE OF THE PATIENT

The general appearance of the patient often has given the first evidence suggesting that a latent hyperthyroidism, long overlooked, was present. The skin takes on a peculiar appearance, rather difficult to describe, that I have called a salmon-colored hue. It is warm, moist, hyperemic, and slightly pigmented. The eyes, in the absence of gross exophthalmos, may show a peculiar stare. Sometimes this stare is unilateral. There is also a certain quickness of motion, an alertness, and even an attractiveness to the behavior of many of these patients that one is not accustomed to find in the ordinary patient with heart disease. In fact most patients suffering from heart failure, particularly when more or less bedridden, are sluggish both in mind and body, whereas with the same degree of decompensation those who also have hyperthyroidism often retain this peculiar alertness and comeliness. It is also common to learn that these patients prefer cold to warm weather. In addition many have premature gray hair. Often this has preceded by many years the development of the major circulatory symptoms. Incidentally the appearance of premature, rather striking, grayness of the hair has often been an important clue in the diagnosis of other conditions. Early graying occurs in four main groups of individuals. First there is a group of perfectly normal people who begin to have gray or even white hair in the twenties or thirties. Often they have a family history of a similar tendency. Among these will be a considerable number who also have a tendency to premature arteriosclerosis. Then there are three diseases with which it is not infrequently associated, i.e., asthma, hyperthyroidism, and pernicious anemia. Although the exact causal relationship is obscure it may turn out that early graying of the hair is due to one common abnormality of the endocrine system. Needless to say, such features will not be ascertained or appreciated unless the physician has already been suspecting the thyroid gland. It is very striking in hospital records how the history and physical findings change after the routine admission notes have been made, when the same observer is told that the patient may have masked hyperthyroidism. Only then do the observations appear that the skin is moist and somewhat pigmented and that the patient has preferred cold weather, or that there has been hyperactivity of the bowels. In other words, one has to seek the evidence, for the patient may be interested only in his breathlessness.

It is to be expected that patients with thyrotoxicosis would be prone to avitaminosis. Even with a normal dietary intake, which is not adequate because loss of weight occurs, increased metabolism demands still greater amounts of vitamins. The result is that deficiencies are common. This may manifest itself in the form of a red sore tongue, skin changes, or red palms. Possibly some of the cardiac abnormalities in hyperthyroidism are actually the result of vitamin B deficiency.

CIRCULATORY CHANGES

Examination of the circulation and especially of the heart is of the greatest importance in these cases, for not only are there peculiarities to be found that help in arriving at the correct diagnosis, but there are also the abnormalities that are associated with the common forms of heart disease with which hyperthyroidism is confused. It is necessary to repeat that transient auricular fibrillation is very common, but many patients even develop the permanent form of this irregularity. The heart sounds are very apt to be hyperactive. An accentuated first heart sound is common in mitral stenosis, in anemia, in some cases of hypertension, in cases of nervous or unstable hearts, but especially so in cases of hyperthyroidism. With this hyperdynamic contraction, often detectable on fluoroscopic examination, there is a diffuse and snapping apex impulse. The vibration of the chest wall resulting from this hyperactive heart makes the impulse diffuse and often creates the impression that the heart is larger than it actually is. Furthermore, a vibration is set up in the chest wall which on palpation feels like a thrill.

When in addition one appreciates the fact that in many cases of hyperthyroidism there is a systolic murmur either at the apex or base of the heart, one can readily see how easily this condition may be confused with mitral stenosis. This mistake has often been made by most competent physicians. In hyperthyroidism the x-ray may even show a slight prominence in the region of the left auricle similar to that which occurs in early mitral stenosis, although the prominence is the result of dilatation of both the pulmonary vessels and the left auricle. In both conditions symptoms of cardiac disease exist, auricular fibrillation is common, there are an accentuated first heart sound and a systolic murmur, and in both there may be a palpable thrill. To be sure the thrill occurs during diastole in mitral stenosis and during systole in hyperthyroidism, but when the heart rate is rapid it is often impossible to time the palpable thrill with any accuracy. The preconception that the condition ought to be mitral stenosis often leads the observer into falsely timing the thrill as presystolic. The one difference between the two conditions is that no murmur will be heard during diastole in cases of hyperthyroidism. This differential point is of the greatest importance. The difficulty becomes greater still when both conditions exist in the same patient, as not infrequently occurs, for one then finds ample evidence of mitral stenosis and has to rely on other criteria to make the additional diagnosis of hyperthyroidism.

There are further peculiarities of the circulation in hyperthyroidism that require mention. It is often difficult and sometimes impossible to slow the heart rate by the use of digitalis when auricular fibrillation is present. Ordinarily with auricular fibrillation, especially when there is no fever, one expects a specific slowing to an essentially normal rate when adequate doses of digitalis are administered. In fact, when such slowing does not occur one is justified in suspecting that the drug is not of normal potency or that the patient has hyperthyroidism. The failure to obtain the expected slowing of the apex rate of the heart in cases of auricular fibrillation following appropriate digitalis dosage has been, in several instances, the first clue that a masked hyperthyroidism was present. Slowing is promptly obtained if the basal metabolic rate is reduced or brought to normal by the use of iodide medication or surgery.

In some puzzling cases the determination of the velocity of blood flow helps to decide whether the cardiac symptoms are due to thyrotoxicosis or not. In most cases of ordinary congestive failure the circulation time is slow, i.e., over 20 seconds. In hyperthyroidism the velocity is apt to be fast, even in the presence of congestive failure. The only other conditions in which the velocity of blood flow is rapid are beriberi heart, arteriovenous fistula, anemia, and fever. If, therefore, a cardiac patient in failure has a reading of 12 to 15 seconds it is strong evidence in support of the diagnosis of thyrotoxicosis. One other laboratory test may be helpful, i.e., the cholesterol content of the blood. This is frequently decreased to about 130 to 150 mg. per 100 cc., whereas most ordinary cardiac patients will show readings of over 200 mg.

BLOOD PRESSURE

Another aspect of the circulation in hyperthyroidism is the blood pressure. The systolic reading may be normal or slightly elevated. In the cases that are occupying our particular attention at present, the so-called "masked thyrocardiacs," the systolic pressure is frequently elevated. This is due to an independent vascular hypertension for it remains essentially unchanged when the hyperthyroid state is eliminated. What is more characteristic is an increase in the pulse pressure, not so striking but similar to that observed in aortic insufficiency. Readings of 160 mm. systolic and 75 mm. diastolic are not uncommon. There may be other features resembling aortic insufficiency such as a capillary pulse, Corrigan pulse, pistol shot in the femoral artery, and even the Duroziez's sign. These are all the accompaniments, if not the result, of the high pulse pressure and the peripheral vascular dilatation.

It may at times be difficult, on bedside examination, to distinguish malignant hypertension from thyrotoxicosis. In both conditions there may be tachycardia, sweating, palpitation, loss of weight, and elevated basal metabolism. The finding of a diastolic blood pressure over 120 mm. would point strongly against the diagnosis of hyperthyroidism.

HEART RATE

Finally the heart rate itself is generally rapid. At times it is difficult to distinguish the tachycardia of hyperthyroidism from that of neurocirculatory asthenia. One helpful distinction lies in the fact that during sleep the rate in the latter condition is normal, whereas in the former the tachycardia, although less pronounced, will still persist. Another peculiarity of the heart rate in hyperthyroidism is the rarity of sinus arrhythmia even on deep breathing and the infrequency of ventricular premature beats.

It must not be expected that a rapid heart will be found in all cases of hyperthyroidism. The rate may be under 80 and even under 70, especially in males, in the presence of thyrotoxicosis. I have repeatedly seen such cases where because of the slow heart rate hyperthyroidism had previously been entirely overlooked.

BASAL METABOLISM

When the possibility of hyperthyroidism has arisen the basal metabolic rate should be determined. Unless the patient is in great distress this can generally be accomplished satisfactorily. The greater difficulty is to interpret the readings. If it is found to be distinctly below normal an active hyperthyroidism can be ruled out. If the figures range from zero to

+10 or +15 per cent it is extremely unlikely that the gland is toxic. There are rare instances, however, in which an active hyperthyroidism is going on, in the sense that cardiac disturbances take place as a direct result of the thyroid gland, while the basal metabolic rate is perfectly normal. I know of two patients in whom transient attacks of auricular fibrillation were taking place who had a perfectly normal basal metabolic rate. During the course of the subsequent several months, while the attacks of palpitation were recurring, the rate gradually rose to +20 per cent and later to over +40 per cent. Then, after subtotal thyroidectomy, the metabolic rate fell to normal and the paroxysmal fibrillation disappeared. It is evident in such rare cases that the thyroid was "toxic," as far as its effect on the heart was concerned, at a time when the metabolic rate was normal. May it be that patients such as these actually had an original metabolic rate of --20 per cent, plus or minus (which many healthy individuals have), and when an elevation of 20 per cent occurred they were already "toxic" and yet showed normal readings?

When the readings are +20 to +30 per cent, it may be no simple matter to decide whether this slight elevation in rate is due to the thyroid gland or is the result of the cardiac failure itself. Slight to moderate elevation in the metabolic rate has occasionally been found by some observers in cases of cardiac failure. These borderline readings may be very difficult to interpret. When properly conducted and repeated metabolism determinations show an elevation of +35 or more, in the absence of fever or leukemia, one can be fairly certain that they indicate hyperthyroidism. There is a small group of cases, especially associated with hypertension, in which even this degree of elevation in the basal metabolism will be associated with a normal thyroid gland. An elevation of the metabolism in a hypertensive patient should also make one think of the possibility of an adrenal tumor (pheochromocytoma), especially if the blood pressure falls and the pulse rate rises on standing. In the ordinary hypertensive patient the pressure rises somewhat on standing. I have also seen four patients with aortic stenosis who had readings persistently over +20 to +40 per cent and yet whose thyroid glands were found to be normal when examined grossly and microscopically. Tests need to be repeated, since not infrequently, without specific medication, the elevation disappears when a second or third test is made. The specific reduction of the basal metabolic rate following iodine administration can serve as a valuable aid in diagnosis. Properly conducted and properly interpreted this laboratory test proves to be of indispensable value in the diagnosis of many of these obscure thyrocardiac patients.

OTHER TESTS

Another test that would indicate hyperthyroidism is the finding of an elevation of protein-bound iodine in the blood (normal range is 4–8 micrograms per 100 cc.).

The most recent test for thyrotoxicosis is determination of the radioactive iodine uptake of the thyroid gland. This is performed by the use of a Geiger counter, which determines the amount of iodine that accumulates in the thyroid gland during a given interval of time after the administration of a given amount (10–15 microcuries) of radioactive iodine. Cases of myxedema will show strikingly low figures and those of hyperthyroidism will show high uptakes (60 per cent or more in 24 hours). This test is very helpful because it requires very little cooperation on the part of the patient and the result is obtained directly. The test is invalid and may lead to a false diagnosis if the patient has had iodine in his food or as a medication before it was done. In fact, I have seen a patient in whom the clinical diagnosis of thyrotoxicosis was confirmed by operation, and yet the iodine uptake test was normal. If inorganic iodine such as potassium iodine or an organic compound like lipoiodine has been taken, some months should elapse before the test may be regarded as valid.

On very rare occasions hyperthyroidism may be associated with Addison's disease. The diagnosis is then difficult. It may be suspected on the basis of the following features. The absence of hypoglycemic attacks, which are frequent in Addison's disease, would make one think of thyrotoxicosis. The heart will not be small and the basal metabolism will be relatively elevated, i.e., more than −5 per cent. Furthermore, the clinical manifestations of hyperthyroidism will be atypical and not prominent.

Treatment

Until several years ago the choice of treatment for this group of patients was a fairly simple matter. It consisted of all the usual procedures employed in the treatment of the common forms of heart disease, but included in addition the giving of iodine. After a period of ten to fourteen days on this management a subtotal thyroidectomy would be performed and the patient would do well. The details of this program will be discussed below. The situation is now changed because of two non-surgical methods that are available, i.e., thiouracil preparations and radioactive iodine. There is abundant experience with the earlier type of treatment, extending over a period of many years. It will take some time before a comparable experience will be accumulated in order to determine the relative efficacy of these newer methods of treatment.

Radioactive iodine has already been successfully employed in thyrotoxic states. The procedure is simple and inexpensive, would require very little hospitalization and carries no immediate risk. The principle involved is clear. The iodine is taken up by the thyriod gland and only to a very small extent by any other organ. There the radioactivity takes place in intimate relation to the thyroid cells to produce their destruction or decreased activity. The result is similar to the effects of x-rays, except that no other organs are appreciably involved. Cures have been obtained, and in fact myxedema has been produced when the dose was excessive. How permanent the cures will be and what late complications in the thyroid gland or other organs may ensue remain to be seen.

The other nonsurgical method is the use of propylthiouracil or

Tapazole (methimazole). Since the introduction of thiouracil by Astwood as a method of decreasing thyroid function newer less toxic preparations have become available. These drugs block the formation of thyroid hormone within the gland. The one most commonly employed at present is propylthiouracil. With this drug serious complications such as agranulocytosis are very rare. Furthermore, there has been considerable experience with its use, although the time covered is still far short of that available from the older method, i.e., iodine and surgery.

It has also become clear that the underlying cause of hyperthyroidism is not likely within the thyroid gland itself. The thyrotropic hormone of the pituitary gland has much to do with the thyrotoxic state. It is also thought that exophthalmos is determined by some control of the pituitary gland. Certain patients may be cured of hyperthyroidism and yet progress with malignant exophthalmos. In these cases the administration of thyroid gland tablets and iodine may be helpful. Adrenal steroids have also been used with some success. It is therefore not surprising that attempts at therapy should develop which involve a direct attack at the production of hormones by nonsurgical measures.

After the diagnosis has been established propylthiouracil is given orally. The dose employed ranges from 100 to 200 mg. three times daily. The condition is followed particularly by repeated basal metabolism determinations. Generally it requires several weeks and sometimes much longer to lower the metabolism to normal. Occasionally the drug is partially or totally ineffective. Medication needs to be continued for some months. If a satisfactory result is obtained the question will then arise whether to omit the drug entirely or to decrease the dose. This can only be determined by trial and error. In some cases the condition appears to be arrested even months after complete withdrawal of the medication. In others symptoms recur.

With the passage of years, some of the early enthusiasm has waned as more and more of these patients have required ultimate operation. As I have watched this development it has appeared that many patients under propylthiouracil treatment have required more lengthy hospitalization and observation than with the older method of treatment. There can be no doubt, however, that a large number can be successfully treated in this way, if careful observation is carried out. I have had patients with auricular fibrillation and congestive failure regain compensation with restoration of a normal sinus rhythm. Likewise I have witnessed dramatic relief of angina from the use of propylthiouracil alone. It is striking that in several of such cases the anginal attacks, which were recurring as often as ten or more times daily at rest, disappeared within a few days after the onset of drug therapy. This striking change took place, therefore, before there was any appreciable fall in the basal metabolism. This makes one think that the effect was produced by a neutralizing action on some toxic product rather than by a decrease in the work of the heart. In general, it is clear that propylthiouracil or similar compounds have great value in a selected group of patients suffering from thyrotoxicosis and even in thyrocardiac patients, and will spare some patients the need of surgery.

I now come to the discussion of the older method of treatment. This consists of giving 10 drops of Lugol solution three times daily in addition to the measures ordinarily employed in the particular cardiac case. Digitalis and diuretics should be used if there is auricular fibrillation or congestive failure, as well as thoracentesis and other procedures as necessary. In most cases a period of seven to ten days will be required to prepare the patient for subtotal thyroidectomy. Occasionally, because of the severity of the complicating heart disease, a longer period will be necessary. The diet should be abundant and it is well to add vitamins, especially vitamin B_1. The preoperative medical treatment should be continued as long as there is evidence of a progressive improvement as shown by a fall in the metabolism, slowing of the heart rate, and a diminution in congestion. It is useless to wait for the auricular fibrillation, if present, to disappear, or to use quinidine preoperatively. The type of anesthetic does not seem to be of any great importance. Many of my patients were given a general anesthetic although others had local anesthesia. The surgeon should be urged to take out more rather than less of the gland, as too frequently an insufficient amount is removed.

The postoperative care consists of continuing iodine therapy for about two weeks, and whatever other measures the cardiac problem requires. If the rhythm of the heart had been regular before the operation, an attack of transient auricular fibrillation the first day or two after the operation is not uncommon. If there had been persistent auricular fibrillation, in many instances the heart will be found to resume its normal rhythm spontaneously during the first week or two after surgery. The basal metabolic rate should be determined from time to time with the hope that it will be normal within two weeks after the operation. In most cases in which satisfactory results are obtained the metabolic rate is already normal by that time, although in some it is still appreciably elevated only to fall to normal more gradually several weeks later. If the rate remains elevated the operation has not been a success, and some of the troublesome features such as auricular fibrillation may persist. If the metabolism has returned to normal and this irregularity is still present one should seek for other causes of auricular fibrillation, especially mitral stenosis. Sometimes the murmur of mitral stenosis or aortic insufficiency may become audible only after the metabolism has been brought to normal after the operation. On the other hand, a systolic murmur, so frequent during active hyperthyroidism, often disappears with a return of the metabolism to normal. On several occasions I have found definite evidence of mitral stenosis which was previously unsuspected in patients who had been operated upon for hyperthyroidism, where auricular fibrillation persisted despite a normal metabolism. If this irregularity has not disappeared by a fortnight after the operation one may give quinidine with the expectation that a normal rhythm will be re-established. It is advisable to do this, bearing in mind that, if mitral stenosis is also present, quinidine therapy will entail the same limitations and same dangers that obtain in cardiac patients without thyroid disease.

The results obtained by the above method of treatment are nothing short of miraculous. Patients previously invalided and apparently hopelessly so have been restored to good health and frequently to a state of complete recovery. When it is appreciated that in many of these patients, those included by the term "masked thyrocardiacs," proper diagnosis could not even have been made up to a few decades ago and that they would finally have succumbed to heart failure, one can then fully sense the progress that has been made. This progress has been the combined result of the pioneer physiologic work in bodily metabolism, the wonderful development of surgical technique, and finally the careful bedside clinical observations that brought to light this hitherto unrecognized group of thyrocardiac patients.

The surgical mortality in these cases since the introduction of the preoperative use of iodine has become almost nil. There is practically no cardiac patient too sick to be helped or too sick to undergo the operation. Not only is the immediate risk very slight, but the improvement obtained is quite lasting. Unlike other forms of chronic heart failure, where the improvement after careful treatment is apt to be only too temporary, here permanent relief is obtained and the patients often are able to carry on full duty without further medication. To be sure, they are left with whatever independent form of heart disease happened to be present, be it valvular, hypertensive, or coronary, but now the previously embarrassed heart resumes its compensated state and is able to continue so for years. In no other group of patients who suffer from chronic intractable heart failure despite good medical management have the members been able to resume varying degrees of physical activities for as long a time as those in this group under discussion. It is this difference in outlook and in treatment that makes the problem of thyrocardiac disease so important.

One of the advantages of surgery is the detection and extirpation of any neoplastic process that might be present in the gland. Occasionally one finds such cancerous tissue unexpectedly. One never needs to worry about cancer of the thyroid in the presence of diffuse hyperplasia or classic Graves' disease. Malignant lesions occur exclusively in an adenomatous goiter, most commonly in a single nontoxic adenoma, and only very rarely with the toxic type.

There is no better way of crystallizing the above problem than to cite briefly some personal experiences. One of the first patients of this type that I had the good fortune to examine in 1921 was a woman in the sixties who had had progressive hypertensive heart failure for two and one-half years, during the last six months of which she had been bedridden. Despite excellent care under the supervision of competent consultants she had been progressively losing ground. The clues in this case were a history of transient auricular fibrillation progressing into the permanent form of the irregularity, a recurrent glycosuria, and the failure of the rapid irregular heart to slow on adequate digitalis dosage. In addition there was a certain quickness of motion that the patient manifested despite the fact that she was orthopneic, showed free fluid in the chest and abdomen, and had generalized anasarca. The basal metabolic rate was found to be +71 per cent and eventually, after a subtotal thyroidectomy, all signs of congestion disappeared, the thythm of the heart became regular spontaneously, the metabolic rate became normal, and during a subsequent period of twelve years she never had return of the heart failure. After a long and useful life she finally developed dyspnea and hypertensive heart failure and died about fourteen years after the operation. Her condition remained long overlooked because of the absence of thyroid enlargement and exophthalmos.

Another dramatic result was obtained in the case of a man 60 years old suffering from angina pectoris. During a period of six years there had been increasing occurrence of the attacks so that finally they came very frequently while the patient was at rest, even awaking him from sleep every half hour or so. The condition remained refractory to all medical methods of treatment although the attacks were always temporarily relieved by nitroglycerin. In desperation the patient wanted to undergo some form of surgical operation such as cervical sympathectomy or alcohol injection of the dorsal roots to obtain relief. He was in this state when I first saw him. The physical examination revealed no abnormalities. The heart rate ranged between 70 and 80. After a period of observation of a week during which time I was at a loss as to what to do, for he was having forty attacks of angina a day, it suddenly struck me that his skin was somewhat moist and slightly pigmented. He also moved rather quickly and jerkily in bed. This led to the suspicion of masked hyperthyroidism. The basal metabolic rate was found to be +45 per cent and on Lugol's solution it fell to +5 per cent. With this fall came a striking improvement with no attacks at night and only about four during each day. No evidence of an enlarged thyroid gland could be made out by palpation or x-ray examination. Despite this a very small adenoma was found and removed from behind the manubrium. This emphasizes the importance of x-ray examination in searching for a mediastinal goiter when none can be felt in the neck. Often one which would otherwise be overlooked can be discovered in this way. All attacks of angina disappeared after operation and he was able to resume his normal activities for many years thereafter. He experienced anginal attacks only if he hurried up hill. In other words, the anginal state was actually present but was held in abeyance as the metabolism was kept normal.

The following experience illustrates the difficulty of recognizing hyperthyroidism in the presence of mitral stenosis. This man, 40 years old, had a history of rheumatic fever and was known to have mitral stenosis. He gradually developed increasing dyspnea and over a period of eighteen months became bedridden with advanced congestive heart failure. His physician and the consultant in attendance had observed that it was impossible to slow the heart rate below 100 even when full doses of digitalis were given. When I saw him it was this rapid irregular heart rate in the face of constant administration of digitalis, together with a "salmon-colored skin," that first made me suspect a latent hyperthyroidism. While the patient was in a state of advanced congestive heart failure with an apex rate of 170 to 180, the basal metabolic rate was found to be +40 per cent. On the same dose of digitalis (0.1 gm. twice daily) but with the addition of 10 drops of Lugol's solution three times a day, the heart rate quickly fell from 180 to about 60, the basal metabolic rate fell to +6 per cent, and there took place an extraordinary diuresis. Within ten days the patient felt perfectly well. It was believed, however, that the improvement would only be temporary if the toxic gland were not removed. There was no exophthalmos or palpable thyroid gland. It was difficult in this case, as in so many others, to convince the patient that he should undergo an operation. In fact it was not simple in some instances to prevail upon the surgeons to perform the operation, for often they did not believe the gland was diseased. However, after the operation in this case the striking improvement that had taken place on Lugol's solution was maintained despite the fact that the patient still had mitral stenosis and auricular fibrillation. He was able to resume his work which he had been forced to give up two years previously.

In another case a middle-aged woman was seen in advanced congestive failure. She had been quite sick and bedridden for several months and had had repeated tappings of the right chest, each time with removal of a liter or more of fluid. The findings strongly pointed to the diagnosis of mitral stenosis. The heart was quite rapid and grossly irregular, and the sounds were hyperactive. There were a slight apical systolic murmur and a questionable faint diastolic murmur. In addition there was a short vibration or thrill at the apex, difficult to time because of the rapid rate. The electrocardiogram showed definite right axis deviation, and x-ray examination showed the left auricle to be moderately enlarged. One can see that all the features of mitral stenosis were present except for a clear-cut diastolic murmur. After a week had elapsed our studies revealed that the blood cholesterol was low (140 mg.) and the circulation time was fast (12 sec.) despite the presence of marked right hydrothorax and enlarged liver. The condition improved somewhat on iodine therapy and the metabolism fell from +47 per cent to +12 per cent. After a subtotal thyroidectomy further improvement occurred, but auricular fibrillation continued. Two weeks after the operation quinidine restored the rhythm to normal and the patient recovered completely. Even the dilated left auricle and the right axis deviation returned to normal. The patient remained well and showed no signs of heart or thyroid disease for many years.

One could go on at great length and describe numerous other instances in which apparently hopeless cardiac invalids were resurrected by, first, the detection of suspicious evidence of masked hyperthyroidism and then by the institution of proper treatment. The important lesson from all this is constantly to suspect an undetected toxic thyroid gland when treating patients with cardiac disease. Although a very few such patients will be sufficiently improved by the use of iodine therapy alone, the vast majority will do better to undergo a subtotal thyroidectomy.

The question of x-ray treatment for hyperthyroidism deserves a word of comment. I have had little experience with it because it is time-consuming and too often ineffective. The fact that operation is so safe nowadays makes surgery the method that still has merit. In a series of ninety-nine patients with thyrocardiac disease, many of whom were critically sick, even still showing congestive failure at the time of operation, there was no surgical mortality whatever. These figures speak for themselves.

The reader may appear confused as a result of the above discussion of the treatment for thyrocardiac disease. The truth is that the author is also somewhat in the same position. Now that we have several possible methods of therapy the choice is difficult. Obviously, if a physician works in a locality where there is an appreciable surgical mortality from thyroid surgery or where aphonia, hoarseness, and tetany are not infrequent complications, or if incomplete operations are performed and recurrent hyperthyroidism is common, it would be preferable to advise nonsurgical procedures. However, in these thyrocardiac patients, most of whom are elderly, it has appeared to me that postoperative thyroid storms are almost unheard of and that the fear of progressive exophthalmos is extremely slight. Furthermore, the cosmetic aspect of surgery is unimportant in this group. The choice will also be influenced at times by economic considerations. Hospital patients under propylthiouracil treatment have required more lengthy periods of observation and were away from their work for a longer time than those subjected to operation. Finally, the therapeutic use of radioactive iodine has been very successful. Only future experience will clarify the ultimate place this method will occupy in our choice of treatment. It must be said that good results are not restricted to one method of treatment. In the course of the coming years, with increased experience, the criteria for the selection of one course of treatment or another will become established.

Syphilitic Heart Disease

Syphilis affects the circulation in one of several ways. There is a very rare condition in which it involves the peripheral blood vessels, producing a picture of malignant arteriosclerosis and hypertension. The more important lesions are aortitis and aneurysm, aortic insufficiency, and involvement of the coronary arteries and of the myocardium. It is much more common in males than in females, and in the colored race than in the white race.

AORTITIS AND ANEURYSM

Although the spirochetes no doubt localize in the aorta a short time after the initial infection, clinical evidence of syphilitic disease of the aorta ordinarily does not become apparent for many years (fifteen to twenty on the average) after appearance of the primary lesion. However, in occasional instances this does occur within one to two years. The favorite site is the first portion of the ascending aorta, although any part may become affected. For many years, therefore, a syphilitic process may be going on in the aorta without any impairment in health or any abnormalities on physical examination. When syphilitic aortitis first becomes detectable it will do so by producing a slight dilatation of the ascending aorta. It will be difficult to elicit this by percussion. X-ray examination will be necessary, and even then it is no simple matter to differentiate a syphilitic dilatation from one that accompanies hypertension or one that is due to arteriosclerosis.

For the most part syphilitic aortitis of itself produces no symptoms. When it does, there is pain in the chest that resembles somewhat that seen in the disease of the coronary arteries. The resemblance, however, is only superficial, for the pain is not particularly brought on by walking and is not so characteristically constricting in type as it is in angina pectoris. Here the pain is more boring and more steady. It is frequently more troublesome when the patient is at rest, or in bed at night, or when he lies in certain positions. Physical examination for the most part reveals no essential abnormalities. A localized systolic pulsation may be seen or felt at the base of the heart, particularly in the second right interspace. On auscultation there need be no murmurs or irregularities whatever, or only a slight systolic murmur is present. The aortic second sound often takes on a peculiar accentuated or metallic quality. When there are no other more definite evidences of syphilis it is extremely difficult to make a clinical diagnosis. As has just been mentioned, the x-ray may be very helpful but often still leaves us in doubt. It is now thought that the finding of calcification of the wall of the ascending aorta on x-ray examination is strongly suggestive of a syphilitic process. This sign has proved to be correct in a few cases, even when the serologic test of the blood was negative. Similar calcification of the arch or descending portion of the aorta, however, does not have this same significance. The Wassermann test will be found positive in only about 75 to 85 per cent of the cases, so that negative findings cannot satisfactorily rule out the diagnosis and positive results may not establish that the process in the aorta is syphilitic.

When the syphilitic process in the aorta produces a true aneurysm the diagnosis is more readily established. This takes the form of diffuse or sacculated dilatation. When the latter is present one can safely assume that syphilis is the cause. Aneurysm of the aorta produces symptoms mainly by pressure on neighboring structures, and this will in a large measure depend on the portion involved and the direction that its enlargement takes. It may press on the trachea or either bronchus and produce cough (often with a brassy quality), a tracheal tug, or atelectasis of the lung. It may expand backward and cause erosion of the vertebrae and ribs. This then becomes quite painful. On the other hand, it may erode bone anteriorly through the manubrium and clavicles and present itself as a pulsating tumor in the front of the chest. Inequality of the pupils and pulses or aphonia may result from pressure on nerves or large arteries. Aneurysms may attain a considerable size and produce no noticeable symptoms, merely because their growth does not happen to cause pressure on any of these important structures.

Apart from the findings just mentioned, an aneurysm often produces local pulsations in unusual sites. Such pulsations are to be sought for by inspection and palpation over the base of the heart and in the upper back between the scapulae. All the points referred to should be gone into when an adult complains of a boring pain in the chest and careful x-ray examination should be made. It has been said that there are two types of aneurysm of the aorta—those with signs and those with symptoms. One should add a third type, i.e., those with neither signs nor symptoms. I have seen patients with syphilitic aortic aneurysms the size of an orange, when there were no symptoms and no abnormal physical findings (except by x-ray) even after the exact location of the aneurysm was known.

The efficiency of the general circulation is not materially affected by syphilitic aortitis with or without aneurysm. If the valves, the coronary arteries, and the myocardium are spared there will be no evidence of congestive heart failure. The largest syphilitic aneurysm I ever saw occurred in a patient who had a perfectly normal heart. There never was evidence of cardiac failure, and on postmortem examination the weight of the heart was less than 300 gm. and the valves and myocardium were normal in every way. The aneurysm was almost as large as a football, and originated from a hole in the aorta 1.5 cm. in diameter. When congestive heart failure is present with luetic involvement of the aorta, some added factor will be found which acts deleteriously on the heart.

The syphilitic process may extend downward and involve the orifices of the coronary arteries, which open just at the root of the aorta. This is not a rare complication, and when it does occur all the possibilities exist that attend an inadequate coronary circulation. Anginal attacks may occur and sudden unexpected death result. Syphilis, therefore, produces angina pectoris by narrowing the orifices of coronary vessels. It hardly ever involves the main course of the arteries, as occurs in ordinary cases of angina. A few cases have been reported in which the mouths of both the right and left coronary arteries were completely occluded by a gradual syphilitic process. The circulation through the heart had apparently been adequately maintained, although no flow through the coronary arteries was possible. The work of Wearn has emphasized the possible role that may be played by the thebesian vessels in maintaining the health of the heart. Compensatory circulation through these small channels that open directly into the ventricular cavities probably explains how such patients could have carried on in life, and may also account for the compensatory mechanism that goes on in nonsyphilitic cases of coronary artery disease.

AORTIC INSUFFICIENCY

Of greatest importance is the effect of the syphilitic process on the aortic valves, as this accounts for most of the disability and mortality in syphilitic heart disease. The disease often extends downward and destroys the integrity of the aortic orifice. It then produces aortic regurgitation just as occurs in rheumatic fever but, unlike the latter, it never results in stenosis of the aortic valve. The appearance of the aortic cusps also differs in the two conditions. In the syphilitic form the commissures become separated, whereas in the rheumatic they become fused. When aortic insufficiency is present the heart may become enlarged and in time congestive failure results. Cardiac enlargement does not occur because of the aortitis but as a direct result of the valvular insufficiency. When dyspnea and other evidence of circulatory failure intervene the prognosis is apt to be quite grave, as response to treatment is on the whole unsatisfactory.

The diagnosis of syphilitic aortic insufficiency will depend on eliciting evidence of this type of valvular defect (Chap. 4). It is most important to appreciate that, during the early stages, the aortic diastolic murmur which is so important may be very faint and only audible with the patient upright and after a forced expiration. At times it is difficult to determine whether aortic insufficiency is part of a syphilitic, rheumatic, hypertensive, or arteriosclerotic process, and all the means available will be required to help in the differentiation. The difficulty may be particularly great because an Austin Flint murmur resembling mitral stenosis may be present in syphilitic aortic insufficiency. In general, luetic aortic incompetency occurs at about the age of 40 to 60, is much more common in males than in females, is only rarely associated with auricular fibrillation, and never results in stenosis of valves. It is compatible with good general health and vigor for many years, but when cardiac decompensation first develops the downward progress from then on is apt to be rapid. Cheyne-Stokes breathing and nocturnal dyspnea are common.

SYPHILITIC MYOCARDITIS

Direct syphilitic involvement of the heart muscle is very rare. When it does occur it may take one of two forms. There are isolated instances of localized gumma of the heart. When such a process involves the conduction apparatus, complete heart block may result. There are rare instances in which a myocardial gumma becomes calcified or causes a localized aneurysm. Under such circumstances, x-ray and kymographic examination may help in diagnosis. The other form is a diffuse luetic myocarditis. This is also quite rare and produces a rapid development of congestive heart failure that fails to respond to the customary methods of treatment. Syphilitic disease of the heart muscle has been regarded by some observers as being quite common. It used to be looked upon as a common cause of angina pectoris, especially in younger people. The opinion has gradually changed, and now it is thought that syphilis is a rare cause of heart disease apart from its effect on the aorta or the aortic valves.

Treatment

When congestive failure develops from syphilitic heart disease the response to treatment is rather unsatisfactory. The hope, therefore, lies entirely in the preventive aspects of this disease. All the efforts that are being made to diminish the incidence of the primary infection will naturally prevent the subsequent development of this form of heart disease. Likewise the early detection of syphilitic infection and the careful and thorough treatment of syphilis in its early stages will do a great deal to prevent these late complications. In fact it is already apparent, since the introduction of the Wassermann test, the discovery of salvarsan and penicillin, and the present public health campaigns against venereal disease, that syphilitic heart disease is becoming much less prevalent.

If syphilitic cardiovascular disease is detected before either anginal or congestive symptoms have developed treatment is directed in the hope of preventing or delaying such complications. In the past, a course of potassium iodide and a heavy metal such as mercury or bismuth would be given for one month and then followed by arsenic intravenously. In general, this would consist of 10 to 20 drops of saturated solution of potassium iodide three times daily and 0.013 to 0.026 gm. ($\frac{1}{5}$ to $\frac{2}{5}$ grain) of mercury succinimide intramuscularly three times weekly. After one month, weekly injections of neosalvarsan would be given intravenously, increasing the dose gradually from 0.2 to 0.45 gm. Instead of mercury, or as an adjunct to it, bismuth salicylate (0.2 gm. in 2.0 cc. of oil) might be employed intramuscularly. At present a course of penicillin has become preferable. Because of the rare possibility of a Herxheimer reaction one begins with a small dose and rapidly increases the amount. It is too early to know what the ideal program should be. The following would seem to be a reasonable course. The first day 10,000 units may be given intramuscularly six times daily at four-hour intervals. The dose then is doubled each day until each dose is 160,000 units, then continued at that level. The entire period of treatment might extend over ten to fourteen days. The total amount of penicillin would be about 7,000,000 to 10,000,000 units. This program could be altered as to dosage or intervals of injections, or one might see fit under certain circumstances to give single daily injections of long-acting procaine penicillin. It is not the purpose to push antisyphilitic therapy to the point of making the Wassermann test negative. Although one would welcome this reversal it often is impossible to change the reaction of the blood, and continued vigorous therapy may do more harm than good. After a period of treatment has been carried out as outlined above, it may be repeated once or twice a year.

When congestive failure is present all the customary methods of treatment are employed, such as digitalis and diuretics (Chap. 20). I have seen practically no evidence that antiluetic therapy has been useful at this stage of the disease, except in a rare case of localized gumma of the left ventricle with aneurysm which promptly disappeared on treatment. However, penicillin might be given in the hope of delaying further progression. It is particularly inadvisable to use arsenic intravenously if the coronary arteries are involved and anginal symptoms are present, for I know of two instances in which sudden and unexpected death occurred a few minutes after an intravenous injection of salvarsan.

When pain is due to disease of the aorta, especially when a definite aneurysm is present, antiluetic therapy can be very efficacious. The pain may disappear entirely. This type of pain should be carefully distinguished from anginal pain, for intravenous therapy should be avoided in the latter condition. If aneurysmal pain is very troublesome and refractory to medical treatment, surgical measures might be considered.

In a few isolated and properly selected cases of sacculated aneurysm of the aorta, wiring has been performed apparently with some success. The cases in which this operation may be applicable are those in which the heart is essentially normal and the aneurysm is both large and localized. The purpose is to produce a firm clot in the aneurysm and thereby prevent or retard its continued enlargement. More recently the operation of wiring has been superseded by wrapping the aneurysm with cellophane. This is more applicable to the descending arch and thoracic aorta. The purpose is to prevent further dilatation or rupture and to relieve pain.

Finally, the surgeons have now been making a direct attack at threatening aneurysms of the aorta. Excision and insertion of grafts or artificial plastic tubes are being employed. Progress in this field is only in its infancy, but much may be expected in the near future. As syphilitic involvement of large vessels is decreasing, similar lesions of arteriosclerotic origin are on the increase, as a result of the greater life expectancy that now prevails. This latter problem will therefore demand greater attention in the coming years.

CHAPTER 10

Bacterial Endocarditis

There has been considerable confusion in the minds of physicians concerning the term "endocarditis" and its clinical significance. When the valves are involved by acute rheumatic fever there occurs an acute endocarditis which often leads to valvular deformities and eventually to what is called chronic rheumatic valvular disease of the heart. The original endocarditis under these circumstances is nonbacterial. If the heart is examined post mortem at the acute stage of the disease the valves will show only slight alterations. Pinhead vegetations may be found, and slight irregularities of the valve margins may be present. Bacteria will be found only very rarely either in the blood stream or on the valves. In other words, until the actual cause of rheumatic infection is discovered, acute rheumatic endocarditis is regarded as a nonbacterial endocarditis. Rheumatic endocarditis is therefore an affection from which clinical recovery takes place in the great majority of cases and as a result of which there develop years later chronic valvular deformities that may lead to congestive failure and other complications of rheumatic valvular disease. The condition which engages our attention in this discussion, on the other hand, is a bacterial affection of the valves which, before the discovery of penicillin, was almost always fatal. Therefore, when discussing "endocarditis," two forms should be considered. The first form is the nonbacterial endocarditis which is mainly rheumatic. The second form is bacterial endocarditis which for purposes that will become evident can be conveniently subdivided into two subgroups, acute and subacute.

Acute Bacterial Endocarditis

Most of the clinical features of acute bacterial endocarditis are similar to those seen in subacute bacterial endocarditis, except that they occur more rapidly, the whole illness is more violent, and it lasts a much shorter time. The cause of the brevity and the fulminating nature of the disease is the type of microorganism that is concerned and the particular disease of which the endocarditis is only a part. The more common organisms responsible for acute bacterial endocarditis are hemolytic streptococci, pneumococci, staphylococci, gonoccoci, and influenza bacilli. There are rare instances in which other bacteria cause this same disease. Occasionally an infection with one of the above organisms may run a prolonged course and would rightly belong to the type designated as subacute. This is particularly true of *Bacillus abortus* infection (undulant fever, or brucellosis). The subacute type, however, is so common and so distinct that for practical purposes it deserves to be distinguished from those designated as acute endocarditis.

Acute bacterial endocarditis is a part of an overwhelming general infection with involvement of the blood stream. It is always secondary to some other primary disease process. The patient may have an acute or subacute gonorrheal infection and during a phase of bacteremia, if the valves of the heart become involved, acute bacterial endocarditis due to the gonococcus develops. Another has an ordinary lobar pneumonia, and in a similar fashion a pneumococcus infection of the valves develops. (Virus pneumonia is not associated with endocarditis.) In this way almost any infectious process can at times become the primary cause of involvement of the valves.

It is often difficult and at times impossible to diagnose this condition. The evidence of endocardial involvement is apt to be overshadowed by the severe septicemia and the underlying disease. A patient is very ill with pneumonia or with streptococcus septicemia, and the fact that the valves are affected may be overlooked unless significant murmurs develop or embolic phenomena occur. These are not invariable, however. There is present a considerable fever with or without chills, rapid pulse, and the general appearance of a severe acute infection. The spleen becomes enlarged, petechiae and emboli are common, and meningitis is not rare. Many of these features merely indicate a severe infection and do not necessarily point to a disease of the valves. The finding of a positive blood culture establishes the fact that there is a septicemia but does not prove that bacteria are lodged on the valves. This accounts for the fact that many such cases are first detected on postmortem examination.

It is of some interest that although pneumococcus endocarditis is quite common among fatal cases of bacterial pneumonia, it cannot be regarded as a cause of chronic valvular diseases. I have seen only one case in which it seemed that an attack of pneumonia was the cause of a chronic valvular disease. In this instance there were no murmurs or other evidence of heart disease before the illness, and definite signs of aortic insufficiency appeared directly after the pneumonia. When the physician is inquiring into the past history of a patient and is told that there was some leak in the heart ever since an attack of pneumonia, he has reason to doubt the assumed relationship. On closer scrutiny it may be found that the murmur antedated the attack of pneumonia and was due to a previous rheumatic infection or that the alleged pneumonia was in itself rheumatic in type or actually an instance of rheumatic pericarditis with signs of compression of the lungs, which cannot be distinguished from the signs of pneumonia. However, in the future the situation may be different. As some recoveries may now be expected following the use of the newer drugs, we will undoubtedly see cases of chronic valvular disease resulting from cured instances of acute pneumococcus endocarditis.

Unlike subacute bacterial endocarditis, the acute form frequently affects valves that were previously normal. Both sides of the heart are vulnerable to this infection. Although the aortic and mitral valves are more commonly involved, the pulmonary and tricuspid valves may also be affected. The disease runs a course of several days to a few weeks and was formerly almost always fatal.

TREATMENT

In the past, many chemicals and sera have been used without success. With the discovery of sulfonamides some cures were obtained, and with the introduction of penicillin and related drugs many more recoveries take place. The actual details of this treatment will be discussed under subacute bacterial endocarditis for it is essentially the same in the two conditions. Suffice it to say that, because the illness may run a short and stormy course, the exact microorganism should be identified as quickly as possible and the dosage of the drug employed should be larger rather than smaller than might have been needed. However, it would hardly be wise to delay treatment in a suspected case merely because a definitive diagnosis had not yet been established or the blood cultures were still sterile. As a result of this point of view we may now see recovered cases with compensated chronic valvular disease, not rheumatic in origin, that we have never seen before. Furthermore, bacterial endocarditis is now being prevented as a result of the liberal use of these preparations during febrile illnesses before the valves have been involved, as well as being cured after such involvement. In fact, cases are being cured that have not and could not have been diagnosed.

The entire problem of treatment has changed since the discovery of the new antibacterial agents, i.e., sulfonamides, penicillin, streptomycin, and other similar drugs. Physicians are so prone to use these drugs for febrile illnesses, even if the exact diagnosis is not established, that undoubtedly many patients who formerly would have ended up with bacterial endocarditis now recover. The result is that at present this disease is seen more rarely, and when it is already present it need not progress to the full-blown clinical picture formerly seen. Both the acute and subacute types of bacterial endocarditis are now so responsive to treatment that it is becoming rare to observe all the dramatic complications and developments that previously occurred which were so disastrous and fatal. The situation is not unlike the disappearance of the ravages formerly witnessed in the course of pernicious anemia before the discovery of liver therapy.

Subacute Bacterial Endocarditis

PREDISPOSING CAUSES

As a result of considerable accumulated experience it has seemed that there are certain individuals who are more prone to develop this disease and others who are much less so. As a rule patients who develop subacute bacterial endocarditis have had some sort of heart murmur for years but otherwise have been fairly well. The heart is only slightly or moderately enlarged, the rhythm is regular, and there is no hypertension. They have had little if any dyspnea and have been able to carry on usual activities. When the original infection was rheumatic fever, they have probably had one or only two bouts of this, thereafter remaining free from recurrent rheumatism. In other words, those patients with valvular deformities who on the whole are in comparatively good health are most vulnerable. In contrast to this, it is rare indeed to see the disease develop in patients who have had chronic persistent auricular fibrillation or who have previously had congestive heart failure or hypertension. In fact, it is not very common in outspoken cases of mitral stenosis, particularly in those in which there is marked constriction of the valve. It is frequent in patients with well-compensated aortic insufficiency or stenosis or mitral insufficiency. It practically never develops in a previously normal heart, but rather in those which have some abnormality of the valves or endocardium, either rheumatic or congenital in origin. In general it may be said that 20 to 25 per cent of all patients suffering from valvular disease formerly succumbed to bacterial endocarditis.

In an analysis of 111 cases of subacute bacterial endocarditis it was found that a past history of rheumatic fever was obtained in forty-two instances, of chorea in three, and of both in six cases. Eleven other patients had a history of scarlet fever. There is an indirect association between scarlet fever and rheumatic fever in that the latter may follow in the wake of the former. Some patients who develop a heart murmur after an attack of scarlet fever will be found on close scrutiny to have had mild limb or joint pains during their convalescence, and it can be surmised that they actually had an attack of mild rheumatic fever which was precipitated by the scarlatina infection. Recently it has been found that those children who had cardiac involvement supposedly as a result of an attack of scarlet fever have had the same high familial incidence of rheumatic heart disease as occurred in ordinary cases of rheumatic fever. This leads one to believe that scarlet fever produces a chronic endocarditis only in those susceptible individuals who are already potentially rheumatic. Of the entire group of 111 cases, in only one could no other cause but a syphilitic aortic insufficiency be found to account for the previous valvular injury. In eight other cases there was a positive Wassermann reaction in the blood, but in all there was stenosis of the aortic or mitral valve or a past history of rheumatic fever which made it likely that a rheumatic rather than a syphilitic lesion was the predisposing cause. Congenital lesions were the site of the bacterial endocarditis in five cases.

Among the known specific precipitating causes of subacute bacterial endocarditis extraction of teeth or even simple dental manipulation, such as filling or cleaning of teeth, is the most common. Such a history can be obtained in at least 20 per cent of the cases.

Bacterial endocarditis is rather rare during pregnancy but is more likely to develop during the first few months after delivery in those women who have the appropriate cardiac background. This may be due to the increased amount of dental work done in these months or to the presence of bacteria in the uterus and vagina. Streptococci have been found in the uterus in many cases for some days after delivery. Prophylactic administration of penicillin for several days after the beginning of labor would therefore be advisable.

The time elapsing between the original injury to the valve and the development of bacterial heart disease is difficult to ascertain accurately. In a group of sixty cases the average interval between the first time the patients knew they had "heart disease" and the development of this final disease was about twelve years. The shortest interval was one year, and the longest was forty-five years.

INCIDENCE

Males predominate over females in the proportion of three to two, despite the fact that among all cases of mitral stenosis the proportion is two to one in favor of females. This reflects the relative antagonism between mitral stenosis and subacute bacterial endocarditis. The most prevalent decade is 20 to 29, although the disease occurs in individuals at all ages from childhood to old age. It is curious that although males strongly predominate after the age of 30, the reverse is true under the age of 20.

CLINICAL FEATURES

Subacute bacterial endocarditis or endocarditis lenta is a fairly common condition and is mainly due to the *Streptococcus viridans*. The infection becomes implanted almost invariably on previously injured valves. Generally there has been some rheumatic valvulitis from which a satisfactory recovery had taken place or, much less frequently, there has been some congenital defect like patent ductus arteriosus, ventricular septal defect, or bicuspid aortic valves. Even when evidence of an early rheumatic infection cannot be elicited it will be found that some sort of heart murmur was present before this final infection developed.

The onset of the disease is rather gradual. It generally is initiated by a so-called "simple cold" or sore throat or not infrequently by the extraction of a tooth or the removal of tonsils. Rarely a local septic infection such as is seen after a simple abrasion of the skin may be the precipitating cause. Bacterial endocarditis due to *Escherichia coli* and staphylococcus has occurred following urethral manipulation, such as the passing of a sound. It may occur post partum or postoperatively if there has been some minor secondary infection. When these causes usher in the disease it must be borne in mind that if the heart were originally normal subacute bacterial endocarditis would have been less likely to develop. It is because the patient already has some old abnormality of the endocardium, especially if he belongs to the vulnerable group, that a few stray bacteria in the blood stream start growing on the valves. Very frequently the onset is griplike or may resemble that of typhoid fever. The patient may have complained originally of a "cold" and state that since then he has not felt well. Malaise, anorexia, sweats, and chills gradually develop. There is a slow loss of strength and weight, although during the early few weeks many are able to do and some actually continue at their usual work. Fever is practically always present and generally is of the swinging type, about 98 to 99° F. in the morning and 101 to 103° F. in the evening. Occasionally the fever is very slight, hardly rising above 99° F. for some time.

Although many of the clinical features commonly seen in previous years are now often lacking because of early treatment, it is helpful to describe them in some detail as they may appear in an untreated case. They will still occur in neglected cases or in those that do not respond to therapy. The various important features of this disease occur in no constant order. In some, only the symptoms listed above develop for a long time; in others, complications that ordinarily come late may be the initial event, calling attention to the gravity of the situation. I recall an instance in which a young dentist suddenly developed blindness in one eye due to a retinal embolus. Although he had not felt exactly well for a week or two, he was at work when the visual accident occurred. The significant points to bear in mind are petechiae, splenic enlargement, red blood cells in the urine, clubbing of the fingers, painful finger tips, emboli, and a positive blood culture. These are particularly important because they help to distinguish this disease from an active rheumatic infection of the heart or its valves.

The petechiae are small oval hemorrhagic areas, about 1 to 2 mm. long, which on close inspection will show a gray or white center. They are commonly found in the conjunctival sac, the mucous membrane of the mouth, or on each side of the neck, although they may occur anywhere over the body. They are almost pathognomonic of a bacterial endocarditis. The spleen gradually becomes enlarged, the change at first being suspected on percussion and finally being determined by palpation. The enlargement is due both to embolic infarctions and to the general septic process. A palpable spleen is rarely found in rheumatic fever itself or in well-compensated valvular disease of the heart. The liver often becomes markedly enlarged during heart failure, but only occasionally the spleen.

The presence of a considerable number of red blood cells in the urine is also distinctive because they are not found in ordinary heart disease unless there is an active nephritis as well, and are found only very rarely during simple rheumatic fever. Acute pericarditis is common with rheumatic infections and very rare with bacterial endocarditis. Clubbing of the fingers is common after the first few weeks of this disease. It is not seen in rheumatic fever or in ordinary heart failure. It does occur in congenital heart disease when there is chronic cyanosis, in chronic pulmonary infections, and in some other cardiac states associated with cyanosis. Its presence as a constitutional or hereditary condition at times makes its interpretation difficult. Apart from the clubbing, there is also a peculiar type of pain in the finger tips that deserves attention. Patients often complain of sudden pain in the balls of their fingers. It comes, lasts a few days, and then completely disappears. During this time one may see, at the tip of the finger or under the nail, a somewhat purplish spot which gradually fades entirely. Because of the unusual location, pains of this type are highly distinctive of a bacterial endocarditis. Similar pains and discoloration of the skin can occur elsewhere, of course, but their interpretation is not so simple, although splinter hemorrhages anywhere in the skin are fairly distinctive.

The recovery of bacteria from the blood stream by culture methods is the most important evidence of bacterial endocarditis. The ease with which they are recovered varies considerably in different cases and does not necessarily depend on the height of the fever. At times repeated blood cultures may be negative, although other aspects of the case indicate a severe infection, whereas in some instances in which the afternoon temperature is less than 100° F. a positive culture is readily obtained. The organism that is found is generally the *Streptococcus viridans* or the nonhemolytic green-producing streptococcus. These bacteria may be slow to grow in artificial media, so that the cultures should be kept for a week or two. Bacteria are very rarely found in blood culture during rheumatic fever, but will be found in most cases of subacute bacterial endocarditis if repeated search is made.

Finally one of the characteristic features of the disease is the occurrence of emboli. They are common in the spleen, producing acute sharp pain over the lower lateral aspect of the left chest, in the kidney causing pain in the loin or in the abdomen with radiation to the groins, in the limbs, or in the brain with the necessary consequent complications. Emboli to the intestines sufficient to produce significant symptoms are rare, although occasionally gangrene of the intestines may result. The tissues involved in these various infarctions rarely break down or suppurate. When the vegetations involve the right side of the heart pulmonary emboli occur.

In a small group of cases, as the disease progresses, the active stage, as expressed by fever and chills, quiets down and a picture of chronic progressive renal insufficiency develops. These patients appear to have chronic nephritis with nitrogen retention and marked anemia. They may have little or no fever for long periods of time, show no bacteria in the blood stream, and die a renal death. In such cases the clinical diagnosis will have to rest on the presence of cardiac murmurs, clubbed fingers, anemia, and other general peculiarities of the illness. Hypertension is apt to be absent or only slight in these patients.

Rarely one may see what can be called "silent" bacterial endocarditis. I recall overlooking such a case which I regarded as being either neurocirculatory asthenia or mild rheumatic fever. This young soldier had a mitral systolic murmur from a previous rheumatic bout and complained of weakness and mild atypical discomforts in the precordium. There was no dyspnea or evidence of cardiac inefficiency. For many weeks there was no fever, leukocytosis, or increased sedimentation rate. No clubbing, hematuria, or embolic phenomena developed. Only during the last days of his life was it apparent that he had any infection, when his condition rapidly deteriorated and he died. At autopsy bacterial endocarditis of the mitral valve was found.

There is a type of case in which the vegetations may be confined to the right side of the heart and in which peripheral arterial emboli are striking by their absence and the blood cultures prove negative for most of the course of the illness. Small emboli, however, become dislodged and produce multiple pulmonary infarctions. Such cases may resemble pneumonia and be wrongly diagnosed as such. This state of affairs is apt to occur when a bacterial endocarditis develops on the defect of a patent ventricular septum or patent ductus arteriosus. I have seen an instance in which on postmortem examination a ring of vegetations encircled the aperture of the septum on the right ventricle while there were no vegetations in the left ventricle. It seemed that the flow of blood from left to right ventricle prevented the growth of the bacteria against the stream. The presenting symptoms in this case were pulmonary, and the peripheral arterial phenomena were lacking.

The course of the illness, if untreated, is gradually downhill. It may be suddenly altered or terminated by peculiar accidents such as rupture of a valve, the ventricular septum, or the ventricular wall, or by a gross cerebral embolus. There is even a recorded instance in which an embolus into the coronary artery from a vegetation of the aortic valve caused instant death in an individual who was well enough to be playing golf when he was stricken. Ordinarily, however, the disease lasts several months or longer, with slow wasting such as one might expect with a prolonged septic process. The symptomatic complaints may be very few for long periods of time. In fact, some would hardly think there was anything wrong and wonder why they are regarded as sick and kept in bed. During the early weeks or even months there may be no dyspnea or evidence of cardiac failure. These do occur later in the disease, and heart failure may be regarded as the final cause of death in a considerable portion of cases. Other patients merely waste away with increasing anemia. In a small number a major embolus brings to a close this lingering disease. In a very few the end result is a glomerular nephritis with uremic manifestations.

THE VALVES INVOLVED

It is frequently found on postmortem examination that the vegetations of subacute bacterial endocarditis involve more than one valve. When they are confined to one valve they are almost as common on the mitral as on the aortic leaflets. Much more rarely is the pulmonary or tricuspid valve affected. A correlation of postmortem findings with the presence of heart murmurs enables one to predict fairly accurately the location of the vegetative process. When the original defect is a congenital lesion the vegetations will be centered about the area involved. In acquired heart disease (almost always rheumatic and only rarely syphilitic), if there is an apical systolic murmur and no diastolic murmur the vegetations will be confined to the mitral valve. Occasionally there is only a systolic murmur but one that is best heard at the base of the heart due to aortic stenosis without evidence of aortic insufficiency. Under these circumstances there will be vegetations on the aortic valve. When an aortic diastolic murmur is heard there will always be found an active bacterial endocarditis of this valve either alone or with extensions on the mitral valve. When there are typical signs of mitral stenosis without evidence of aortic insufficiency the growths will be found on the mitral valve, but when an aortic diastolic murmur is also present it will be difficult to draw any conclusion for the murmur at the apex may prove to be an Austin Flint phenomenon. In this way one can fairly well predict the location of the vegetative process.

There are very rare occasions when it is definitely known that no murmurs were present before the infection occurred. Then as the disease developed an aortic diastolic murmur became audible. Under these circumstances one may strongly suspect that congenital aortic bicuspid valves were present and bacterial endocarditis developed on these valves.

DIFFERENTIAL DIAGNOSIS

During the early days this disease offers considerable difficulty in diagnosis. The insidious onset with vague nonlocalizing symptoms may lead to a diagnosis of grip. Later as the fever continues and sweats develop tuberculosis will be suspected or because of spots on the skin and enlarged spleen typhoid fever will be considered. More frequently, because of the presence of a heart murmur, fever, and some vague pains, the condition will be regarded as rheumatic fever. The absence of any murmur is a very reliable clue in eliminating the diagnosis of subacute bacterial endocarditis. I have seen only two instances of this disease in which either a systolic or diastolic murmur was not heard on careful auscultation. Generally the murmur is of more than very slight intensity and in most cases does not change over long periods of time. The sudden development of a new murmur or the accentuation of an old murmur occurs but rarely. This indirect method of ruling out the diagnosis has proved helpful on several occasions. I recall two instances in which the diagnosis of subacute bacterial endocarditis was made by competent physicians on the basis of some of the clinical features discussed above. In the absence of any murmurs I expressed the definite opinion that some other cause would be found for the fever and sweats. In a few days tubercle bacilli were discovered in the sputum.

The presence of a murmur, on the other hand, does not necessarily mean that there is an active bacterial endocarditis. It obviously is a common finding in rheumatic heart disease, and the new infection with fever, sweats, and various aches and pains may be a recurrent rheumatic bout with or without rheumatic carditis. This differentiation between rheumatic fever and subacute bacterial endocarditis is sometimes very difficult and always most important. No matter how ill the patient suffering from the former condition may be we are hopeful of a recovery, and no matter how well one with the latter condition may appear we fear a fatal outcome unless treated vigorously with specific drugs. Apart from the specific and more characteristic features previously discussed there are some more general differences between the two diseases. The heart rate is apt to be more rapid in relation to the degree of fever in rheumatic than in the bacterial infection. Although both may show a moderate degree of anemia it becomes eventually more marked in the latter condition. Although both show a slight leukocytosis this may be absent in the presence of fever more often in subacute bacterial endocarditis. Salicylates do not alter the fever or the symptoms in the one and generally do so in the other. Pericarditis, arrhythmias, and alterations in the electrocardiograms (especially prolonged P-R time) are common in rheumatic and rare in bacterial infections.

The presence of a distinct murmur and its proper interpretation, however, may be the main clue to the diagnosis. I recall an instance when a man was taken while at work with severe pain in the left loin radiating to the genitals. He also noticed grossly bloody urine. It seemed like a definite case of stone in the left kidney or ureter and was so regarded by all the physicians who saw him. There was a moderately loud apical systolic murmur which he had known about for many years. On close questioning I learned that he had not felt really well for several weeks. Although there was no fever at this time, to explain both the murmur and the sudden pain in the kidney a diagnosis of subacute bacterial endocarditis with left renal embolus was made. This was confirmed by the finding of *Streptococcus viridans* in the blood stream, although the culture was made when the patient's temperature was only 99.2° F. This eventuality is by no means rare in patients who have had a so-called "benign" systolic murmur for many years.

Finally, skin tests may help to differentiate rheumatic fever from bacterial endocarditis. In 80 to 90 per cent of cases of rheumatic fever, if dead cultures of *Streptococcus hemolyticus* or *Streptococcus viridans* (0.1 to 0.01 cc.) or the split protein products of these bacteria are injected intracutaneously, a positive reaction consisting of a definite wheal will result in twenty-four hours. In a fairly large series of cases of subacute bacterial endocarditis such tests have proved entirely negative except in rare instances. This is a simple test and the reading can be made in twenty-four hours. With our present experience, if the skin test is positive, one may incline to the opinion that the condition is not a bacterial endocarditis. If it is negative one may suspect this diagnosis, but it must be remembered that in about 50 per cent of normal individuals and 10 per cent of rheumatic patients the reaction is also negative. These differences in skin reactions and other suggestive clinical evidences of a certain incompatibility between the rheumatic state and bacterial endocarditis have led me to think that those individuals who lose their rheumatic predisposition or allergic type of response are the ones who become more susceptible to the development of bacterial endocarditis. The more immune they become to the one, the more susceptible they are to the other. It is known that patients who already are suffering from *Streptococcus viridans* endocarditis are highly immune to streptococci. This is evident from the skin test and from the presence of immune bodies in their blood. In fact I have injected living virulent streptococci in considerable quantities, subcutaneously, in such patients without producing any local reaction or producing only a very slight one. The simultaneous presence of rheumatic carditis and bacterial endocarditis on postmortem examination in a few cases is not in conflict with the view that there is an antagonism between the two diseases. The bacterial infection, just like any infection, may stir up rheumatic fever, and the bacterial infection may have preceded rather than followed the rheumatism. In any event, the skin test has proved of some value in differentiating doubtful cases.

It is generally regarded that emboli and a positive blood culture are the two outstanding and determining evidences of a bacterial endocarditis. This really needs some qualifications. Emboli occur in rheumatic and other types of heart disease in which there is no vegetative endocarditis. In such cases, sterile mural thrombi are generally present in the auricles, from which bits may become dislodged producing peripheral emboli either into the systemic circulation or to the lungs. When such emboli occur, recovery is likely to take place. Likewise, streptococci may occasionally be found in the blood stream by culture studies when there is no reason to believe they are coming from the valves of the heart. It follows, therefore, that although these points are extremely important the rest of the clinical picture is essential to validate the diagnosis of subacute bacterial endocarditis. Because of the grave prognosis that the diagnosis of subacute bacterial endocarditis entails, most careful consideration must be given to other possibilities, such as tuberculosis, undulant fever, rheumatic heart disease, and the like.

PROGNOSIS

Bacterial endocarditis was formerly one of the most fatal of the common types of cardiovascular disease. Its duration varies considerably, from a few months to a year or more. Recoveries, however, have been very rare in the past, if the diagnosis is reserved for those cases that display the complete clinical picture. Very likely in mild cases in which the fever does not rise above 101° F., and in which one might hesitate to make a positive diagnosis, spontaneous recovery does take place. On the other hand, if a fatal outcome is regarded as essential to the diagnosis, there obviously can be no recoveries. There have been instances of spontaneous satisfactory recovery in which a careful review of the data forces one to accept the diagnosis. It is curious that on very rare occasions a patient may recover symptomatically and yet continue to harbor the streptococci in the blood stream for a long time. Now with use of antibiotic drugs the expectation is that 75 per cent or more of the patients will recover.

TREATMENT

When sulfonamides came into general use the first real therapeutic advance took place. The mortality fell from 99 or 100 per cent to about 90 per cent. Definite recoveries resulted, especially with preparations like sulfadiazine, combined with fever therapy. The entire outlook changed dramatically with the discovery of penicillin and other drugs like streptomycin and Aureomycin. The results will depend on how early treatment is instituted and how carefully the exact therapy is chosen for the particular microorganism involved. There have been reports of small series of cases (numbering twenty or more), in which no fatalities at all occurred.

A search of the older literature and a glance at the earlier editions of this book will quickly reveal an amazing variety of therapeutic procedures that were formerly tried in the hope of obtaining cures. Various chemicals, dyes, vaccines, sera, transfusions, and other more fanciful procedures were employed. None of them met with any success. Formerly there was no advantage, except an academic one, in making an early diagnosis of bacterial endocarditis, for treatment was no more effective then than late in the course of the disease. Now it is imperative to make as early a diagnosis as possible, for if it is too long delayed not only may cures be less attainable but irreparable damage such as congestive failure or hemiplegia may result.

Once the clinical diagnosis is suspected the patient should be sent to a hospital. The care, both diagnostic and therapeutic, of such a case is too involved to be carried out adequately at home. Chemotherapy should not be instituted immediately, not until one and preferably several blood cultures have been taken. Inasmuch as the contemplated diagnosis involves a long and expensive course of treatment, it is very desirable to be on certain ground and especially to determine what microorganism is the cause of the infection. There will be times when much delay may be disastrous. This may not permit more than one or a few blood cultures being taken. If a physician has already given chemotherapy for a few days when the diagnosis is still obscure, it may render blood culture studies unreliable for some while thereafter. Inasmuch as at this time the case is in its early stage, one may properly hesitate to embark on a long course of treatment and prefer to await developments for a short while. In the long run much confusion and trouble may be avoided, at times, by patience and intelligent observation.

Another advantage of taking blood cultures is that when the organism is identified it will be possible to choose the appropriate type of chemotherapy and its dosage. Whenever possible the laboratory should determine the concentration of the antibiotic required to inhibit the growth of the specific germ. Likewise, the concentration of the drug in the blood stream on a particular course of treatment can be measured. In that way the physician can feel more certain that the infection will be controlled, or learn that the dose needs to be increased or the type of drug changed. At times, even frequent blood cultures prove to be negative, but if there is sufficient clinical evidence to render the diagnosis likely or if there is a fair suspicion of it, a regular course of treatment should be carried out.

In most cases of bacterial endocarditis, acute or subacute, penicillin is the drug of choice at present. There are differences of opinion as to the dosage and the method of administration. No doubt in future years the accepted procedures will change. At one time constant intravenous drip was used. Others employed repeated intramuscular injections of penicillin. Still others tried continuous intramuscular injection. The method in most common use and the one I employ is repeated intramuscular injections of penicillin at three- or six-hour intervals throughout the day. The dose will vary, but a satisfactory one to start with in the average adult is 2,000,000 to 4,000,000 units daily. In many cases it will become apparent in a few days that therapy is effective. The fever will quickly subside, the general well-being and appearance of the patient will improve, and blood cultures will become sterile. The latter finding, though comforting, is not altogether reliable, because under chemotherapy the cultures may be negative even while the infection remains active. A positive blood culture is more decisive in indicating that the treatment is not effective. It is rare for bacterial resistance to develop during active treatment, particularly when the infection is due to the alpha hemolytic streptococcus. Development of resistance to penicillin of enterococci during therapy is not uncommon. If the clinical progress is favorable the same dose is continued for a minimum of four weeks and possibly one or two weeks longer. If the cultures remain positive or fever and symptoms persist, the dose probably needs to be increased or the drug changed.

When the offending organism is the enterococcus, as may occur after genitourinary trauma or in patients who have been edentulous, very large doses of penicillin will be necessary, i.e., 10,000,000 to 20,000,000 units daily. It will also be advisable to add 1 or 2 gm. of streptomycin daily. If the organism is a staphylococcus, often resistant to penicillin, other broad-spectrum antibiotics will be indicated, such as Aureomycin, Terramycin, Erythromycin, etc., 1 to 2 gm. daily. Careful observation, including the in vitro determination of the relative sensitivity of the causative organism to the various antibiotics, will be necessary in treating some of these difficult cases.

Now, as these preparations have become less expensive, it is wiser to err on the side of excessive rather than of inadequate amounts. Furthermore, laboratory studies may show that a sufficient concentration of the drug in the blood stream has not been reached. It has seemed that some cases of well-compensated free aortic insufficiency with a hyperactive heart beat have required larger doses than would be expected.

One wonders whether, under such circumstances, with a rapid velocity of blood flow, more of the drug is washed out of the blood stream through the kidneys. Some have advised continuing treatment for six to eight weeks, even if everything appears favorable. It is difficult to be dogmatic about this. Practical considerations will inevitably influence the decision, such as the cost of medication, the expense of hospitalization, and the discomfort of the patient from such prolonged course of intramuscular injections. Others have felt that similar results may be obtained by giving the penicillin three times daily rather than six or eight times. The suggestion that simultaneous administration of heparin is valuable has not generally been accepted. I not only do not advise it but fear that it adds further risks.

After treatment has been carried out for four or six weeks and the condition is apparently satisfactory, penicillin is omitted. If all goes well, nothing untoward develops. Further blood cultures should remain sterile, and fever should not return. Occasionally embolic phenomena which are worrisome occur during these early subsequent weeks. They do not always indicate that the infection is still active. At times, even without further treatment, all goes well and we conclude that they were sterile emboli. The streptococcus skin test which generally was negative in the early stages of the disease often becomes positive as recovery takes place. In fact, it is supporting evidence that the infection has been controlled if this change in skin reaction takes place. Occasionally a bout of fever occurs during the penicillin therapy that is due to the drug itself. It may be difficult to differentiate this from fever due to the underlying disease.

If the case is progressing favorably the temperature will remain normal, the blood culture negative, the white blood count and sedimentation rate will be normal, and the patient will give evidence of a sense of well-being. If the clinical and laboratory features point to a persistence of the infection, further treatment is necessary. At this point the dose of penicillin may need to be doubled or quadrupled. If the original organism was gram-negative, or, as occasionally happens, if a mixed infection occurs or a second microorganism becomes involved, supplementation with the combination of streptomycin and dihydrostreptomycin in a dose of 0.5 to 1.0 gm. of each daily intramuscularly is advisable, or Aureomycin 0.5 to 1.0 gm. four times daily by mouth would be indicated. Sometimes it is appropriate to administer more than one of these antibiotics simultaneously.

Methods have been used to increase the blood level of penicillin. For this purpose benzoic acid, 2.0 gm. four times daily, has been employed. Another and preferable drug is probenecid (Benemid), 0.5 gm. every six hours, which diminishes renal excretion of penicillin and thereby results in a high concentration in the blood. These procedures are generally not necessary and may upset the patient's digestive tract. However, at times they may be useful adjuncts to penicillin therapy, especially when one is forced to give very large doses.

The most common offending organism in this condition is the alpha hemolytic streptococcus (viridans). Other organisms isolated in different cases are the enterococcus, *Staphylococcus albus*, gamma streptococcus, pneumococcus, brucella organisms, the *Escherichia coli* group, and para-influenza.

Throughout this period of treatment very little else in the way of specific medication is necessary. The patient may be kept in bed during the early days, but if he appears fairly well and essentially symptom-less, as many do, he may be allowed out of bed during the latter part of this period. There are no restrictions in diet, with the possible excep-tion of salt if there is any fear of congestive heart failure. If the latter is present treatment is given as one would with any case of heart failure. In a few cases heart failure is present as a result of the prolonged infec-tion, before chemotherapy is effective. It also may appear during the early weeks or months afterthe infection has been controlled. It appears that in some cases the actual endocarditis precipitates a reactivation of rheumatic fever. In other cases the prolonged illness, the possible increase in the mechanical deformity of the valves, or injury to the coronary arterial tree by small emboli results in a deterioration of myo-cardial function and definite congestive heart failure.

It is wise to investigate the condition of the teeth while the patient is under active penicillin therapy. X-rays should be taken and if any infected teeth are found or even if it is suspected that a tooth may need to be removed at a later time it is best to do all the operative work at once. Because of the risk of reinfection following tooth extrac-tions, there is no better time to do the necessary operative work on the teeth than while the patient is on full doses of penicillin. In some instances I had all teeth removed during the active treatment with penicillin, as a preventive of further attacks of bacterial endocarditis. This may seem to be a drastic step. It must be realized, however, that recurrences are possible, and simple dental manipulation of the teeth or even the act of chewing may be followed by a transient bacteremia, which is not always inhibited by the customary prophylactic measures that are employed. Whenever the cosmetic effect of total dental extrac-tion is not important, this procedure has much in its favor.

PREVENTION

Now that we have effective chemotherapy and know fairly well which patients are most likely to develop bacterial endocarditis, pre-ventive measures should be taken whenever possible. It has been found that in about 20 per cent of cases, subacute bacterial endocarditis was observed to follow within one to several weeks after a tooth extraction. There is ample bacterial evidence to show that in a considerable pro-portion of normal individuals the simple extraction of a tooth is immedi-ately followed by a bacteremia, generally due to alpha nonhemolytic streptococcus. Similar, but less frequent, bacteremia has been found after other dental manipulation such as filling a cavity or prophylactic cleaning of the teeth. Unfortunately the same bacteremia has occasionally followed massage of the gums or the ordinary act of chewing. Therefore it is imperative to advise all patients who have rheumatic valvular disease or congenital heart disease to receive prophylactic penicillin treatment.

The routine course of prophylactic treatment has been changing. The earlier methods must have had some value, but failures did occur. I have had a patient who developed subacute bacterial endocarditis after a tooth extraction, although she received 300,000 units of penicillin in beeswax intramuscularly one hour before the extraction and again several hours later. Fortunately she recovered after a prolonged course of antibiotic therapy. One would prefer to outline a course of oral therapy so that patients might be able to carry out the program more readily. It will be some time before the very best and most practical method of prevention will be determined. At the present time two courses are recommended. If the oral method is to be used a tablet of 250,000 to 500,000 units of penicillin-V is to be taken four times daily the day before the extraction and for the following four days. An additional tablet may be taken just at the time of the extraction. The second method, and one that is probably preferable, is to give an intramuscular injection of 600,000 units of aqueous penicillin and an injection of 600,000 units of long-acting procaine penicillin in oil with 2 per cent aluminum monostearate one-half hour before the extraction. More prolonged and troublesome methods of penicillin prophylaxis for routine dental care that some would advise will defeat their own purpose as they will not be followed. Theoretically, the above courses of treatment should be carried out for any visit to the dentist that involves manipulation of the teeth or gums, such as a filling of a tooth or a prophylactic cleaning of the teeth. If there is a history of penicillin sensitivity other broad-spectrum antibiotics should be used in comparable doses. The above applies with equal force to procedures like catheterization of the bladder or cystoscopy, but here it would be well to add 1 gm. of streptomycin twice daily for a few days and to give very large doses of penicillin, such as 10,000,000 units twice daily, because the enterococcus is a frequent offender in genitourinary problems and is quite resistant.

Prophylactic measures should also be employed for vulnerable individuals who are to undergo any surgical procedure that involves the possibility of a spreading infection, such as lancing a boil, tonsillectomy, appendectomy, or termination of pregnancy. This can easily be done when the condition requires hospitalization, but should be carried out even in office or house practice. Finally, prompt antibiotic treatment of sore throats and "colds," especially if there is any fever or if the infection can be identified as streptococcal in origin, will help to prevent the subsequent development of either rheumatic fever or bacterial endocarditis.

GENERAL COMMENTS

It is premature to tell what the ultimate outcome will be in treated cases of bacterial endocarditis. The immediate mortality should be not more than 25 per cent. This figure can be improved if cases are recognized early and treated adequately. The main causes of death after recovery from the bacterial infection are cerebral embolism, congestive failure, or renal insufficiency. The great majority of recurrences of infection (80 per cent) appear within the first four weeks after treatment has been stopped. Generally, bacterial evidence of this appears before clinical manifestation. It therefore is wise to perform weekly blood cultures for a while after cessation of specific treatment. If positive cultures are obtained further treatment is indicated.

When the patient has done well and convalescence has progressed favorably, he should gradually resume whatever duties his cardiac status will permit. Many appear to be quite fit and about as well as they were before and able to perform essentially normal duties. I have had a patient who has since gone through two pregnancies without mishap. Others, although in satisfactory health, have not been quite so well as they were before the infection. It is reasonable to suspect that the valvular deformity may be greater after than before the infection. Furthermore, all the circumstances that predisposed the patient to the original bacterial endocarditis remain, so that recurrences of the same type of disease in the future are not unlikely. I have already seen one instance of a second bout after a satisfactory recovery from a first attack. In an appreciable minority of cases progressive congestive failure has developed during the first year after recovery.

CHAPTER 11

Congenital Heart Disease

By ALEXANDER S. NADAS, M.D.

Congenital heart disease is a structural abnormality of the heart present from birth. These malformations, although extremely important in children, are of less significance in adults. The reasons for this are twofold: obviously, many patients with congenital malformations of the heart die before they reach adulthood, and degenerative diseases of the circulation become more important in the later years of life. Nevertheless, enough of these patients survive into adulthood to make this discussion well worth while in a text principally aimed at the general practitioner and the internist. Furthermore, the operative techniques for correction of these lesions, which have been developed within the past fifteen years, have made most of these conditions surgically correctable today.

Incidence

No accurate figures on the frequency of congenital heart disease in adults are available. British authors place the over-all incidence at about 3 per 1000 at birth; this figure drops to 1 per 1000 in children ten years of age, the difference presumably representing infants and children who died before they reached the tenth birthday.

The frequency of individual lesions is hard to determine; published figures vary considerably, depending on the particular interests of the author and on whether the data are based on clinical or postmortem observations. However, I think that the statement probably can be made with assurance that patent ductus arteriosus, coarctation of the aorta, ventricular septal defect, atrial septal defect, pulmonary stenosis, and the tetralogy of Fallot each represents 10 to 15 per cent of the total number of patients having congenital heart disease who live to be at least two years old.

Etiology

In the vast majority of cases, the etiology of congenital heart disease is unknown. Certain contributing factors may be mentioned, however.

Heredity obviously plays a definite role in a small number of instances. Siblings of patients with congenital heart disease have an appreciably greater chance of having congenital heart disease than do children in the general population. The increase has been quoted by some to be tenfold. This means that a mother with one child who has congenital heart disease would still have less than a 2 per cent chance of having a second youngster similarly affected. This is an important point, and should enable the physician to encourage the parents of patients with congenital heart disease to have more children if they so desire. Some lesions (patent ductus arteriosus, coarctation of the aorta, and pulmonary stenosis) are more likely to occur in siblings than are others. The same lesion is prone to appear in siblings, particularly those of the same sex.

Associated congenital malformations may offer a diagnostic clue to the nature of the congenital cardiac malformation present. Mongolism is usually associated with a foramen primum type of atrial septal defect; patients with arachnodactyly or with Turner's syndrome are prone to have coarctation of the aorta.

Environmental influences, such as anoxia, vitamin deficiencies, and the like, have induced pregnant rats to give birth to litters with congenital cardiac anomalies. In humans, the effects of German measles during the first trimester of pregnancy are well documented; these infants are likely to be born with patent ductus arteriosus, although almost all of the other types of congenital heart disease have been seen and reported. The correlation is close enough, however, to make the physician strongly suspect the presence of patent ductus arteriosus in any child with congenital heart disease born from a mother who had German measles in the first trimester of pregnancy. On account of the seasonal incidence of German measles, more patients with patent ductus arteriosus are born between October and January than at any other time of the year. The effect of other viral diseases has not been well documented. That anoxia may also be effective in humans in the production of congenital cardiac anomalies is suggested by South American studies revealing a higher incidence of patent ductus arteriosus among Indians living at high altitudes than among those living at sea level.

Clues Suggesting the Diagnosis of Congenital Heart Disease

CYANOSIS

Patients with heart disease who show definite cyanosis of the fingers, toes, and mucous membranes probably have congenital malformation of the heart. Although acquired heart disease (mitral stenosis), pulmonary disease, methemoglobinemia, and even argyria may be mentioned as possible causes, in most instances of really severe and generalized cyanosis, the underlying disease is a congenital heart lesion.

More than 30 years ago Lundsgaard and Van Slyke pointed out that the absolute amount of reduced hemoglobin is the determining factor in the causation of cyanosis; they stated that at least 5.0 gm. of reduced hemoglobin per 100 cc. of blood must be present in the capillaries before cyanosis becomes visible. Although this figure is considered somewhat high today, the general principle certainly is still valid. If one remembers the fact that, in an individual with a normal circulation the capillaries contain about 2.5 gm. of reduced hemoglobin per 100 cc. of blood, it may be clearly seen that the addition of only another 2.5 gm. per 100 cc. is needed to produce visible cyanosis. This 2.5 gm. (or more) may originate basically from two sources: (1) The aortic blood may carry reduced hemoglobin, in which case arterial unsaturation is the cause of the cyanosis (central cyanosis). (2) The oxygen extraction at the capillary level may be so extensive that more than 5.0 gm. of reduced hemoglobin is present in a patient whose arterial blood is fully saturated (peripheral cyanosis).

Central cyanosis (that accompanied by arterial saturation of less than 91 per cent) may be the result of either poor oxygenation of the blood in the lungs (pulmonary cyanosis), with unsaturation of the pulmonary venous blood, or of an admixture of unoxygenated blood to arterial blood within the heart or great vessels (shunt cyanosis), with fully saturated pulmonary venous blood. The vast majority of the individuals with cyanotic heart disease have shunt cyanosis. This may be differentiated from pulmonary cyanosis by the facts that, as a rule, it is more severe, it gets worse on straining or crying, and it improves only moderately, if at all, with the inhalation of pure oxygen.

In peripheral cyanosis the arterial blood is fully saturated, but the oxygen extraction, mostly due to slow circulation time (shock) or low cardiac output (pulmonary stenosis, mitral stenosis) is so high that more than 5.0 gm. of reduced hemoglobin per 100 cc. is present in the capillaries. This type of peripheral cyanosis may be differentiated from the central type by its generally mild nature, by the lack of involvement of the mucous membranes, and, of course, by the presence of full arterial saturation (more than 95 per cent).

CLUBBING

In its fully developed form, clubbing consists of widening and thickening of the terminal phalanges, with convex nails. It is noted best and earliest over the thumbs. Clubbing always accompanies severe cyanotic congenital heart disease. Rarely it may also be caused by pulmonary disease, subacute bacterial endocarditis, or liver disease, and it may even be familial in origin.

SQUATTING

This characteristic posture, assumed after exertion by patients with cyanotic congenital heart disease, usually first appears when the child is about one and a half or two years old, and social pressure commonly abolishes it by adolescence. Squatting helps to return the arterial oxygen saturation to its pre-exercise level, probably by increasing the peripheral venous return. Another possible mechanism is that with this position a larger portion of the ventricular output may go to the head and less to the lower part of the body.

UNDERDEVELOPMENT

Although many patients with congenital heart disease are well-developed, well-nourished individuals, the majority are undersized and poorly nourished.

LEFT-SIDED CHEST PROMINENCE

Cardiac enlargement and active pulsations may easily cause bulging of the elastic thoracic cage of young children. Although patients with rheumatic heart disease may also have marked left chest prominence, its presence should make the physician suspect congenital cardiac malformation. Conditions associated with left-to-right shunt are more prone to cause this deformity.

MURMUR

Congenital heart disease is usually accompanied by a loud murmur, and even a thrill. As a matter of fact, some of the loudest murmurs are found in patients with congenital malformations of the heart.

The localization of the murmur is of some interest, in that, on the whole, the presence of a murmur around the apex is likely to suggest rheumatic heart disease, whereas loud murmurs at the xiphoid process, the left sternal border, or the second left interspace usually indicate congenital heart disease.

Frequently, the character of the murmur suggests the accurate diagnosis. A continuous machinery murmur at the second left interspace is pathognomonic of patent ductus arteriosus. There are rare exceptions to this general rule, as a somewhat similar murmur may be present with an arteriovenous aneurysm of the mammary or coronary artery or branches of the pulmonary artery, with a high ventricular septal defect, and with an aortic septal defect. The rasping and stenotic murmur at the left upper sternal border indicates pulmonary stenosis; the presence of a low frequency mid-diastolic rumble at the apex or lower left sternal border suggests the presence of a left-to-right shunt.

The time of appearance of the murmur is of prime importance. If it was noted at birth, or even within the first five years of life, the diagnosis of congenital heart disease may be made with assurance. In this regard, it is interesting to note that stenosis of the semilunar valves gives rise to a murmur which is usually noted soon after birth, whereas the atrial septal defect murmur may not be heard until later in childhood.

Individual Lesions

It is not intended to discuss in great detail all the various congenital anomalies of the heart. Whole textbooks should be and have been written on the subject. The lesions to be discussed here are those which are common, which are likely to present themselves to the general practitioner or internist, and for which surgical assistance either is presently available or is near realization. The defects will be discussed under the following headings:

1. The Left-to-Right Shunt Group
2. The Right-to-Left Shunt Group
3. Vascular and Valvular Lesions

THE LEFT-TO-RIGHT SHUNT GROUP

The principal anatomic abnormality in this group of defects is the presence of a communication between the systemic and the pulmonary circulation. Their principal physiologic characteristic is that, because the pressure in the systemic circuit is relatively higher than it is in the pulmonary circuit, the direction of the blood flow is from left (systemic) to right (pulmonary). This does not mean that the shunt is from left to right all the time; under certain acute situations (straining, crying, or shock) or chronic conditions (development of pulmonary vascular obstruction), the pressure relationship between the two circuits may change to the extent that the blood flows from right to left. Nevertheless, the dominant and original shunt is from left to right in all lesions to be discussed at this time.

The group as a whole is characterized by one or more of the following features: (1) absence of cyanosis, (2) underdevelopment, (3) left chest prominence, (4) apical diastolic rumble, (5) cardiac enlargement, (6) hyperdynamic impulse, and (7) pulmonary vascular enlargement, as shown on the roentgenogram.

Atrial Septal Defect. An atrial defect is an opening in the interatrial septum at least 1 cm. in diameter, not completely covered by a valve. This excludes patent foramen ovale, by itself a functionally insignificant lesion.

Anatomically there are two types of atrial defects with very different clinical significance. The so-called "ostium primum" defect is usually single and is low in the septum and posterior. It commonly involves an associated abnormality of the mitral or tricuspid valve, or both, or even the ventricular septum. In contrast, the ostium secundum defect may be single or multiple; it is high in the atrial septum, and frequently anterior.

Physiologically, atrial septal defect of the secundum type is characterized by a large shunt from the left to the right atrium; this is the result of the difference in volume-pressure characteristics of the two ventricles. The shunt may be demonstrated at cardiac catheterization by slipping of the catheter from the right atrium into the left atrium and even down to the left ventricle or by the presence of a higher oxygen content in the blood in the right atrium than in that of the superior vena cava. For this difference in oxygen content to be significant, it must be at least 1.5 volumes per cent. The right atrial pressure is slightly elevated and approximates the left atrial pressure. Right ventricular and pulmonary arterial pressures in young individuals are usually normal; in older individuals with pulmonary vascular disease, both may be elevated to systemic levels. In such an individual, of course, the size of the left-to-right shunt will be small or negligible. The foramen primum type of lesion is frequently associated with pulmonary vascular disease and mitral regurgitation of an appreciable degree.

The symptomatology may be negligible in childhood. In adults in their twenties or thirties, progressive exertional dyspnea, and even congestive failure, appears.

At physical examination, these patients usually appear frail. There is a hyperdynamic impulse at the xiphoid process, and left chest deformity is seen. A thrill at the lower left sternal border is palpable in the foramen primum defect only.

On auscultation, the foramen secundum defect is characterized by a soft systolic murmur at the second left interspace, whereas in individuals with foramen primum, a rasping systolic mumur is heard at the lower left sternal border and apex. Low frequency diastolic murmurs (rumbles) are heard only in atrial defects with large shunts; these may follow either the second sound or the third sound and are heard best at the lower left sternal border or the apex. It should be emphasized that the presence of an apical diastolic murmur in a patient with atrial septal defect does not necessarily indicate associated mitral stenosis. The second sound is widely split in both the ostium primum and ostium secundum defects.

The roentgenologic findings are enlargement of the right atrium, right ventricle, and pulmonary artery, with a considerable degree of pulmonary vascular engorgement and even "hilar dance." In addition, patients with foramen primum defects show left ventricular enlargement.

The electrocardiogram reveals complete or incomplete right bundle branch block in practically all cases. The degree of right ventricular hypertrophy varies with the pressure in the right ventricle. Additional evidences of left ventricular hypertrophy are noted in individuals with ostium primum defects. Prolonged atrioventricular conduction is noted in at least 25 per cent of the patients.

The course and prognosis of atrial septal defect depends on the size of the opening and its location. Small defects are tolerated without difficulty for many years. Larger defects with big shunts may cause congestive failure and may predispose toward the development of pulmonary vascular obstruction in the late twenties or thirties. The average life expectancy of all patients with atrial septal defect is about forty years.

Among the complications of atrial defects, rheumatic heart disease and auricular fibrillation should be mentioned. Subacute bacterial endocarditis is extremely rare.

Medical management of patients with atrial septal defect includes the vigorous use of chemotherapeutic and chemoprophylactic measures to prevent the development of rheumatic fever. Anti-congestive measures are successful in prolonging the life of these patients for many years after failure first appears. There is no effective treatment at present for pulmonary vascular disease. Asymptomatic patients should be encouraged to lead normal lives.

Surgical treatment, by any of the well-accepted approaches (Gross, Björk, Bailey, or Swan), is indicated in all patients who have a large shunt and significant cardiac enlargement, particularly if they have symptoms. The operative risk in patients with uncomplicated foramen secundum type of defect is no higher than 10 per cent. Surgery of patients with ostium primum defects and those with pulmonary vascular obstruction carries a prohibitive risk today.

Partial Transposition of the Pulmonary Veins. If one or more, but not all, of the pulmonary veins enter the right atrium instead of the left, partial transposition of the pulmonary veins exists. Almost without exception, only one lung is involved. If the veins from the right lung drain anomalously, an ostium secundum type of atrial septal defect is frequently also present. The point of entry of these veins into the right atrium may be at the superior vena cava, the inferior vena cava, or the atrium itself.

For all practical purposes, the clinical and physiologic pictures and the prognosis are the same as those presented by a moderate-sized atrial septal defect. There are only two ways—neither of them foolproof—that a partial transposition of the pulmonary veins may be distinguished from an atrial septal defect. One is by clearly observable entrance of the catheter into the lung field from the right atrium, and the other is by dye-dilution curves obtained from the two main pulmonary arteries.

Surgical repair may be accomplished on the basis of the indications and by means of the techniques mentioned in the section on atrial septal defect. Most thoracic surgeons are able to cope with one or the other or both situations from the same operative approach.

Ventricular Septal Defect. Defects of the interventricular septum vary in size from 0.5 or 3.0 cm. to complete absence of the septum. Most of the defects are high in the membranous septum; only rarely are they low in the muscular portion.

The principal factors determining the physiologic effect of a ventricular septal defect are the size of the opening and the pressure gradient between the two ventricles. If the defect is small the right ventricular pressure is usually considerably lower than that found in the left ventricle, hence the flow of blood across the defect is also relatively slight. In contrast, if the defect is large, the pressure in the right ventricle is practically identical with the left ventricular pressure. The size of the shunt through the large ventricular defect depends on the relationship of the pulmonary to systemic vascular resistance. If the resistance in the lungs—because of the presence of pulmonary vascular disease—is high, little blood flows from the left to the right ventricle. It may even take a right-to-left course. In contrast, if the pulmonary resistance is low, a tremendous left-to-right shunt through a ventricular septal defect may occur.

Two other physiologic variants of ventricular septal defect should be mentioned briefly; one is the association of pulmonary stenosis with a ventricular septal defect and a left-to-right shunt, the other the combination of aortic regurgitation with ventricular septal defect.

SMALL VENTRICULAR SEPTAL DEFECT (ROGER'S DISEASE). Small defects of the ventricular septum (approximately 0.5 cm. in diameter), without significant right ventricular hypertension, are usually referred to as examples of Roger's disease.

Individuals with this type of lesion are generally asymptomatic, and only the discovery of a murmur leads them to the doctor.

At physical examination they seem normal in all respects except for the presence of the murmur. This is usually noted best at the lower left sternal border, is grade 3 to 5 in intensity, is frequently accompanied by a thrill, and transmits relatively poorly. This latter point is particularly important in differentiating this murmur from the one associated with infundibular pulmonary stenosis. The heart sounds are normal.

Roentgenologic examination shows a normal-sized heart with right ventricular contour. The pulmonary vasculature may be slightly engorged.

The electrocardiogram is usually within normal limits.

At cardiac catheterization, the only abnormal finding is the presence of at least a 1 volume per cent increase in oxygen content of the blood in the right ventricle, compared with that in the right atrium.

Small ventricular defects are benign lesions, usually compatible with a normal life expectancy. The only complications which need to be mentioned are rheumatic fever and subacute bacterial endocarditis.

No specific medical or surgical treatment is indicated for patients with small ventricular defects. Chemotherapy and chemoprophylaxis should be employed in the usual fashion. The patient should be encouraged to lead an entirely normal life.

LARGE VENTRICULAR SEPTAL DEFECT (EISENMENGER'S DISEASE). A defect of 0.5 to 1.5 cm. in diameter in the membranous portion of the interventricular septum results in the clinical picture of large ventricular septal defect. As indicated before, the pressure in the two ventricles is practically identical, under these circumstances. Whether or not there is overriding of the aorta seems to be of relatively minor importance. The flow through the defect depends on the status of the pulmonary vasculature.

In contrast to patients with Roger's disease, these individuals are sick from early infancy. Dyspnea, exercise intolerance, repeated severe respiratory infections, and episodes of congestive failure dominate the picture.

At physical examination there is usually a significant degree of underdevelopment. Moderate or slight cyanosis is seen in at least half of the patients. The left chest is prominent and the cardiac impulse is hyperdynamic, involving the xiphoid process as well as the apex. A loud, rasping, systolic murmur is heard at the lower left sternal border and is frequently accompanied by a thrill. A diastolic rumble or early diastolic blow may be present at the apex or lower left sternal border. The pulmonary second sound is booming. In patients with associated pulmonary stenosis, a stenotic murmur is heard at the second left interspace, and the pulmonary closure is normal or diminished. If free aortic regurgitation is present with a large ventricular septal defect, a murmur closely resembling that of patent ductus arteriosus is heard at the lower left sternal border; the pulse pressure is also widened in these individuals.

Roentgenologic examination reveals moderate or marked cardiac enlargement involving the left and right ventricles, the left atrium, and the pulmonary artery. Pulmonary vascular engorgement with hilar dance is present.

The electrocardiogram reveals combined ventricular hypertrophy, occasionally with right bundle branch block and atrial hypertrophy.

At catheterization, the right ventricular and pulmonary arterial pressures are elevated to the systemic range. A jump in oxygen content of at least 1 volume per cent is noted in the right ventricle, compared with the right atrium. In advanced cases, the systemic arterial sample is unsaturated.

The course in these individuals is a very stormy one. Their infancy is characterized by repeated episodes of pneumonia and congestive failure which often prove fatal. If they weather the first two years of life, they usually do fairly well throughout the first and second decades, at which time increasing cyanosis and breathlessness appear. Hemoptysis may be a prominent symptom at this stage. Death usually occurs in congestive failure in the third or fourth decade.

Medical treatment of patients with large ventricular defects is symptomatic, along the lines indicated previously in the section on atrial septal defect. Surgical treatment by means of open heart surgery with the aid of a pump oxygenator has been successfully accomplished in several centers throughout the United States. It is too early to outline definite indications for operation. Speculations based on the experience gathered from other lesions would suggest that patients with large defects, large flows, and relatively little pulmonary vascular disease, will be the best subjects for corrective surgery.

SINGLE VENTRICLE.   From the anatomic viewpoint, no vestige of the ventricular septum should be present in patients with a single ventricle. From the physiologic viewpoint, however, one speaks of a single ventricle if both the systolic pressure and the oxygen content are the same in the right and left ventricles and the systemic artery; the oxygen content in the pulmonary artery is identical with that in the systemic artery, but the pressure may vary considerably, depending on the presence or absence of pulmonary stenosis. Thus, it may be seen that there is no sharp distinction, physiologically speaking, between a large ventricular septal defect and a single ventricle.

The effects of a single ventricle on the circulation depend to a large extent on the presence or absence of pulmonary stenosis. If there is severe stenosis of the right ventricular outflow tract, the clinical picture of severe cyanotic congenital heart disease—not greatly different from the tetralogy of Fallot—results. If, on the other hand, there is free communication between the common ventricular cavity and the pulmonary vascular bed, the picture will be one of a large left-to-right shunt, without cyanosis, but with chest deformity, systolic and diastolic murmurs, and pulmonary plethora.

The prognosis for these individuals is poor; most of them die within the first few weeks of life. Others, in whom a salutary balance between systemic and pulmonary circuits is established, may be practically asymptomatic for several decades. Finally, a third group of patients having dominant but not an overwhelming degree of pulmonary stenosis may show severe limitations of exercise and marked cyanosis, partially correctable by a shunt operation (Blalock or Potts).

Communications between the Great Arteries.   The defects to be discussed in this section may be either the result of persistence of a normal fetal structure (patent ductus arteriosus) or the outcome of a profound developmental anomaly (persistent truncus arteriosus).

TYPICAL PATENT DUCTUS ARTERIOSUS.   The ductus arteriosus connects the pulmonary artery, at its bifurcation, with the arch of the aorta, just beyond the origin of the left subclavian artery. In fetal life, this structure is necessary to supply the descending aorta with blood. Within a few hours after birth, functional closure of the duct occurs—anatomic closure follows in 90 per cent of all individuals, by the end of the first or second month. In the condition to be discussed here, the duct remains anatomically and functionally patent beyond the neonatal period and is also considerably larger than normal.

In extrauterine life, because the pressure in the aorta is higher throughout the entire cardiac cycle than it is in the pulmonary artery, a left-to-right shunt from systemic to pulmonary artery occurs. Under these circumstances, the left atrium, left ventricle, and pulmonary artery handle an appreciably larger volume of blood than do the right atrium, right ventricle, and the descending aorta.

Many individuals who have typical patent ductus arteriosus are completely asymptomatic; in others, underdevelopment, fatigue, or an increased number of severe respiratory infections are noted.

At physical examination, a thrill at the second left interspace is commonly palpable; left chest prominence is usually present. The cardiac impulse is hyperdynamic and is maximal at the cardiac apex. The peripheral pulses are bounding and, the larger the ductus, the wider the pulse pressure will be. At auscultation, the pathognomonic finding is the presence of a continuous systolic-diastolic, machinery murmur at the second left interspace. This murmur starts with the first sound, assumes a crescendic configuration, reaches its maximal intensity at the time of the second sound, and thereafter trails off in a decrescendo fashion. The heart sounds may be completely obscured by this roaring murmur, but occasionally a distinct loud second sound may be heard at the pulmonary area.

The roentgenologic picture depends a great deal on the size of the ductus and the volume of blood shunted through it. Patients with small shunts may have entirely normal roentgenograms; in contrast, large ductus are characterized by considerable enlargement of the left ventricle, left atrium, and pulmonary artery. The pulmonary vasculature is engorged in these cases, and a hilar dance is usually present.

The electrocardiographic changes also depend on the size of the ductus. Small ductus are accompanied by normal tracings; large shunts show left ventricular and, occasionally, left atrial hypertrophy.

Cardiac catheterization reveals an increase in oxygen content of at least 0.5 to 1.0 volumes per cent at the pulmonary arterial level, as compared with that of the right ventricle. Occasionally the catheter may pass from the pulmonary artery, through the ductus, into the aorta. The pressures in the right ventricle and pulmonary artery are usually within normal limits or only slightly elevated.

For reasons not completely clear, a typical ductus murmur is seldom if ever heard during the neonatal period. However, in most patients the typical machinery murmur is clearly noticeable by the end of the first or second year. The average patient is asymptomatic throughout childhood, but fatigue, dyspnea, and even congestive failure may occur in the second to fourth decades. This is obviously not a rule without exception, and many instances are known where a patent ductus arteriosus was compatible with a normally active life for fifty to sixty years. The major dangers for these patients are congestive failure and subacute bacterial endocarditis.

The treatment of choice for the patient with typical patent ductus arteriosus is surgery. Operation, consisting of ligation or division of the ductus, is recommended for every child between the age of two and twelve years who has a typical patent ductus arteriosus. It is somewhat more difficult to advise an adult in regard to operation. If the patient is not completely symptom-free, surgery is recommended without hesitation. If the individual is asymptomatic, and if all the clinical evidence points to a small ductus, one may refrain from advising operation.

The surgical mortality in patients with asymptomatic patent ductus, at a favorable age period, in the hands of a competent surgical team, should not be more than 1 per cent. In a study of over 700 cases operated on by Gross it was found that 95 per cent had no other cardiac abnormalities. The other 5 per cent had small septal defects, bicuspid aortic or pulmonary valves, or mitral stenosis. One per cent of all cases had an aortic pulmonary window.

The results of surgery should be excellent. Patients are restored to perfectly normal health. Subsequent bacterial endocarditis is extremely rare. Gross had one case which occurred early in his work after the ductus had been ligated and had recannulized, and another which developed seven years after operation was cured by antibiotics. Should a patient present himself with the problem of bacterial endocarditis and patent ductus the infection should be treated first with appropriate antibiotics and two or three months later operation can be performed. If the infection cannot be readily controlled by medication or if the situation is otherwise urgent, operation can still be performed without undue risk. In fact surgery alone was curative in the early days before penicillin was discovered.

ATYPICAL PATENT DUCTUS ARTERIOSUS (Patent Ductus Arteriosus with Pulmonary Hypertension).   The pulmonary arterial and the right ventricular pressure in patients with typical patent ductus arteriosus are elevated only slightly or not at all. There is, however, a small group of individuals—many of them infants—in whom a patent ductus arteriosus is accompanied by appreciable pulmonary hypertension. This clearly changes the pressure relationship between the two circuits and thus alters the clinical profile of the condition, based on a continuous flow of blood in the left-to-right direction. The majority of these individuals have moderate or severe symptoms—dyspnea, fatigue, or spells of cyanosis.

On physical examination they seem poorly nourished. Frank cyanosis and even clubbing may be present in 15 per cent of the patients. Sometimes this is more marked in the left hand and in the feet than it is in the right hand. The cardiac impulse is usually maximal at the xiphoid process, suggesting right ventricular enlargement. Left chest prominence is common. The pulse pressure may or may not be widened. At auscultation the second left interspace murmur is not as typically machinery-like as it is in patients with patent ductus arteriosus who do not have pulmonary hypertension. Either the crescendic element of the systolic component is missing, or the diastolic element is shorter or even absent. In a few patients only a faint systolic murmur can be heard at the second left interspace. The pulmonary closure is always booming.

Roentgenologic examination always shows some enlargement of the right ventricle and the pulmonary artery, with or without left ventricular enlargement. The pulmonary vasculature, particularly in the middle third of the lung field, is engorged, with or without hilar dance.

The electrocardiogram shows right ventricular hypertrophy and incomplete right bundle branch block, with or without left ventricular hypertrophy.

Cardiac catheterization reveals an increase in the oxygen content in the pulmonary artery of at least 0.5 volume per cent, compared with the right ventricle. Moderate or severe pulmonary arterial hypertension is present, due either to a tremendous flow through the ductus or to pulmonary vascular disease. Arterial unsaturation in the femoral arterial sample may be noted; if this is present and the right brachial arterial sample is fully saturated, the diagnosis of a "reversed ductus" (with blood flowing from pulmonary artery to aorta) may be made without hesitation. Under these circumstances the lower part of the body may be cyanotic while the upper part is not.

Pulmonary arterial hypertension may well develop in later adulthood in patients who in their early years had a perfectly "typical" patent ductus arteriosus; this is presumably the end result of the wear and tear on the pulmonary vessels, due to the large pulmonary flow through the years. In other instances, however, the ductus is "atypical" from early childhood; thus, one must assume that these children are born with pulmonary hypertension due either to an unusually large pulmonary flow or to congenital pulmonary vascular changes.

The adult in whom pulmonary vascular changes and, later, pulmonary hypertension develop probably is in a pretty difficult situation. Even assuming that he survives an operation on the duct, it is doubtful that the pulmonary vascular changes are reversible. Furthermore, the operative risk in these individuals is nearer the 25 to 50 per cent range than to the 1 per cent range quoted for asymptomatic patients with typical patent ductus.

The infant or child whose pulmonary hypertension is based primarily on congenital pulmonary vascular obstruction faces almost the same dilemma as the adult with a similar situation.

The infant or child whose pulmonary hypertension is based on a tremendous left-to-right shunt through the ductus is in a much better situation. Operation, at a somewhat increased risk (about 10 per cent), may result in complete elimination of the pulmonary hypertension and restoration of a normal circulation.

Because of these considerations, I believe that patients with patent ductus arteriosus—children or adults—who have a large left-to-right shunt should be operated on even when appreciable pulmonary hypertension is present. Conversely, surgery is not recommended for patients with patent ductus arteriosus and pulmonary hypertension who do not have an appreciable left-to-right shunt or in whom the shunt through the ductus is predominantly in the right-to-left direction.

AORTICOPULMONARY FENESTRATION. A rare anomaly, to be mentioned only briefly, is aorticopulmonary fenestration, or aortic septal defect. Embryologically, this is caused by incomplete division of the bulbus cordis. The result is a defect situated immediately above the semilunar valves and connecting the aorta with the pulmonary artery. The proximity of the lesion to the valves and the coronary arteries makes surgical closure extremely difficult or even impossible.

The physiologic consequences and the clinical profile are practically indistinguishable from those of atypical patent ductus arteriosus. The only clinical clue in the differential diagnosis is that the continuous murmur is usually maximal at the lower left sternal border rather than at the second left interspace.

The prognosis of these patients is guarded—operation should be attempted if possible, with full awareness of the high risk involved.

PERSISTENT TRUNCUS ARTERIOSUS. Complete failure of the bulbar ridges to develop results in the persistence of the fetal common arterial trunk; the pulmonary artery and the aorta form a common vessel separated from the ventricular chamber by two to four semilunar valves. Thus, invariably, a high, large ventricular defect—or even absent septum—is associated with this anomaly.

Physiologically, the principal feature of the common truncus arteriosus is that the entire circulation is supplied with blood from the same source, with identical pressure and having the same oxygen content. Whereas in the majority of instances the aorta and the coronary arteries are functionally adequate, the pulmonary arteries may or may not be of satisfactory size. If the pulmonary arteries are hypoplastic, pulmonary blood flow and pulmonary venous return are small and the patient has severe arterial unsaturation. Conversely, if the pulmonary arteries are normal in size, cyanosis is barely evident.

The clinical picture varies tremendously, depending on the size of the pulmonary blood flow. On the whole, these patients are sick infants, with congestive failure and some cyanosis. The only characteristic auscultatory feature—not consistently present—is a continuous machinery murmur heard over the left and right sides of the chest, both anteriorly and posteriorly. Such a murmur associated with cyanosis, an electrocardiogram showing right ventricular hypertrophy, and a radiogram revealing a large supracardiac shadow with absent main pulmonary artery segment should immediately raise the suspicion of common truncus arteriosus.

Most patients with this condition die in infancy; however, some live through adolescence, and even early adulthood.

No treatment is presently available for these individuals.

THE RIGHT-TO-LEFT SHUNT GROUP

The principal abnormality in this group of defects is also the presence of a communication between the systemic and pulmonary circuits, but, in contrast to the left-to-right shunt group, this abnormality is associated with a second anomaly resulting in higher than normal pressure in some or all of the compartments of the right side of the circulation. This arrangement results in the shunting of blood from right to left, causing arterial unsaturation. As mentioned previously, an initially left-to-right shunt may become temporarily or permanently a right-to-left shunt (atrial septal defect, ventricular septal defect, or patent ductus arteriosus); the conditions to be discussed here, however, are associated with dominantly right-to-left shunt throughout their natural course.

As a whole, this group is characterized by one or more of the following features: (1) cyanosis, (2) clubbing, (3) squatting, (4) anoxic spells, (5) absence of apical diastolic rumble, and (6) absence of hyperdynamic impulse.

Tetralogy of Fallot. Anatomically the tetralogy of Fallot consists of four principal features: (1) pulmonary stenosis or atresia, (2) dextroposition of the aorta, (3) ventricular septal defect, and (4) right ventricular hypertrophy. The stenosis is usually infundibular, although various authors have described the occurrence of valvular stenosis in a minority of their patients. The degree of dextroposition—or overriding—of the aorta is difficult to determine accurately; as a matter of fact, because of the nature and position of the ventricular septal defect, a certain amount of overriding is inherent in the defect itself. The degree of right ventricular hypertrophy depends on the severity of the pulmonary stenosis.

Physiologically this syndrome may be defined as consisting of pulmonary stenosis with a ventricular septal defect and a right-to-left shunt. Two principal handicaps result from these physiologic facts: (1) central cyanosis, and (2) limited pulmonary blood flow, resulting in more or less exertional dyspnea.

Most patients with the tetralogy of Fallot show evidences of dyspnea, cyanosis, and squatting. In infancy and childhood they may be subject to attacks of unconsciousness and convulsions (anoxic spells).

At physical examination one is impressed by the cyanosis and clubbing. The cardiac impulse is heaving and maximal at the xiphoid process. A thrill at the mid or lower left sternal border is noted in more than half of the patients. The second sound is almost invariably single and diminished at the pulmonary area; a normal or even accentuated second sound is heard at the lower left sternal border. A stenotic systolic murmur, grade 3 to 4 in intensity, is usually heard at the lower left sternal border. In general those with the loudest murmurs have the least cyanosis and are less likely to be incapacitated. But older individuals who have no cyanosis, who are in fairly good health, and who have no murmurs do not have tetralogy of Fallot. A minority of the patients, with the severest degree of pulmonary stenosis, may have no significant systolic murmur at all, but a vague continuous murmur originating from the extensive bronchial collaterals may be heard at any point over the chest.

The roentgenologic picture is characterized by a relatively normal-sized heart with a coeur en sabot (or sheep's nose) contour. The main pulmonary arterial segment is absent or hypoplastic, and the pulmonary vasculature is diminished. The aortic arch is on the right side in 25 per cent of the patients.

The electrocardiogram shows moderate or marked right ventricular hypertrophy, with varying degrees of P pulmonale.

Cardiac catheterization reveals a pressure drop when the pulmonary artery is entered from the right ventricle. The right ventricular systolic pressure is practically identical with systemic arterial pressure. Arterial unsaturation of varying degrees, and exaggerated by exercise, is noted.

Patients with the severest type of disease show deep cyanosis at birth or shortly thereafter. Many of these infants die in spells of unconsciousness before they reach their first birthday. Individuals with slightly less severe pulmonary stenosis become noticeably cyanotic during the first few months of life; the anoxic spells (unconsciousness) in these patients are not as severe or as numerous as those noted in the patients with the severest disease. When they learn to walk, dyspnea on exertion and squatting are noted; when they reach school age, their difficulties increase—they can walk barely one or two blocks and cannot play with their contemporaries. Without surgical assistance, death occurs in the teens or twenties from inadequate oxygen supply, cerebrovascular accident, or subacute bacterial endocarditis. A third group of patients—no more than 10 to 15 per cent of the total—may not show symptoms until they are one or two years old. These patients never have anoxic spells, but suffer from gradually increasing exertional dyspnea and cyanosis; they may not show the classic picture of tetralogy of Fallot until they are nearly ten years old. In these individuals life expectancy, without operation, may be placed at 20 to 30 years, although individual instances of longevity have been noted in the literature. It may be worth emphasizing that congestive failure practically never occurs in children with tetralogy of Fallot.

Among the complications of the tetralogy of Fallot syndrome, one should mention brain abscess. This diagnosis should be thought of and the help of a neurosurgical consultant should be sought immediately if a patient with tetralogy of Fallot exhibits signs and symptoms pointing to the central nervous system. Headaches, vomiting, or personality changes are the commonest presenting symptoms. Papilledema, as well as changes in the motor and sensory spheres, may be noted. The electroencephalogram may indicate a localizing lesion. Hemiplegia without any evidence of a space-occupying lesion is probably due to profound anoxia or cerebral thrombosis.

Medical management of patients with the tetralogy of Fallot is extremely important and may be of considerable assistance. The hematologic status deserves careful attention. Patients with hematocrit levels higher than 85 per cent should be considered for venesection. Individuals with hypochromic anemia, even when the erythrocyte level is high, should be given iron. Anoxic spells may be combated by the administration of morphine (1 mg. per 5 kg. of body weight) or by inhalation of 100 per cent oxygen. Antibiotics should be given prophylactically as well as therapeutically, according to the principles outlined earlier. Perhaps most important of all, one should give emotional support to these patients and encourage them to live the fullest life possible within their limitations.

The optimum time for operation is between the age of five to ten years. The operative approach to the tetralogy of Fallot is twofold. One group of procedures aims at symptomatic relief and does not attack with finality the underlying structural abnormality. Among these palliative procedures three should be mentioned: (1) The Blalock-Taussig procedure increases the effective pulmonary blood flow by establishing a shunt from the subclavian artery into the low pressure pulmonary artery. (2) The Potts procedure accomplishes the same purpose by establishing a direct connection between the aorta and the pulmonary artery. (3) The Brock procedure increases the pulmonary blood flow by opening up the right ventricular outflow tract directly through a transventricular incision. The ventricular septal defect, however, is not corrected.

A totally different approach—one of complete correction of the pulmonary stenosis and the ventricular septal defect by open heart surgery—has been advocated within the past year by Lillehei and his associates at the University of Minnesota and by the Mayo Clinic group. This procedure poses considerable technical difficulties and involves the use of cross circulation or a pump oxygenator.

Unquestionably the desired result is the complete correction of the defect; thus the second group of procedures should be advocated when they become safe enough. At present, however, the mortality is still within the 25 per cent range; also, there is some question about the ability to completely close the ventricular septal defect in all cases. In short, then, this is the operation of the future, but not necessarily of the present.

In view of the near perfection of the open heart approach to this problem, is one justified in recommending a palliative procedure? In my experience, the symptomatic operation should be advocated only if the individual really needs it and needs it immediately. As an example, one can cite the small baby whose life is threatened by severe anoxic spells or the youngster who cannot go to school because of his disabling exertional dyspnea or socially embarrassing squatting. I do not believe it is wise or humane to withhold palliative surgery from these patients and impose several years of suffering on them until the perfect operation is available. This is particularly true since the palliative surgery gives excellent symptomatic relief for at least ten years at a mortality risk of 8 per cent or less. Which of the shunt procedures (the Blalock or the Potts) should be employed depends on the preference of the individual surgeon; both have their advantages and disadvantages, and both give excellent results in about 90 per cent of the survivors.

In my opinion—not shared by everyone—the Brock procedure, at present, offers less advantages than any of the shunt operations. The mortality is definitely higher, the postoperative complications are more harassing, and perhaps the future approach to a ventricle once incised may be more difficult.

One of the beneficial results after a successful operation is that the erythrocyte count and hematocrit value decrease toward normal. In fact, this change to a large extent is a guide to the efficacy of the operation and goes hand in hand with the more obvious general improvement of the patient. Occasionally bacterial endocarditis may develop some time after an operation such as the Blalock procedure. Fortunately this complication can then be cured medically.

Tricuspid Atresia. No direct communication between the right ventricle and right atrium exists in patients with tricuspid atresia. The right atrial blood is shunted through a foramen ovale or an atrial septal defect into the left atrium, where complete mixture with the pulmonary venous blood occurs. Consequently, the right ventricular cavity is hypoplastic in most instances; it either receives no blood at all or only a very small amount through a ventricular septal defect from the left ventricle. The pulmonary blood flow is obviously considerably diminished. If the ventricular septum is intact and there is no opening between the right atrium and right ventricle, a small amount of blood may still reach the lungs for oxygenation through small branches coming from the aorta to the bronchial arteries.

All these patients, from infancy on, are severely sick with cyanosis, dyspnea, anoxic spells, and even congestive failure.

At physical examination, marked underdevelopment and severe cyanosis with clubbing are noted. Hepatomegaly, occasionally with presystolic pulsation, is commonly present. The first and second sounds are loud and *single* at the lower left sternal border; pulmonary closure is diminished. A grade 3 to 4 systolic murmur at the left lower sternal border is present in most, but certainly not all, of the patients.

The roentgenologic findings vary considerably. In some cases the picture cannot be distinguished from that of tetralogy of Fallot; in other instances, a dextrocardia-like image is presented; in still others, the right border in the posteroanterior view and the anterior border in the left anterior oblique are sharply cut. The pulmonary vasculature is almost invariably diminished.

The characteristic electrocardiogram shows left axis deviation with left ventricular hypertrophy and marked P pulmonale.

At cardiac catheterization, the catheter fails to enter the right ventricle. It commonly passes from the right atrium to the left atrium. The right atrial pressure is higher than the left atrial pressure; the left atrial oxygen content is identical with the systemic arterial oxygen content and shows definite arterial unsaturation.

Seldom do these individuals survive the first year of life, but instances of survival through the first and second decades have been reported. The cause of death is either anoxia or congestive failure.

Medical management offers little but temporary symptomatic relief to these children. Those who survive the first year of life may be benefited by a Potts or Blalock procedure, although the risks are high (at least 25 per cent), and the results in the survivors are not nearly as satisfactory as they are for patients with tetralogy of Fallot.

Single Ventricle.   See pages 233–234.

Persistent Truncus Arteriosus.   See pages 237–238.

Eisenmenger's Complex.   See Large Ventricular Septal Defect, pages 232–233.

Complete Transposition of the Great Arteries.   If the aorta originates from the right ventricle and the pulmonary artery from the left, complete transposition of the great arteries is present. This results in two separate circulations—systemic and pulmonary—without obligatory admixture of venous and oxygenated blood. Survival is possible only if there is some means of communication between the two circuits to insure the entry of oxygenated pulmonary venous blood into the systemic circulation. A persistence of the fetal pathways—foramen ovale and ductus arteriosus—usually serves this purpose, although additional communications in the form of ventricular septal defects or atrial septal defects may also be present. The origin of the aorta from the right ventricle is commonly unobstructed, whereas pulmonary stenosis is present in a sizable percentage of cases.

Most of these patients are sick from birth. Deep cyanosis, poor development, dyspnea, and congestive failure dominate the picture.

Physical examination usually reveals severe cyanosis, a large heart, and congestive failure. The pulmonary second sound is commonly absent. In approximately a third of the patients, no significant murmurs are heard. In the others, a grade 2 to 4 systolic murmur is heard at the lower left sternal border.

The roentgenologic picture is strikingly abnormal in all but the youngest infants. There is usually diffuse cardiac enlargement, involving principally the right ventricle, with pulmonary plethora and absent main pulmonary artery segment. The supracardiac vascular shadow may be narrow in the posteroanterior view, but widens considerably if the patient is turned to the left anterior oblique position.

The electrocardiogram shows right ventricular hypertrophy, with a moderate degree of P pulmonale.

There are only a few detailed reports of cardiac catheterization in these severely sick infants. Typically, the catheter enters the aorta from the right ventricle, and the oxygen saturation of the blood in the pulmonary artery is higher than it is in the aorta.

The outlook for these patients is grim. Probably less than 10 per cent survive the first year.

No adequate medical or surgical treatment is available for these individuals. In selected patients who survive the first few years of life and in whom pulmonary stenosis is present, a combined operation consisting of a shunt procedure and enlargement of the atrial defect may be performed.

Complete Transposition of the Pulmonary Veins.   In complete transposition of the pulmonary veins, the pulmonary venous blood enters the right atrium; there it is mixed with the caval flow. In order for the individual to survive, some of this right atrial blood must be transferred from the right atrium to the left atrium (through a foramen ovale or atrial septal defect); hence, the discussion of this malformation is included among the right-to-left shunt group. This is in marked contrast to the patients with partial transposition of the pulmonary veins, where the shunt is exclusively or dominantly left to right, carrying oxygenated pulmonary venous blood into the right atrium. Almost invariably the pulmonary veins enter the right atrium by means of one common trunk; in more than 50 per cent of the patients this enters into the superior vena cava, in about 30 per cent into the coronary sinus or the right atrium directly.

Most of these youngsters are brought to the doctor with symptoms of dyspnea, fatigue, or congestive failure.

At physical examination, underdevelopment is noted. Cyanosis in these patients is usually slight, in contrast to the deep cyanosis of patients with transposition of the great arteries. Severe right-sided failure is evident in the majority of them. The cardiac impulse is usually heaving and maximal at the xiphoid process. A thrill is only rarely palpable. On auscultation, a triple or quadruple rhythm, giving the impression of a gallop without tachycardia, is commonly heard. Phonocardiographic analysis reveals the multiple rhythm to be composed of a late first sound, a well-split second sound, and a third or third and fourth sound. In most patients a systolic murmur is heard at the lower left sternal border. In addition, a diastolic murmur, in the form of a mid-diastolic–presystolic rumble or even a continuous venous hum, is commonly observed.

The roentgenologic picture is pathognomonic in the individuals whose anomalous veins enter the superior vena cava; here a large supracardiac shadow is observed, giving the cardiac silhouette a "figure-of-8" appearance. If the pulmonary veins enter elsewhere on the right side of the heart, the picture is not nearly as characteristic and consists only of marked right-sided enlargement and pulmonary plethora.

The electrocardiogram shows marked right ventricular hypertrophy. P pulmonale of a severe degree, comparable only to that found in tricuspid atresia, Ebstein's disease, and severe isolated pulmonary stenosis, is the rule.

Cardiac catheterization reveals the oxygen content to be the same in the blood from the right atrium, left atrium, aorta, and pulmonary artery. Pulmonary arterial pressure may show some elevation. A mild degree of arterial unsaturation is present.

Probably 80 per cent of these patients die before the end of the first year of life. In spite of this, greater familiarity with the syndrome has uncovered an increasing number of individuals in their teens and twenties who have this anomaly with only mild limitations.

Medical treatment of congestive failure often improves these patients significantly for a matter of months. Surgical treatment, performed infrequently, and then only in patients who live beyond infancy, may proceed along two general lines. One approach approximates the common pulmonary venous trunk to the left atrium and establishes an anastomosis. The other technique, using open heart surgery, shifts the atrial septum in such a way that the veins enter the left atrium. No clear-cut indications for these operations have been worked out, and the mortality figures are not known. It is probably safe to say, however, that surgery is dangerous and difficult, to be advocated only because of the generally hopeless prognosis of the anomaly.

Coarctation of the Aorta.   Coarctation is a narrowing of the lumen of the aorta, usually situated beyond the origin of the left subclavian artery, at the insertion of the ligamentum arteriosum.

The principal physiologic problem in coarctation of the aorta is to insure adequate blood flow and pressure in the part of the vascular system beyond the coarctation. This is achieved by one or more of three mechanisms: (1) elevation of the left ventricular pressure; (2) by-passing the coarctation by means of collaterals; or (3) by-passing the coarctation by a patent ductus arteriosus conducting blood from the pulmonary artery to the aorta. In a simple or "adult" type, mechanisms 1 and 2 are operative. In the so-called "fetal type," a combination of 1 and 3 is observed; this anomaly is also referred to as coarctation of the aorta with systemic left and right ventricle, since the upper half of the body is supplied by the left ventricle and the lower half receives blood from the right ventricle through the pulmonary artery and the ductus arteriosus. The adult type of coarctation usually represents a sudden narrowing of the aortic arch, whereas in the fetal or preductal type the coarctation commonly involves a rather long segment.

Most children with simple coarctation of the aorta are completely asymptomatic and the condition may be first suspected when the school physician tries to account for the hypertension found on routine physical examination. In contrast, all patients with "fetal" coarctation are seriously sick, with cyanosis, dyspnea, and congestive failure in infancy. A small number, certainly less than 10 per cent, of the patients with simple coarctation may also go into cardiac failure in infancy. Some of the adults complain of fatigue or aches in the legs on effort. Others may have pain in the mid-back from aneurysmal dilation of the aorta and intercostal arteries beyond the constriction.

On physical examination these patients (usually males) are found to be well developed and well nourished. A thrill may be palpable at the suprasternal notch and the second right interspace. The cardiac impulse is maximal at the apex and is heaving. With the patient leaning forward, the tortuous intercostal arteries may be palpated over the back. The radial pulses, especially the right, are powerful. The femoral pulses are either absent or weak and are always asynchronous with the radial pulses. Blood pressure determination always reveals a relative, but not necessarily an absolute, hypertension of the upper extremities. In other words, the systolic pressure in the arms may not be but generally is elevated, but it is always higher than that in the legs, whereas normally the reverse is true. The second sound in the aortic area is loud. In the majority of cases a stenotic systolic murmur is heard at the second left or right interspace, the neck, and, sometimes loudest, over the back. A continuous murmur originating from the collaterals may be heard over the second right or second left interspace, or the back. Occasionally there may be an early diastolic blow at the lower left sternal border or a mid-diastolic rumble at the apex.

There is a very small group of cases in which rupture of the aorta may occur during pregnancy when coarctation of the aorta is present. This may be associated with only a very minimal degree of hypertension, i.e. a systolic level of 140 mm. There is some relationship between the pregnant state and the tendency of the aorta to rupture.

The patients with "fetal" coarctation do not present the classic picture just described. They are usually small infants in severe failure whose only distinguishing feature may be the presence of hypertension of the arms or the particular pattern of cyanosis, involving the lower half of the body and perhaps the left arm.

In adult practice the diagnosis of coarctation will frequently be overlooked unless the physician develops the habit of deliberately palpating the femoral arteries in all patients and particularly in any one who has hypertension, even if the blood pressure in the arms is only slightly elevated. This is especially imperative if there is a slight systolic murmur in the pulmonary area. If the femoral arterial pulsations are vigorous one can fairly safely dismiss the diagnosis of coarctation. If these pulsations are feeble or absent, pulsations of the abdominal aorta should be sought for. Occasionally the femoral pulses are difficult to feel, especially in obese individuals, when the abdominal aorta pulsates normally. If the femoral pulsations are decreased the blood pressure of the legs should be determined. If these readings are lower than those of the arms, a presumptive diagnosis of coarctation of the aorta can be made and then the other features of the condition may be investigated. A simple "blanching test" is of interest. The time for the return of the normal pink color of the skin after firm pressure over the tip of one of the fingers and that of one of the toes is determined. It will be found to be very much greater in the toes than in the fingers in cases of coarctation, i.e., 4 to 8 seconds, compared with 2 to 3 seconds.

Roentgenologically, simple coarctation of the aorta is characterized by left ventricular enlargement with a small aortic knob. In severe cases, left atrial enlargement is noted. Scalloping of the ribs, due to erosion by collaterals, is usually seen in patients more than ten years of age. An E sign is observed on the barium-filled esophagus at fluoroscopy; the first arc of the E is the precoarctated part of the aorta, and the second arc is the post-stenotic dilatation. Patients with "fetal" coarctation show marked cardiac enlargement involving both the left and the right ventricle.

The electrocardiogram in the adult type of coarctation shows left ventricular hypertrophy of varying degrees. If right ventricular hypertrophy is present in a patient with suspected coarctation of the aorta, the anomaly is almost certainly of the fetal type.

Cardiac catheterization in the adult type reveals essentially normal cardiodynamics in the right side of the circulation. Clear-cut differences between the systolic pressure of the right brachial artery and that of the femoral artery will be noted, however. Patients with coarctation of the aorta and "systemic left and right ventricle" invariably show marked pulmonary arterial hypertension; occasionally the catheter may pass through a patent ductus arteriosus into the descending aorta, where the oxygen content is identical with that found in the pulmonary artery and lower than that in the right brachial artery. The term "systemic left and right ventricle" here connotes that in case of a ductus below the coarctation the right ventricle, as well as the left ventricle, is helping to maintain the pressure below the coarctation.

The course of patients with simple coarctation of the aorta—with the rare exception of those having congestive failure—is uneventful throughout childhood and adolescence. However, if operation is not performed, only 25 per cent of them can be expected to live beyond the fourth decade. The others die as a result of subacute bacterial endocarditis, ruptured aorta, or hypertensive cardiovascular disease. Most patients with the fetal type of coarctation die in congestive failure within the first weeks of life.

Patients with coarctation of the aorta should be treated surgically. The operation consists of wide excision of the narrowed segment and direct suturing of the two ends or interposition of an aortic graft. The operative risk in asymptomatic patients between ten and twelve years of age is less than 5 per cent in the hands of competent surgeons. Postoperatively, in 90 per cent of the patients the blood pressure in the arms returns to normal, and the femoral pulses become easily palpable. Infants with coarctation of the aorta who go into congestive failure should be treated medically (with digitalis and mercury) before operation. Practically all of those who have the adult type of coarctation respond favorably to this regimen, and surgery may be postponed until a more appropriate time. A few of these patients with the adult type of lesion and all of those with the fetal type fail to respond to medical management; for these patients, operation in infancy is advocated, with only slim hope of success. Surgery is almost always fatal in individuals with coarctation of the aorta with "systemic left and right ventricle," even if it is performed in older children who manifest no evidence of congestive failure.

The insertion of an aortic graft is necessary when the isthmus of the graft is long or when there is extensive thinning of the aneurysmal wall beyond the constriction. It is of interest that a follow-up study has revealed no instance of aneurysmal formation of the inserted grafts, although a few became calcified some months after operation. The latter change might possibly have been the result of the particular pH of the fluid in which the graft had been kept.

Aortic Stenosis. Although the principal etiologic factors in the causation of aortic stenosis in adults are probably rheumatic fever and arteriosclerosis, there is reason to assume that a certain percentage of the adults and the majority of the children with pure aortic stenosis have, in effect, congenital disease. In children the argument is based simply on the fact that arteriosclerosis does not occur at this age and that rheumatic fever almost never occurs in children less than three or four years of age, while aortic stenosis takes many years to develop. In adults with pure aortic stenosis, the principal argument in favor of a congenital lesion is the observation that a much smaller number of patients in this group have a history of rheumatic fever than is true if aortic stenosis is found in combination with aortic regurgitation or with involvement of the mitral valve.

Congenital aortic stenosis in children is rare. Nevertheless, about 70 patients with this disease have been seen at The Children's Medical Center in Boston in the past five years. What percentage of the adults with aortic stenosis and without a history of rheumatic fever have, in fact, a congenital anomaly, is hard to estimate, but I think it may well be a higher portion than has been believed heretofore.

Anatomically, the deformity may be divided into valvular and subvalvular types. In the valvular type, the cusps are fused to form a dome-shaped diaphragm. Subaortic stenosis, on the other hand, is caused by a fibrous ring encircling the left ventricular outflow tract, about 5 to 10 mm. below the aortic ring.

The clinical picture, including the physical examination, x-rays, and electrocardiograms, is barely distinguishable from that of acquired aortic stenosis. Males are more commonly affected than females. The characteristic harsh stenotic murmur is heard well at the second right interspace, the neck, and over the back. Often a loud systolic click is observed at the aortic area. The pulse pressure is normal or narrow. A wide ascending aorta may be observed on the x-ray film. Severe degrees of left ventricular hypertrophy with strain may be seen in young children, although many have normal electrocardiograms.

The physiologic data collected at right and left heart catheterization are similar to those described in acquired aortic stenosis. It is interesting to note that valve sizes of 0.05 to 0.2 sq.cm. are not uncommon in children and may be accompanied by left ventricular peak systolic pressures of more than 200 mm. of mercury.

Most patients with congenital aortic stenosis are asymptomatic throughout childhood and early adulthood. In rare instances, congestive failure, and even death, has occurred in infants with aortic stenosis; it may be assumed that a considerable amount of endocardial fibroelastosis was present in these cases of utmost severity.

Almost more disturbing than the death of an infant with fibroelastosis, aortic stenosis, and congestive failure are the not too rare instances when a completely asymptomatic, athletically built adolescent with aortic stenosis suddenly drops dead while playing basketball or riding a bicycle. This may occur with some frequency in the group of youngsters whose electrocardiograms show the severest type of left ventricular strain. It almost never happens if the electrocardiogram is normal or shows only moderate left ventricular hypertrophy.

The differentiation of valvular from subaortic stenosis is almost impossible by clinical means; there is some suggestion, however, that patients with the severest types of congenital aortic stenosis almost invariably have a valvular lesion.

In the management of patients with congenital aortic stenosis, it is fairly important to restrain them from severe competitive sports. Although they may pursue normal activities, it is wise to direct their interests to a way of life not dominated by physical competition. They should take part in sports only as long as they can stop without embarrassment if and when they feel fatigue. Interscholastic athletics should be forbidden.

Indications and techniques for surgical treatment of youngsters with congenital aortic stenosis have not yet been crystallized. However, only those patients with the severest degree of left ventricular hypertrophy, as shown on the electrocardiogram, should be considered for operation. Surgery should always be preceded by the most careful physiologic evaluation, including right and left heart catheterization.

In adults surgery for congenital aortic stenosis should be considered in the same light as surgery for the acquired lesion.

Vascular Rings. Vascular rings are congenital anomalies of the aortic arch and its tributaries causing varying degrees of compression of the trachea and the esophagus. This is almost exclusively a pediatric problem.

One part of the ring surrounding the trachea and the esophagus is always the arch of the aorta. The second component may be (1) a second aortic arch (double aortic arch), (2) left ligamentum arteriosum, (3) anomalous right subclavian artery, (4) anomalous innominate artery, or (5) anomalous left common carotid artery. The first one of these anomalies is the commonest; the latter two are comparatively rare.

The anomalous right subclavian artery usually causes no respiratory symptoms, but occasionally swallowing difficulty occurs; double aortic arch is one of the severest anomalies, causing dysphagia, cyanosis on feeding, and respiratory embarrassment in early infancy. The other defects cause principally respiratory symptoms.

The clinical picture consists of a great deal of wheezing and stridor; these babies often lie in opisthotonus. Feeding exaggerates the stridor and causes cyanosis; vomiting is frequent. The lungs may be full of crepitant rales. Physical examination, x-ray, and electrocardiography reveal no abnormality of the heart.

The encroachment of the vascular ring on the esophagus may be demonstrated by x-ray of the barium-filled esophagus: the compression of the trachea may be revealed by a tracheogram.

Operative relief of the obstruction is indicated if it causes symptoms. In patients who have double aortic arch, left ligamentum arteriosum, or anomalous right subclavian artery, this is accomplished by means of severing the appropriate vessel. In the case of anomalous innominate or left common carotid artery, the vessel is pulled to the side and anteriorly, and fastened to the chest wall.

Pulmonary Stenosis with Intact Ventricular Septum.   Variously described as "pure pulmonary stenosis" or "isolated pulmonary stenosis," this entity has been recognized with increasing frequency within the past ten years. Undoubtedly because of the clear-cut definition of the clinical profile, or on the basis of cardiac catheterization data, this anomaly is recognized today as one of the most frequent ones encountered, whereas in 1945 Currens and his associates were able to collect only eleven examples of the disease. One wonders under what diagnoses these anomalies were classified before the introduction of cardiac catheterization. Probably most of them were diagnosed as small atrial or small ventricular defect.

Approximately 4 of 5 patients with isolated pulmonary stenosis have a valvular lesion; the stenosis in the rest of them is subvalvular, with the formation of an infundibular chamber. The pulmonary artery, when the lesion is valvular, is dilated and thin. The foramen ovale may or may not be patent; the ventricular septum is intact.

The principal physiologic consequence of pulmonary stenosis is that the right ventricle must exert a higher than normal systolic pressure in order to produce the pulmonary flow necessary for any given situation. Since the ventricular septum is intact, the right ventricle is able to produce pressures, if necessary, in excess of the systemic pressure. This is in marked contrast to the situation in tetralogy of Fallot, in which the right ventricular pressure can never exceed systemic pressure. In other words, adequate pulmonary flow can be established in most patients with pulmonary stenosis and intact ventricular septum, but sometimes it is accomplished at the price of a very high right ventricular pressure. Corresponding to the high right ventricular pressure seen in some, but by no means in all, individuals with isolated pulmonary stenosis is the elevated right atrial pressure which may result in a right-to-left shunt through a foramen ovale.

The clinical picture varies with the severity of the stenosis. Approximately a third of the patients are asymptomatic; the others show varying degrees of dyspnea, fatigue, and even cyanosis. The murmur is usually discovered in early infancy.

On physical examination, the patients are well developed and well nourished with only slight if any cyanosis. A thrill is frequently palpable at the second left interspace; the cardiac impulse is maximal at the xiphoid process. A stenotic, grade 3 to 5 systolic murmur is heard at the second left interspace. A systolic click, much like that heard in aortic stenosis, may be heard at the pulmonary area. The second sound in the pulmonary area is generally decreased. An atrial sound may be audible at the apex in patients having the severest degree of pulmonary stenosis with marked right atrial hypertrophy. Evidences of congestive failure, including an enlarged liver with presystolic pulsations, are seen only in individuals with the severest disease.

Roentgenologically, slight or moderate right ventricular enlargement, with a dilated pulmonary artery segment and diminished pulmonary vasculature, is seen. Marked cardiac enlargement is rare, and indicates extremely severe stenosis with failure.

The electrocardiogram reveals right ventricular hypertrophy in all patients with moderate or severe pulmonary stenosis. One or more of the following electrocardiographic features indicate a right ventricular systolic pressure higher than 100 mm. of mercury: (1) RV_1 of more than 20 mm., (2) P pulmonale of more than 3.5 mm., or (3) definite right ventricular strain pattern in leads V_1 to V_4.

Cardiac catheterization reveals right ventricular hypertension with a gradient across the pulmonary valve. The pressure in the right ventricle may vary from 50 to as much as 220 mm. of mercury, whereas pressure in the pulmonary artery is only 10 to 30 mm. In patients with valvular stenosis, the transition from the low pressure pulmonary artery to the high pressure right ventricle occurs within one cardiac cycle. Arterial unsaturation of mild degree is seen in patients with severe stenosis and is due to the right-to-left shunt through the foramen ovale.

The course of the disease depends on the severity of the stenosis. Infants with pinpoint pulmonary orifices may die in congestive failure within the first few months of life. Conversely, patients with only mild stenosis may live a normal life for a long time. In between these two extremes, all shades of severity may be found.

All patients with pulmonary stenosis and intact ventricular septum who show symptoms and whose right ventricular pressure is at least 100 mm. of mercury should be treated surgically. Whether asymptomatic individuals with high pressure should be operated on, and, if so, when, is a much harder problem to decide. If the heart shows progressive enlargement one is more inclined to advise surgery. My own belief is that probably all individuals with right ventricular pressures of 100 to 150 mm. of mercury probably will need surgery at some time. In this instance the Brock transventricular approach to the pulmonary valve is practiced, with good results in most instances, at a mortality risk of considerably less than 5 per cent in patients without congestive failure. In the presence of decompensation, the risks are much higher. In other centers, open heart surgery by means of hypothermia or a pump oxygenator is recommended; the relief of the stenosis by these methods is more complete, but it introduces a number of new operative hazards.

The Pulmonary Vascular Obstruction Syndrome. Significant elevation of the pulmonary arterial pressure may be the result of either a marked increase in pulmonary blood flow or a significant increase in pulmonary arteriolar resistance, with normal or even diminished pulmonary blood flow. In the pulmonary vascular obstruction syndrome, the pulmonary arterial systolic pressure is elevated to levels closely approximating the systemic arterial pressure, because of a marked increase in pulmonary vascular resistance. The syndrome, thus defined, may be associated with intrinsic congenital heart disease (ventricular septal defect, patent ductus arteriosus, or atrial septal defect) or may be present as so-called "primary pulmonary hypertension," without structural abnormality of the heart. Not included in the syndrome are instances where the increase in pulmonary resistance is clearly secondary to parenchymatous pulmonary disease, kyphoscoliosis, or mitral stenosis.

The small or medium-sized arterioles of the lung are the site of maximal involvement, showing varying degrees of intimal and medial thickening, plaques, and thrombi.

The clinical picture of the pulmonary vascular obstruction syndrome is well defined and essentially homogeneous, regardless of whether it is associated with congenital heart disease or not. The symptoms vary from the mildest degree of exertional dyspnea to severe incapacity, cyanosis, hemoptysis, syncope, and chest pain.

On physical examination, mild cyanosis and clubbing are noted. A powerful xiphoid impulse is palpable. At auscultation the most striking finding is the presence of a booming, relatively narrow pulmonary second sound; systolic murmurs of grade 2 to 3 intensity may be heard at the left sternal border. Individuals with maximal pulmonary vascular obstruction show an early diastolic blow at the lower left sternal border.

The roentgenologic picture is characterized by mild or moderate right ventricular enlargement, a prominent main pulmonary artery, and diminished peripheral pulmonary vasculature, commonly contrasting with the increased hilar markings.

The electrocardiogram shows varying degrees of right ventricular hypertrophy with P pulmonale.

Cardiac catheterization reveals elevated pulmonary arterial and right ventricular pressures with moderate or mild arterial unsaturation.

The course and prognosis in these individuals varies a great deal. There is reasonably good evidence to suggest that pulmonary vascular obstruction may exist in some patients from early infancy to early adulthood and may be compatible with a reasonably normal life. In others, signs and symptoms begin in the twenties or thirties and may lead to death within two or three years. It is worth remembering that chest pain and syncope are particularly ominous prognostic symptoms. I have the distinct impression that patients whose pulmonary vascular obstruction is associated with intrinsic congenital heart disease may have a longer life expectancy after the development of the vascular changes than do individuals with "essential pulmonary hypertension." One further point to be emphasized is the general "brittleness" of these individuals; they represent increased risks for any procedures, i.e., for cardiac catheterization, angiography, or even anesthesia.

Unfortunately, no treatment for this syndrome exists today. A number of palliative measures (Dicumarol, antispasmodics, or inhalation of 100 per cent oxygen) have been suggested without good evidence of success. The avoidance of fatigue and prevention of respiratory infections are about as much as can be done. If an operable congenital cardiac defect is associated with this syndrome, surgery is advocated only if a sizable left-to-right shunt still exists; even under these circumstances, the operative hazard probably increases five- or tenfold.

Ebstein's Anomaly.   The downward displacement of the posterior, and frequently of the septal, leaflet of the tricuspid valve is known as Ebstein's anomaly. This anatomic situation results in the upper part of the right ventricle being incorporated into the right atrium. Thus, the portion of the right side of the heart above the apex of the tricuspid valve is huge, while the true right ventricular cavity is small and consists only of the outflow tract. The walls of the atrial cavity are thin and flabby; the infundibulum is thick and narrow. The tricuspid valve is usually incompetent, and the foramen ovale is patent.

Symptoms consist of varying degrees of cyanosis, dyspnea, fatigue, and right-sided failure. Attacks of paroxysmal tachycardia may occur.

At physical examination, mild cyanosis and clubbing are noted. The cardiac impulse is diffuse and feeble. At auscultation one is impressed by a triple or quadruple rhythm, similar to that heard in complete transposition of the pulmonary veins. Pulmonary closure is diminished. A grade 3 systolic murmur is heard at the lower left sternal border and a mid-diastolic–presystolic rumble is present at the apex.

The roentgenograms show marked cardiac enlargement. The silhouette in the posteroanterior view simulates that of a pericardial effusion or pure pulmonary stenosis with failure. The enlargement involves principally the right atrium; the pulmonary vasculature is diminished.

The electrocardiogram in the typical case reveals incomplete or complete right bundle branch block without right ventricular hypertrophy. The P-R interval may be prolonged and arrhythmias may be demonstrated.

Cardiac catheterization, because of the tendency to arrhythmias, is more than usually dangerous in these people. The sparse data in the literature reveal mild arterial unsaturation and high right atrial pressure, with evidence of tricuspid regurgitation. The pressure tracings in the right ventricle and the right atrium are often almost indistinguishable in contour.

The prognosis of patients with Ebstein's anomaly is poor. Symptoms commonly start in infancy and childhood, but occasionally they do not manifest themselves until much later. Death in congestive failure usually occurs in the second or third decade.

Only symptomatic medical treatment is available.

Anomalous Origin of the Left Coronary Artery.   If the left coronary artery originates from the pulmonary artery rather than from the aorta, owing to anomalous division of the common arterial trunk in the embryo, evidences of coronary insufficiency may be noted in infancy. This is a most uncommon condition, less than fifty cases being described in the literature so far.

Symptoms usually begin between the second and sixth months of life and consist of episodes of pallor, cyanosis, colicky pain, tachycardia, tachypnea, and perspiration. These spells tend to occur at feeding time and last for only a few minutes. Between attacks the baby is relatively well, although obviously underdeveloped. Congestive failure is rare.

Roentgenological examination reveals nonspecific cardiac enlargement. Auscultatory findings are also non-contributory; in fact, it is rather striking to note a very large heart without a murmur. The electrocardiogram may be the most significantly abnormal finding; it commonly shows the typical pattern of anterior myocardial infarction with ST and T wave changes in the limb leads and a QS pattern in the left chest leads.

No effective treatment is available at present, although operative attempts at transplantation of the coronary artery have been proposed.

DEXTROCARDIA

In dextrocardia, the heart is in the right chest cavity, with its apex pointing to the right. There seems to be general agreement that dextrocardia not accompanied by transposition of the abdominal viscera is, as a rule, associated with severe malformations of the heart. There is no unanimity of opinion, however, in regard to the frequency of associated anomalies in cases of dextrocardia with abdominal situs inversus. It probably can be stated that in the latter situation a structurally normal heart may frequently be present.

In cases of "mirror-image" dextrocardia, with a structurally normal heart and transposition of the abdominal viscera, no symptoms referable to the cardiovascular system are present. However, bronchiectasis may be associated with the anomaly (Kartagener's syndrome). Palpation of the apex beat may be the best way to discover dextrocardia at physical examination, although the faintness of the heart sounds in the left side of the chest may raise suspicion of its presence. Cardiac fluoroscopy and electrocardiography are the only conclusive evidences on which to base the diagnosis of dextrocardia. The electrocardiogram shows inverted P and T waves in Lead I, with upright P and T in aVR.

Patients with "isolated" dextrocardia, without abdominal situs inversus, and almost invariably with congenital heart disease, are usually sick children. The associated anomaly usually involves defects in septation, transposition of the great arteries, or pulmonary stenosis; the aortic arch is frequently on the left side. The most common lesions associated with "isolated" dextrocardia are: single ventricle with pulmonary stenosis, persistent truncus arteriosus, and transposition of the great arteries. The nature of the congenital heart disease is almost impossible to diagnose clinically, even with extensive catheterization and angiographic studies.

The prognosis and treatment of dextrocardia depend on the presence and nature of the associated anomaly.

Miscellaneous Lesions

GLYCOGEN STORAGE DISEASE OF THE HEART

Glycogen storage disease of the heart is a rare condition, not more than forty cases having been reported altogether. It is almost exclusively a disease of young infants. Familial occurrence is noted; it is usually seen in children of the same sex within one family.

The principal histochemical abnormality is the presence of unusually large glycogen deposits in the heart and the skeletal muscles. It should be emphasized that, in contrast to the hepatic form of the disease, the glycogen content of the liver is not significantly increased. The two conditions are not known to occur simultaneously.

Clinically these infants appear wasted, pale, and slightly cyanotic; dyspnea is occasionally noted. The heart is tremendously enlarged, causing signs and symptoms of pulmonary compression. By striking contrast, evidences of congestive failure are rare. If they occur, they do so only terminally. The heart sounds are "muffled," and murmurs are absent.

Roentgenologically diffuse cardiac enlargement is noted. The electrocardiogram reveals evidences of left ventricular hypertrophy with ST and T wave changes. Results of clinical laboratory tests aiming at evaluating the carbohydrate metabolism, glucose tolerance, Adrenalin tolerance, etc., are usually within normal limits.

No treatment is available. Sudden death, probably due to arrhythmia, usually occurs before one year of age.

ENDOCARDIAL FIBROELASTOSIS

Endocardial fibroelastosis is a relatively common cause of congestive failure in infants and children, but occasionally it has also been reported in adults. There is some evidence to the effect that, although the cases occurring in the very young may be "primary," i.e. developmental in nature, those encountered in adults may be "secondary" to myocardial disease, coronary insufficiency, or metabolic defect.

The characteristic histologic finding is the presence of a thick subendocardial accumulation of elastic fibers, much like the finding in "collagen disease." The most common localization of accumulation is under the parietal endocardium of the left atrium and left ventricle, giving these structures a "milky" appearance at autopsy. Frequently there is additional involvement of the mitral and/or the aortic valve in the process, giving rise to functionally significant stenosis.

Usually the onset of symptoms occurs before the patient is one year old, but instances are known where the patient was completely asymptomatic until the age of six or seven years, and even adulthood. Evidence of left- and right-sided failure dominate the clinical picture. The heart is large; murmurs are present only if there is appreciable valvular involvement. Some of the sickest patients have no murmurs at all.

Roentgenologically enlargement of the left ventricle and left atrium are commonly noted; the lung fields show passive congestion. The electrocardiogram reveals left ventricular hypertrophy with ST and T wave changes, but without a QS pattern in the left chest leads. Occasionally low voltage is present in all leads.

Cardiac catheterization studies show results quite similar to those encountered in patients with constrictive pericarditis. There are mild elevation of the "pulmonary capillary" and pulmonary arterial pressures, an early diastolic "dip" in the right ventricle, and elevated right atrial pressure.

Treatment of the symptoms of congestive failure with vigorous anti-congestive measures is obviously indicated. The use of steroids has also been proposed in the treatment, as was the surgical approach of increasing the myocardial blood supply by abrasion of the epicardium. Whether any of these efforts at treatment are effective is well nigh impossible to tell, since the diagnosis cannot be made with absolute certainty except post mortem. Consequently I feel that, although the use of steroids, because of its success in some instance of rheumatic fever, may be condoned as a last resort in desperately sick children not responding to the conventional anticongestive measures, surgical approach is probably not justifiable at present in these patients in whom a certain diagnosis is not possible. In addition, I believe that there are serious doubts about the efficacy of this type of surgery even in people with well-recognized coronary disease.

CHAPTER 12

Functional Heart Disease

For practical purposes it seems convenient and helpful to classify all patients having abnormal signs or symptoms of heart disease but no structural disease of the heart as suffering from functional heart disease. This will naturally include a great variety of conditions. In general there will be two groups of such patients, those having some abnormal physical findings in the heart and others with symptoms but without abnormal findings. There will be many, of course, who will manifest both symptoms and signs. Numerous terms are used to designate these conditions and, although they may connote slightly different states, they all may properly be used to specify functional heart disease in the sense described above. Among the current terms are "neurocirculatory asthenia," "effort syndrome," "disorderly action of the heart," "soldier's heart," "cardiac neurosis," and "nervous heart." It will be seen in the succeeding paragraphs that other designations may well be used in this same group of patients, such as "benign cardiac irregularity" and "benign systolic murmur."

Let us first consider the group of patients who have either no symptoms whatever or insignificant ones, who show abnormal signs. During the course of an insurance examination or any other routine examination the physician may detect a faint systolic murmur in the absence of any other evidence of heart disease. This signifies the absence of hypertension, cardiac hypertrophy, diastolic murmurs, or any other cardiac symptoms. If there is no history of any previous rheumatic infection, under these circumstances, a slight systolic murmur can be disregarded and called functional or benign. Such a patient, for purposes of classification, may be said to have functional heart disease (benign systolic murmur). This applies only to a faint systolic murmur.

It will be found useful to estimate the intensity of systolic murmurs just as we do the amount of albumin in the urine. It is also necessary to confine the term "systolic murmur" to a bruit that has an appreciable duration and lasts for a definite interval after the first heart sound. Many mistaken diagnoses are made in designating as murmurs a prolonged first heart sound, frequently detected in hyperactive hearts and thin-chested individuals, when the interval between the first and second heart sounds is entirely clear. A more detailed discussion of the systolic murmur will be found in Chapter 17. Suffice it at this point to bear in mind that one should hesitate in considering loud murmurs as insignificant, benign, or functional.

Apart from the heart itself, the more important factors that seem to be responsible for systolic murmurs are anemia, hyperthyroidism, hypertension, fever, tachycardia, and the emotional state of the patient. In general it has been found that faint systolic murmurs, although present in only a small percentage of people, should be regarded as having no significance. Systolic murmurs of moderate intensity occasionally occur as a functional manifestation, but they may also indicate some organic disease in the heart or elsewhere; murmurs of greater intensity practically always signify some obvious organic disease.

In an extensive study of systolic murmurs it did not seem to matter whether faint systolic murmurs were heard at the apex or base of the heart or whether the patient was examined in the upright or in the recumbent position, although the frequency of benign systolic murmurs varied somewhat under these different circumstances. It is of no importance whatever that a systolic murmur, previously not present, is brought out by effort, for it was found that in practically all normal individuals systolic murmurs appeared directly after a brief brisk effort. The important point in this regard is that systolic murmurs of greater than the faintest intensity deserve investigation. This simple finding may be an important clue to the diagnosis of otherwise unsuspected hyperthyroidism or bacterial endocarditis. Although in some cases no adequate explanation will be found for the presence of a systolic murmur and such an abnormality is consistent with a long and active life, there is a tendency at present to pay too little attention to systolic murmurs and consider them all as benign. Apart from the conditions just mentioned, this type of "benign" systolic murmur often proves to be a manifestation of rheumatic heart disease; it frequently is associated eventually with stenosis of the aortic or mitral valve and occasionally is an evidence of myocardial disease or of congenital heart disease. Notwithstanding these considerations there remain some individuals with faint systolic murmurs who must at present be regarded as having no organic disease and in whom the diagnosis of functional heart disease (benign systolic murmur) must be made.

Further physical findings frequently regarded as benign or functional are certain arrhythmias. Almost all the arrhythmias that are met with in general practice can at times occur in patients who have no organic heart disease. The presence of sinus arrhythmia and of extrasystoles of any type is frequently the cause of apprehension and sometimes of discomfort when the condition is entirely functional. The same is true of paroxysmal auricular tachycardia. As our experience has broadened we have come to realize that even auricular fibrillation and flutter, paroxysmal or permanent, may occasionally be unassociated with any other disease. On rare occasions ventricular tachycardia has been observed in otherwise normal individuals. All these irregularities of the heart, of course, do occur with organic disease as well and it becomes very important to use every reasonable means to exclude organic conditions before making the diagnosis of functional heart disease (benign irregularity). It is particularly important not to overlook hyperthyroidism when auricular fibrillation is present, as this may be the sole manifestation of a toxic goiter.

If any of the above irregularities are present without symptoms of angina or congestive heart failure, and if other features like hypertrophy of the heart, hypertension, a diastolic murmur, significant changes in the electrocardiogram, a past history of rheumatic infection, abnormal configuration of the x-ray shadow of the heart and aorta, or a positive Wassermann reaction are absent, the condition must be regarded as functional. It does not follow that all these investigations are necessary to arrive at this conclusion, but these are the various factors to be considered in the study of such cases in which the primary complaint is apt to be palpitation of the heart.

The sensations that develop from benign extrasystoles are so peculiar and at times so distinctive that one should be familiar with them, as often the description of the symptoms given by the patient establishes the diagnosis even without any further examination. They are frequently described as a "flop of the heart," "the heart turns a somersault," "it skips or hesitates," there is "a sudden thump or jump or choking sensation in the throat," "the heart suddenly sinks," or "a wave passes over me." Although the actual terms used are varied, they are all characteristically descriptive of what is going on. Some compare the sensation to "the sudden flapping of a bird's wings" or to "a fish suddenly turning in the water." The sensations produced by the extrasystoles appear to come from the premature beat itself, though they have often been thought to result from the forceful beat that follows the pause. These disturbances are most apt to occur when the patient is at rest, especially while quietly seated or while trying to fall asleep. This is explained either by the fact that the mind is not occupied with other things or, more likely, by the fact that while the subject is at rest the heart rate is slower and the opportunity is greater, during the longer diastolic pauses, for premature beats to arise. At any rate, the sensations are generally absent while the patient is active, walking, or busily engaged in his affairs, although there is one rarer type that is brought on particularly by effort.

Although it has long been known that extrasystoles frequently are of no serious significance and that perfectly well individuals may have them, only more recently has it been possible to ascribe a definite neurogenic origin to them. Beattie and Brow made animal experiments reproducing persistent ventricular extrasystoles and found that, if certain nerve tracts coming from the hypothalamic region were cut, the irregularity disappeared. It is of some interest that the hypothalamic region is concerned with the control of our emotions. They also found that if these tracts were cut beforehand the extrasystoles could not be produced by the same technique which always brought them out in animals not subjected to this treatment. In other words, there is a center in the brain that can initiate or that is intimately connected with the formation of premature heart beats. This work has firmly established a structural anatomic basis for conditions that have long been regarded as functional or nervous.

Treatment for patients with extrasystoles varies considerably. When the extrasystoles come infrequently, all that is needed is an explanation that nothing serious is going on. The patient should be encouraged to carry on normal physical duties. It will only rarely be necessary to restrict the use of coffee or tobacco. When the irregularity is very disturbing, quinidine sulfate in doses of 0.2 to 0.3 gm. two or three times daily, or even less, is often effective. Procaine amide (Pronestyl), 0.25 gm. three to four times daily, may be more effective if the extrasystoles are of the ventricular type. Papaverine (0.1 gm.) administered three times a day by mouth has been advised. At times the patient learns that a certain medication is effective but only necessary just before the palpitation is expected to occur.

It has been stated that auricular fibrillation which generally is associated with organic heart disease can be at times a purely functional disturbance. This is particularly true of the paroxysmal type of auricular fibrillation, but I believe it also occurs in a few cases when the arrhythmia is permanent. In the absence of rheumatic heart disease, especially mitral stenosis, and of coronary artery or hypertensive heart disease, one must always suspect that there is an underlying hyperthyroidism when auricular fibrillation, either transient or permanent, is present. If the basal metabolic rate is normal the possibility of a toxic thyroid gland as the cause of the auricular fibrillation is ruled out for the most part. This is not invariably true, however, for it is believed that even some of these patients with a normal basal metabolic rate already have disease of the thyroid gland and will subsequently show an elevated rate, and that the auricular fibrillation may disappear after subtotal thyroidectomy. It has seemed that some such patients have been improved without surgery by taking Lugol's solution. It is also interesting that most of these apparently normal patients whom I have seen with auricular fibrillation and a normal metabolic rate have looked alike, have been males, and resemble in some ways patients with active hyperthyroidism. There are also instances of auricular fibrillation in which an adenoma of the thyroid is present and all tests fail to show evidence of hyperthyroidism. Despite this the recurrent paroxysms of auricular fibrillation have disappeared after a subtotal thyroidectomy.

When hyperthyroidism alone is the cause of the auricular fibrillation, the irregularity may still be regarded as functional, for it disappears under appropriate treatment of the thyroid gland and there remains no evidence of organic heart disease. Some work has been done showing that in hyperthyroid animals transient auricular fibrillation can be reproduced by the injection of Adrenalin. It was found that without Adrenalin such animals would never show auricular fibrillation, and that

Adrenalin in normal animals produced only ventricular irregularities and not auricular fibrillation. One might infer that in patients with hyperthyroidism the secretion from the adrenals has some relation to the production of auricular fibrillation. This would explain the occurrence of transient spells of this irregularity following emotional shocks and fright. At any rate, it has become clear that permanent structural disease of the heart is not a prerequisite for auricular fibrillation.

The other general type of patients comprises those who have various symptoms in whom abnormal physical signs like irregularities may or may not be present. Such patients are often young, and they complain of palpitation, weakness, giddiness, pain in the region of the heart, and frequently shortness of breath. The palpitation generally is associated with a normal heart rhythm. They merely feel the pounding of the heart which has either a normal rate or is slightly accelerated. When the rate is found to be rapid while the patient is awake it will be normal during sleep. The pain is almost always apical rather than sternal, and it may be of a dull, constant aching character or momentary and stabbing. When there is shortness of breath it may be merely of the type that accompanies a state of fatigue, as if it were a greater burden to lift the chest, or it may be a peculiar "sighing type" of breathing. This latter phenomenon is sufficiently common and characteristic to require special emphasis. We frequently see patients, often young women, who complain of shortness of breath without any other evidence of heart disease. On questioning them it will be found that the dyspnea occurs particularly at rest. It is obvious that true cardiac dyspnea at rest indicates a very grave condition, and yet these individuals appear quite well. On further questioning they will describe the sensation as air hunger, and say, "I just can't get enough air." During the examination the physician is apt to catch them in the act, so to speak, and see them occasionally take a very deep breath like a sigh. At that very instant it is well immediately to ask the patient if that is what is troubling her. This enables one to identify this primary complaint as functional, for the patient actually overventilates the lungs for some peculiar reason and still does not feel that sufficient air is obtained. Even minor changes in the electrocardiogram, such as very slight inversion of the T waves in any of the leads and slight depression in the S-T segment, have been observed in some cases. When this condition is marked and maintained it may result in sufficient overventilation to produce symptoms of tetany. The patients may complain of tingling and numbness of the extremities, and may show carpopedal spasm and a positive Trousseau (spasm of the fingers on squeezing the forearm) or Chvostek (contraction of the face on tapping the facial nerve) sign. A proper explanation and assurance that nothing serious is happening is often sufficient to cure the patient.

Other features that are present in these functional cases deserve attention. Sweating, tremulousness, and nervousness, together with palpitation, make one think of the possibility of hyperthyroidism. At times the differential diagnosis is not simple and will require basal metabolism studies. Although a somewhat increased heart rate is commonly present, if observations are made while the patient is asleep it will be found to be slow. At times the entire picture resembles incipient tuberculosis, and constant care should be taken to avoid overlooking a tuberculous process by having roentgenograms taken of the lungs when any doubt exists.

Scherf has reported a group of cases that would ordinarily be classified as cardiac neurosis or neurocirculatory asthenia, in which he regards the cause to be some disturbance in the endocrine system. In these cases there may even be minor changes in the electrocardiograms with flat or slightly depressed S-T intervals. Scherf believes these patients can be helped or cured by the administration of estrogenic hormone.

NEUROCIRCULATORY ASTHENIA

The functional cardiac disease that is often designated "neurocirculatory asthenia" is sufficiently important to merit more detailed discussion. This condition, first described during the war between the states, was very prevalent in the First World War. It was interesting to observe the different circumstances under which the symptoms developed. Some of the soldiers first began to show evidence of an unstable neurocirculatory apparatus when they first appeared before the examination boards, when they were not yet drafted into the army. The very thought of becoming a soldier and enduring all the hardships that it entails was sufficient to produce palpitation, weakness, chest pain, tremulousness, sweating, giddiness, and dyspnea. Others first showed these symptoms while they were training in the camps. Still others did well until they were sent overseas. At the other extreme, there were men who carried on sturdily for two or three years, going through terrible experiences in the trenches without showing any evidence of neurocirculatory asthenia, and then finally the nervous reserve would become exhausted. As a last straw it might be a simple event that had never previously disturbed them, such as a shell explosion, which precipitated the symptoms. It is not surprising that all these different gradations were found during the First World War. If this condition was more frequent among the British soldiers than among the American, and from my own observations I believe this was true, it probably was due to the fact that the British had to undergo the terrific strain of warfare longer than the Americans, and that in another year or two after we entered the war we would have had to equip special hospitals to look after these functional cardiacs as did the British.

Probably the most important factor in predisposing to this disease is the constitutional factor. Many have a subnormal nervous makeup. It is common to elicit a story of nervous breakdown, fainting spells, psychosis, neurasthenia, epilepsy, and the like in the past or family history of the patient. With this background, it may then be necessary to have a precipitating cause to bring to the surface the symptoms of functional heart disease. The relative importance of those two factors—

predisposing and precipitating—will vary in different individuals. No doubt if one factor is sufficiently prominent the other need be very slight to produce the symptoms. During the war, when the psychic trauma of combat was most intense and prolonged, individuals without any detectable evidence of a constitutional defect in their nervous stability finally developed "soldier's heart." Others with a marked background of nervous instability would break down at the slightest provocation. During the First World War the precipitating causes were linked up primarily with fear and less frequently with infection. Gunshot wounds, shell explosions, being buried, gassing, "trench fever," and rheumatic fever made up the common direct causes that precipitated the symptoms of neurocirculatory asthenia. In civil life the same hereditary constitutional factors are present, but the direct precipitating causes are anxiety following the loss of one's fortune, the death of some friend or relative, a love affair, or any state conducive to fear or emotional and nervous tension.

The symptoms previously enumerated as accompanying neurocirculatory asthenia mainly concern the cardiovascular and nervous systems. Because for the most part these symptoms are the very ones that are brought on by effort in normal people, the condition has also been called "effort syndrome." The difference is that in these patients the effort required to produce the symptoms is inordinately slight, compared with that necessary to produce them in normal individuals. Easy fatigability, breathlessness, palpitation, and precordial pain are the most common complaints. Those afflicted cannot stand much physical or mental activity. On examination very little of importance is discovered. Some have a peculiar expression of fatigue in their faces. They may show cyanosis of the face and hands which is due to local sluggishness of the circulation. The heart shows nothing abnormal except occasionally a slight systolic murmur. Not only is the heart not enlarged but there is a tendency for it to be small as determined by x-ray examination. In most, the electrocardiograms are normal but occasionally slight flattening or even inversion of the T waves in Lead I or II may be found. There may be a tremor of the hands and a moist skin. All that has been said concerning neurocirculatory asthenia or soldier's heart, which is so prevalent in soldiers, is applicable to civil practice, only the clinical manifestations are less prominent in civil life.

The importance of this condition is that it must be recognized and not confused with organic heart disease. So often the physician errs and makes a "cardiac cripple" out of one who is structurally sound. A patient with only minor functional complaints may become much worse and even invalided unnecessarily as a result of a mistaken diagnosis. The physician, believing that he is dealing with some valvular or myocardial disease, cautions the patient against overactivity or may even direct that he stay in bed. This convinces the sufferer that his heart is diseased and from then on he becomes more and more introspective and the symptoms become aggravated. It may subsequently become very difficult or impossible for some other physician to convince him that his heart is sound.

Even patients having organic heart disease or some other organic disorder may have in addition some form of functional heart disease. In some, the latter may be the cause of the primary complaints, and the heart may be in a perfectly compensated state. It then may be more difficult to appraise the situation, but it is very important to identify those features that are purely neurogenic, for digitalis, diuretics, and other treatment for heart failure may make things worse rather than better.

Having made the diagnosis of functional heart disease one should speak with emphasis and assurance. It is not sufficient to tell the patient "Your heart is normal, but don't overdo." Or, in reply to the question "May I play tennis?" if the physician says "No, I think that is too strenuous," any intelligent patient has a right to feel that the physician is holding something back from him or is not certain of his ground. One should reply "You can do anything you please; even if you overdo and feel tired no harm will come." From this he may become convinced that there is nothing to fear and thereby make the most important step in his recovery. Apart from this assurance it is well to try to disentangle any disturbing psychic factors that may be playing a role. All other general hygienic influences conducive to good health should be gone into, such as graded exercise, and particularly the question of nutrition. In those who are underweight a gain of weight proves very helpful. Although digitalis is of no use and may be harmful in neurocirculatory asthenia, and drugs in general are of little value, one might try one of the tranquilizing preparations such as Equanil.

A few words may be appropriate concerning the relation between neurocirculatory asthenia and warfare. My own personal experience in the first and second world wars leads me to the opinion that soldiers with this condition added very little to our efforts as actual fighting men. Once symptoms were present it is unlikely that any were able to carry on front line duty. Some men with milder symptoms who improved under a course of graded exercises were returned to duty. Not many were able to carry on. More often, after a few days of shelling, back they would appear in one hospital after another and occupy bed space for months. The obvious inference is that when the diagnosis is made such a man should not be accepted for military service at all or only for limited duty. This policy would be wise until the need for men is so great that second rate soldiers have to be drawn. It must also be appreciated that, in making the diagnosis, symptoms are more important than signs, for it is the complaints they have, such as breathlessness, syncope, weakness, palpitation, and precordial pain, that incapacitate them.

A wrong opinion prevailed among most physicians concerning prognosis. It was thought that the moment war ended and the fear of suffering or death was over the symptoms would all disappear. Follow-up studies showed that not to be the case. Although many men improved, many others retained their symptoms to a greater or lesser extent indefinitely. This could not be explained entirely on the desire of these veterans to receive pensions, for some who did not need or accept pensions continued to be handicapped.

Prognosis

Prognosis in cases of functional heart disease is uncertain with regard to the symptoms but excellent as to life. Although one does not fear any serious complications and there is no mortality due to this condition, cures are not readily obtained. Often the underlying fear or psychic disturbance cannot be removed, or the symptoms go through cyclic changes, improving and then reappearing as periods of nervous stress and strain come and go. Even without any obvious cause some patients will continue to be bothered by one or another of these functional symptoms as evidence of some neurocirculatory instability. Because of the great fear of heart disease that prevails among the laity, patients with functional heart disease need constant reassurance and encouragement to carry on.

CHAPTER 13

Paroxysmal Rapid Heart Action

The heart action may suddenly become rapid in a variety of ways. Several different types of disturbances in the heart mechanism are responsible for these paroxysms. It is important to distinguish one from the other because, as we shall see later, the treatment and the prognosis differ considerably in the various types. Furthermore, there are occasional instances in which proper treatment must be instituted quickly, otherwise disastrous results ensue. This whole subject, therefore, has many very practical aspects, and it is surprising how intelligent management of these disturbances can be carried out by the use of very simple means.

Paroxysmal rapid heart action comprises those conditions in which the heart suddenly becomes rapid. The termination of such a paroxysm is likewise sudden. If one had the opportunity of observing the actual transition either at the onset or the conclusion of these attacks, one would notice that the change takes place instantly. A heart rate which is found to be 70 at one moment may suddenly, in one second, jump to 200 a minute, and at the termination of such a paroxysm the rate falls in one beat from the high level to a normal one. The abruptness of the change is an important point that distinguishes it from a rapid heart in which the mechanism is normal, i.e., normal tachycardia. If a patient is seen with a normal sinus tachycardia of 170, for instance, as might occur in surgical shock, hemorrhage, certain fevers, hyperthyroidism, and other conditions, it generally will be possible to ascertain that the heart rate rose gradually to this high level. It may have taken minutes, hours, or days to change from the normal to the rapid rate. In true paroxysmal heart action no such gradual transitions occur.

The cause of these paroxysms is the inception of a new cardiac mechanism. In the ordinary normal rapid heart the rhythm is really not disturbed. The impulses arise in the normal pacemaker (sino-auricular node) and travel through the heart normally. The only change is that the rate of impulse formation is rapid. In these abnormal paroxysms, on the other hand, the ordinary pacemaker of the heart no longer controls the rhythm and in its place some abnormal mechanism in the auricles or ventricles controls the heart beat. The types of disturbance that may result are paroxysms of auricular tachycardia, auricular flutter, auricular fibrillation and ventricular tachycardia. Although paroxysms may also

266

arise in the auriculoventricular node or the bundle of His (so-called nodal tachycardia), they are rare, and are impossible to recognize without the use of special apparatus.

The following conditions are also considered from the standpoint of electrocardiography in Chapter 21.

Paroxysmal Auricular Tachycardia

Paroxysmal auricular tachycardia is one of the more common of these disorders. It occurs much more often in patients who have no heart disease than in those with organic disease. In this sense it may be regarded as a functional disturbance. The heart rate during an attack will generally range between 150 and 250 a minute. The attack begins and ends abruptly. It may last minutes, hours, days, or, rarely, weeks. During the paroxysms the heart rate is perfectly regular and the sounds are all alike in quality and intensity. The regularity is so precise that on careful measurement contiguous heart cycles will be found to differ in length by no more than $\frac{1}{100}$ second. The rhythm not only is regular but seems to be constant and fixed at the same level for long periods at a time. If an attack were to continue for some hours the heart rate might be found to be 196 at one time and ten minutes later it would still be 196. It is also impossible to disturb this rate by such simple means as having the patient hold his breath or change his position, which measures generally will alter the rate of a normally beating heart. This constancy of rate is an important distinguishing characteristic which enables one to recognize the condition at the bedside. To obtain this the apex rate should be counted accurately for sixty seconds. This can be done with a stethoscope in human beings, when the heart is regular, even when the rate is as rapid as 250 a minute. The error in the count need not be greater than two, one at the beginning and one at the end of the minute, while trying to synchronize the observation with the second hand of the watch. During the intervening beats there need be no inaccuracy whatever. Accurate counting of a rapid regular heart may be facilitated by simultaneously tapping with the foot or the finger. This matter deserves some emphasis because one often hears the expression that the heart was too rapid to count. If the rhythm was regular this generally means that the observer made no real attempt to count accurately. Let us assume that in a given case the rate of 164 was found. Some minutes later the count should be repeated, having the patient change his position, hold his breath, or go through any maneuver which ordinarily affects the heart rate. On the recount the rate will again be found to be 164 or 163. If the second rate were 170 or 160, one might fairly safely assume that the patient did not have paroxysmal auricular tachycardia. A normally accelerated heart, however, might alter its rate to that extent. Thus we have a simple means which helps to characterize this condition. Expressed in other terms, while ausculting the heart not even the slightest alteration in the rhythm will be noted as a result of those measures which generally produce acceleration or retardation under normal circumstances.

SYMPTOMS

The clinical features in this condition are variable. The attacks may occur rarely, one every several years, or frequently. I have seen instances in which the patient had as many as ten paroxysms every day. He will generally complain of sudden palpitation of the heart and become nervous and agitated. Fainting and actual loss of consciousness may occur at the onset of any form of paroxysmal rapid heart action. This probably results from the sudden decrease in the cardiac output with resulting relative cerebral anoxia. Adjustments in the circulation take place, however, so that syncope does not last very long. During the first time or two, not knowing what it all means, he may actually fear that he is going to die. Usually there is no dyspnea with the paroxysm, and after a variable length of time the attack ends as suddenly as it commenced. There frequently is a sensation of gaseous distention of the abdomen or belching of gas during and particularly at the end of the paroxysm. Occasionally a cessation of the attack comes with a vomiting spell. These features make the patient think that the paroxysm is due to "indigestion" or that it is in some way related to his diet. The causes that precipitate the attack are numerous and inconstant. Frequently a sudden movement of the body, such as bending to tie one's shoe or a quick turn of the head, initiates the attack. Much less frequently violent effort brings on a spell. Emotional factors also come into play. Sudden thoughts or even dreams may be the precipitating cause. There remains a great number of instances in which the attack seems to occur spontaneously without any known cause. In some cases there is heart pain during a paroxysm which is more apt to occur after the paroxysm has lasted some time. In its description it may resemble the pain of angina pectoris but it has by no means the same prognostic significance, for when the heart rhythm is normal and slow there will be no chest pain whatever and, in fact, no other evidence of heart disease.

Physical examination of the patient during an attack is apt to reveal no essential abnormality except the rapid heart rate. The patient may seem pale and agitated, and the skin may be moist. When an attack develops in one who is otherwise normal there will be no evidence of circulatory insufficiency except in very rare instances. This is also true in some cases in which there is associated organic heart disease, either valvular or muscular. In fact, there is no other condition in which the heart may be so rapid with so little apparent embarrassment to the circulation. The patient may have no dyspnea or cyanosis and yet show a heart rate of 200 or more.

Under certain circumstances symptoms of considerable gravity develop, such as peripheral thromboses and congestive heart failure. The factors that determine the development of these complications are the following: the duration of the attack, the heart rate during the attack and the condition of the heart before the onset of the attack. It is obvious that a normal heart might stand the rate of 240 a great deal longer than a heart with mitral stenosis, or one with a poor degree of compensation. I have seen a patient with mitral stenosis develop marked dyspnea, edema of the lungs, cyanosis, and engorgement of the liver within a few hours after the onset of tachycardia in which the heart rate was 190. On the other hand, if the rate is extremely rapid and the attack of long duration, even if the heart is structurally normal, disastrous results may develop. This was well illustrated in a case I observed many years ago. A man of 40 who was otherwise perfectly well had had three attacks of tachycardia during the previous few years. Each attack lasted uninterruptedly for five to eleven days. During the first one he developed a hemiplegia, from which he gradually recovered in the course of a few months with a slight residual spasticity of one side of the body. During the second attack he developed aphasia, which gradually disappeared in four months. During the third attack, dry gangrene of the left arm developed, necessitating amputation at the shoulder. I saw this man in 1914 during the fourth attack and found the heart rate to be 250 a minute. After obtaining certain data on this patient the attack was immediately ended by ocular pressure. It was the first time his attacks had been controlled, for the others had stopped spontaneously after lasting many days. In fact this may have been the first instance in which ocular pressure was ever effective as a treatment for paroxysmal tachycardia.

The explanation of the complications that occurred in this case was quite obvious. While the heart was beating 250 times a minute the pulse pressure was extremely low. During several attacks in which the patient was observed the systolic pressure was around 94 to 96 and the diastolic around 88 mm. Therefore, this patient had an effective pulse pressure of no more than 6 or 8 mm. One can readily see from this how thrombosis in peripheral vessels could easily develop. This must have occurred in the cerebral vessels during two of the attacks and in the vessels of the left arm at the time gangrene occurred. The process essentially consisted of stagnation of the blood. The value of proper therapy in such cases is evident, for this patient lived for more than thirty years thereafter.

In general, the changes in blood pressure that occur during paroxysmal tachycardia consist in a tendency for the systolic level to fall and the diastolic to rise, with a diminution in the pulse pressure. The degree of such changes will depend upon the three factors mentioned, namely, the heart rate, the duration of the attack, and the structural condition of the heart. Such attacks have at times been called acute dilatation of the heart. This is a misnomer, for in a series of twelve such instances x-ray measurements of the heart before, during, and after attacks failed to show an appreciable dilatation except in one instance (the case cited in the preceding paragraphs in which the heart rate was 250). In some patients the heart was actually smaller during the attack. Other interesting features that may develop during attacks of tachycardia are a slight fever and a slight leukocytosis. I do not think that these features indicate infection. They are rather the result of congestion.

One can readily see how a simple attack of any type of paroxysmal rapid heart action may be confused with acute coronary thrombosis. A patient has a "heart attack." The heart rate is found to be very rapid. There may be some collapse, a fall in blood pressure, and even chest distress of the anginal type. Fever and leukocytosis may follow. After the attack has ended the electrocardiograms may even show inversion of the T waves, suggesting coronary thrombosis. These changes are probably the result of myocardial fatigue and local relative anoxia and gradually disappear in subsequent days or weeks. All this can occur in a structurally normal heart and also leave the heart entirely intact. The confusion becomes even greater when one considers the possibility that actual coronary thrombosis may result in vulnerable individuals if a low blood pressure and a state of shock persist for a long time. One important distinction is that in simple paroxysms of tachycardia the very rapid rate comes first and then the above signs and symptoms follow, whereas in coronary thrombosis the abnormal tachycardia follows the attack and generally does not appear for one to several days.

TREATMENT

The development of paroxysmal tachycardia may present a serious situation and require immediate and effective treatment during labor or during a surgical operation. I recall an experience in which a woman was being operated on for gallstones. While she was under ether, just as the operation was to be started, respiration ceased, the radial pulse became imperceptible, and extreme cyanosis quickly developed. Artificial respiration had to be instituted and had already been carried on for about ten minutes when I saw the patient. The heart rate was 212 and perfectly regular. Carotid sinus pressure stopped the attack immediately, the heart returning to a normal rate of 80. Normal breathing was immediately restored, and the cyanosis disappeared. The patient was subsequently operated on, and the gallbladder containing stones was removed. In two other cases in which attacks likewise occurred during anesthesia but in which the symptoms were not so alarming, carotid sinus pressure was not effective but ocular pressure promptly restored the heart to its normal rate. Such experiences are not common. The urgency and gravity of the whole situation are so great when it does occur that it deserves this emphasis.

There are two phases to the treatment of paroxysmal tachycardia; the first concerns the treatment of the attack, and the second the procedures that may prevent or diminish the incidence of future attacks. A great many measures have seemed to be successful at one time or another in stopping attacks. They all produce their beneficial effects by stimulating the vagus nerve in one way or another. The act of vomiting is one of these, produced either spontaneously or by the use of an emetic, such as apomorphine, ipecac, and the like. One to 4 teaspoonfuls of syrup of ipecac often is effective when other methods fail, and the dosage may be repeated in one-half to one hour. Inducing the gag reflex by inserting a finger in back of the tongue is another method. I knew one patient who stopped several of his attacks by drinking ice-cold water or swallowing bits of ice. Occasionally lowering the head, or raising the foot of the bed has proved successful. One simple and most helpful measure is holding a deep breath. Many patients have found that this simple experiment can stop their attacks very effectively. It is well to tell such patients to take a deep breath and hold it as long as they can. In normal individuals, holding a forced inspiration produces a slight vagal slowing of the heart, but in this condition it will frequently bring an attack abruptly to an end with restoration of a normal slow rhythm (Valsalva experiment).

Finally, there are three methods which stimulate the vagus nerve more effectively. The first of these is irritation of the carotid sinus, the second is pressure over the eyeball, and the third is the use of drugs. The first of these procedures consists of palpating with one hand for the bulge in the common carotid artery as it divides into external and internal branches while supporting the patient with the other hand placed behind the neck. Pressure is then exerted backward, completely compressing the artery and massaging it for several seconds. This should be done first on one side of the neck, then on the other, but not on both sides at the same time. Pressure should be released after a few seconds and repeated after an interval if necessary. In rare cases hemiplegia has resulted which was due not to an asystole of the heart but rather to obliteration of the circulation to one side of the brain for too long a time. The cerebral accident in these cases always involved the side compressed. If the paralysis had been due to a cessation of the heart beat one side *or* the other would have been affected. The second method consists of exerting rather firm pressure with the thumb over the eyeball. This will be painful. Here again the pressure should be exerted over one eye at a time. This pressure sends a stimulus up the fifth cranial nerve and by a reflex (oculocardiac reflex) down the vagus nerve. When ocular pressure is effective it is not a result of the pain, for pain produced elsewhere in the body causes no such slowing, and I have several times stopped attacks while a patient was under anesthesia. Its use is limited to some extent but there are instances when this will prove successful after other methods have failed.

The distressing feature of arresting attacks of paroxysmal heart action is that on very rare occasions the attack stops but the heart never restarts beating. This experience makes one think that the abnormal rhythm is inhibited but the normal pacemaker, which has not been functioning throughout the attack, fails to initiate any impulses. It is as if the sinus node, which has been asleep, fails to wake up. I have been told of two instances of sudden death, one following carotid sinus pressure and the other after ocular pressure, in which the tachycardia stopped but the heart beat never was resumed.

Attacks of auricular tachycardia can generally be arrested by one or another of the procedures just described. There are instances, however, when the tachycardia is resistant to all these measures. Drugs which have proved valuable in stubborn cases may then be used. On several occasions in which the tachycardia persisted for a long time and could not be stopped by the ordinary means, and the patient's condition seemed rather critical, the intravenous injection of quinidine sulfate immediately restored the normal rhythm. For this purpose one would generally need 0.3 gm. or more of quinidine sulfate. It is best to inject this slowly while someone is listening to the heart over the precordium. Just as soon as the break in the rapidity occurs, injection should be stopped. In two cases I found that after 0.2 gm. of the drug was injected, and while the hypodermic needle was still in the vein, the attack suddenly came to an end. There is some danger in the use of quinidine, therefore this treatment should not be used until other measures fail and the patient's condition is critical enough to warrant it. Another drug that has been used with great success is acetyl-β-methylcholine. The average adult dose is 20 mg. given subcutaneously. Infants have responded favorably to doses of 5 mg. This is a powerful vagal stimulant. Occasionally untoward results occur, particularly in allergic individuals, for which $\frac{1}{60}$ to $\frac{1}{30}$ grain of atropine should be used. Other drugs have been used successfully to stop attacks. Among these are calcium gluconate (10 to 20 cc. of 10 per cent solution given slowly intravenously), parathormone subcutaneously, magnesium sulfate (15 cc. of 20 per cent solution intravenously), and neostigmine methylsulfate (0.5 to 1.0 mg. intramuscularly). There is reason to believe, however, that calcium might be dangerous in ventricular tachycardia. Neosynephrine intravenously has stopped attacks of paroxysmal supraventricular tachycardia within one minute. The mechanism probably depends on increasing the blood pressure. It might be hazardous in cases with hypertension or coronary disease. The dose is 0.5 to 1.0 mg. Curiously enough, I observed one patient who had typical angina pectoris and in addition classic attacks of paroxysmal auricular tachycardia. The two conditions were independent of each other. This patient found that nitroglycerin not only relieved the attack of anginal pain (when the heart rate was normal) but stopped his attacks of tachycardia. Finally, large doses of digitalis (0.5 to 1.0 gm.) often prove successful. Probably any form of digitalis preparation will do, although excellent results have been reported by the intravenous use of Cedilanid (0.8 to 1.6 mg.) or digoxin (1.0 to 2.0 mg.). Atabrine also has been effective in arresting various forms of tachycardia. This is given in doses of 0.1 gm. intravenously (1 per cent solution) or 0.3 gm. in 1 per cent Novocain solution intramuscularly.

Methoxamine hydrochloride (Vasoxyl), given in doses of 5 to 10 mg. intravenously or intramuscularly, may stop paroxysmal auricular tachycardia in a few seconds to a few minutes. The dose may be repeated in ten minutes if the first treatment is ineffective. One can see that numerous drugs are available. In general, some digitalis preparation given intravenously, if the patient has not already been digitalized, would be the first choice if the simpler vagal measures have been ineffective.

It must be understood that in most cases of paroxysmal tachycardia the attacks eventually cease spontaneously and that the patient is none the worse for the spell. It is only occasionally that any heroic treatment would be indicated, but there are instances in which it might prove life saving.

When it comes to preventing the return of such attacks, the problem becomes more difficult. The patients themselves often feel that if treatment were directed at the gastrointestinal tract they might be cured. The physician frequently alters the diet in one way or another, and advises medical treatment for gas, indigestion, or constipation, with the hope of preventing these attacks. In other instances courses of sedatives have been prescribed to diminish the general nervous irritability. In patients who use tobacco excessively the attacks may be attributed to this. Treatment along these lines, however, has always proved practically useless. It has been suggested that Carbachol (carbamylcholine chloride), 4 mg. orally daily, may prevent recurrences of supraventricular tachycardia. I have had no experience with this drug. The two drugs that are helpful in preventing recurrent tachycardia are quinidine and digitalis. Either one or the other, if properly administered, will often either inhibit the attacks entirely or diminish their frequency and severity. In several instances I have found digitalis to be effective after quinidine had failed. In only a portion of the cases is this treatment indicated. If attacks come only on rare occasions, such as once in six to twelve months, it would hardly seem wise to prescribe a course of preventive treatment. Not knowing when an attack is to be expected, such a patient would have to be constantly under the influence of quinidine or digitalis in order that the heart might be prepared on that distant day when the attack otherwise would be due. This would necessitate the constant use of a medicine for the possible prevention of a rare attack. Even if months elapsed and the patient were free from attacks, because of the infrequency of such spells, it would still remain doubtful whether the therapy had anything to do with the result obtained. Under these circumstances it is best to explain the entire situation to the patient, assuring him that nothing serious will develop, to institute no constant drug therapy, but to be prepared to meet each spell as it arises.

When the attacks occur frequently, treatment should be specifically directed at their prevention, for then they may be actually incapacitating and it becomes a simple matter to decide whether or not therapy is effective. Quinidine sulfate may be given in doses of 3 to 5 grains three times a day. If the patient ordinarily has attacks every few days a particular dose should be continued long enough to be certain whether it is effective or not. If attacks continue despite the medication the dose may be increased. Although some patients may tolerate larger doses without showing toxic symptoms, such as ringing in the ears, diarrhea, fever, or skin rash, as a practical matter if attacks continue while 5 grains three times a day are taken it is best to omit the drug entirely.

It was formerly thought that digitalis was of no use in the treatment of paroxysmal tachycardia. This opinion was held mainly for two reasons. (1) It seemed true that the ordinary administration of digitalis during an attack had little influence in stopping it. (2) Its use in preventing the recurrences seemed disappointing, because complete and constant digitalization was generally not carried out. Some years ago I had opportunity to observe four patients who had had courses of quinidine and digitalis therapy without success. The digitalis in these cases was inadequate and when the drug was administered in quantities similar to those used in heart failure, the attacks ceased. One of these patients was having several attacks a day so that he had to quit his work. He had no organic heart disease, and except for these attacks he was well. Under full doses of digitalis all attacks ceased and he was able to return to work. Another patient was a woman aged 60 who had had attacks about every two weeks for the previous three years. They grew increasingly severe so that finally they were absolutely prostrating. When she was seen during one of these spells she was found to be pulseless, no blood pressure reading could be obtained, and the heart rate was 240. She was cold and it looked as though she might die. Ocular pressure instantly brought the heart rate to normal. She had previously taken quinidine at one time, and at another 5 drops of digitalis three times a day for some months without success. She had also taken sedatives and various medicines for indigestion. After the spell just described she was given $1\frac{1}{2}$ grains of digitalis leaves three times a day for one week and thereafter $1\frac{1}{2}$ grains daily. There were no attacks for fifteen months. It was then decided to stop digitalis to see whether or not it was needed any longer. About one week after the drug was omitted a similar attack occurred and digitalis was then reinstituted and the patient had no further attacks. This case was a very striking one, for the patient remained perfectly well for over fifteen years, whereas formerly for three years she was in constant fear of these attacks, had had to live a very confined life, and required constant nursing attention.

There is a rarer variety in which block is present, and which is called paroxysmal auricular tachycardia with block. It was suggested by Wilson that this type of auricular tachycardia and possibly others as well are due to a circus movement in the auricles in which the pathway goes through the auriculoventricular node. In the more common type of paroxysmal auricular tachycardia just described, there is no heart block, the ventricles responding to every auricular impulse. Paroxysmal auricular tachycardia with block occurs in some cases as an isolated disturbance in the cardiac mechanism unassociated with any organic heart disease or as an accidental arrhythmia with some form of structural disease. Much more commonly, however, it is observed as a direct manifestation of digitalis intoxication. As a result of both direct experiments in animals and observations in patients, Lown and his co-workers have shown that paroxysmal auricular tachycardia with block is related to the action of digitalis when there has been a loss of potassium from cells. Because of the great use of mercury diuretics, low sodium diets, and other procedures that drain the body of potassium, this peculiar cardiac irregularity is being observed more and more frequently. Patients with congestive failure now live longer than they formerly did. As a result, a period is now frequently reached when digitalis is administered in ordinary or in larger doses hoping to reverse the downward progress. Thus toxic effects of the drug are more readily produced.

This toxic arrhythmia is frequently overlooked or misdiagnosed. It may be wrongly called normal sinus tachycardia, paroxysmal auricular tachycardia, or auricular flutter or fibrillation. It has fairly definite electrocardiographic features (see Chap. 21), which distinguish it from other arrhythmias. The auricular rate ranges from 150 to 220, the P waves in lead II are small, and generally upright with flat isoelectric intervals between them. Although partial A-V block is present, in most cases there are stages in the development and recession of the arrhythmia which do not exhibit block. The auricular rate is not always absolutely constant, and the ventricular rhythm may be regular or irregular, depending on the presence and degree of the accompanying block.

The condition is frequently precipitated by an active diuresis following a mercury diuretic. This appearance of digitalis intoxication following a diuresis was formerly thought to be due to redigitalization. It now has been clearly shown to be caused by the enhanced action of digitalis that resulted from the loss of potassium. The toxic effect can be prevented by the previous administration of adequate potassium and can be eliminated after it has developed by giving potassium or Pronestyl, which has a similar effect. For this purpose, especially if the situation appears critical, 2.0 to 4.0 gm. of potassium chloride in 500 to 1000 cc. of 5 per cent dextrose in water may be given intravenously in the course of two to three hours. Electrocardiograms should be taken throughout the procedure. The auricular rate will be observed to slow, and frequently a point is reached where partial heart block, previously present, may disappear, with a resultant 1:1 mechanism. At this point the ventricular rate will suddenly become rapid. The infusion should not be stopped, but on continuation of the treatment the auricular rate will slow more and more until a normal mechanism is restored. When the electrocardiograms show a return of a normal sinus rhythm with normal appearance of "P" waves, the infusion is promptly stopped. An oral dose of 5.0 gm. of potassium chloride may also be effective in one to two hours. After the administration of potassium as outlined above, if the auricular rate has slowed but a normal mechanism has not been established, it is advisable to continue potassium therapy. In the presence of a rapid ventricular response when the situation may be more critical, reversion may be expedited by the addition of Pronestyl.

Procaine amide (Pronestyl), intravenously in doses of 0.25 to 1.0 gm., may have an effect similar to that of potassium, and can be given intravenously and under constant electrocardiographic control at the rate of 50 mg. every three minutes.

When paroxysmal auricular tachycardia with block occurs unassociated with digitalis therapy, quinidine is rarely of value, nor is potassium or Pronestyl. It is then best to administer digitalis in doses adequate to maintain a satisfactory slowing of the ventricles even if the rapid auricular rate continues. A normal sinus rhythm may be resumed either spontaneously or as a direct result of digitalis action.

The recognition of this arrhythmia is difficult and generally will require careful electrocardiographic study. It resembles auricular flutter in many respects, but should be regarded as a separate and distinct entity. The ventricular rate though generally rapid may be slow, regular or irregular, and the heart sounds may vary in intensity in different cycles. Carotid sinus stimulation often temporarily slows the ventricular rate and may in this way uncover the rapid auricular beats with the characteristic form of the "P" waves which are otherwise not detectable.

Surgical procedures have been employed in stubborn cases of recurrent paroxysmal auricular tachycardia and in other types of paroxysmal rapid heart action. Either the right or the left or both sympathetic chains from the lower cervical through the upper four or five dorsal ganglia have been removed. It is too early to be certain of the results but they seem promising, although it is already evident that failures will occur.

Paroxysmal Auricular Flutter

Another form of paroxysmal heart action is auricular flutter. Although this condition, once established, is likely to be persistent, occasionally it occurs in paroxysmal form. Here the auricular rate generally ranges from 250 to 350, and the rate of the ventricle is one half of the auricular rate or less. In very rare instances the ventricular and auricular rates are the same. When the condition is first seen, before any treatment is instituted, there is apt to be a 2:1 heart block, so that whatever the auricular rate may be the heart rate as counted at the apex is half as great. The former may be 340 per minute, whereas the ventricular rate is 170. It should be borne in mind that the rate of the auricle is really inferred, for the auricular contraction cannot be heard. The rhythm in untreated patients is generally regular, because every second impulse coming from a regularly beating auricle reaches the ventricle. Occasionally in untreated cases, and frequently after treatment has been started, the rhythm is irregular. Here the degree of block is changing in different heart cycles, so that for a short time every second auricular beat gets through to the ventricles, then only the third or fourth beat gets through, and so the regularity is disturbed from time to time. The resultant irregularity may occasionally be gross enough to resemble auricular fibrillation very closely. There may even be an appreciable pulse deficit. The essential difference between the two conditions is that in auricular fibrillation the irregularity is actually complete, whereas in flutter it follows some definite law; i.e., different groups of ventricular beats will have the same length if accurately measured and properly selected, as they will correspond to the same number of regularly occurring auricular cycles (Chap. 21, Fig. 75).

This type of paroxysmal rapid heart action occurs generally in patients who have organic heart disease, either valvular or myocardial, but may also occur in those with no other evidence of heart disease. Unlike paroxysmal auricular tachycardia, it is apt to persist for long periods at a time or even to remain permanent if untreated. Therefore it is important to try to restore the normal mechanism or at least to control the ventricular rate. There are two purposes in the treatment of patients with this condition. It would be desirable to do away with the mechanism of auricular flutter entirely or to prevent the ventricles from becoming rapid if the flutter persists. In general the two drugs that are used for these purposes are digitalis and quinidine. In about one third of the cases the heart is restored to normal rhythm if digitalis is properly given. At first, as has been mentioned, the ventricular rate is often rapid and regular with a coexisting 2:1 heart block. After the customary dose of digitalis is administered the ventricular rate slows and may become irregular as a result of an increase in heart block, so that a 4:1 or 6:1 auriculoventricular block results. If the ratio between ventricular and auricular beats is constantly 4:1 or 6:1, the rhythm is regular; if this ratio is changing in different cycles the rhythm is irregular. The ventricular rate may now be 60 or 80 but the auricular rate during this time remains unchanged, as the flutter so far is not disturbed. At this point in some cases, auricular fibrillation may suddenly develop with the appearance of a gross irregularity. If digitalis is now omitted, during the course of the next day or so the heart may return to a normal rhythm. In fact, regularization may take place even if the maintenance dose of digitalis is continued. In general, therefore, digitalis may change the auricular flutter into auricular fibrillation and permit the auricles to return spontaneously to a normal rhythm. When this treatment is ineffective, auricular flutter may persist even though the ventricular rate has been slowed by digitalis, or having produced a change to auricular fibrillation this may continue indefinitely, or again return to the original state of flutter. When digitalis does not restore the normal rhythm it may still serve an important therapeutic purpose in maintaining a slow ventricular rate, whether the original flutter or the subsequent fibrillation persists. Inasmuch as the most important purpose of treatment is the prevention of a rapid ventricular rate, no matter what the auricles are doing, digitalis is of distinct value in this condition.

The best treatment of auricular flutter is actually to restore a normal rhythm. It is known that quinidine increases the refractory period of auricular muscle. By so doing it may actually stop the continuous circus which exists in the auricle and which tends to perpetuate the flutter. The dose of quinidine for this purpose is not fixed. In general, from 5 to 10 grains three to four times a day may be given. The procedure I have used is, after digitalis has slowed the ventricular rate and the abnormal rhythm persists, to start with a dose of 0.2 gm. and to increase it by 0.1 gm. with each dose, giving the medication four times a day. During the quinidine therapy a daily dose of 0.1 gm. of digitalis may also be given. At times I have had to increase the single dose of quinidine to 1.0 or even to 1.5 gm. before reversion to normal rhythm was obtained. It is desirable to have the patient under close observation during this time so that frequent electrocardiograms may be taken. It will be noted that during the quinidine administration the actual auricular rate will slow while the ventricular rate accelerates. I have seen the auricular rate of flutter drop from about 300 to 150 as a result of quinidine. At any time during this treatment the normal mechanism may suddenly be restored. The drug is by no means effective in all cases, and, unlike digitalis, has no value in slowing the ventricular rate except when it restores the normal rhythm. The disadvantages of quinidine apart from its frequent ineffectiveness are that it has certain toxic actions that occasionally are serious. On the other hand, there are instances of auricular flutter that are helped greatly by this drug when digitalis has been ineffective.

Paroxysmal Auricular Fibrillation

Paroxysmal auricular fibrillation is a much more common condition than it was thought to be not so long ago. In fact, the term "auricular fibrillation" is applied to a condition that was formerly called "perpetual arrhythmia." It was then believed that once this became established it remained so permanently. We now know that the transient form is quite common. It occurs occasionally in patients with mitral stenosis before it takes on the permanent form. It is also frequently met with in hypertensive heart disease or in so-called "chronic myocarditis." It occurs in some cases of rheumatic fever and in a small proportion of cases of pneumonia. It has been frequently observed during acute coronary thrombosis. Rarely it is seen under a variety of circumstances that seem to have no very definite relations to the heart, e.g., acute angioneurotic edema or chronic gallbladder disease, or as a complication of any surgical operation requiring general anesthesia, especially in operations on the lungs and mediastinum. Possibly the most common condition with which transient auricular fibrillation is associated is hyperthyroidism. This is a frequent event during the ordinary course of the disease and particularly during the first day or two following an operation on the thyroid gland. There remains a small group of patients in whom transient fibrillation occurs and in whom there can be detected no other evidence of heart disease or disease of any important organ. It must be regarded in these isolated cases as a purely functional derangement and not indicative of any disease. It is evident from the great variety of conditions in which transient fibrillation may occur that the symptoms resulting from this disorder and the appropriate treatment must vary a great deal. It is obvious that the sudden inception of a rapid irregular rate can produce very distressing symptoms in a patient who already has serious organic heart disease, whereas if it occurs in a heart that is essentially sound very little embarrassment may result. As will be seen later, in some cases this paroxysmal arrhythmia needs no treatment whatever or treatment may be entirely useless until the underlying cause is removed, whereas in other instances the attack itself presents a therapeutic problem of major importance.

When auricular fibrillation develops the rhythm of the heart becomes grossly irregular. Almost invariably the rate as counted at the apex is quite rapid, 130 to 170 or more. If the patient is digitalized or if, as rarely happens, there is a concomitant defect in the conduction apparatus the apex rate may be slow. With a rapid heart rate there generally is an appreciable pulse deficit, i.e., the pulse rate is 10 or more less than the heart rate. Occasionally when there is hypertension or when the pulse pressure is great, as in hyperthyroidism, or when the heart rate is not very rapid there may be very little if any pulse deficit. The bedside diagnosis, however, is not very difficult in the great majority of cases. The most important feature in the diagnosis is the character of the irregularity. It is a complete, absolute, and tumultuous arrhythmia that one hears. Only in rare instances may it be confused with other conditions.

The symptoms that result from an attack of auricular fibrillation depend in a great measure on the state of the circulation before the onset of the attack. In most cases there is palpitation. This is produced by the rapid agitated contractions of the heart. If cardiovascular disease already exists, dyspnea of a mild or marked degree may quickly develop. In fact some cases may present the picture of acute pulmonary edema. Occasionally an attack of transient auricular fibrillation is associated with the dislodgment of an embolus from an auricular thrombus. If the thrombus is dislodged from the right auricle a pulmonary infarct develops and if from the left auricle hemiplegia or other arterial infarction may occur. If auricular fibrillation develops in a patient already very sick with pneumonia sudden collapse may occur. I recall one such case in which the heart rate suddenly rose to about 200 and the pulse became imperceptible. The patient seemed to be *in extremis*. Twenty minutes after an intravenous dose of strophanthin he quickly revived, the heart rate fell to about 110, the pulse returned, and the patient eventually recovered. There are other instances of transient fibrillation in which the circulation is in such good condition that the patient will have no complaints whatever, except a slight degree of palpitation. One can readily see how varied the picture may be.

TREATMENT

There are two therapeutic aspects to this condition: one concerns itself with the underlying disorder, whether it be pneumonia, exophthalmic goiter, or some other condition; the other is the treatment of the specific attack of fibrillation. In hyperthyroidism it is useless to treat the patient for auricular fibrillation in the ordinary way, as attacks will tend to recur as long as the hyperthyroid state persists. When the treatment of hyperthyroidism is effective in restoring the metabolism to a normal level the tendency to fibrillation will generally disappear spontaneously. In most other types of transient fibrillation direct therapy for the arrhythmia itself is indicated. The two drugs that have distinct therapeutic value in the treatment of this arrhythmia are digitalis and quinidine. The action and the purpose of these two drugs are quite different and so are the results obtained from their use. Digitalis may bring an attack of auricular fibrillation to an end. When such a spell ceases while the patient is taking digitalis it is thought to do so spontaneously. In fact, there is reason to believe that digitalis might tend to perpetuate the condition. The value of digitalis, however, is to slow the ventricular rate while the fibrillation continues. On the other hand, quinidine may even cause an acceleration of the ventricular rate while fibrillation is present, but its main value lies in the fact that it tends to do away with the arrhythmia entirely and restore the heart to a normal mechanism. If it is known that the patient has had previous spells of this arrhythmia of short duration lasting only a few hours, and the general state of the circulation is quite satisfactory, it is just as well to give neither digitalis nor quinidine, but rather to administer some sedative or possibly morphine, for in a few hours the attack may be over. If, on the other hand, the patient already has sufficient organic cardiac disease so that the rapid irregular ventricular rate has already produced or may readily produce generalized congestion or alarming symptoms of circulatory insufficiency, rapid digitalization is indicated. The reason for this is that it cannot be known how long the attack is going to last or whether or not the fibrillation will become permanent. Whether digitalis shall be given by mouth, intramuscularly, or intravenously depends upon the urgency of the situation. The following is an illustration of this problem. A middle-aged woman with fairly well compensated mitral stenosis had, during the course of several years, a few transient attacks of auricular fibrillation, each lasting about an hour or two. During these years dyspnea had been slowly increasing. Finally she had a spell which had already lasted about five hours when I saw her. In this brief time her condition had become alarming. She was semistuporous, had marked acute pulmonary edema, striking generalized cyanosis, and extreme dyspnea. The heart rate was about 190 and the pulse was practically imperceptible. The situation seemed desperate. Inasmuch as she had not been taking digitalis, 8 cc. of digifolin (0.8 gm. digitalis) was immediately given intravenously. In about twenty minutes, although the auricular fibrillation still continued, the heart rate fell from 190 to about 100. The change in the appearance of the patient was most dramatic. The dyspnea, cyanosis, and pulmonary edema all quickly improved and she fell back into a comfortable sleep. As it happened, fibrillation from then on persisted. She continued on digitalis by mouth and later became ambulatory. To be sure, in most cases no such alarming symptoms result. In general, palpitation is the prominent complaint and under such circumstances digitalization by mouth is sufficient. In a case of moderate severity 0.5 gm. of digitalis may be given by mouth in one dose, and if none has been previously given this same dose may be repeated in several hours and again the following day if the heart rate is still rapid. Such a procedure will be effective in relieving the symptoms of circulatory insufficiency. Nowadays preparations that act more rapidly and are less lasting may be preferable, such as Cedilanid 0.8 mg. or Digoxin 1.0 to 2.0 mg. intravenously. It is evident from the foregoing discussion that digitalis should be used to slow the ventricular rate when that rate is rapid, when the attack seems to be persisting, and when embarrassment to the circulation results.

The second phase of the treatment of paroxysmal auricular fibrillation is the prevention or diminution in the frequency of further attacks. In most cases it is best to try the effect of quinidine sulfate. This may be given in doses of 0.3 gm. three times a day. It should be continued for a sufficient time to ascertain whether attacks are being inhibited or not. If they had been coming once or twice a week and if, while the patient is taking quinidine, none occur for several weeks, it is fair to say that the attacks were specifically inhibited by quinidine. The drug might then be continued for several months. If, however, the attacks persist with equal frequency on this dose, it generally means that quinidine was of no value, although a larger dose might be tried. Occasionally attacks have a tendency to recur at certain times of the day or night. In these cases the dose of quinidine may be given an hour or so before the expected attack and prove helpful. If quinidine sulfate is ineffective as a preventive and the attacks are troublesome or frequent, the patient should be digitalized thoroughly and kept on maintenance doses constantly. This need not prevent the return of the spells, but will so prepare the heart that when they do occur the ventricular rate will not be rapid. In one such case when the attack occurred before digitalis was given the heart rate was about 140. A few days later, after only 1 gm. of digitalis had been taken by mouth, a similar attack occurred and the heart rate was about 100. The following week when the patient was completely digitalized, on routine examination the rhythm, which previously was regular, was found to be grossly irregular with a rate of 70. The patient was entirely unaware that she was having a spell, whereas previously spells had caused considerable palpitation. This experience clearly illustrates the effect of digitalis, for the spells continued but the resultant symptoms were eliminated. It is also a good example of the slowing effect of digitalis on the ventricular rate in the absence of heart failure, for there was no evidence of congestion in this case. There will be occasional instances in which digitalis may be used in the treatment of one specific attack and later quinidine could be given to prevent occurrences. It must be borne in mind that many spells pass off without therapy.

In some troublesome instances of recurrent auricular fibrillation and in other forms of paroxysmal rapid heart action, successes have been obtained by the use of radioactive iodine even in the absence of other evidence of thyrotoxicosis.

Paroxysmal Ventricular Tachycardia

The last type of paroxysmal rapid heart action to be considered is paroxysmal ventricular tachycardia. In this condition the beats arise in the ventricle itself and the auricles either contract at a different rate or in some instances there is reversed conduction so that the impulse that arises in the ventricle travels upward to make the auricles contract. There are several important differences between this type of tachycardia and those arising in the auricles. This condition in the great majority of cases is associated with serious structural heart disease, generally coronary thrombosis. There are occasional instances of its occurring with chronic valvular heart disease and rare cases in which the heart is structurally normal. In fact, instances have been reported in which this arrhythmia would develop in the upright position and disappear on lying down (orthostatic paroxysmal ventricular tachycardia). It may also be precipitated by excessive digitalis therapy, but this is more likely to occur when there is already considerable structural damage to the heart. Unlike auricular tachycardia, which is often unassociated with any serious heart disease, it may generally be assumed that ventricular tachycardia indicates a serious heart disorder.

It formerly was thought that one could not possibly distinguish at the bedside the ventricular from the auricular type of tachycardia. It was considered necessary to have electrocardiograms to identify them. During recent years, however, some simple clinical criteria have been discovered which enable one to make fairly accurate diagnoses using only those means that every physician can readily employ in the sickroom. It has been emphasized that in auricular tachycardia the rhythm is perfectly regular. There are no interruptions in the rhythm. In fact, the differences in length of contiguous heart cycles, if measured accurately, would not be more than one-hundredth of a second. In ventricular tachycardia, although the rhythm may seem to be absolutely regular for stretches of many seconds or even of minutes, one may, in many cases, on careful auscultation detect occasional irregularities. Secondly, in auricular tachycardia the heart sounds of the consecutive regular rapid beats are all alike, whereas in ventricular tachycardia every now and then the first heart sound will vary in intensity or quality. It will become accentuated or muffled or reduplicated. This is due to the inconstant relation between the time of ventricular and auricular systole. Another distinguishing feature is the jugular pulse. Here one may see fewer auricular beats than the ventricular rate as counted over the precordium, and some of the jugular waves are often prominent because the auricles may be contracting while the ventricles are in systole. Finally, the various measures employed to stimulate the vagus nerve which may end an attack of auricular tachycardia will never influence the rhythm of ventricular tachycardia. These criteria, together with the general clinical differences, such as the association of the one with functional heart disease and of the other with grave coronary disease, should make it possible to recognize ventricular tachycardia fairly accurately even without special apparatus.

The beginning and ending of an attack of ventricular tachycardia are abrupt and instantaneous just as in other forms of abnormal rapid heart action. The rate during the attack is usually between 150 and 200, but occasionally a higher rate is reached. When it occurs without organic heart disease these individuals may complain merely of palpitation, although even this may be incapacitating. When, as more frequently happens, it develops during the days that follow an attack of acute coronary thrombosis, it presents a serious complication of an already grave condition. This complication may of itself prove fatal. Proper recognition of the condition becomes very important, inasmuch as treatment may be effective in restoring the heart to a normal rhythm.

In any extensive experience one occasionally comes upon unexpected or rare situations. On two or three occasions the apical heart rate was counted by experienced observers as being one-half its true rate. I recall one instance in which the patient was moribund and pulseless but the heart rate was thought to be about 110. When I first listened to the heart I also counted it about 115. The sounds alternated in intensity and in character as the first and second sounds usually do. Something puzzled me about the heart beat. I began to wonder whether there were two sounds to each cycle, in which event the rate was 115, or there was only one sound to each beat (without an audible second sound), in which event the rate was 230. If the latter were true, there must also be alternation in intensity of the first sound, which does occasionally occur. This dilemma was resolved by the electrocardiograms, which readily showed a heart rate of 230 due to paroxysmal ventricular tachycardia. The heart slowed only slightly following magnesium sulfate intravenously, but promptly returned to normal when quinidine sulfate (0.6 gram) was given intravenously. The patient made a splendid recovery.

In another instance an infant had a paroxysm of auricular tachycardia. At first the heart rate was thought to be regular and 150, assuming that there were two sounds to each cycle. When electrocardiograms were taken the ventricular rate was found to be 300. Here, again, there was only one audible heart sound to each beat and what was at first interpreted as the second sound was in fact another ventricular contraction. This condition was readily controlled by digitalis.

In a third case heart sounds were entirely inaudible because of the noisy breathing from pulmonary edema and the feeble heart beat. The rate was assumed to be about 90 because the pulse, though feeble and irregular, was 90. This patient was also moribund several days after an acute myocardial infarction. The true state of affairs was only deciphered by very careful auscultation. During the very brief periods of apnea (Cheyne-Stokes breathing was present), on listening very carefully at the apex, very distant heart sounds could be heard at the rate of about 190. Obviously paroxysmal ventricular tachycardia had been overlooked for several days by relying on the radial pulse rate and not utilizing simple auscultation to its fullest extent. This experience occurred in a patient's home before portable electrocardiographs were available. He responded promptly to quinidine after all other drugs failed to check his downward progress. The inference from all this is that careful auscultation is extremely important and occasionally even life saving.

TREATMENT

It has been mentioned that measures like carotid sinus pressure or ocular pressure are ineffective in arresting ventricular tachycardia. Likewise, digitalis has no beneficial effect on this condition. In fact, there is evidence that digitalization may tend to prolong such attacks and accelerate the rate further. I studied one instance in which the heart rate rose from 145 to 180 as the patient was given full doses of digitalis. However, there are very rare instances when digitalis might prove beneficial. If the patient has congestive heart failure and has received no digitalis, or is underdigitalized and develops paroxysmal ventricular tachycardia, digitalis may sufficiently improve the circulation and help to abolish the tachycardia. In this connection it also must be appreciated that auricular fibrillation with a rapid ventricular rate may result in aberration of the ventricular complexes to such a degree that they resemble tachycardia of the ventricle.

The drugs that can restore a normal mechanism when ventricular tachycardia is present are quinidine and Pronestyl. There is reason to believe that the mechanism involved in the condition is a circus movement, just as it is in auricular fibrillation and auricular flutter, only in the former the circus is in the ventricles and in the latter it is in the auricles. It is logical to infer that the action of quinidine in breaking up this circus is likewise the same in those two conditions. It has been my experience that quinidine has been effective in a larger proportion of cases of ventricular tachycardia than in those of auricular fibrillation.

The therapeutic dose of quinidine in this condition is variable and has to be determined individually in different cases. One patient who had no organic heart disease but complained of frequent attacks of palpitation, which were proved to be due to ventricular tachycardia, remained entirely free from attacks as long as she took 0.3 gm. of quinidine three times a day. Other instances, in which the attacks occurred during coronary thrombosis, were controlled by doses of 0.4 and 0.6 gm. three times a day. One patient with mitral stenosis, auricular fibrillation, and ventricular tachycardia required 0.8 gm. to stop the tachycardia and doses under 0.8 gm. three times a day failed to prevent a return of the condition. He maintained a normal rhythm for many months while taking the larger dose (0.8 gm.). Finally, in one very striking case of coronary thrombosis in which this treatment was actually life saving 1.5 gm. five times a day for several days was required both to stop an attack and to prevent its return, smaller doses having proved to be ineffective. In the last instance we dared to give such large doses because the condition of the patient seemed otherwise hopeless, and it was found that smaller doses had had a partial effect in slowing the ventricular rate from 200 to about 150. This slowing of the ventricular rate on increasing doses of quinidine is almost a constant finding. At times the rate keeps slowing with each large dose, only to return to the original level as the effect of the drug wears off. On rare occasions a large dose of atropine given subcutaneously while the rate was partially slowed by quinidine promptly restored the heart to a normal rhythm. In selected cases quinidine may be given intramuscularly or even intravenously. Quinidine hydrochloride (Brewer) and quinidine gluconate (Lilly) may be used for this purpose. It has been suggested that Atabrine given intramuscularly in doses of 0.3 to 0.6 gm. in 10 cc. of 1 per cent Novocain has caused regularization in cases of auricular fibrillation and flutter and in ventricular tachycardia in one or two hours when quinidine has failed. The physician will have to weigh the circumstances carefully before employing methods of therapy that entail some risk. It is, therefore, evident that the judicious use of quinidine in ventricular tachycardia may be of considerable value and on rare occasions life saving.

Magnesium sulfate (2.0 to 4.0 gm. intravenously) may also stop ventricular tachycardia instantly. I have seen patients in whom the attack stopped within one minute. In others it failed when quinidine administered intravenously was successful. Another treatment suggested is the intravenous use of morphine. The dose given is about 0.015 gm. and may be repeated in one-half to two hours. The effect is supposed to take place in thirty to sixty minutes. I have had little experience with this treatment. Potassium salts on very rare occasions may be helpful. I saw a patient who had ventricular tachycardia for six weeks. He had failed to respond to large doses of quinidine given orally and intravenously. Finally, reversion to a normal rhythm occurred after three doses of potassium acetate (2.0 gm. each) given orally at two-hour intervals. Following regularization this patient lost 12 pounds of edema.

The most recent drug to be used for paroxysmal ventricular tachycardia is procaine amide (Pronestyl). This may be given intravenously in doses of about 1.0 gm. in a volume of 10 cc. It is probably preferable, although less convenient, to dilute the vial of 10 cc. to 100 or 200 cc., using 5 per cent dextrose in water and administering the drug at the rate of 0.1 gm. per minute, or more slowly. It is well to record the electrocardiogram continuously during the procedure, so that the infusion may be stopped just as soon as the desired result has been obtained. The required dose may be less or more than the expected 1.0 gm. Reversion to normal rhythm may occur in several minutes and is generally preceded by gradual slowing of the ventricle. It can also be used orally in capsules or in tablets of 0.25 gm., giving one or two doses four times daily. The oral method is preferable to prevent recurrences and is particularly applicable in the treatment of ventricular extrasystoles. It has very little value in supraventricular arrhythmias.

Like many other valuable medications there are occasional untoward side-effects from Pronestyl. Hypotension is frequent, and therefore careful blood pressure determinations are advisable during its administration. Elderly patients with advanced decompensation are more susceptible to toxicity. This is also true of patients with chronic bronchial asthma. When ventricular tachycardia develops in the course of Adams-Stokes disease, Pronestyl is contraindicated, for it is likely to induce ventricular fibrillation.

Diagnosis of Types of Paroxysmal Rapid Heart Action

As an aid in the diagnosis of the various types of paroxysmal rapid heart action a composite figure of the effect of vagal stimulation on these arrhythmias has been constructed (Chap. 21, Fig. 81). A study of this figure will enable the physician to visualize the results obtained by simple physical examination. The first tracing shows the effect of right carotid pressure in a normal heart. There is a gradual slowing and a smooth return to the original rate. The second curve shows a similar slowing effect when normal tachycardia is present. This patient had an acute coronary thrombosis and the rapid heart rate made me wonder whether he had flutter; in fact the appearance of the electrocardiograms on first glance suggested this diagnosis. The gradual slowing of the heart with a smooth return to its original rate eliminated this diagnosis. The third curve illustrates a typical arrest of an attack of auricular tachycardia. One observes the abrupt cessation of the rapid rate with a prompt resumption of normal beats. Interruptions during the transition due to extrasystoles or vagal effects are common. No other type of rapid heart action is completely controlled in this fashion.

The fourth tracing shows the effect of carotid pressure in auricular flutter. The ventricular rate is promptly slowed (although the auricular rate remains unaffected), but there follows an "irregular" return to the previous rapid rate. The point that distinguishes flutter from normal tachycardia is that, as the vagal effect subsides, the ventricles return to their original rate in a jerky fashion. After a short cycle a longer one may appear, then another short one, until finally the constant rapid rate is resumed. This is to be compared with the second tracing where it may be seen that after the cessation of carotid sinus stimulation each beat becomes shorter and shorter until the original rate is restored. The fifth set of electrocardiograms illustrates the events in auricular fibrillation. The rhythm is grossly irregular at the start, becomes slower during the vagal stimulation, and then returns to its original absolute arrhythmia.

The sixth curves are those of ventricular tachycardia. Here no effect whatever is produced. Very slight irregularities which are fairly characteristic of this condition continue throughout the tracing. The lowest set shows the effect of vagal stimulation on paroxysmal auricular tachycardia with block.

When the changes that have been described are translated into corresponding auscultatory findings obtained over the precordium, it is striking what accurate diagnoses can be made by simple bedside methods. The one confusing aspect of this problem is paroxysmal auricular tachycardia with block. In some ways this resembles auricular flutter and it may be difficult, if not impossible, to diagnose this condition by simple clinical or bedside methods. Electrocardiographic studies will then be necessary.

CHAPTER 14

Acute Cardiovascular Emergencies

A practicing physician is often confronted with apparent or real circulatory emergencies and needs to have some basis for making quick decisions. One of the most important of these decisions is whether or not the situation is serious. A fainting spell may be quite benign or indicative of a very grave disorder. A sudden severe pain may be a simple cramp or a spasm or may be due to an embolus. An attack of suffocation at night may be due to a spasm of bronchial asthma, which will shortly leave the patient none the worse, or it may be one of acute pulmonary edema. The purpose of the following discussion is to consider some of the more common cardiovascular upsets in which the patient or his family are apt to call the physician suddenly because they believe a serious emergency exists.

BENIGN SYNCOPE

One of the commonest sudden circulatory upsets is a fainting spell. Simple syncope is not very frequent in organic heart disease. There are many patients with valvular or myocardial disease who never faint and when a brief loss of consciousness occurs it is not always related to the organic lesion found in the heart. The only valvular disease in which syncope occurs with any frequency is aortic stenosis. This complication was discussed previously (Chap. 4). Occasionally the onset of any form of paroxysmal rapid heart action (Chap. 13) is associated with syncope. In most cases a simple fainting attack is a benign event occurring in otherwise healthy individuals. The precipitating factors for this are varied. The sight of blood, an overheated or crowded room, a sudden fright or the prick of a needle at the time of a vaccine injection or as blood is withdrawn for a Wassermann test, all may make some people faint. Another common cause is standing erect and fairly motionless for a considerable length of time. A sudden change of posture from the recumbent to the upright position is another cause. Persons who have marked postural or orthostatic hypotension may faint on quickly standing up. All these factors are intimately related to the nervous control of the vasomotor apparatus. In most of these instances loss of consciousness would not have occurred had the individual been recumbent. There is apt to be a splanchnic dilatation and a temporary cerebral anemia which naturally becomes aggravated if the body is in the upright position. For this reason it is customary to lower the head between the knees to revive one who has fainted.

If a person is seen during a faint it will be observed that he quickly grows pale and at the outset there is a fall both in the heart rate and in the blood pressure. Generally these early changes are not noted because by the time a physician arrives the heart rate has risen and the normal blood pressure level has been restored. There is much in this upset that resembles a vagal explosion or a temporary hypervagotonic state. In fact I recall once seeing a young man who could faint at will. After suddenly changing his position from recumbent to upright several times he would always faint. For an hour or so after a subcutaneous injection of 2.0 mg. ($\frac{1}{30}$ grain) of atropine sulfate, he could not be made to faint. It appeared that atropine paralyzed the vagus and prevented the reflex from taking place. This need not be the only or even the most common mechanism that controls benign syncope. The sympathetic nervous system may be involved in some reflex way that permits changes in blood pressure. From a therapeutic point of view it is wise to try tincture of belladonna, 10 drops after each meal, or ephedrine sulfate, 0.025 gm. three times a day, when such attacks recur with sufficient frequency to merit medication. Wearing a tight abdominal corset may also be of some value. It is hardly necessary to recall that sudden massive internal hemorrhage needs to be thought of as a possible explanation of a fainting spell. When no organic disease is present, a patient having benign syncope should not be restricted in his activities and he should be assured that his heart is sound.

There are frequent instances in which syncopal attacks remain unexplained, even showing nothing abnormal during the attack except for the state of unconsciousness. The heart, pulse rate, and blood pressure may remain unchanged. Subsequent postmortem examination may fail to throw light on the mechanism of such episodes. I have seen frequent attacks of unconsciousness of this type in a patient who eventually showed three old coronary thromboses. Syncopal attacks may also occur for some unknown reason in cases of cortical atrophy or cerebral sclerosis. In these cases one can assume that transient cerebral spasm takes place.

EPILEPSY

Obviously benign syncope of the type just described needs to be distinguished from petit or grand mal. The difficulty is not great if one witnesses the attack, for there is no change in the pulse rate in epilepsy. I have made the error of confusing the two conditions when judgment had to be made from the history alone. The family history of epilepsy, the occurrence of an aura, the loss of sphincter control, the occurrence of convulsions and the postparoxysmal headache or sleep may help to differentiate the two. It is obvious that cardiac therapy would be of no avail in syncope due to epilepsy, but that instead phenobarbital or Dilantin would be used.

ADAMS-STOKES SYNCOPE

There is one condition in which syncope is a major and characteristic event and is the result of serious disease of the heart, i.e., Adams-Stokes disease. Here sudden unexpected painless unconscious spells occur with or without convulsions. These attacks are due to a sudden failure of the ventricles to contract or to a sudden marked slowing of their rate. The severity of the paroxysm will in a large measure depend on the duration of ventricular asystole. If this only lasts several seconds, the patient merely feels a "light wave" come over him. If it is longer he will lose consciousness and fall. If it lasts still longer convulsions occur, and if the beat is not resumed after a few minutes death ensues. When the attack ends the patient may feel perfectly well and be ready immediately to resume his former state. These attacks come suddenly, generally without warning or aura and with varying frequency. In some the spells are rare; in others there may be many during the same day, even producing a "status epilepticus."

The treatment for the syncopal attacks of Adams-Stokes disease, apart from that for whatever underlying condition may exist, is ephedrine or Adrenalin. The former is given in doses of 0.025 to 0.05 gm. ($\frac{3}{8}$ to $\frac{3}{4}$ grain) by mouth two or three times a day, and the latter subcutaneously in doses of about 0.3 to 0.5 cc. of 1:1000 solution. Adrenalin in oil (1 cc. contains 2 mg.) may be used and repeated every 12 to 24 hours. Propadrine may be substituted for ephedrine, the dose being the same. For oral administration Isuprel sublingually in doses of 10 to 20 mg. three or four times daily may be more effective than ephedrine. I had one patient with Adams-Stokes disease who took three Isuprel tablets (10 mg. each) three times daily for several years with what appeared to be excellent control of his syncopal attacks. When the situation seems urgent and immediate effects must be obtained Adrenalin should be used and repeated as often as seems necessary, even every two hours in some cases. When attacks recur at very rare intervals, it is hard to evaluate any therapy, but ephedrine may be tried by mouth. There are rare instances in which Adrenalin has been injected directly into the heart during a prolonged period of asystole with recovery of the patient (Chap. 21, Fig. 115). It is obvious that under such circumstances a subcutaneous injection would be useless as blood flow has already ceased and no absorption would take place. There is also suggestive clinical and fairly sound pharmacologic evidence in support of the value of barium chloride (0.03 gm. four times a day) in the prevention of recurrent attacks of this sort. Other measures that seem occasionally to be useful are inhalations of 1:100 Adrenalin solution, full doses of atropine, Metrazol intramuscularly or by mouth, thyroid extract, and complete digitalization.

Bellet has had beneficial results in increasing the ventricular rate of complete block and favorably influencing the frequency of recurrent syncopal attacks by the intravenous injection of molar solution of sodium lactate. This is given at the rate of 15 to 60 cc. per minute. The amount and speed of injection is decreased as the ventricular rate rises and reaches a suitable level. It must not be forgotten that a brisk blow over the precordium or the prick of a hypodermic needle into the ventricle may at times initiate the heart beat when asystole has suddenly developed.

All the above procedures are inadvisable when the syncopal attack is initiated by ventricular acceleration, because they enhance ventricular irritability and thus would sustain or worsen the situation. Ventricular standstill or undue slowing is the one condition in which their application is useful. When syncopal attacks result from increased irritability of the ventricle then the treatment of choice is quinidine or magnesium sulfate. The latter may be given intravenously in a dose of 4.0 gm. over several minutes. It is obvious that in order to treat Adams-Stokes attacks intelligently, it is necessary to distinguish these two types of onset. This can be best accomplished by an electrocardiographic study.

Quite recently a mechanical cardiac pacemaker has been devised by Zoll which has been of value and occasionally life saving in cases of Adams-Stokes disease or under other circumstances in which there is sudden cardiac arrest. External electrodes are applied on the surface of the chest and an electric current is passed through the body at a fixed given rate. This may artificially maintain the heart beat for a certain length of time until the heart itself takes over. The same apparatus includes a defibrillator, which may be effective if ventricular fibrillation rather than asystole is present.

Apart from medications that are used in the hope of preventing repeated syncopal attacks, there is a surgical aspect that needs consideration. A considerable number of patients with Adams-Stokes disease also have gallbladder disease, generally with stones. In fact, it would appear that gallstones are quite common in this condition. It is also known that there are reflexes from the gallbladder to the heart. With this background, I have had cholecystectomy performed on seven patients with syncope without any operative mortality. Although it is extremely difficult to appraise the long-range value of any therapeutic procedure in this condition, in which the course is so unpredictable, it has seemed that the attacks of syncope have been dramatically controlled and inhibited in some of these patients. I have enough assurance of this relationship first to carry out routine roentgen examination of the gallbladder in all cases of Adams-Stokes disease and to advise cholecystectomy if the gallbladder is found to be definitely abnormal.

VENTRICULAR FIBRILLATION

Another type of syncope that results from a disturbance of the mechanism of the heart beat is one due to ventricular fibrillation. Although this is generally a fatal condition and very likely one of the causes of sudden death in patients with coronary artery disease, rarely it is a transient phenomenon. When it occurs the ventricles actually stop beating and fail to eject blood into the circulation. If contractions are not quickly resumed death results. This mechanism is apt to follow a preliminary period of ventricular tachycardia or frequent ventricular extrasystoles (Chap. 21, Fig. 114). When it can be established that syncopal attacks are due to such disturbances, quinidine sulfate (0.2 to 0.3 gm. three times a day) should be tried, as from both a theoretical and a practical point of view such medication may do away entirely with the attacks or at least diminish their frequency or severity. An electrical defibrillator, if available, should be tried for the specific attack, or, when possible, even direct massage of the heart.

CAROTID SINUS SYNCOPE

Quite a different type of syncope that has been particularly studied is that which results from carotid sinus irritability. Soma Weiss and his co-workers discovered a considerable group of people with hypersensitive carotid sinus reflexes, some of whom are prone to fainting attacks. It has long been known that pressure over the carotid artery can often slow the heart beat, and this mechanism has been used to stop attacks of paroxysmal tachycardia (Chap. 13) and to study certain cardiac arrhythmias, especially auricular flutter and heart block. It previously was thought that the method of action of this manipulation was by direct stimulation of the vagus nerve which lies beneath the carotid artery. Hering, however, showed that this is not the correct explanation, but that it is a reflex effect (carotid sinus reflex) produced by irritation of nerves surrounding the carotid artery at its bifurcation into the internal and external branches. Although under normal conditions the carotid sinus undoubtedly serves an important role in regulating certain bodily functions related to the blood pressure level, the heart rate, the effect of changes in posture, and other cerebral phenomena, in some individuals the sensitivity of this region is increased and results in a tendency to dizziness, syncope, and convulsions. This occurs more frequently in patients with arteriosclerosis or hypertension but may be present without such changes. Increased sensitivity of the carotid sinus may also result from local irritation produced by a neighboring gland or a tumor in the neck. In some cases syncope is apt to occur as a result of a twist of the neck to one side or the other or to a peculiar position of the head from wearing a high collar.

Whenever a problem of syncope arises that is not readily explained by some other cause the patient should be tested for carotid sinus sensitivity. The proper part of the carotid artery should be sought for and will generally be identified by the finding of a local bulge or prominence at its bifurcation. First light and then more firm pressure and irritation should be applied, preferably with the patient sitting rather than recumbent. The pressure should be exerted for several seconds, first on one side and then on the other. Pressure should not be continued for more than a few seconds at a time because if the carotid circulation is shut off for too long hemiplegia may result. When a positive result is obtained the primary complaint of syncope will be reproduced and there is apt to result a fall of blood pressure or a slowing of the heart, although syncope may even take place without these effects. When the attacks of syncope can be ascribed to an increased sensitivity of the carotid sinus, it has been shown that the administration of daily doses of ephedrine sulfate (25 to 50 mg. two to four times a day) may be effective in preventing such attacks. Occasionally atropine or tincture of belladonna (10 drops three times a day) may also inhibit the attacks. On the rare occasions in which a local tumor or gland is responsible for the attacks, removal of the cause is curative. Furthermore, Weiss and his collaborators obtained some permanent cures in a small number of cases by resecting the nerve plexus from the carotid artery. Ray and Stewart reported some cures in cases of carotid sinus syncope by intracranial section of the glossopharyngeal nerve. Finally, roentgen irradiation over the carotid sinus has been recommended and cures have been reported. However, I have had no experience with this form of treatment.

CEREBRAL ACCIDENTS

Sudden prolonged unconsciousness is commonly due to cerebral hemorrhage or thrombosis, subdural hematoma or cerebral embolism. With all these there is apt to be paralysis of one side of the body and if the speech centers are involved aphasia also results. It is important to realize that cerebral hemorrhage occurs in older persons with hypertension. When a sudden hemiplegia develops with or without unconsciousness in one who has not a significant hypertension there are several conditions to bear in mind. One must think of rupture of a cerebral aneurysm, carotid artery thrombosis, syphilis of the brain, polycythemia, Buerger's disease, and brain tumor. When sudden paralysis occurs in younger people, especially when ocular muscles are involved, a rupture of a small intracranial aneurysm must be suspected. Such aneurysms are thought to be due to congenital deformation and not to syphilis. Finally embolism to the brain may cause sudden unconsciousness or hemiplegia. Some evidence of previous heart disease will then be discovered. It occurs mainly under four sets of circumstances—mitral stenosis, auricular fibrillation, cardiac infarction, and bacterial endocarditis. When it is associated with the first two an embolus becomes dislodged from a sterile mural thrombus in the left auricle. When it develops from the third condition the embolus arises from a mural thrombus in the left ventricle that resulted from an infarction of the musculature following a coronary thrombus. Sterile mural thrombi may be present in the cardiac cavities for years without doing any harm, and at present there is no way of detecting their presence or of predicting whether embolism will result. In bacterial endocarditis septic emboli are dislodged from the vegetations on the affected valves.

There is one aspect of cerebral embolism which has not been explored but which may be of interest. It has impressed me that most patients with mitral stenosis complicated by cerebral emboli have little or no dyspnea. In general they have fairly good function and have been able to lie quite flat in bed. On the other hand, cerebral emboli are very rare in cases of mitral stenosis with advanced cardiac failure or with orthopnea. One wonders whether or not the upright position of the neck and head makes it more difficult for small thrombi, dislodged in the blood stream, to go up the carotid arteries. If the clot is heavier than blood it would remain in the lower portion of the stream and spare the cerebral circulation. Other possible explanations are that with advanced failure the velocity of blood flow is decreased, and this would tend to diminish the likelihood of emboli, or that emboli are dislodged soon after mural thrombi develop. If the latter is true it would account for the occurrence of emboli early rather than late in the progress of mitral stenosis or auricular fibrillation. This problem needs further investigation.

In recent years, as a result of a greater interest in disease of the circulation and the introduction of angiography, thrombosis of the carotid arteries is being more frequently found to be the cause of "cerebral accidents." This x-ray technique is equally useful in detecting small cerebral aneurysms that often rupture with disastrous results. These thromboses may be "chronic," with repeated bouts of paresis of a limb or dysphagia or dysarthria. The symptoms may become manifest after any fall in blood pressure in a vulnerable individual. This may occur during sleep, after a brisk hemorrhage, or following a lumbar puncture. The rupture of a cerebral aneurysm may be accompanied by a sudden severe headache and present the picture of an acute subarachnoid hemorrhage.

It has been stated that cerebral hemorrhage occurs with hypertension. It is important to realize that the elevation in blood pressure is very apt to persist after the rupture of the cerebral vessel even if the patient is unconscious. Therefore, one should hesitate to regard the condition as due to cerebral hemorrhage if the blood pressure is normal. It may be found to be due to one of the other causes previously mentioned. At times one is thereby led to suspect the presence of a mural thrombus in the heart or cardiac infarction. Finally, sudden paralysis of one side of the body may take place only to disappear in a few hours. This may even be repeated. I have seen complete temporary hemiplegia recur several times during the course of a week in a man with hypertension. This very likely is due to transient spasm of the cerebral arteries and not to any permanent occlusion or rupture of a vessel. It is clear, therefore, that sudden cerebral accidents present a problem in differential diagnosis and that they should not be too readily regarded as instances of an ordinary apoplectic stroke.

The prognosis for patients having these cerebral accidents will naturally vary considerably. These hemorrhages or thromboses are almost never instantly fatal. In this respect they differ from coronary attacks, which often kill instantly. When coma develops and continues for more than a day or so the outlook is grave. A slight fever and leukocytosis are common findings and are merely the result of the cerebral infarct or of the extravasated blood. A hypostatic bronchopneumonia is a frequent complication during the early days following a cerebral accident in elderly people and is apt to prove fatal if not treated. If the patient survives the first week he generally recovers. When paralysis has occurred some recovery of function is the rule, and on the whole improvement in the power of the leg is greater than that of the arm. In some, although physical recovery may be satisfactory, permanent mental impairment may result.

If the diagnosis of cerebral embolism is made promptly it may be worth while to try an injection of the stellate ganglion with procaine. Some prompt beneficial results have been reported. Inasmuch as this is a fairly simple procedure and there is little else that one can do therapeutically it seems justifiable.

The treatment for cerebral vascular accidents is supportive. Occasionally lumbar puncture is performed or hypertonic salt solution or magnesium sulfate is given by mouth, by rectum, or intravenously to diminish intracranial pressure. The results from these methods of treatment have not been very impressive, and the same may be said of phlebotomy. If the spinal fluid is bloody or it is under increased pressure, repeated punctures may be helpful. Caffeine sodium benzoate given intramuscularly in full doses (0.5 gm.) may be useful as a respiratory stimulant, and digitalis may be given if there are indications for its use, such as auricular fibrillation or congestive heart failure. When a localized subdural hematoma is suspected trephining the skull or surgical exploration would be indicated. At times x-ray examination may reveal dislocation of the pineal gland and thereby guide the surgeon to the correct side for operation. Even exploration of both sides of the brain may be necessary to find the localized blood clot.

PAROXYSMAL DYSPNEA

A common cause for sudden alarm and one for which the physician may be hurriedly called is a paroxysm of dyspnea or palpitation. Paroxysmal dyspnea is most apt to occur at night and is often associated with Cheyne-Stokes breathing. It is common in hypertensive heart disease, in syphilitic aortic insufficiency and in disease of the coronary arteries. It occurs much less frequently in rheumatic valvular disease. The patient is awakened from sleep with suffocation and air hunger. He is agitated and develops a cough and a wheeze. The typical picture of acute pulmonary edema, with abundant pink frothy sputum, may follow. The patient often has a cold sweat and struggles for air. The attack when mild may last only fifteen minutes to a half hour and be followed by a fairly comfortable sleep. When it is more severe the dyspnea continues uncontrolled and the patient's life seems to be at stake. It is generally wise for the physician to administer a hypodermic injection of 0.010 to 0.015 gm. ($\frac{1}{6}$ to $\frac{1}{4}$ grain) morphine and 0.6 mg. ($\frac{1}{100}$ grain) atropine. Within fifteen minutes after such treatment most of the attacks subside. Occasionally a phlebotomy of 500 cc. is extremely valuable. This is more beneficial if hypertension is present. The same result may be approximated by applying tourniquets to the extremities, thereby producing peripheral venous stasis. After the acute emergency is over adequate digitalis should be given to control future attacks. Another therapeutic measure that is often effective is the intravenous injection of aminophylline (0.24 to 0.48 gm.). This may stop an attack in five to ten minutes. It is also valuable in spells of acute bronchial asthma.

There is a growing impression that peripheral vasoconstriction plays a significant role in acute pulmonary edema. With this in mind one would be justified in expecting beneficial effects from nitroglycerin. Sarnoff has recently suggested use of a new preparation for this purpose. This is Arfonad, which is a ganglionic blocking agent that increases cardiac output without increasing cardiac work in congestive heart failure. Some favorable results have already been reported from the use of this drug. Furthermore, hexamethonium, about 2 mg. intravenously, by its ganglionic blocking action may abort acute pulmonary edema in 15 minutes when the blood pressure is elevated. Another procedure that may be tried is carotid sinus stimulation.

Paroxysms of dyspnea occur in still other conditions and for other causes than those just described. Occasionally dyspnea and even acute pulmonary edema is the initial event in acute coronary thrombosis, and treatment will then have to be directed accordingly. A patient may have a pulmonary embolism or infarct of the lung and be taken with sudden breathlessness and generalized pulmonary edema. It must be remembered that hemoptysis or bloody sputum frequently is absent in these conditions. Furthermore, a sudden increase in heart rate due to paroxysmal rapid heart action of one form or another may quickly produce air hunger, especially if it develops in one who already has significant organic cardiovascular disease. The differential diagnosis and treatment for these paroxysms have already been discussed (Chap. 13). Suffice it to say that such disturbances in the mechanism of the heart beat must be sought for because the proper treatment, which is generally very effective, will depend on accurate diagnosis. In the ordinary case of paroxysmal dyspnea (so-called "cardiac asthma") the heart rhythm remains normal and the rate is only slightly accelerated. In these other conditions the rate is very rapid and the rhythm may be either regular or irregular. Some patients will require large doses of digitalis, others may be readily controlled by pressure over the carotid sinus or the eyeball, and a third group will require quinidine or Pronestyl therapy, depending on whether the paroxysm is due to auricular fibrillation or flutter in the first, to auricular tachycardia in the second, or to ventricular tachycardia in the final instance.

PULMONARY EMBOLISM AND INFARCTION

Sudden dyspnea or pain in the chest or both may be due to a pulmonary embolus. The condition may closely simulate an attack of coronary thrombosis. The clinical features of the latter have already been discussed (Chap. 6) and need not be repeated. A large pulmonary embolus may cause death within five or ten minutes. It rarely kills as suddenly (in seconds or a minute) as does a coronary attack. Frequently the agony lasts longer, and in many instances recovery occurs. Infarction of the lung need not take place during the early minutes or hours of such an attack, as a longer time is required to produce these changes. The clinical features will vary considerably, depending on the size of the pulmonary embolus and upon the suddenness of the occlusion. It must also be borne in mind that pulmonary thrombosis can occur because of local changes in the lung that is congested and is not always due to embolism.

The most alarming and sudden cases are due to emboli dislodged from peripheral veins, especially those of the leg and the pelvis. Such venous thrombosis is common after surgical operations on the abdomen, and embolism may occur whether there has been clinical evidence of phlebitis or not. These accidents are most common about ten days postoperatively, but may develop any time. Attention has been called to the fact that fatal pulmonary embolism may result from deep-seated phlebitis following apparently innocent accidental injuries of the legs. In patients with organic heart disease pulmonary embolism follows the dislodgment of bits of mural thrombi from the right auricle, especially when mitral stenosis or persistent auricular fibrillation has been present. These are not so apt to be massive or fatal but are more likely to be accompanied by pulmonary infarction.

Pulmonary embolism or thrombosis may cause sudden dyspnea with or without chest pain. The breathing may have a peculiar character, as if the patient has a foreign body in his throat—a gasping struggle with the mouth wide open, like a fish out of water, but very little air is inspired. When pain is present it rarely has the radiation to the arms that characterizes coronary thrombosis. Cyanosis is also variable. Sudden faint feeling or actual loss of consciousness without any pain is a common initial symptom. Frequently it will be observed that the pulse and temperature had been rising for a few days before the more dramatic acute manifestation of pulmonary embolism took place. These premonitory features are probably due to the underlying thrombophlebitis. The picture of shock is frequently present, as in coronary thrombosis. If the patient survives the first twelve hours, fever and leukocytosis develop. When infarction of the lung results hemoptysis can occur. Bloody sputum, however, is not at all necessary to the diagnosis of pulmonary infarction. Jaundice is common with pulmonary infarction whether hepatic engorgement is present or not. The heart rate is apt to increase, the pulmonary second sound may be accentuated, and the blood pressure may fall. Dilatation of the pulmonary artery occurs. This may be discovered by percussion or by x-ray examination, or be revealed by a pulsation in the second left interspace. At times a systolic murmur or a to-and-fro rub appears at the pulmonary area. Even changes in the ventricular complexes of the electrocardiograms resembling those seen in myocardial infarction may be found. The characteristic electrocardiographic pattern consists of deep S_1, prominent Q_3, clockwise rotation with a shift of the transitional zone to the left, a vertical electrical axis, and tachycardia, S-T segment depression in leads I and II, and in the left precordial leads, as well as T wave inversion in V_1 to V_3 or V_4 may be found. Significant Q waves or loss of R wave amplitude other than that accounted for by rotation of the electrical axis does not occur. The differential diagnosis may be extremely difficult, but a survey of all the data and particularly a search for the focus from which an embolus may have arisen and the relation of the attack to a previous operation may enable one to arrive at the correct diagnosis.

CORONARY THROMBOSIS AND SUDDEN CHEST PAINS

The lay public has now become quite aware of the significance of pain in the chest and its relation to coronary artery disease. This leads to many hurried calls for a physician. Many such emergencies turn out to be false alarms. Bearing in mind that coronary thrombosis is very common one must not forget that there are other causes of severe pain or distress in the chest. Some of the more important conditions that may simulate coronary thrombosis, such as pneumothorax and dissecting aneurysm, were discussed previously (Chap. 6). Besides these conditions, other and milder disorders at times turn out to be the cause of such attacks. I have been called to see numerous cases diagnosed as coronary thrombosis in which later events showed that the whole disturbance was due to neurosis, herpes zoster, bronchial spasm, arthritis of the spine, acute pyelitis, acute hemorrhage from a peptic ulcer, or other conditions. Great care, therefore, must be exercised in the interpretation of chest pain.

PERIPHERAL EMBOLI

Peripheral embolism furnishes further examples of sudden circulatory emergencies. These occur under the same circumstances as those mentioned above for cerebral embolism. The embolus may affect the kidney, spleen, intestine, or limbs. When the abdominal viscera are involved the diagnosis may be quite difficult. More usual surgical conditions like acute appendicitis or perforated peptic ulcer will need to be considered, but occasional unnecessary surgery will be inevitable. Splenic or renal embolism is best treated medically, whereas involvement of the mesenteric arteries when recognizable is apt to require an intestinal resection. A sudden severe pain in the arm or leg with blanching and coldness of the limb and disappearance of the arterial pulsation usually means an embolus. Many physicians still confuse arterial occlusion and venous phlebitis. In the latter condition the limb is not cold and there eventually develops swelling, whereas in the former there is no swelling and the temperature of the affected part falls. Some patients with embolism recover on symptomatic treatment. Embolectomy, together with heparin therapy, has been practiced at times with excellent results and at other times without success. It is best performed during the first six hours after the onset and certainly before twenty-four hours have elapsed. The use of an apparatus which produces artificial alternate suction and compression of the limb may be of aid in this problem and make embolectomy unnecessary. When gangrene has already developed in a limb, amputation will be necessary. Other methods are being tried, such as procaine hydrochloride injections in the lumbar sympathetic system and freezing the limb involved.

PAROXYSMAL RAPID HEART ACTION

Any of the forms of paroxysmal rapid heart action discussed in the previous chapter may be the cause of a cardiovascular emergency. When organic heart disease already is present, although compensation may be excellent, or even if the heart is structurally normal, a sudden change of rate from 80 to 160 or 200 may produce a state of collapse or shock or sudden acute pulmonary edema. At times with the onset of such a rapid rate actual syncope may take place, and in some cases anginal pain may occur. The physician should make every effort to examine the heart during the attack in order to establish the exact type of abnormal rhythm that is responsible, for the treatment (see Chap. 13) will vary with the different forms.

ACUTE HEMORRHAGE

Many instances of acute hemorrhage have obvious causes and present an emergency situation. A massive nosebleed, or a large hemoptysis or hematemesis presents individual problems. Treatment is then directed at the underlying condition, whether it is hypertension, pulmonary tuberculosis, cirrhosis of the liver, or peptic ulcer. Occasionally with extensive internal bleeding diagnosis may become very difficult. Hypertensive patients may have acute hemothorax or hemoperitoneum. Of particular interest are cases of acute and massive gastrointestinal bleeding. Because of the sudden shock and collapse these patients may resemble those with coronary thrombosis. Only in a day or so, when a dark or tarry stool is passed, may the true nature of the disease become apparent. Furthermore, during the state of shock accompanying severe hemorrhage, coronary thrombosis occasionally develops as a complication. This increases the difficulty in differential diagnosis. When threatening hemorrhages develop as a result of the administration of anticoagulants prompt measures are indicated. Vitamin K_1 oxide is then recommended in doses of 50 to 75 mg. intravenously (each ampule of 1 cc. contains 50 mg.) at a rate of about 10 mg. per minute. This is to counteract dicumarin preparations. If heparin was the agent used the excess bleeding time can be controlled by intravenous injection of 50 to 100 mg. of protamine sulfate.

EXCESSIVE TRACHEAL SECRETIONS

There are frequent conditions in which the patient seems to be drowning in his own bronchial and tracheal secretions. This may occur during pulmonary infections, congestive heart failure, or postoperative states. The use of a suction tube inserted through the nose into the trachea or even through a tracheotomy tube may be very helpful and at times even life saving.

AIR EMBOLISM

On rare occasions, during the performance of therapeutic pneumoperitoneum, thoracentesis, or other manipulation, air emboli may develop. The froth may become trapped in the pulmonary artery. There is experimental and some clinical evidence to support the view that placing the patient on his left side may permit the air to ascend to the right pulmonary vessels, freeing the left and thereby preventing an otherwise fatal outcome.

"CO₂ NARCOSIS"

In some cases of severe pulmonary emphysema or of chronic advanced pulmonary disease with difficulty in perfusion, inhalation of concentrated oxygen by tent, mask, or catheter may precipitate coma.

In chronic pulmonary disease the respiratory center becomes relatively insensitive to CO_2; the only stimulus therefore sustaining ventilation is hypoxia. When O_2 is administered the arterial oxygen tension increases. The sole stimulus for respiration having been removed, ventilation becomes depressed, with a rise in CO_2 concentration. When the pCO_2 exceeds 100 mm. of mercury, CO_2 narcosis ensues. This may follow even after brief periods of O_2 breathing of one to two hours. Intravenous salicylates may be of benefit in overcoming this type of CO_2 narcosis. A dose of 6 to 8 gm., given over a 60-minute period, may enhance the sensitivity of the respiratory center to CO_2 with a resulting decrease in the arterial pCO_2, and a rise in the pH and arterial oxygen concentration. The inference is that cases of this sort need careful watching during oxygen therapy and therapy should be discontinued if suggestive evidence of stupor appears. Some may require an artificial respirator for a while until the critical period is passed. When respirations are depressed by an excessive dose of morphine in pulmonary cases intravenous caffeine and artificial respiration are indicated.

PARALYSIS FROM POTASSIUM

Derangement in potassium metabolism may of itself threaten the life of a patient. Paralysis of both striated and cardiac muscles may result from either an excess or a deficit of potassium in the cells. If there is potassium accumulation in the body, i.e., hyperkalemia, as may occur in marked or prolonged anuria or oliguria, the artificial kidney if available is the most efficient method of treatment. Lacking this the prompt rapid intravenous injection of 100 to 200 cc. of 3 per cent sodium chloride solution is recommended. Once improvement has been obtained this can be followed by the intravenous infusion of 50 to 100 gm. of 25 per cent dextrose in distilled water. The solution should also contain $\frac{1}{2}$ unit of crystalline zinc insulin for each gram of dextrose.

The opposite condition, i.e., hypokalemia, may occur in insulin treatment of diabetic acidosis, or result from the loss of body fluids that accompanies vomiting, diarrhea, fistulas, gastrointestinal suction, excessive diuresis in congestive failure, in cases of "potassium-losing" nephritis, and in patients with familial periodic paralysis. The treatment of potassium depletion, apart from correction of its cause, is the administration of potassium chloride, 1.0 gm. three times daily, in the form of enteric-coated tablets or intravenously, depending on the circumstances.

GENERAL COMMENTS

It can readily be seen from the foregoing discussion that the emergencies in cardiovascular disease are numerous. Sudden events and changes in the clinical condition of the patient are found to have a limited number of causes. They require a mechanism that can produce a sudden alteration in the blood supply of an individual part of the body or that suddenly changes the mechanism of the heart beat. A blood vessel can rupture or become partially or completely occluded. The heart may suddenly take on too rapid or too slow a beat as a result of a disturbance in the normal rhythm. Finally, certain sudden nervous influences or reflexes may be set at work, producing vasomotor changes or alterations in the blood pressure resulting in syncope. They all require individual analysis for, without this, intelligent treatment cannot be carried out.

CHAPTER 15

Medicolegal Aspects of Heart Disease

Physicians have become more and more concerned with the relation of trauma to heart disease. The decisions that need to be made by courts, industrial accident boards, and insurance companies often require medical opinions as to the existence of heart disease, or as to the possible development of heart disease or the aggravation of pre-existing heart disease following trauma or accidents. We physicians have had little to do with the formulation of the existing laws and may believe that some are imperfect or even unwise. That is not our present concern. It is expected that we should offer intelligent and honest opinions as to the medical problems involved, leaving it to the judge and jury to interpret the law in the light of these facts and opinions.

As an illustration of a situation that seems unfair or at least unwise, the following may be mentioned. Two men were injured in the same way while working and died several months following the accident, as a result of the injuries received. One was a 25-year-old man who was perfectly well, and the other was a man 68 years of age who was known to have had hypertension and angina pectoris. In the first instance, the young man's life expectancy was shortened forty years or more, while in the second it was shortened possibly two or three years. In the eyes of the law in many courts or of industrial accident boards the damages for the death of the two individuals would be identical. It would seem more just from a sociologic point of view to differentiate the total amount of harm done to an individual by a specific accident according to the life expectancy, when a known organic condition exists. This and other aspects of the problem are making it difficult or impossible for patients with heart disease, even when the cardiac abnormality is trivial, to obtain employment in industry.

There are many circumstances in which a physician is unable to answer questions of cause and effect if heart problems arise after accidents. The experience of most of us is confined mainly to the ordinary progress of heart disease. Our knowledge concerning the effects of trauma on the circulation is limited. Because of this lack of knowledge, the honest physician is often compelled to say he does not know whether a certain blow to the leg or chest or a fright can cause myocardial injury or any given arrhythmia. He may reason to the best of his ability and decide that the particular abnormality could not be or was a very unlikely result of the accident. He might state that the cardiac condition was a coincidence or was present before the accident, or was the result of the natural progress of disease. He would be influenced by his limited theoretical knowledge and by the fact that he had not encountered such a causal relationship in his general practice. Similar points of view have been taken in the past concerning certain matters, only to find that years later such opinions were wrong. A good example of this is pain in the back following severe injuries. When such pain continued for months or years and physical examination including x-ray studies revealed no abnormality, the condition was often called neurosis or "railroad spine." In some cases it would even be inferred that the patients were malingering. No doubt many of these cases were functional or neurogenic, but we know now that some were due to a dislocated and compressed intervertebral disk. Only in recent years has this condition been recognized.

The same situation exists in relation to heart disease. Formerly it was difficult to understand how a patient might develop angina pectoris or symptoms of coronary artery disease following trauma. If a man complained of anginal symptoms after an accident, I previously took the position that he must have had symptoms of this before but was not telling about them. The most that one could admit was that the condition was aggravated by the accident. Through the interest of Warburg in Denmark and of Beck and Boas in this country, we have learned that direct blows to the chest, even without fractures of ribs or actual abrasion of the skin, can traumatize the heart muscle or coronary arteries so as to produce symptoms of coronary insufficiency. The "steering wheel" accidents that have become so common are good examples of the type in which contusion of the heart muscle occurs. There are now well-authenticated cases in which, after an accident, definite angina pectoris or coronary thrombosis developed. Even instances of rupture of the heart or of a valve have been observed. These cardiac conditions may result not only from direct trauma of the chest, but also from severe injuries to other parts of the body or as a result of very severe and unaccustomed strain. I recall seeing an instance of a ruptured mitral valve which resulted from the severe strain of rowing a boat in a storm. The ruptured valve was found on postmortem examination. In this case increasing dyspnea and congestive failure developed, the man dying several months after the strain.

Of considerable importance from a medicolegal point of view is the differentiation of pulmonary embolism and coronary thrombosis. This problem has already been discussed in Chapter 6. It may be emphasized that after traumatic accidents, especially those involving fractures or bruises of the legs and the application of casts, thrombophlebitis and subsequent pulmonary emboli are common and that they are often misdiagnosed as posterior myocardial infarction. Occasionally disinterring the body even months after death has clarified the situation (see pp. 141–142).

Arrhythmias of the heart may also result from unusual physical or mental strain. Many such cardiac irregularities produce no significant ill effects. Others are of more importance. I remember seeing a man who developed auricular fibrillation directly after falling down an elevator shaft. In another case, a man who had been operated upon for hyperthyroidism and had been symptomatically cured had a recurrence immediately after being held up in the street by a burglar. The symptoms of hyperthyroidism with auricular fibrillation promptly returned.

The most important point in many of these cases is the time relation between the accident and the cardiac abnormality. If the exact status of the patient before the accident is known, it is reasonable to assume that new objective or subjective evidence of disability occurring within minutes, hours, or several days is due to the accident. Objective evidence is obviously more reliable than subjective. It therefore is important to record findings such as heart rate and rhythm, blood pressure, electrocardiograms, the presence of rales in the lungs, roentgen findings, and the like, as soon as possible after an accident. When the physician has to depend on symptoms, due regard must be had to functional and emotional reactions and to the possibility of malingering. However, the courts and some physicians have had a tendency to minimize the importance of post-traumatic neurosis. Many of the soldiers of the First World War who suffered severe neurocirculatory asthenia have ever since been much more handicapped than others who had fractures of bones or gunshot wounds of the abdomen or chest. In some of these cases the nervous symptoms have continued indefinitely, even when the question of war compensation did not enter into consideration. This has been found to be true in a follow-up study in England and has its counterpart in civil practice.

The following experience is illustrative. A man of 40 who had always been well and strong had worked steadily for many years. He had been accustomed to manipulating very heavy steel beams. One day he was hit by a swinging beam and sustained a violent crushing blow to the body. An arm and ribs were fractured, and it took a few months for physical recovery. When the patient became ambulatory he complained of weakness, palpitation, dyspnea on effort, and tremulousness. These are the classic symptoms of neurocirculatory asthenia. I found no evidence of organic heart disease or any other significant organic disease. I regarded this working man as being in a worse condition than if he had recovered with a permanent limp in a leg or a contracture of an arm, but without any nervous symptoms. I felt certain that he would never be able to do the strenuous physical work to which he was formerly accustomed. I am afraid that such patients, when we feel that they are honest, receive poor treatment in medicolegal controversies.

The time relation is also very important when the question of aggravation of a pre-existing condition comes up. If a new chain of symptoms or findings develops a few hours or a few days after an accident and the clinical status before the accident appears to have been stationary, it is fair to assume that some degree of aggravation occurred. On the other hand, if examination reveals that there was no change for a few weeks and certain disabilities resulted thereafter, it is extremely unlikely that the accident was the cause of the change. In a case of this sort a very minor accident was supposed to have aggravated a preexisting mitral stenosis and auricular fibrillation. I had reliable data before and after the accident which showed no change whatever. The patient claimed his breathing was worse, but I knew that the vital capacity of the lungs was in no way affected. This enabled me to maintain that the state of cardiac efficiency was not altered by the accident.

The main difficulty is in interpreting symptoms. When the problem of angina is involved, we are so dependent upon the subjective complaints that errors can easily be made, either for or against the interest of the patient. We must first be certain of the diagnosis and then we should try to get some proof that the anginal pain is more frequent, more severe, of greater duration, or brought on by less effort. If there is reason to doubt the veracity of the patient, he may need to be "shadowed" in order to check his statements. This does not come within the province of a physician, as we are not detectives, but rather guardians of the health of our patients. It may be the work of a lawyer or the insurance company. In all these matters scrupulous care and honesty on the part of the examining physician are paramount.

Finally, the troublesome question of "total and permanent disability" will be discussed. From a purely sociologic point of view, this provision in insurance policies has often proved to be a great blunder. It has undermined the morale of many an honest citizen and has forced some physicians into practices which, from an ethical point of view, are at least open to question. Many of us would be happier if no such insurance policies had ever been written. Insurance companies are suffering tremendous losses which must be borne by all policyholders. This is due partly to the unexpected increase in chronic cardiovascular disease that has taken place during the past decades and partly to the economic depression of previous years. Added to this is the fact that many unrighteous claims have been granted because of the dishonesty of policyholders, occasionally with collusion of unscrupulous physicians.

The first difficulty comes in interpreting the term "total and permanent disability." Some totally blind or deaf people support themselves. A man could be bedridden and yet earn something reading proof or translating foreign medical publications, as I know one physician did for two years. It is the duty of the court to make a legal interpretation of this phrase. When a person takes out such insurance, he probably has in mind a protection against his inability to continue his accustomed work. If a man is an active obstetrician and has to climb stairs to get to his patients' homes, and must be able to exert himself vigorously when using forceps, then increasing breathlessness from cardiac weakness or from emphysema of the lungs renders him unfit to continue his occupation permanently. However, if he is a dermatologist with mainly an office practice, he may be able to carry on for some months or years longer.

Now, are we to say that one or both are totally and permanently disabled? Many a disabled individual could carry on some mild or sedentary occupation, if he were trained differently and if such a position were available. But we cannot make a dermatologist out of an obstetrician overnight. Likewise, a day laborer cannot easily be trained to be a cashier. The best we as physicians can do is to express an honest opinion as to whether or not a given occupation is an added hazard to the comfort or life of the patient concerned.

It is not our duty to help insurance companies undo losses that they have sustained. If we make an unwise investment in a home or in business, we have to suffer the loss. Insurance companies made what have proved to be unwise contracts and must inevitably pay for their mistakes. On the other hand, we must protect them against any false claims, by a most painstaking medical analysis, keeping in mind the interest of the patient and the company. Unfortunately, the final decision may depend on the amount of insurance involved. If a physician in general practice has insurance protection of $4,000 a year against total and permanent disability, his position may be different if he earns $10,000 rather than only $4,000 yearly. When he develops angina pectoris and finds it hard to climb stairs or drive his motor car in wintry weather, he may well prefer to carry on because of a greater income, even if he may shorten his life or have more attacks of angina. If his income is no greater than his insurance, he is much less likely to want to suffer any more than necessary. A physician may quite reasonably urge one man to carry on and another to quit work when the physical disability is the same in both cases. At times it seems that the advantages of retiring are not great enough to warrant the financial loss involved. In some cases the joy and satisfaction of working compensates for the increase in discomforts. Some physicians would choose to have more attacks of angina but continue their practice. I believe that a man has a right to choose whether he will have more suffering and keep at work, or less suffering and accept his insurance protection, provided there is no doubt about the diagnosis and the reality of the symptoms or disability.

There has been a move on the part of some insurance companies that seems wise and should be extended. When a patient has coronary artery disease and his condition seems fair, it may be advisable to permit him to try to resume some work. If such an individual has been receiving total permanent disability benefits, some companies will give him a trial period of three months, during which time full compensation is continued while he resumes some or all of his duties. If at the end of that time it is clear that he cannot carry on, he again retires and continues to receive disability payments. If his progress is favorable after this three months' period, he then discontinues receiving the disability benefits and carries on with his work. This is a wise and useful provision, both for the insurance companies and for the policyholders, for it may save the former expense and may help to rehabilitate the patient. Physicians should cooperate in this plan with the understanding that the insured will not jeopardize his interests by making an honest effort to return to work.

To return to the difficult problem of angina in which subjective complaints are so important, it may be necessary to perform pecial tests for diagnostic purposes, such as a Master two-step test or a ballistocardiographic examination. "Shadowing" this patient may also be necessary, to determine whether he actually is unable to walk or work. It must be remembered, however, that detecting a man walking a mile or two in Florida in the winter does not necessarily mean that he can walk one block in New England. Many individuals who can do very little in cold climates can exert themselves a great deal in warm ones. One should try to check the statements that are made in direct relation to the individual's ordinary working activities. Furthermore, it is fair for the physician to assume that his patient is honest, until he knows otherwise. This is particularly true when the family physician has known the patient for many years and has always found him to be honorable. I have known instances in which men were receiving insurance for total disability which I thought was entirely unjustified, and I have informed the companies to that effect. Unfortunately, too, I have seen instances when patients were disbelieved and had their insurance discontinued, only to prove their honesty by dying of a coronary thrombosis. The physician has a difficult task. Only by great care and wise and honest regard, for both the interest of our patients and the protection of insurance companies, can the high standards of our profession be maintained and the services expected of us be rendered.

CHAPTER 16

The Significance of Bronchial and
Other Factors in the Production of Dyspnea

Breathlessness is the most important symptom of heart disease. In the early stages of cardiac failure it may be the only evidence that the cardiovascular apparatus is inefficient. This is true whether the problem is one of valvular or of nonvalvular heart disease. The physical findings at this time may be entirely negative or may be very insignificant, showing only those alterations which are commonly present in patients without any heart disease. It becomes very important, therefore, to be able to interpret intelligently the significance of this primary complaint—shortness of breath. Other factors beside heart failure play their respective roles in the production of dyspnea, and some of these, especially the bronchial, deserve consideration.

Inasmuch as heart disease is extremely common and asthmatic bronchitis is also very prevalent, it is not surprising that the two conditions are frequently present in the same individual. From a purely statistical point of view it would be expected that a considerable number of people might suffer from both diseases. In point of fact, however, I have seen so many patients with organic heart disease, especially rheumatic valvular disease, who were also suffering from asthma that I have been led to believe that the relationship is not merely coincidental. It may be that the prolonged pulmonary stasis which accompanies heart failure, of itself, in some way renders the bronchial tree more susceptible to the asthmatic state. Another relationship which seems to be important is that other allergic stigmata, such as a previous history of hay fever, urticaria, or chronic eczema, or a family history of such diseases, are frequently detected in rheumatic cardiac patients. One may suspect that such individuals are allergic in two different senses. In the first place, they are sensitive to the proteins that bring about bronchial asthma, hay fever, and urticaria. In the second place, they may be regarded as allergic in the sense that many manifestations of rheumatic fever are now looked upon as allergic reactions. These considerations may explain the undue frequency of asthmatic bronchitis in cardiac patients.

Bearing in mind that shortness of breath is the outstanding complaint in both conditions, it is most important to distinguish how much of the disability is due to each, for the prognosis and treatment will depend a great deal upon this distinction. This differentiation is obviously most important, because, although dyspnea due to asthmatic bronchitis is distressing, it comes and goes and is compatible with a long and fairly useful life, whereas when it results from cardiac failure, especially when it is of the paroxysmal type, the outlook is very grave. Furthermore, digitalis is helpful for cardiac dyspnea and useless for bronchial dyspnea, and medication like ephedrine, Adrenalin, and potassium iodide, which often is beneficial for bronchial dyspnea, is practically of no avail in cardiac failure.

Such problems are best illustrated by actual practical experiences. Some years ago I was called to see a woman 60 years of age who was suffering from attacks of dyspnea, especially at night. She was the mother of a physician and had been seen by a most competent consultant who regarded the condition as hypertensive heart disease with paroxysmal nocturnal dyspnea, or so-called "cardiac asthma." This diagnosis carries with it a very ominous prognosis, for such patients do not live on the average more than a few years. I found that the dyspnea was only of several weeks' duration. Physical examination showed the customary amount of arteriosclerosis for a woman of her age. There was slight hypertension, the readings being 180 mm. systolic and 100 mm. diastolic. The heart was slightly enlarged, the action was regular with a rate of 90, and there was a slight systolic murmur at the apical and basal regions. There was no peripheral pitting edema and no hepatic or venous engorgement. Up to that point the findings were compatible with the diagnosis previously made, for many patients with paroxysmal cardiac dyspnea show very little of significance on examination, except cardiac enlargement. The signs in the lungs, however, gave the clue to the proper diagnosis. Rales were heard generally distributed throughout both lungs and were readily audible over both sides anteriorly. They were inspiratory and expiratory and of the squeaking type, such as are found in asthma or emphysema. There were no moist rales at the bases of the lungs. When rales are due to cardiac failure they are almost invariably moist and inspiratory and limited to the bases of the lungs. When they are generally distributed, as occurs in acute pulmonary edema, they are also moist or bubbling and may occur in both phases of respiration, but the patient is then obviously in an acute serious state. Such was not the case here. The conclusion, therefore, was that the patient, although elderly, hypertensive, and somewhat arteriosclerotic, had no heart failure whatever, and that the dyspnea was entirely due to asthmatic bronchitis. Subsequent developments confirmed this opinion. The digitalis she was taking was omitted, and instead she was told to take 10 drops of saturated solution of potassium iodide three times a day, $\frac{3}{8}$ grain of ephedrine morning and night, and to use steam inhalations. Either as a result of the medications or because of the changes in weather which often have an effect on an asthmatic state, she quickly improved and remained ambulatory for many years. Congestive heart failure never developed, although she lived more than ten years after this experience, occasionally having recurring bouts of bronchial dyspnea.

The above experience illustrates the misinterpretation of the cause of dyspnea in a patient who proved to have no element of cardiac failure whatever. The following case illustrates the importance of differentiating the various factors involved when there is known organic heart disease. This patient was a man about 40 years old who had been coming to the heart clinic for some years. He had rheumatic mitral stenosis and auricular fibrillation. There was a past history of hay fever. He had remained fairly well compensated, taking 0.1 gm. of digitalis daily, and was able to attend his little grocery shop. One day he was taken into the hospital and was found to be desperately sick. He had extreme dyspnea, the heart rate was accelerated and grossly irregular, there was a fever of 101° F., and he was irrational. Extreme dyspnea and orthopnea were the outstanding features. His condition was regarded sufficiently serious so that he was put on the dangerous list. What amazed the physicians in attendance and comforted the family was that I held out a fair hope for his recovery. I did so because a good bit of the respiratory distress could be accounted for on the basis of bronchial dyspnea. Although there were many moist congestive rales at the bases of the lungs, there were also numerous asthmatic squeaks throughout both lungs. He not only recovered but was able to continue at his light occupation for several years. I have had numerous other similar experiences in which the proper interpretation of the various factors producing dyspnea served as the main basis for offering a better prognosis than might otherwise have been made and in instituting more intelligent treatment.

The detection of a bronchial factor in cardiac patients is of considerable importance in treating ambulatory cardiac patients in an outpatient clinic. Here we have a group of individuals belonging to the lower economic strata of life and if they are gainfully employed it is imperative to keep them so whenever possible. Picture a married man 40 years of age who has mitral stenosis and auricular fibrillation, who works indoors as a salesman and is able to carry on fairly satisfactorily. The occupation is not laborious, and he manages to keep on the job and support himself. We all know that if such a man takes sick leave very often he will lose his job and that he may never be able to find another. He has been taking digitalis constantly and thereby the heart rate is kept fairly slow. Under these circumstances there will come a time when congestive failure will supervene, requiring a period of rest in bed. This will generally be ushered in by increasing dyspnea. On the other hand, if the increase in dyspnea were due to asthmatic bronchitis we would not only be justified in permitting this man to keep at work but we probably would advise him to do so, in order that he might not jeopardize his earning power. Furthermore, increasing the dose of digitalis in these cases is generally of no avail, while a combination of ephedrine and potassium iodide often improves the condition. A familiarity with the bronchial factor in the production of dyspnea and the detection of the asthmatic type of rales have formed the background for the proper treatment of these patients. This has enabled patients to continue at work who would otherwise have been put to bed and has saved many of them their jobs.

There is a serious form of dyspnea, really bronchial in origin, which results from chronic emphysema of the lungs (chronic cor pulmonale). This generally is a slowly progressive process maturing into its severe stage later in life. Occasionally, however, it may appear in its advanced form at middle age. The patient often has a characteristic slightly bluish suffused appearance to his face. The chest is increased in its antero-posterior diameter, cyanosis develops early and may become quite marked, and there is progressive dyspnea. The breath sounds are diminished in intensity, expiration is prolonged, cardiac dullness diminishes because of the overlying expanded lungs, and the heart sounds become distant. The intercostal spaces are increased, the diaphragm is depressed and liver dullness is diminished. In a pure case there is right ventricular enlargement. Electrocardiograms often show right ventricular hypertrophy and complexes of low amplitude. An x-ray of the chest may show a prominent pulmonary conus. Objective signs of congestive heart failure, like pitting edema and enlarged liver, come late in the disease. There often is a marked reduction in the vital capacity of the lungs because they are already fully distended and the enlarged chest cavity cannot expand much more. What is even more important is that the entire respiratory cycle lasts much longer than normal and it is difficult to increase the number of breaths per minute.

Furthermore, although in a normal individual 90 per cent of the total vital capacity can be expired during the first one or two seconds, in cases of emphysema it will take much longer. This type of dyspnea in association with cardiac failure is not dramatically helped by digitalis, but when it is used in conjunction with other measures directed at the bronchial condition digitalis may be of some benefit. These measures include bronchial dilators, antibiotics, expectorants, etc. The use of morphine is dangerous, especially when the condition is advanced and the vital capacity of the lung is very low. The condition can be ameliorated by a properly fitted abdominal belt. This belt can actually elevate the diaphragm and thereby aid its mechanical movements, increase the vital capacity of the lungs, and improve the breathing. Isuprel inhalations are often very beneficial or 5 to 8 drops of Vaponephrin in a hand nebulizer three to four times daily may help. Tracheal suction may be advisable. Potassium iodide, ammonium chloride, aminophylline, and sodium salicylate are also employed. Phlebotomy is indicated if the hematocrit level is elevated. Inhalation of oxygen may be helpful but must be administered with caution. It is quite striking that in the early stages and often for many years patients with chronic emphysema may be quite short of breath on effort and yet have no orthopnea, being able to lie flat quite comfortably.

A much neglected and overlooked group of cases is one in which there is emphysema and a mediastinal goiter. The latter may be benign or toxic, and generally has been present for many years before it is detected, because no enlargement of the thyroid gland need be detected on ordinary physical examination and there may be little if any evidence of thyrotoxicosis. Such patients have increasing breathlessness and often display a peculiar suffused appearance of the face. Roentgenologic examination will reveal the thoracic goiter and often will show a compressed or deviated trachea. If discovered early enough, operation may afford great relief or at least arrest the progress of the condition.

Closely related to pulmonary emphysema is a condition in which the primary pathologic process is in the fine pulmonary arteries. It has been called Ayerza's disease, and the patients with the condition have been called black cardiacs. Although it was first thought to be syphilitic in origin, most of those cases now recognized have been found to be nonsyphilitic. The striking feature is the intense cyanosis with increasing severe dyspnea and weakness. This is a type of chronic cor pulmonale similar in its manifestations to the severe forms of "emphysema heart." Not infrequently in cases of this sort the disease is not primary in the pulmonary vessel wall itself but is rather the result of multiple miliary pulmonary emboli coming from some distal focus or in fact the result of local thromboses of the small pulmonary branches. Rarely miliary carcinomatous metastases present the same clinical picture.

Patients with advanced pulmonary arterial disease often suffer syncopal attacks. In the late stages peripheral edema may be present. Examination of the heart may show little abnormal except for an accentuated pulmonary second sound. X-ray reveals evidence of right-sided enlargement and a dilated pulmonary artery. The electrocardiograms will almost invariably display complexes indicative of right ventricular enlargement. Catheterization studies by Dexter showed that pressure in the pulmonary artery and right ventricle is considerably increased but is normal in the left auricle and in the pulmonary capillaries. These circulatory findings are similar to those obtained in compensated well-marked mitral stenosis, except that in the latter "pulmonary capillary pressure" is increased when heart failure is present. It is of significance that in marked pulmonary vascular disease exercise does not produce an increase in cardiac output.

There are several other factors to be considered in interpreting breathlessness, such as anemia, functional dyspnea, and obesity. The first of these can quickly be dismissed. An appreciable degree of anemia is rarely of importance in patients who have cardiac failure from organic heart disease. Occasionally dyspnea is present solely as a result of anemia in patients whose cardiovascular apparatus is essentially normal. Moreover, appreciable dilatation of the heart may also be caused by anemia. Such patients may be erroneously treated for heart disease when liver or iron properly administered is all that is needed. It must be borne in mind that when the hemoglobin content of the blood is sufficiently reduced, dyspnea, especially on effort, can develop because of the diminished oxygen-carrying power of the blood. It is needless to say that digitalis cannot correct this defect. Furthermore, if the anemic state and dilatation of the heart persist for a long time, irreversible cardiac hypertrophy may take place.

A more important problem is dyspnea due to neurotic or functional factors. This frequently takes the form of "sighing breathing" and has been discussed in Chapter 12 and need not be gone into in detail here. Let it suffice to mention that it is common in those who have no organic circulatory disease and is not at all rare even in those with definite structural changes. When this condition is marked and maintained it may result in disturbing hyperventilation. Symptoms of tetany develop with tingling and numbness of the extremities. It is not difficult to interpret properly this type of dyspnea, especially if the physician observes the patients taking these deep breaths (overventilation) when they complain they cannot get enough air. It often has been helpful in my experience to find that, after an individual has complained bitterly of not being able to breathe even while at rest, the vital capacity of the lungs proved to be normal. It is almost impossible for an individual to have distressing breathlessness from cardiac failure and yet have a normal vital capacity of the lungs. These considerations apply with equal force even when definite organic heart disease is present. Many patients with well-compensated valvular disease have dyspnea of neurogenic origin. The vital capacity of the lungs may be normal, the prognosis will be good, and treatment must be directed at the functional state. Here also it is obvious that the proper interpretation of functional dyspnea will avoid errors in diagnosis, prognosis, and treatment.

There is still another type of functional or neurogenic dyspnea that is different from that called "sighing breathing." It takes on a variety of forms. I once saw a young girl who appeared well, had very few complaints, and merely showed a very faint systolic murmur. The respiratory rate, however, was about 55, although there was no dyspnea and the mother was not aware of the rapid rate of breathing. In another case a hysterical man had a respiratory rate of 120 with otherwise normal findings. He had very few complaints and could lie flat. During sleep, however, the rate of respiration was normal. In two other cases there were marked dyspnea and orthopnea with very noisy and rapid breathing. One case was first regarded as due to serious heart disease, then to bronchial asthma. The patient was cured by psychotherapy. The other was a most extraordinary case featured by terrific attacks of suffocation. The patient even had an exploratory operation on the mediastinum in one hospital and a tracheotomy in another. He also seemed to be cured, at least temporarily, by psychotherapy. These may be regarded as instances of hysterical dyspnea.

Consideration must also be given to the weight of the patient who complains of breathlessness. Mention has been made of the fact that dyspnea may be the only early manifestation of cardiac failure. It is also well known that obese individuals frequently suffer from organic cardio-vascular disease, especially hypertension. What is not fully appreciated is that obesity itself in an otherwise healthy individual can produce shortness of breath. The stout person cannot breathe as freely as the lean. The diaphragm does not descend so readily, and when the adiposity particularly involves the abdominal region the diaphragm is apt to be held in a high position and the vital capacity of the lungs is diminished. It follows, therefore, that not all obese patients who have dyspnea have heart failure, and that even when there is definite evidence of organic heart disease, the dyspnea may be only partly, if at all, the result of weakening of the circulation. There are many obese patients whom I have seen who had been treated for heart disease when I felt convinced they were not suffering from anything more than obesity. Such patients will do better on a dietary regimen judiciously followed, directed at a slow reduction in weight, than they will on digitalis therapy. In fact, even if the obesity is permitted to continue they do well, as this form of dyspnea is not progressive and is apt to be elicited only on effort, particularly climbing of stairs. It is evident that the converse of this is true; i.e., other things being equal, shortness of breath is more serious in a thin individual, for here despite the freedom of diaphragmatic movement there still is limitation in expansion of the lungs.

Because breathlessness is the primary evidence of heart failure, whenever this is a major complaint either the patient or the doctor will quickly suspect the heart as the cause. It must not be forgotten that there are other causes of shortness of breath. Many diseases, particularly of the thoracic cavity, may produce dyspnea and occasionally they are overlooked when a weakened myocardium is thought to be present. Some of these conditions are pneumonia, tumors of the lung, miliary carcinomatosis of the lung, Hodgkin's disease, silicosis, sarcoid of the lung, pulmonary fibrosis, aortic aneurysm, pulmonary tuberculosis, bronchiectasis, pneumothorax, and septicemia. Under one set of circumstances or another the possibility of these diseases will need serious investigation, especially if the heart is found to be normal in size.

In this connection mention should be made of deformity of the chest as a cause of true myocardial insufficiency. The condition is called cardiorespiratory failure. The thoracic cage is occasionally so deformed as a result of early infantile paralysis or tuberculosis of the spine, or because of congenital and developmental deformities such as "trichterbrust" or "funnel chest," that the position of the heart is markedly distorted. Dilatation and hypertrophy of the cardiac chambers with congestive heart failure may result. This is produced by mechanical factors such as kinking or constriction of the large vessels leading to or from the heart, or by changes in the lung. It is now believed that the difficulty in respiratory function is much more important than the cardiac status. Such cases progress like severe forms of chronic cor pulmonale from pulmonary emphysema, pulmonary artery disease, or chronic pulmonary fibrosis. Although this type of heart failure is quite rare it calls attention to the desirability of correcting as much as possible all chest deformities during the early years of life.

The foregoing discussion amply justifies the point of view that the mechanism of dyspnea needs careful appraisal. Various possible factors have different prognostic and therapeutic implications. Only in this way will serious practical errors be avoided.

CHAPTER 17

The Clinical Significance of the Systolic Murmur

There has been a great deal of discussion concerning the causes and significance of a systolic murmur. There has been much speculation on the physical and mechanical factors involved in the production of murmurs, and considerable effort has been made to correlate the presence of systolic murmurs with anatomic diagnoses. Despite this, much confusion remains, especially in the clinical interpretation of such findings. Not so very long ago the detection of a systolic murmur meant heart disease and many an innocent, perfectly healthy person was condemned as a chronic cardiac cripple, treated as such, restricted in his activities, and made to live his life in the constant fear that so commonly characterizes the life of an organic cardiac. Others, as a result of such a mistaken diagnosis, developed the full-blown picture of cardiac neurosis and thereafter lived with the handicaps that accompany this condition. Some in defiance led a normal and active life for a great many years, to the amazement of the physician who originally made the diagnosis and who either openly or implicitly gave a grave prognosis.

This point of view was quite prevalent before the First World War. The presence of a systolic murmur was often regarded as meaning mitral regurgitation, and this diagnosis carried with it the inference that the mitral valve was diseased. During the war, however, so many young soldiers had systolic murmurs and yet were apparently well that much doubt was cast on its organic significance. The result of this experience was that the pendulum gradually moved to the diametrically opposite position. Whereas formerly all systolic murmurs were regarded as serious, a teaching developed that systolic murmurs had no clinical significance whatever. One authority went so far as to say "throw the stethoscope away," emphasizing the importance of eliciting the early symptoms of heart failure. Another expressed an extreme point of view that organic mitral insufficiency did not exist, that there was stenosis of the mitral valve or the valve was normal. This latter opinion was based primarily on postmortem experience, in which it was found that when the diagnosis of mitral regurgitation was made the valve was found to be either normal or stenosed. There is every reason, however, to believe that a middle course is much nearer the truth. Systolic murmurs cannot be entirely disregarded, nor do they always mean heart disease. They deserve our most careful consideration, for only in this way will those

316

of importance be distinguished from the insignificant ones. Furthermore, as will become evident in the following discussion, the proper interpretation of a systolic murmur may occasionally serve as the main clue to a diagnosis that otherwise would be entirely overlooked.

It must be conceded that on examining most normal people no murmurs will be heard over the precordium. Furthermore there is ample proof of the fact that disease of the mitral valve or a loss of the normal integrity of the valve leaflets can result in a systolic murmur. If the mitral valve of a dog is cut there will immediately develop a systolic murmur that previously was not present. The reverse of this, however, is not true, for apical systolic murmurs can be present when the mitral valve is normal. Apart from other factors to be considered later, a systolic murmur best heard at the apex of the heart can be due to regurgitation of blood through the mitral valve whether the valve is structurally normal or diseased. If we have reason to believe that the valve is diseased the condition is regarded as "organic mitral insufficiency." If we believe that the valve is structurally normal the term used to designate the condition is "relative mitral insufficiency." This is a valid conception because there are numerous states in which for one reason or another the left ventricular cavity is enlarged or dilated and in this process of dilatation the mitral ring is sufficiently stretched so that normal leaflets can no longer completely close the orifice during ventricular systole and there results a regurgitation of blood. There are, therefore, two conditions in which the mitral valve can be regarded as incompetent, one organic and the other functional.

Organic mitral insufficiency generally results from a previous rheumatic infection. Under these circumstances the valve is actually distorted, the free margins are apt to be thickened and retracted, and, although the slow process of stenosis has not as yet manifested itself, so that there still is free flow of blood during diastole from auricles to ventricles, there is regurgitation through the incompetent valve during systole. It is often difficult to be certain whether or not a true organic mitral insufficiency exists because there need be no symptoms referable to the circulation and no other evidence of cardiac disease, not even hypertrophy of the heart. However, when a patient has had a previous history of rheumatic fever or chorea, and there is an apical systolic murmur of greater than slight intensity, especially if there is some cardiac hypertrophy and an accentuated pulmonary second sound, it is a fair presumption that the mitral valve is organically diseased and insufficient. It is no disproof of this contention to find a stenosis of the mitral valve on postmortem examination ten, twenty, or thirty years later. When such a patient lives his span of life and dies of cardiac failure, mitral stenosis is very likely to be present. Fatalities from heart failure occur but rarely during the stage of mitral insufficiency so that ordinarily we have no opportunity to confirm the diagnosis at the autopsy table. One circumstance did occur which enabled us to see the mitral valve during the stage of organic insufficiency without stenosis, i.e., subacute bacterial endocarditis. In this way a fatal disease develops in a patient who has only a systolic murmur long before congestive heart failure would otherwise have occurred and we are permitted to examine a mitral valve that is diseased but not stenotic. I have seen numerous such instances which have convinced me of the validity of making the diagnosis of organic mitral insufficiency.

There seems to be two types of organic rheumatic mitral insufficiency. One which was just described is well tolerated, shows no evidence or very little evidence of functional disability, has little or no cardiac hypertrophy, and merely displays an apical systolic murmur of moderate or loud intensity. Such patients carry on well for a great many years, although they are vulnerable to bacterial endocarditis. The other presents an entirely different and opposite kind of clinical picture. The heart becomes markedly enlarged, with huge dilatation of the left auricle, auricular fibrillation is present, there may be a fairly loud apical diastolic rumble of the type seen in mitral stenosis even with a striking diastolic thrill, the electrocardiogram may show left ventricular enlargement, and gross evidence of both right- and left-sided congestive failure is present. In a word the patient with the one type is doing very well while that with the other is gravely ill. It is not clear to me whether the latter is merely the end-result of the former, whether active myocarditis is the determining factor that produces the progressive deterioration of the condition, or whether the degree of incompetency of the valve is the determining factor. In these very sick patients, although there are physical findings of well-marked mitral stenosis, on postmortem examinations the valve may be found to be quite patulous with a large diaphragm-like appearance, producing only a slight degree of anatomical constriction but permitting a striking degree of reflux. There really is some relative mitral stenosis as the left ventricular cavity is enlarged and the left auricle is huge. But the type or degree of mitral stenosis is not the mechanically significant factor, nor is the condition suitable for the present methods of mitral surgery. These cases may present difficult problems both in diagnosis and in the selection of cases for mitral valvuloplasty.

There is another type of structural mitral insufficiency that is very difficult to diagnose which may result from calcification of the annulus fibrosus. This can readily be seen on fluoroscopic examination, but produces no characteristic physical findings. A moderate mitral systolic murmur is present in most but not in all cases. It generally occurs in older persons and may be present without any other significant evidence of disease or disability, although it also is found associated with organic disease of the mitral valve itself. This type of calcification of the mitral ring (in contrast to the leaflets) may or may not be associated with mitral regurgitation. I am apt to suspect the presence of calcific mitral annulus under the following circumstances: the finding of a moderately loud apical late systolic murmur, a negative past history of rheumatic fever, and the absence of congestive failure, in an elderly individual, especially a female with striking gray hair.

Relative mitral insufficiency, on the other hand, is a common occurrence in a variety of conditions. When the heart is enlarged and the left ventricle is dilated in patients with hypertension, syphilitic aortic insufficiency, or myocardial disease from any cause, a systolic murmur of varying intensity is frequently heard at the apex. There results a relative incompetency of the valve without any true progressive disease of its structure. It is of some importance to bear in mind the distinction between organic and relative insufficiency, for in the former we fear the eventual development of mitral stenosis or the subsequent complication of bacterial endocarditis, whereas in the latter neither of these conditions will develop no matter how long the patient lives.

Unfortunately many systolic murmurs cannot readily be classified in either of the two groups just mentioned. It is this which has led to so much confusion and has given rise to such terms as accidental, cardiorespiratory, hemic, or functional murmurs. It is not the intention here to explain or analyze all these murmurs but rather to present some points of view that have developed from an extensive clinical study of the systolic murmur and which have proved useful in a practical way.

At the outset progress will be impeded if we do not start with clearly defined terms. By definition a systolic murmur, no matter how faint, must have duration; it must last an appreciable interval into systole between the first and second heart sounds. Because systolic murmurs have been so generally regarded as benign and inconsequential, medical students and young house officers have developed the habit of finding many systolic murmurs that never exist. They know that nothing will be said about it if some one else fails to hear it, especially as we know that faint murmurs may come and go, but they fear missing a murmur if it is present. The result has been a looseness and carelessness in examination and in terminology. Frequently I have failed to hear any murmur whatever on most careful auscultation when others have described a systolic murmur. One additional reason is that with the definition just given, a prolonged or impure first heart sound that frequently is heard, especially in thin-chested individuals with hyperactive hearts, will not be called a murmur for there is no true bruit extending into systole. With this definition in mind it is surprising how often classic instances of mitral stenosis will show no systolic murmur. The characteristic diastolic or presystolic rumble will be heard ending with a snapping first heart sound, but no murmur will be heard during systole.

The other essential in this discussion is that we must indicate the intensity of the systolic murmur. Quantitative descriptions have become useful in describing other findings, for example, the amount of albumin or sugar in the urine, the degree of jaundice or of peripheral edema. A very large trace of albumin, for instance, is not customarily seen in the simple albuminurias accompanying fevers, whereas it is suggestive of nephrosis; on the other hand, a slightest possible trace of albumin does occur with the former and not with the latter. Similar notations are applicable in describing systolic murmurs. For some years I have used the following terminology and, although at first glance it may seem cumbersome, within a very short time those who have tried to use it have found it simple and reasonably accurate, so that different observers would coincide very closely in their descriptions. Systolic murmurs are divided into six gradations. Grade I intensity is the faintest that is audible on the most careful auscultation. Although faint it must have an appreciable duration. This type of murmur is frequently overlooked if the examination is only casual. It is generally not heard at all during the first few seconds of auscultation but then becomes audible. In fact, if a faint murmur is heard immediately it generally means that it is grade II. Grade VI intensity is the loudest murmur that one ever hears. These murmurs are rare and are such that they can be heard with the stethoscope away from the chest wall. The other four gradations (II to V) fall in between these two extremes. They may be called "very slight," "slight" "moderate," "loud," "very loud," and "loudest possible" murmurs.

In fact, one can call a murmur grade II if it is slight but heard immediately, whereas a grade I murmur is not. Furthermore, a grade V murmur is very loud, cannot be heard if the entire stethoscope is removed from the chest, but is audible if one edge of the stethoscope is in contact with the chest wall. With a short period of practice, different observers will find that they generally will use the same notation and almost never will vary more than one gradation in intensity.

With the foregoing as a background, it was found that on examining over one thousand so-called "normal" or noncardiac individuals, systolic murmurs of grade I intensity were fairly common, those called grade II were less frequent, and those of grade III were quite rare. The interesting point was that in every instance in which a systolic murmur of grade III intensity was heard, although such patients were in the hospital primarily for some condition unrelated to the heart, such as prostatic disease, hernia, or hemorrhoids, definite evidence of organic heart disease was found. In fact, this was also true of many patients who had grade II murmurs. Several factors were undoubtedly involved in the production of some of the murmurs of grade I and II intensity, and in interpreting such murmurs these factors need to be carefully considered. These are fever, anemia, tachycardia, hypertension, hyperthyroidism, and possibly nervous excitement. The last of these probably produces its effects primarily through its increase in rate. It does not follow that these conditions invariably produce systolic murmurs. Other influences which are at present poorly understood are involved and determine whether a murmur will result or not. However, it is fairly certain that the conditions named can be the specific cause of a murmur and therefore need to be carefully considered in estimating the significance of such murmurs, although they alone will not account for murmurs of grade III intensity or louder. It is obvious that when the above six conditions are known not to exist, then the presence of a systolic murmur of more than grade I intensity is likely to be due to organic heart disease.

There is one possible mechanism in the production of a systolic murmur, which is common to some of the conditions, that I wish to discuss. This is the velocity of blood flow. The rate at which the blood flows around in the circulation (not the heart rate) is increased in hyperthyroidism, anemia, fever, and exercise. An increase in the basal metabolic rate of the body will be accompanied by a speeding up of the velocity of blood flow. It is interesting that many patients with these conditions also have systolic murmurs. I have frequently observed grade I or II systolic murmurs in patients with hyperthyroidism and found that they disappeared after the basal metabolism was brought to normal by subtotal thyroidectomy. Likewise, perfectly normal young men who show no murmur will almost invariably develop a grade I or II systolic murmur directly after a short brisk effort, such as running. These murmurs will also disappear as the heart quiets down. These murmurs have often been explained on the basis of temporary dilatation of the heart with relative insufficiency of one valve or relative stenosis of another. X-ray examination of the heart in some of these conditions has failed to show any dilatation and in fact, at times, such as directly after a brisk effort, the heart seems to be a bit smaller than it is at rest. May it not be that the murmur is produced because the blood is ejected with a snap? It has been shown that there is a speed with which a fluid running through a tube does so without producing eddies and bruits and beyond which such disturbances do arise. This explanation seems logical when measurements of the velocity of blood flow show it to be accelerated. However, even when this is normal, a systolic murmur can result from the same mechanism if we assume that the rate of ejection from the heart is accelerated for a short distance up through the aorta and pulmonary arteries, although the rate of flow through the entire circulation is unaltered. In any event there seems to be some relationship between the rate of ejection of blood from the heart and the development of a systolic murmur.

One by-product of this study was the finding of a transient systolic murmur developing almost invariably in normal persons after a brisk effort. This is of some importance, for it has become the habit of physicians who examine for insurance companies or civil service commissions to make such an exercise test and to draw certain inferences from the appearance of a systolic murmur. Although such a test can be of great value in uncovering mitral diastolic or presystolic murmurs that otherwise might be entirely overlooked, it is obvious that no significance whatever can be attached to the appearance of a systolic murmur after effort.

When a deliberate and careful attempt is made to interpret the significance of a systolic murmur, eliminating the factors discussed in the foregoing paragraphs, we are still left with a considerable number that are difficult to explain. Let us suppose that the heart is slow, there is no fever, hypertension, anemia, or hyperthyroidism, and a systolic murmur is present. If it is a grade III murmur, one is almost certain to find other evidence of organic disease such as cardiac enlargement, a systolic thrill, a diastolic murmur, or significant electrocardiographic abnormalities. If it is of grade I intensity, unless other evidence of heart disease is present, no significance can be attached to it, although even some of these I believe eventually prove to be rheumatic or organic. If, however, the intensity of the murmur is grade II a most careful investigation must be made for a possible rheumatic background. Apart from the past history of rheumatic fever and chorea, which will often be lacking, inquiry should be made of a family history of rheumatic fever or valvular disease and one should try to elicit a history of early nose-bleeds, vomiting spells, undue nervousness or sweats or some unexplained illness in childhood. The point is that many rheumatic infections mask themselves in such obscure fashion and show no more than a systolic murmur. In this way patients with grade II systolic murmurs will often be identified as having some form of rheumatic valvular disease. Others will be found to be suffering from some form of congenital heart disease, such as ventricular septal defect, pulmonary stenosis, atrial septal defect, patent ductus arteriosus, or coarctation of the aorta.

Having such indefinite evidence, it is not easy to convince oneself and much more difficult to convince others that a heart showing hardly anything more than a systolic murmur is not normal. This is particularly so because in some such cases, even those followed for a great many years, nothing further happens to incriminate the heart. This unfortunately is not true in all cases. I have seen numerous instances in which patients with so-called "benign systolic murmurs" later developed conditions which proved that the original murmur, although in no way impairing the efficiency of the circulation, was due to an inherent structural defect. In some, a later bout of typical rheumatic fever serves to indicate that the early murmur probably was also rheumatic. In many the subsequent development of subacute bacterial endocarditis also proves that the original murmur was due to a minor rheumatic valvulitis or to some congenital defect because this complication is almost never superimposed on a previously normal heart. In still others, as years go on, a systolic murmur that was regarded as functional or insignificant becomes readily identified as due to aortic stenosis, when a systolic thrill develops over the upper or mid portion of the precordium. This has proved to be so in cases that I have followed even when the systolic murmur was originally more prominent at the apex than in the aortic area. In some the eventual appearance of the signs of mitral stenosis indicates that the early murmur was due to a mitral valvulitis. I have frequently followed patients who were well but showed a systolic murmur and found ten years later that a basal thrill and even x-ray evidence of calcification of the aortic valve developed. This is to be expected because long before a degree of stenosis of the valve has occurred sufficient to produce the classic signs, there must have been a time when the constriction was slight and the systolic murmur only faint.

A few illustrative experiences will help to emphasize how the proper interpretation of an "insignificant systolic murmur" may lead to a correct diagnosis that would otherwise be overlooked. It was my duty some years ago to make routine examination of forty members of the first year class of the Harvard Medical School. There was only one who showed a systolic murmur. This was of grade II intensity. This young man felt well and did not consider himself sick. There was no previous history of rheumatic infection and no hypertension, and the heart showed no other abnormalities. One might have dismissed this finding as of no importance and called it a benign or functional systolic murmur. On closer scrutiny it was found that his skin was somewhat moist and hyperemic and that there was a very slight tremor of the fingers. The heart sounds were also hyperactive. Although there was no exophthalmos or thyroid enlargement, hyperthyroidism was suspected, for which he was later treated as the basal metabolic rate was found to be +45 per cent. In this case the systolic murmur was the only feature that led to a diagnosis which otherwise would hardly have been suspected.

In the following instance (referred to in Chap. 10) attention to a simple systolic murmur also was the main clue to the diagnosis which had been entirely overlooked. A day laborer was sent into the hospital with a diagnosis of stone in the left kidney. A day or two before, he had been taken with a sudden sharp pain in the left loin extending around the left part of the abdomen and down to the genitals. There was gross hematuria which was noted by the patient himself. He had been working when this occurred and complained of very little else. Examination was essentially negative, except for a grade II apical systolic murmur. The urine showed gross and microscopic blood. The temperature and pulse rate were normal. The same diagnosis of left renal stone was made by the hospital staff, no attention being paid to the systolic murmur. When the patient was shown at a staff conference, in my attempt to explain the presence of the murmur I elicited some additional information by direct questioning. Although he had been working steadily he had not been feeling quite so well during the previous few weeks. He had also known that he had some sort of a murmur for years but had paid no attention to it as it never troubled him. On the basis of this I ventured the diagnosis of subacute bacterial endocarditis with an embolus to the left kidney. This suggestion was rather ill received but that afternoon, although the temperature was only 99.2° F., a blood culture was taken which was positive for *Streptococcus viridans*. Cystoscopic examination which was contemplated was not performed and the progress was typical of subacute bacterial endocarditis. Postmortem examination performed some months later showed typical vegetations engrafted on an old rheumatic mitral endocarditis. This case also illustrates that during the years when the patient felt well and showed nothing more than a systolic murmur, the diagnosis of organic mitral insufficiency would have been justified.

In this final case the interpretation of a systolic murmur was helpful in deciding upon the proper treatment. A retired foreman, 60 years of age, came under my care because of shortness of breath, especially at night. He was evidently suffering from congestive heart failure. The heart was enlarged, the rhythm was regular, and there was a grade II basal systolic murmur. No thrills or diastolic murmur could be detected. There was no hypertension or rheumatic or syphilitic past history, and there was no history of angina pectoris. The Wassermann reaction was negative. The question arose here whether or not we were dealing with a case of syphilitic aortitis. This deserved serious consideration, for in about 15 to 25 per cent of such cases the Wassermann reaction is negative. Although I do not believe that disease of the wall of the aorta (so-called "roughening") is a factor in the production of basal systolic murmurs, this has been the current teaching, and a systolic murmur might be explained in this way. X-ray examination, however, showed definite calcified stenosis of the aortic valve. This finding not only made the anatomic diagnosis but served to rule out syphilis as an etiologic factor, for syphilis never produces stenosis of valves. In this way the patient was spared a course of antisyphilitic treatment which not only would have been useless but might have been harmful. When his clinical condition improved as a result of ordinary treatment for congestive heart failure, a typical systolic thrill of aortic stenosis was felt and the murmur increased in intensity to grade III. It is obvious from this and many similar experiences that a murmur may be faint when cardiac function is poor and louder as the circulation improves. Furthermore, a faint murmur may have greater significance when heard in an obese individual or in a patient with an emphysematous chest than in a thin person. The distance between the origin of the murmur and the external chest wall will necessarily affect the loudness of murmurs.

Finally, there are some general remarks about systolic murmurs that are not out of place. Too much emphasis has been placed on the transmission of murmurs in deciding whether they are "functional" or organic. The louder the murmur, the greater will be its transmission, and very faint murmurs are not transmitted. The location and the loudness are important, not the transmission. A loud aortic systolic murmur is transmitted to the neck and a similar murmur in the mitral area to the axilla because these locations are near the point of maximum intensity of these murmurs. A very loud murmur, no matter of what origin, will be heard over a large area. I question the importance of transmission of murmurs through the blood stream. I have heard grade VI murmurs transmitted down the arms and audible over the olecranon process of the elbow when they could not be heard over the brachial artery. They seemed to be transmitted well through bone. Furthermore, the distinction between organic and relative or functional murmurs often has erroneous connotations. The former sounds more serious than the latter, whereas relative dilatation of cardiac cavities resulting in functional systolic murmurs is apt to signify a graver condition of the heart muscle. There are some nervous persons who show hyperactive hearts and a systolic murmur without other evidence of organic disease who fall into a group of potential hypertensives. They often have a very slight fever, show flushing of the skin of the neck, and as they are followed for years they eventually develop permanent essential hypertension.

It must not be inferred from the foregoing discussion that all systolic murmurs should be regarded with gravity. For the most part we should do as we have been doing in the past. It is often wise to instruct patients with unexplained murmurs to use penicillin prophylactically when undergoing dental extractions or other procedures that involve the possibility of producing bacterial endocarditis. Patients with systolic murmurs and no other evidences of circulatory embarrassment may remain in good health for many years or even indefinitely. If there are no symptoms of cardiac weakness they should be allowed to do as they please. There really are no restrictions that they need. They may be allowed to enjoy the kind of physical activities and sports that produce no ill effects. This advice is proper not because it is felt in all cases that the systolic murmur has no meaning, but rather because there is no advantage in enforcing rest or denying such individuals the ordinary pleasures of life. However, it must be clear that an attempt should be made to ascertain the cause of the murmur. As an aid in this direction proper terminology and estimation of the intensity of murmurs should be employed. In this way diagnosis will become more accurate, treatment in some cases will be directed more intelligently, and vague terminology will become clarified.

CHAPTER 18

The Patient with Heart
Disease as a Surgical or Obstetrical Risk

Heart Disease and Surgery

The physician is frequently asked by a surgical colleague whether a certain patient can stand an operation. This is by no means as simple a problem as it seems, for it requires an answer to three different questions. First, the physician must help in the diagnosis of the condition currently complained of and decide whether the problem is surgical after all. As will be seen, many cardiac affections present features which make them similar to and cause confusion with acute surgical abdominal emergencies. Secondly, when there is an obvious disease that is amenable to surgical treatment one has to decide whether or not the prognosis of the cardiac condition is good enough to warrant subjecting the patient to a major operation. Finally, when an operation is contemplated the physician should have some idea as to the surgical or operative mortality in various cardiac disorders.

With regard to the first problem a physician often can spare a patient an unnecessary operation by making a correct diagnosis when the condition supposedly is an acute surgical abdomen. In children, pericarditis or acute rheumatic fever may be accompanied by abdominal pain and tenderness, slight fever, and leukocytosis, and even nausea and vomiting. When joint pains are absent, acute appendicitis may be closely simulated. Inasmuch as there is no specific test for either condition, at times it will be necessary to perform an abdominal exploration to be sure of the diagnosis, for it is safer to find an occasional normal appendix than to overlook appendicitis that develops into a fatal peritonitis. There will be occasions, however, in which the detection of some of the subsidiary evidences of rheumatic infection, such as epistaxis, or a positive family or past history of rheumatic fever or rheumatic heart disease, will be sufficient to make one doubt the diagnosis of acute appendicitis and delay operation. After a delay of twelve to twenty-four hours it may then become quite clear that there is nothing surgical about the condition.

On very rare occasions the sudden development of auricular fibrillation in one suffering from some form of organic heart disease may be attended by acute pain and tenderness in the epigastrium or right upper quadrant, nausea, vomiting, abdominal rigidity, slight fever, leukocytosis, and slight icterus. The whole picture may resemble an acute cholecystitis. I have seen such a patient upon whom a cholecystectomy had been performed, following which there was satisfactory recovery. About one year later I saw the same patient go through a similar spell, and she recovered on digitalis therapy. Reviewing the data of her previous experience it was clear that she had mitral stenosis and had developed a paroxysm of auricular fibrillation which resulted in abdominal symptoms presumably due to an acutely engorged liver. After the gallbladder, which contained no stones, was removed the auricular fibrillation spontaneously disappeared and recovery was satisfactory. The second attack was like the first and was again accompanied by a sudden paroxysm of a rapid irregular heart action with an enlarged tender liver. This time the symptoms all subsided on appropriate treatment for the cardiac condition. It is obvious that the previous operation was unnecessary.

Another circulatory condition that produces symptoms resembling an acute surgical abdomen is embolism to one of the abdominal viscera. An embolus to the spleen or the kidney can result in sudden pain and tenderness in the abdomen, with fever and leukocytosis. This is apt to occur in those cardiac patients who show evidence of mitral stenosis, auricular fibrillation, or subacute bacterial endocarditis. The treatment is expectant and supportive, and not surgical. When such an embolus involves the mesenteric vessels surgical treatment may be necessary. The diagnosis, however, is by no means simple, and fortunately such a complication requiring operative resection is rare.

Finally, acute coronary thrombosis may resemble very closely an acute surgical condition of the upper abdomen. This has been adequately discussed in a previous chapter (Chap. 6). Suffice it in this connection to recall that all available methods may be necessary to make this differential diagnosis and to avoid the error of operating on a patient who is in the throes of a desperate cardiac affliction. The resemblance may be to acute gallstone colic, perforated peptic ulcer, or acute pancreatitis. An electrocardiographic study may be invaluable and distinctive under these circumstances. Physicians have become aware of this diagnostic difficulty and now must be alert not to make the opposite error and overlook an abdominal disorder requiring immediate surgical intervention.

There are other acute circulatory emergencies that bring up the question of some surgical intervention in which the physician's judgment may aid in determining the proper treatment. At present, for example, it is a matter of careful judgment whether or not to try to remove a peripheral embolus to an extremity. Embolectomy is of value only in the first six to twenty-four hours, and it must be remembered that gangrene rarely develops in the arms. Anticoagulant therapy seems to offer a fairly satisfactory method of treatment. Novocain injection of the sympathetic nerves to the limb involved may help to relieve the additional spasm that occurs with embolism, and refrigeration of the extremities is occasionally employed. It is clear, therefore, from the preceding discussion, that when a physician is asked whether a patient can stand an operation, he should first try to decide whether there is any surgical problem involved at all or whether the cardiac disorder itself and its complication may adequately explain the difficulty.

The second point to determine is whether the life expectancy of the particular patient suffering from heart disease warrants undertaking the surgical procedure that is contemplated. Is it to be expected that the patient will live long enough to enjoy the results of the operation to make the temporary discomfort and risk worth while? This involves an estimation of the prognosis in the type of cardiac disease that is present, frequently a difficult matter. However, it is often fairly obvious that the patient cannot be expected to live more than a year or two and one would then hesitate to recommend an operation that is not urgent or one that is contemplated for a condition which can be treated, even if less satisfactorily, by nonsurgical methods. Too frequently women with hypertensive heart disease or mitral stenosis are subjected to pelvic operations, only to succumb to circulatory failure within a year or so after the operation. For many who survive the procedure there must be some who make up the ordinary surgical mortality that attends such an operation. Patients with fibroid tumors of the uterus who also suffer from advanced heart disease with an accompanying poor life expectancy are much better treated by radiation than by surgery. Similarly, operations such as those for prolapse of the uterus or for pelvic repair might well be avoided in such patients. Instead, nonsurgical methods may be employed. The same may be said for a simple hernia. In a word, whenever possible it is wise to employ simple nonsurgical methods of treatment in patients with advanced heart disease, although one should not hesitate to subject them to operations that are more urgent, such as that for acute appendicitis.

The third consideration is to estimate the surgical mortality in patients suffering from different types of organic heart disease. During the past two or three decades, as a result of the improvement of surgical techniques and of anesthesiology, and because of the advances in the treatment of heart disease, the use of antibiotics, and other discoveries, the mortality from all surgical procedures has fallen markedly. Statistics obtained a generation ago are no longer applicable. In general it may be stated that with the exception of a small and limited group of patients, most cardiac patients tolerate surgical operations almost as well as non-cardiacs. In an extensive review made some thirty years ago it was found that, with the exception of patients suffering from coronary artery disease, the operative mortality among cardiacs was only a little greater than among non-cardiacs. The presence of appreciable nephritis or congestive failure added somewhat to the operative risk. Hypertension or auricular fibrillation was only of very little importance. The results were equally good in valvular and non-valvular cases. The only group in which the surgical mortality was definitely greater included patients suffering from angina pectoris or those who had a previous coronary thrombosis. Even in the coronary cases the risk has diminished sharply in recent years.

It is of interest to analyze the cause of death in cardiac patients who succumb to surgical procedures. In most cases this will be found to be due to the same complications that occur in non-cardiacs, i.e., uncontrolled sepsis, hemorrhage, inadequate or ineffective surgery, postoperative pulmonary emboli, atelectasis, or pneumonia, etc. In others, death is due to the concomitant heart disease occurring at about the same time as it might have occurred if the operation had not been performed. An illustration of such an experience is one in which death occurred forty-eight hours after amputation of a gangrenous leg in a patient who was moribund following an acute coronary thrombosis with a femoral embolus.

Only in a small number will the fatality be found to be a direct result of the heart disease and be hastened or precipitated by the operation. These may be called "unexpected cardiac deaths" and include those in which it seemed that the patient died from some complication of heart disease that would not have occurred had he not been operated upon and had he not had heart disease. When analyzed in this manner certain unpredictable complications will be met with. Occasionally sudden and unpredictable death will occur, especially in those subject to such fatalities, i.e., patients with angina, coronary artery disease, or aortic stenosis. Furthermore, patients with coronary artery disease may develop a coronary thrombosis during or shortly after an operation. This probably results from a temporary fall in blood pressure with its accompanying slowing of coronary flow. For this reason great care must be taken to avoid any prolonged hypotension in cardiac patients, especially in older people and in those suffering from coronary artery disease. Peripheral arterial emboli may be precipitated by operations, particularly when auricular fibrillation or mitral stenosis is present. Pulmonary emboli also occur after operations in cardiacs because they are prone to thrombophlebitis.

Being aware of the hazards that cardiacs are subject to, one can take certain precautions. Patients with congestive failure should be given appropriate treatment preoperatively. This can be carried out rapidly or more slowly, depending on the urgency of the operation. Those with valvular or congenital heart disease who might be prone to develop bacterial endocarditis should receive adequate antibiotic treatment. Measures should be employed to diminish the likelihood of thrombophlebitis of the legs, such as the application of elastic stockings to the legs and leg exercises. Whether the routine use of anticoagulants before and after surgery in vulnerable cases is desirable is an open question and deserves further study. As has been stated above, all available means should be used to prevent the occurrence or abbreviate the duration of hypotension.

The choice of anesthesia to be used in cardiacs is still a debatable subject. Some prefer general anesthesia, others spinal or local anesthesia.

With the rapid development of anesthesiology as a specialty it seems that different methods have been employed by different men with equally good results. It very likely depends on the particular experience and habits that prevail at any one hospital and on the person administering the anesthesia, rather than on the type of patient involved. Discussions between the anesthetist, the surgeon, and the physician will determine the eventual choice. In the past it has seemed that, in general, ether was well tolerated by cardiacs. Where an expert anesthetist is not available it probably still remains the anesthesia of choice.

My own experiences throw light on the safety of major surgical operations in patients suffering from various types of heart disease. In a considerable number of private patients with various forms of organic heart disease, valvular, hypertensive, and coronary in type, some having varying degrees of congestive failure, there has been only two surgical deaths from operations such as cholecystectomy, resection of stomach or intestines, prostatectomy, thyroidectomy, etc. One patient was a woman 60 years old with aortic stenosis, who died instantly just after a subtotal thyroidectomy had been completed. The other died of pulmonary atelectasis several days after a nephrectomy. He was a man about 50 years old who was obese, and had slight hypertension, mild coronary symptoms, and chronic bronchitis. There were no operative mortalities following cholecystectomy in about 40 patients with angina or previous myocardial infarction, or in an equal number of patients with mitral stenosis (most of whom also had auricular fibrillation). Likewise there were no fatalities in patients who had various cardiac arrhythmias, such as paroxysmal auricular tachycardia or auricular fibrillation, or in seven patients with Adams-Stokes disease. All of the latter went through cholecystectomy with recovery. In a word, cardiacs in general tolerate operations surprisingly well and should not be denied the benefits to be derived from surgery, if simple, satisfactory, nonsurgical methods of treatment are not available and if the prognosis of the cardiac condition is good enough to enable them to enjoy the results of surgery a reasonable length of time.

Heart Disease and Obstetrics

There is some similarity between the problems involved when a patient with heart disease becomes pregnant and when one is to undergo a surgical operation. There is one important difference, however, in that the former condition is to a great extent predictable and voluntary. This increases the responsibility of the physician for he will be asked whether pregnancy should be contemplated or, after it has occurred, whether it should continue. The intelligent answer to these questions will require not only a knowledge of diagnosis and prognosis of heart disease but also an insight into the social and economic life of the family involved.

Several cardiac conditions can readily be dismissed as having no influence on the question of pregnancy, for the response of the heart under these circumstances is practically the same as when the heart is perfectly normal. These conditions are all the forms of functional heart disease and well-compensated mitral insufficiency. Patients with benign irregularities of the heart or those showing insignificant faint systolic murmurs may be regarded as taking a normal risk. The same applies to those who have a louder mitral systolic murmur, with or without slight cardiac hypertrophy, in whom a past history of rheumatic fever or some other features indicate that there is an organic mitral regurgitation. Provided there has been no evidence of congestive failure and the patient's response to exercise is satisfactory, such a patient can be regarded practically as undergoing a normal risk in pregnancy.

On the other hand there are some cardiac conditions which make pregnancy highly inadvisable. If a patient is suffering from subacute bacterial endocarditis it is obvious that the seriousness of the underlying disease does not warrant undertaking or continuing with pregnancy unless the infection responds to chemotherapy. If the mother is suffering from active rheumatic fever it is undesirable that she be pregnant at that time. Apart from any ill effects that the pregnancy may have on the mother, and it is not certain that there are such ill effects, the child may be born with a rheumatic carditis, for there have been instances of acquired intrauterine rheumatic heart disease.

The presence of coarctation of the aorta renders pregnancy precarious, because such patients are particularly prone to rupture of the aorta. In fact pregnancy itself may predispose to dissection of the aorta on rare occasions. About 50 per cent of dissecting aortic aneurysms in women under the age of 40 years occur during pregnancy.

The main problem arises in patients with mitral stenosis and aortic valvular disease. Of first importance is the state of compensation of the circulation. If there is any evidence of congestive heart failure or if such failure has once been present in the past, it is best to advise that no further pregnancies be undertaken. Even when an apparently satisfactory state of compensation can be established by appropriate medical treatment, the risk of recurrent heart failure is too great and the life expectancy of the mother is too short to make it advisable for such a woman to go through pregnancy. If it is undertaken, a high maternal mortality must be expected. In general, women with rheumatic heart disease with congestive failure or with auricular fibrillation will have a maternal mortality of 10 to 25 per cent, and only 50 per cent will have viable children. On the other hand, if there is no objective evidence of heart failure or dyspnea is either entirely absent or only of a slight degree, women with mitral stenosis, aortic stenosis, or aortic insufficiency should be permitted to go through pregnancy. The only exception to this is the presence of permanent auricular fibrillation. This latter condition is generally associated with some signs of heart failure, and for that reason alone will contraindicate pregnancy, but even when such has not been the case patients with auricular fibrillation are generally suffering from a disordered circulation that is too far advanced to warrant taking the risk. Women manifesting those conditions that contra-indicate pregnancy, i.e., permanent auricular fibrillation, or present or past congestive heart failure, should therefore be cautioned to avoid pregnancy and should be instructed in the methods of contraception.

There are differences in the advice which the physician should give when the question of the first or of a subsequent pregnancy arises. What has been said above concerning well-compensated cases of aortic or mitral disease applies primarily to those women who contemplate their first pregnancy. Even when there is some doubt as to the exact state of the heart a slight added risk might be hazarded for the joy of having a child, in contrast to a childless life. The situation is not quite the same if the patient already has one or more healthy children. Realizing that there is always a greater risk among pregnant organic cardiac patients than among normal women, no matter how apparently trivial the disease may be, I feel that, if there are already three children, under no circumstances should any more pregnancies be undertaken. It is not pertinent to the question to recall the instances in which women with mitral stenosis have satisfactorily borne eight or ten children. We see as patients only those who have survived. Many of the other multiparas have succumbed, leaving their children motherless.

A distinction is made when there are already three children because that constitutes a satisfactory family from both a social and an indi-vidual point of view. It must be remembered that there is a strong famil-ial factor in rheumatic heart disease and that with numerous pregnancies there is a great likelihood that one or more of the children will eventually suffer from rheumatic heart disease. If precautions are taken in families with stigmata of important hereditary nervous disorders like insanity, why should not similar considerations be given to this disabling form of heart disease? Furthermore, with numerous pregnancies among people of humble or modest means, the task is not ended with recovery from the confinement. The rearing of several infants and children without the aid of nurses and maids may prove to be a greater task than the preg-nancy itself and more than the disabled heart of the mother can stand. The social and economic status of the patient therefore deserves careful consideration.

When there is already one child and further pregnancies are con-templated the physician would do well to encourage a second pregnancy. Both the first and those subsequent pregnancies that are planned should take place during the early years of married life. Some women, either through fear or from improper medical advice, delay this decision and thereby lose valuable years. Unless some acute episode has taken place, the cardiac condition does not generally improve with advancing years, so that a pregnancy will be better borne earlier rather than later. Furthermore, the mother will enjoy the life of the children longer if they are born during the early years of married life. A second pregnancy should be encouraged if there are no contraindications, because a family is not secure with one child. Through some unfortunate accident or illness that child may die. Two healthy children, therefore, consolidate the family and also prevent the difficulties that often arise from a "spoiled" single child. When it comes to the third pregnancy, one may rightly exercise a choice. In a word, I urge the first pregnancy, advise the second, and consent to the third.

The statements made in the preceding paragraphs require certain modifications, now that operations on the valves of the heart are being performed. If a woman with mitral stenosis shows early or more advanced evidence of cardiac limitation and would be suitable for mitral valvuloplasty, this operation should be performed before pregnancy begins. Or the operation can be done during the early months of pregnancy if the cardiac condition appears to be threatening. In this way sufficient improvement in the heart may result to enable the patient to undertake the added burden of pregnancy with greater safety. With the proper selection of patients, the total maternal mortality in pregnant women suffering from rheumatic valvular disease (mainly mitral stenosis) has been reduced to about 1 per cent

Women with organic heart disease should seek medical advice before pregnancy has begun and again at the earliest evidence of pregnancy. During the early weeks tests for pregnancy might be necessary to make intelligent decisions. If the case is one in which the risk is obviously very great, e.g., mitral stenosis, or auricular fibrillation with advanced heart failure and enlarged liver, termination of pregnancy should be undertaken during the first two or three months and can be performed without any undue risk. If the case is neglected and the patient first presents herself in this condition during the last trimester the situation is serious, for the maternal mortality is very high (close to 35 or 50 per cent), and stillbirths are common. Abortion in this severe and late stage is generally inadvisable, and one may then do the best one can with optimum treatment of heart failure and hope for the best.

When it is decided that pregnancy should continue in a patient with well-compensated valvular disease, and particularly in one with some evidence, even if slight, of cardiac insufficiency, the patient should be carefully advised concerning her activities and be observed by her physician at two- to four-week intervals. It generally is unnecessary to administer digitalis unless there is auricular fibrillation or congestive failure. The diet should contain minimal amounts of salt (not more than 2 gm. of sodium chloride daily).

Women should be cautioned against overdoing. Frequent shopping trips may precipitate symptoms of congestive heart failure. There still prevails in the minds of many women and some physicians that an expectant mother must "harden" herself by deliberate exercise for the trial of labor. I have seen such a patient systematically walk three miles a day over hilly ground at the advice of her obstetrician, month after month, until she developed heart failure. A respiratory infection is also a frequent cause of upsetting the state of compensation and in so far as possible it should be avoided. When a minor respiratory infection has occurred more than the usual care and rest should be advised.

The earliest evidence of weakening of the circulation will be a slight increase in the dyspnea, a slight nonproductive cough, and the presence of a few rales at the bases of the lungs. Inasmuch as some subjective dyspnea may have been present before the pregnancy occurred, and many women without heart disease may complain of slight dyspnea during pregnancy, it is no simple matter to appraise this symptom. It has proved very helpful to me in following these patients to watch the vital capacity of the lungs. When the patient progresses favorably it will be found that the vital capacity of the lungs, which is an excellent objective index of the degree of breathlessness, will remain essentially unchanged throughout pregnancy. It is surprising that even at the eighth month, when the abdomen is markedly distended by the enlarged uterus, the movements of the diaphragm are not impeded sufficiently to lower the vital capacity. By this simple determination one can obtain a check on the patient's clinical condition. Obviously the physician should carefully examine the patient during these frequent visits, watching particularly for basal rales, in addition to observing the blood pressure and urinary findings. Pitting edema of the legs, which is such an important sign of congestive heart failure, is not trustworthy during pregnancies, because many women manifest this as a result of pressure of the uterus on the pelvic veins or for other reasons.

If heart failure is present in the first trimester, the question of abortion will need serious consideration. There will be occasional circumstances in which it will seem justified to permit pregnancy to continue with the clear knowledge that the maternal risk will be decidedly greater than for a normal woman. Such a decision might readily be made in the case of a first pregnancy, and especially if the heart failure responds to medical management.

When there are already two or more children and the mother does not want to take the much greater risk that attends all organic cardiac disease, abortion during these early months is indicated if failure is present. All this presupposes that there are no religious considerations that influence acceptance of medical judgment. A conservative policy of medical management may at times even be applicable to the cardiac in the poor risk group, namely those with mitral stenosis and auricular fibrillation, provided the condition can be kept under satisfactory control.

The situation is different in the patient after the fifth month of pregnancy. From then on it seems best to permit pregnancy to continue. The hazard of abortion has now become great, and there is the hope that careful medical treatment will enable the patient to survive to the last month of pregnancy when the cardiac status often improves.

The mode of delivery has been a point of contention. In the past some obstetricians have favored abdominal section as a procedure of choice, while others have preferred normal vaginal delivery. At present the consensus of opinion is that the latter method entails less risk for the mother. Cesarean section is justified for obstetric, not cardiac, indications. In the past, some preferred abdominal section because of the opportunity it afforded of performing sterilization when it seemed indicated. This does not appear to be a cogent justification for carrying out the more serious procedure. Sterilization can be deferred for a later date.

Whenever the problem of sterilization comes up, it should be undertaken only after the most careful consideration. Too often this operation is performed when the cardiac prognosis is entirely misjudged. In such cases the patient continues to carry on in fairly good health for many years but remains childless. It is apparent that she could have borne one or more children without undue hazard. I recall an instance in which sterilization was performed at the time of the first confinement, and the child died during the first twenty-four hours. The mother recovered satisfactorily and remained well compensated, despite a combined mitral and aortic lesion. She probably would have been able to go through one or two more pregnancies, but of course sterilization prevented conception. Modern surgery of the heart is developing so rapidly that the outlook for some of the difficult cases has already improved and may continue to do so in the coming years. This applies not only in the matter of tolerating pregnancy but also in rendering the operation of sterilization less advisable.

When the time of delivery is near at hand it should be a routine procedure to start penicillin therapy, 500,000 to 1,000,000 units four times daily and to continue it for five or six days after delivery. The purpose of this is to prevent the rare complication of bacterial endocarditis, for it is known that streptococci may be present in the vagina for some days after delivery.

There is one type of heart failure that occasionally develops rather suddenly in pregnant women even when the heart was normal before pregnancy. This may take the form of acute pulmonary edema during a toxemia of pregnancy with a rising blood pressure. The mechanism is an acute left ventricular failure. This condition is amenable to cardiac therapy. Complete recovery can take place following the use of morphine, digitalis, and phlebotomy when necessary. In such cases the heart may return to normal and pregnancy may continue in the usual manner. There is another rather rare type of heart failure that may develop directly after pregnancy in some women who never manifested any evidence of heart disease before pregnancy. It is regarded as a type of myocarditis of unknown etiology and seems to be refractory to the customary methods of management.

The intelligent cooperation between the obstetrician and the cardiologist has brought about a tremendous fall in the maternal mortality of those suffering from heart disease. This has been well exemplified in the special cardiac clinics established in lying-in hospitals, such as that instituted by Hamilton and now carried on by Burwell in Boston. We now are able to advise patients whether or not to undertake the hazards of pregnancy and then to guide them along to a successful termination with a surprisingly small risk.

When the above general rules are applied the maternal mortality will be about 1 per cent. This is still ten times as great as in normal women. There will be unexpected instances of congestive failure in some cases of mitral stenosis, or fatalities may occur from gross emboli. In my own experience there has been no mortality whatever except among a few patients who became pregnant against my advice.

Finally, one may ask whether the life span of cardiac patients who recover is shortened by pregnancy. This is a difficult question to answer. Some statistics indicate that women with rheumatic heart disease (not dying in pregnancy) are five years younger at the time of death than women with comparable conditions who have not been pregnant. This difference may be due to the fact that some develop congestive failure, recover partly, and succumb a short time after delivery. If heart failure does not develop it seems unlikely that life has been appreciably shortened.

CHAPTER 19

Factors Concerning Prognosis in Heart Disease

All physicians at one time or another have had the disturbing experience of making an absolutely wrong prognosis while treating patients with heart disease. This occurs even when the diagnosis is correct. Such wrong prognoses are made both when the condition seems hopeless and the patient recovers, and also when the patient has been doing satisfactorily and dies unexpectedly. It is particularly humiliating to the individual physician and harmful to the general medical profession when a hopeless prognosis is given and the attending physician is dismissed, if one of the irregular practitioners is called in and, in the natural course of events, the patient recovers. Such an experience makes an everlasting impression on the parties involved and on their friends, and serves to place in disrepute the entire medical profession. It is not surprising that the lay public should feel as they do under these circumstances. Mistakes in prognosis, more so than mistakes in treatment, are responsible for the growing activities and importance of the numerous unorthodox medical cults that prevail today. The purpose of this discussion is to throw some light on the factors involved in the prognosis of heart disease so that such errors may be minimized.

There are two parts to the problem of prognosis that frequently arises in cardiac patients. The first concerns itself with the immediate and the second with the ultimate outcome. The factors that concern the latter are very involved and difficult to measure. It is almost futile to speculate as to exactly how long a patient with compensated aortic or mitral valvular disease will live. There are so many uncontrolled and unpredictable influences at work that although one can formulate some average figures which roughly guide our concepts of life expectancy it is difficult to apply them to individual cases. Two patients start out at the age of 15 years with apparently similar lesions, e.g., a slight aortic or mitral insufficiency. One carries on in good health to the age of 50 or 60 and the other picks up a minor infection that initiates subacute bacterial endocarditis at the age of 30. This formerly proved fatal. The same marked differences in ultimate outcome characterize disease of the coronary arteries. One patient with angina pectoris has a sudden exitus shortly after the first symptoms develop, and another continues in fairly good health for a great many years. When we realize that there may be such extreme variation in life expectancy among apparently similar

337

cases, for the present it seems idle to try to predict exactly how long many of these patients will live. Perhaps it is just as well that prognosis is no more accurate. It enables both the physician and the patient to be hopeful and not to feel that the day of judgment is absolutely fixed.

The difference between predicting immediate and ultimate results is well illustrated by the influence of the presence of auricular fibrillation with valvular disease. Whereas auricular fibrillation indicates a more advanced state of rheumatic heart disease and, on the average, the life expectancy is shorter in the rheumatic cardiac patients with auricular fibrillation than in those with regular rhythm, the immediate prognosis and expectations for improvement are better if this irregularity is found than when the rhythm is normal and the same degree of cardiac failure is present.

It is obvious that in any form of heart disease, other things being equal, the more ill the patient seems to be, the more dyspnea, the more peripheral congestion and similar symptoms, the more serious will be the outlook. On the other hand, there are many patients with marked symptoms and physical signs of circulatory embarrassment in whom the prognosis is a good deal better than in others with much milder evidences of the same type. This occurs because other less obvious factors are not the same in the two groups of cases. We must try to explain why some patients with heart disease unexpectedly do better and others do worse than predicted, and even why, in some cases that are considered entirely hopeless, recovery takes place.

One simple aid in estimating prognosis is the heart rate at which the patient develops congestive failure. If two patients with mitral stenosis and auricular fibrillation present the same degree of cardiac failure, but one has a heart rate of 130 and the other a rate of 80, in general it may be said that the prognosis is better in the one with the rapid rate. Here it is evident that digitalis and other treatment may be expected to slow the rapid rate and effect a good deal more improvement than when the rate is already slow. In other words, when the heart rate is slow and there is considerable peripheral edema, not so much improvement can be expected as when the rate is rapid. This is especially true when the disturbance is one in which it may be predicted that slowing will be obtained, such as is the case in auricular fibrillation.

The size of the heart is of some importance in judging prognosis. The larger the heart, other things being equal, the poorer the prognosis. This does not mean that one patient with a large heart may not do better than another of a different type with a small heart. I recall seeing a patient with mitral stenosis and auricular fibrillation who had marked congestive heart failure. She improved strikingly on ordinary treatment so that all evidence of congestion disappeared, and in fact the vital capacity of the lungs, which had been very low on admission, rose to a normal level before she left the hospital. She walked up two flights of stairs with one of the physicians and showed less respiratory distress than he did as a result of this effort. One might have predicted that she would do extremely well. Her heart, however, was very large, almost filling the chest, and she died within a year. Such experiences are not uncommon.

One of the most important factors requiring proper appraisal is the role that infection plays in producing symptoms and signs of heart disease. It is evident that infection, although violent, may come to an end. A patient may be desperately ill with respiratory distress, very rapid heart rate, even showing signs of generalized congestive heart failure, and yet recover so that all evidence of circulatory embarrassment disappears. Such a patient may not only feel well and remain well indefinitely, but physical signs of heart involvement, such as murmurs, may disappear entirely. This sort of dramatic improvement is not altogether uncommon in young people. This can occur because under such circumstances almost the entire picture that develops is due to an infection, generally rheumatic fever. This is apt to be accompanied by a pancarditis with involvement of the pericardium, myocardium, and endocardium. This sort of an infection may not only terminate, but recovery from it can be practically complete. I have seen such patients who were ill enough to be on the danger lists in hospitals but who recovered entirely and showed no signs or symptoms of heart disease in subsequent years. If, on the other hand, the same degree of circulatory failure occurred without an infection merely as an end-result of a burnt-out, long-standing chronic cardiac condition, recovery of the type described would be extremely rare. Improvement may occur so that the patient may become ambulatory, but there will always remain a varying degree of disability which is generally considerable. The inference to be drawn is that when infection of the heart is present, although the condition may be very critical and frequently fatal, one has reason to be hopeful, for a satisfactory recovery is always possible.

The role of bronchial dyspnea in heart disease needs special consideration in judging prognosis. There are a great many people with bronchitis of the asthmatic type and emphysema. There are also a great many individuals who have one form or another of heart disease. It would be quite natural, therefore, to find a certain number who happen to have both conditions. Furthermore, dyspnea on effort or at rest and paroxysmal dyspnea are symptoms that are common to both heart disease and asthma. It therefore becomes very important at times to determine how much of the respiratory distress is circulatory and how much is bronchial in origin. The importance of the differentiation lies in the fact that the prognosis in a patient with marked dyspnea of bronchial origin may be excellent whereas if the dyspnea were mainly cardiac, the outlook would be quite grave. There are numerous instances of mistaken prognoses because of the improper interpretation of the mechanism of dyspnea. For cases illustrating this problem and for the details that help in avoiding such errors, see Chapter 16.

Dyspnea may be produced by other factors which have no direct bearing on heart disease but which one must clearly distinguish, because in so far as they are present the prognosis is so much better. Obesity in itself can produce shortness of breath when the heart is normal, and therefore can be responsible for a part of the dyspnea when there is heart disease. The same degree of dyspnea will have less significance in an obese than in a thin individual if the other findings are the same. In fact, there are many obese patients in whom a diagnosis of heart disease is made because they complain of shortness of breath, yet who really have no structural disease of the heart. Likewise patients with nervous weakness and debility complain of shortness of breath and palpitation and often are regarded as having organic heart disease when the entire problem is functional. Furthermore, there are many patients with compensated organic heart disease whose symptoms are in the main functional or neurotic in nature. In so far as that is true the prognosis is so much better. There is one particular aspect of this question that deserves attention. I refer to a group of comparatively young individuals who complain of shortness of breath even while at rest. They are apt to say that they cannot get enough air and will frequently be seen to take deep breaths ("sighing breathing"). They actually overventilate their lungs and still want more air, in contrast to patients with "cardiac asthma" who really cannot take a deep breath and who have true respiratory distress. They will show no signs of cardiac failure and no evidence of serious organic disease and yet feel short of breath without effort. When spontaneous paroxysmal dyspnea is of importance it will generally be accompanied by obvious signs of grave heart disease, whereas in this type of "sighing breathing" examination will reveal no essential abnormality. The distinction between these two types of dyspnea occurring when the subjects are at rest is most important, for the prognosis in one is excellent and in the other it is very grave.

It is obvious that the facility with which the symptoms of heart failure (dyspnea, edema, and chest pain) develop and with which they disappear under treatment is of some help in judging prognosis. Edema of the legs that develops only at the end of the day and disappears overnight is less serious than edema that persists all day. The same is thought to be true of anginal pain coming in some patients only if they hurry up a hill and in others even when they try to shave themselves. Similarly, if the patient improves quickly, one may regard the outlook as better than if it takes many weeks to accomplish the same result. Although there are exceptions to the foregoing principles, in general they will be found to be true.

In following a case of mitral stenosis I have found that the development of hypertension is indicative of a better prognosis than one might otherwise expect. As a group, the majority of patients with mitral stenosis will have died before they reach the age of 50. More recently we have learned that an appreciable number will live to 60 and some to more than 70. It is curious that hypertension is much more common in this older group of patients with mitral stenosis than in the general population for corresponding ages, despite the fact that mitral stenosis of itself in younger people is accompanied by a blood pressure somewhat lower than the average.

What relationship mitral stenosis has with hypertension is not clear. It may be that the original rheumatic infection that produced the mitral stenosis also had some insidious effect on the blood vessels, eventually causing the hypertension. Another possible explanation for the undue frequency of both conditions is that rheumatic valvular disease is more prone to occur in the same vascularly vulnerable individuals who would more likely develop hypertension anyway. Or may it be that prolonged organic heart disease in some way is conducive to hypertension? Finally, is the apparent better prognosis when both conditions are present due to the fact that only those cases with a milder degree of mitral stenosis can develop hypertension? In any event, I have frequently been aided in giving a better prognosis than would otherwise be warranted by finding the blood pressure elevated. For example, the presence of a systolic blood pressure of 140 to 160 during some acute cardiac emergency like an infarct of the lungs with generalized pulmonary edema in a patient with mitral stenosis would lead one to hope for recovery although the patient might appear desperately ill. Similarly, if the blood pressure from year to year gradually rises to 160 systolic or more, a patient with mitral stenosis may progress more favorably than one would otherwise expect. The development of moderate hypertension, therefore, is a favorable sign during the course of mitral stenosis.

It is well to contrast the prognosis of dyspnea and congestive heart failure in cases of mitral disease with that in aortic valvular disease. Many patients have well-marked heart failure with mitral stenosis, recover compensation, and again become ambulatory. They may carry on for many years, going through repeated breaks in compensation. On the other hand, when a patient with aortic stenosis or insufficiency, rheumatic or syphilitic, once has dyspnea and peripheral edema his months are often numbered. However, the aortic patient is apt to be stronger and suffer less from dyspnea than the patient with mitral stenosis, until this final break in compensation does occur. The effect of tricuspid stenosis on prognosis was discussed in Chapter 4. It is of interest that when this lesion is present the length of life after heart failure develops is much greater than it is in any other form of valvular disease.

Of special significance in considering the question of shortness of breath is nocturnal paroxysmal dyspnea. This occurs most frequently in patients with aortic, hypertensive, syphilitic, or coronary artery heart disease. This symptom, even more than pulsus alternans, gallop rhythm, and bundle branch block, carries with it a very poor prognosis. Most patients will not survive the first development of nocturnal dyspnea more than two years. However, I have seen numerous patients with pulsus alternans and gallop rhythm who did well for more than five years. We must try to individualize in our prognosis, and it will be found that if these grave signs were brought to light by some acute episode, which can disappear, they need not have the same hopeless outlook. Many patients will show Cheyne-Stokes breathing, pulsus alternans, and gallop rhythm during the height of a coronary thrombosis or an attack of paroxysmal tachycardia and yet recover and do well for years. In fact, in some of these cases of paroxysmal tachycardia the sign of ill omen disappears permanently and the patient remains well indefinitely. Although there are many exceptions, in general it is true that when nocturnal dyspnea, Cheyne-Stokes breathing, pulsus alternans, gallop rhythm, or block of the left branch of the bundle of His occurs, the prognosis must be guarded.

Thyroid heart disease is unique in that the prognosis almost invariably is much better than it would be with the same apparent evidence of cardiac embarrassment if there were no hyperthyroidism. When the diagnosis of hyperthyroidism and heart disease is properly made and effective treatment is instituted, patients who otherwise could rightly be expected to be incurable and even helpless invalids can generally be restored to comparative comfort or complete health. There is no other condition in which such extraordinary improvement occurs and is so well maintained as in hyperthyroid heart disease. For this reason the diagnosis is most important, although it is still too frequently overlooked. It must be said, however, that the apparently sick patients are those who generally, but not invariably, have an additional and independent form of heart disease as well, such as mitral stenosis, hypertension, or coronary artery disease, and that even here the prognosis is still very good.

In contrast to hyperthyroidism, the presence of chronic nephritis in a patient with heart disease makes the prognosis much worse. Quite often when the term "cardiorenal" is used in describing the clinical condition, there really is no significant nephritis. The urinary findings are those of passive congestion and not of true renal insufficiency. It is quite important to make this distinction from the point of view of prognosis and, ordinarily, simple methods are sufficient to indicate the proper differentiation. Even when the urine contains albumin and casts, if the specific gravity is high, the urine is of high color, and there is no secondary anemia, it is extremely unlikely that the kidneys are involved to any important degree. Renal function studies may also be somewhat depressed as a result of passive congestion and return to normal when the cardiac condition improves. It will be helpful, therefore, to appraise the renal factor intelligently in order to make a proper prognosis when there is congestive heart failure.

There are other rarer forms of heart disease in which the prognosis may be excellent despite a considerable degree of heart failure, because treatment is so effective. This applies to cases of beriberi heart, failure from arteriovenous fistula, constrictive pericarditis, and heart failure accompanying acute nephritis or toxemia of pregnancy.

Finally, several types of complications may occur in heart disease which may be regarded as unexpected "accidents" and which may suddenly change the outlook entirely. It often is impossible to predict which patients will develop these complications or when they will occur.

Certain general principles, however, enable us to divide our patients into those who are more likely and those who are less likely to have these unexpected "accidents." I now refer to the development of subacute bacterial endocarditis, emboli (pulmonary or arterial), the different forms of paroxysmal rapid heart action, heart block, and coronary thrombosis. It is obvious that in a patient with heart disease who has been progressing most satisfactorily, the prognosis may suddenly become grave if one of these complications develops.

As for subacute bacterial endocarditis, one may expect that patients with well-marked mitral stenosis or hypertension as a group will only rarely develop it. If there has been persistent auricular fibrillation or a past history of congestive heart failure, it is extremely unlikely that the patient will ever have subacute bacterial endocarditis, no matter how long he lives. It also may be said that if there is no heart murmur, the patient not only has no subacute bacterial endocarditis but will not develop it in the immediate future. On the other hand, those most susceptible to this disease are the patients who have been fairly strong, comparatively free from dyspnea or recurrent attacks of rheumatism, and able to work, and who have shown an apical systolic murmur of mitral insufficiency or a basal diastolic murmur of aortic insufficiency. In a word, it is the well-compensated patient with valvular disease, generally rheumatic, having the above murmurs and a regular heart, without hypertension, who is most apt to develop subacute bacterial endocarditis.

When it comes to predicting which patients will have emboli the problem is even more difficult. In general it may be said that those with mitral stenosis are much more apt to have emboli either from the right auricle to the lungs or from the left auricle to the systemic circulation, than are those with aortic disease. The presence of auricular fibrillation, with or without mitral stenosis, is also conducive to the production of emboli from either auricle. Emboli from the ventricles (generally the left ventricle) occur almost exclusively following a coronary thrombosis and infarction of the ventricular musculature. I know of no method, however, of foretelling which ones of the above types of patients will actually have emboli. When such an "accident" occurs the prognosis may need to be suddenly changed.

Arterial emboli in cases of mitral stenosis with auricular fibrillation most commonly occur shortly after the onset of the arrhythmia, i.e., within days, weeks, or months. Although they may occur after one or more years of this persistent irregularity they do so much more rarely. One might infer that emboli are more likely to be dislodged soon after they form in the left auricle and are much less likely to be dislodged if they have been present a long time and become well organized and adherent to the auricular wall. These facts need to be considered in estimating the effect of surgery for mitral stenosis. It would appear that cerebral emboli are much less common during a given number of years following a satisfactory mitral valvuloplasty than during the same period of time before the operation. Although this is at least partly true, the natural occurrence of cerebral emboli is much less during these later years without operative intervention. In fact, the favorite time for a cerebral embolism in mitral cases is when the heart is well compensated and there is very little dyspnea. Contrariwise, this complication is much rarer when there is advanced congestive failure, auricular fibrillation, marked dyspnea, and striking hepatic enlargement.

The third type of "accident" in patients with heart disease is the sudden development of a new rhythm of the heart. A patient with complete heart block and a slow rate of 30 to 35 may carry on in good health for a great many years. Attacks of Adams-Stokes syncope, however, do occur unexpectedly and any one of the attacks may be fatal. It is impossible to predict when this may take place. A much more common "accident" in which the rhythm of the heart changes is paroxysmal rapid heart action. This may be due to auricular fibrillation, auricular flutter, auricular tachycardia, or ventricular tachycardia. This is not the place to discuss the differential diagnosis of these arrhythmias except to state that in most cases ordinary bedside methods suffice for their proper differentiation. When the heart suddenly becomes rapid the clinical condition often quickly changes for the worse, but the patient generally does better than the physician anticipates because many of these disturbances are transient and self-limited or respond most satisfactorily to treatment. Furthermore, there are many individuals who have no heart disease whatever who suffer from these paroxysms of rapid heart action and carry on indefinitely with practically no restriction in activities. The important point with regard to these paroxysms is that the outlook is not so grave as it seems, for most of them respond to proper treatment.

Finally, we must consider angina pectoris and the "accident" of coronary thrombosis. There is no other condition in the practice of medicine in which it is so difficult to predict the outcome. Patients who suffer from angina pectoris may die suddenly and unexpectedly shortly after they are first seen, or they may live for over twenty years. Such sudden fatalities may but need not be the result of an acute coronary thrombosis. In some the vessels, although showing atheromata, will not be thrombosed. It is even believed that sudden death may occur in angina pectoris with a normal heart and normal coronary arteries. If this does occur, it must be rare. Patients with angina are also prone to attacks of coronary thrombosis that do not cause sudden death. I know of no way of predicting when these accidents will occur. Furthermore, when a patient has an attack of coronary thrombosis there is no satisfactory method of foretelling whether he will survive or succumb. I have seen patients who were most seriously ill recover and others, who apparently were doing extremely well, suddenly die. The age at which other members of the family died of coronary disease at times is helpful in prognosis. Here the physician should remain hopeful under the darkest circumstances and yet give a guarded prognosis when the progress seems most favorable.

Finally, it is well to realize that as a result of improvement in the care of the cardiac patient, especially the proper use of mercurial diuretics, salt restriction and other procedures now employed, patients with congestive heart failure live a good deal longer than they did a generation ago. We now see patients with congestive failure carry on for years when formerly they died in months. Some of the older statistics of prognosis, therefore, need revision.

It is better if the physician is overly optimistic than if he is pessimistic in making prognoses in heart disease. Less harm is done to the patient, by and large, if he lived in hope but was not able to carry on as long as he might have expected, than if he lived in fear of succumbing shortly and survived for a longer time with the sword of Damocles hanging over his head, provided he received intelligent care. The physician should not try to become a prophet.

The foregoing are some of the general principles that I believe will prove valuable in formulating the prognosis in individual patients suffering from cardiac disorders. It is clear that much remains to be known, but I have found that these generalizations have been extremely helpful and that their use will at least diminish the number of errors in prognosis, which errors are constantly placing the medical profession in disrepute in the minds of the general public and encouraging the work of the irregular pseudomedical cults that pervade our country.

CHAPTER 20

Nature and Treatment of Congestive Heart Failure · Surgical Treatment of Valvular Disease

It is no simple matter to analyze in detail the nature and exact mechanism of congestive heart failure. Despite exhaustive clinical, physiological, and pathological studies, many questions remain unanswered. It may be of some value, however, to review some of the more generally accepted concepts that bear on this subject.

Peripheral Circulatory Failure

At the outset the physician must clearly understand what conditions are not heart failure. The fact that the heart becomes rapid and the blood pressure falls does not necessarily mean that the heart is failing or that there is any heart disease. Patients who die of infections such as pneumonia, puerperal sepsis, and typhoid fever die when the heart stops, but death is not due to heart failure. The enfeebled state of the circulation is due to peripheral circulatory failure. Measures ordinarily employed to help the heart are generally useless and at times even harmful. In this condition the circulating blood volume diminishes; there is an inadequate return of blood from the periphery due to stagnation or pooling of blood in the capillary bed and venules. The heart is not apt to dilate and, unless there are pulmonary complications, the patient has no dyspnea, orthopnea, or significant tissue edema.

Peripheral circulatory failure or shock is common in infectious diseases and is often the presenting problem following hemorrhage, severe trauma, burns, surgical operations, and anesthesia, and in stuporous states such as diabetic coma and cerebral hemorrhage. Generally, patients with peripheral failure will show a cold, moist skin with blotchy cyanosis, rapid pulse, and an anxious facial expression. The blood pressure often is low but the systolic level may at times be fairly well maintained while the diastolic level falls. The cause of this state is not altogether clear, but that the primary difficulty in the circulation lies in the capillaries and the small peripheral vessels seems likely. Studies have shown that the minute output of blood from the heart in this condition is apt to be lowered, and that the venous pressure is decreased rather than increased.

346

As for treatment, digitalis is for the most part useless and probably harmful. It will not slow the heart rate under these circumstances and there is reason to believe that it will actually further diminish an already decreased cardiac output. In fact, none of the drugs we have are of great value. It would be desirable to increase the blood volume. For this purpose injections of 1000 cc. or more of 5 per cent glucose in normal salt solution may be given subcutaneously or intravenously. Sometimes transfusions of blood are indicated. The most effective method at present is the intravenous injection of plasma or human albumin. For acute emergencies caffeine sodium benzoate (0.5 gm., or $7\frac{1}{2}$ grains) or coramine (1 to 5 cc.), administered intramuscularly or intravenously, may be employed. Inhalation of oxygen may also be helpful. There may be rare occasions of acute circulatory collapse in which such heroic intravenous medication will be helpful and possibly life saving. There is hope that some of the newer preparations will be more effective in combating the low blood pressure of circulatory collapse. For no matter what the cause, a maintained low blood pressure is dangerous in that it sets up a vicious circle from which recovery is extremely difficult if at all possible. Oliguria, nitrogenous retention and increasing stupor quickly result. There is some evidence that preparations like Paredrine (10 to 20 mg.) given subcutaneously, or, better still, norepinephrine (Levophed) by continuous drip will favorably counteract this state and produce an elevation in blood pressure without an increase in the work of the heart.

The Nature of Congestive Heart Failure

SYMPTOMS AND SIGNS OF CONGESTIVE FAILURE

It is necessary to mention only briefly the clinical evidence of congestive failure, as it is fairly well understood by most physicians. One should distinguish failure of one ventricle from that of the other, although both are frequently involved. Furthermore, it must be appreciated that subjective complaints generally precede physical signs as evidence of early heart failure. Patients may show murmurs, arrhythmias, and cardiac enlargement for many years and remain well compensated. There are very few physical findings which of themselves would make one infer that heart failure is present or impending in the absence of symptoms. Among these are chiefly Cheyne-Stokes breathing, a diastolic gallop rhythm, and possibly pulsus alternans, which may occasionally be elicited. Most of the other physical findings follow subjective complaints.

The earliest evidence of heart failure is abnormal breathlessness. The patient notices shortness of breath on effort that formerly produced no distress. This is due to failure of the left ventricle. In some, dyspnea may come suddenly at rest, particularly at night. The mechanism of these disturbances will be discussed. With increasing dyspnea the amount of effort that can be tolerated comfortably decreases, finally reaching the point of orthopnea or difficulty in lying recumbent. Cheyne-Stokes breathing is common. In the earliest stages physical examination of the lungs may reveal no abnormality, although the vital capacity of the lungs will already be diminished and x-ray may show some pulmonary congestion. Later, increase in the pulmonary second sound, basal rales, and finally hydrothorax develop. In some cases a slight unproductive cough coming at night or on effort occurs as a result of pulmonary congestion.

The early evidence of right-sided failure is increased venous distention or dependent edema. The ankles begin to swell as the day progresses, the swelling disappearing over night. Later, edema of the legs persists and extends upward, involving the thighs, buttocks, abdomen, and occasionally the upper extremities and face. When there is considerable edema, it may involve the upper part of the body if the patient can lie flat, because of the effect of gravity. As a part of the venous congestion due to right heart failure, the venous pressure increases, the jugular veins become distended, and the liver enlarges. Ascites may be present as a part of the general process of edema and partly as a result of portal obstruction. Due to the congestion of the liver there is often epigastric pain and other abdominal symptoms. In fact, occasionally pain in the right upper abdominal quadrant on walking may be an early or primary complaint, especially in patients with mitral stenosis, even in the absence of dyspnea or noticeable swelling of the legs. In such cases the degree of activity is not great enough to elicit breathlessness, while the increase in right-sided failure is sufficient to cause pain in the liver.

There are other general complaints that accompany heart failure, but they are less distinctive and are met with too commonly in other conditions not associated with heart failure. Weakness, easy fatigability, insomnia, irritability, indigestion, palpitation, and dull ache over the precordium have been emphasized by some authors as early evidence of weakening of the circulation. Although these complaints are frequently found in cardiac patients, they rarely help in establishing the diagnosis of heart failure and in fact are often misinterpreted when due to other causes.

The combination of both right-sided and left-sided failure is seen more often than either one in its pure form. Obviously all degrees of heart failure will be found. In the advanced stage, cardiac patients become cachectic, showing marked loss of flesh and cyanosis of the skin, especially of the distal portions of the body such as the ears, nose, cheeks, hands, and feet. With this cyanosis there is often a slight icteric tint to the skin.

Patients with marked congestive failure have impairment of sweating in hot humid weather. In fact, they have been found to perspire only 25 to 50 per cent of normal and have much greater discomfort with such weather than other people. However, in general, cardiac patients do better with moderately warm and dry weather than with cold.

THE MECHANISM OF CONGESTIVE FAILURE

For generations there have been two diametrically opposed schools of thought concerning the mechanism of heart failure. According to one it is believed that heart failure is due to insufficient output of the heart to the tissues (forward failure), and, to the other, that it is due to congestion of parts of the body or back pressure (backward failure). The arguments pro and con will not be discussed here, but it may serve a useful purpose to mention some of the factors in circulatory dynamics that bear on this question. They will aid in understanding the events we witness in practice and in rationalizing the therapy we employ.

One must distinguish some of the symptoms we often see in cardiac patients that may be looked upon as by-products, complications, or accidents of the condition and not as fundamentally related to the question of heart failure. A patient may have attacks of Adams-Stokes syncope and yet have no evidence whatever of congestive failure, not even experiencing anginal pain or dyspnea on the most strenuous effort. Many cardiac patients suffer from weakness. This may be due to many causes, among which a diminished cardiac output is important. However, such weakness can occur without any congestive failure. This is seen during prolonged paroxysmal tachycardia in which, because of an extremely rapid heart rate, the minute output of blood is markedly diminished. The patient feels quite weak but he may have neither pulmonary nor peripheral congestion. A similar situation in which there is marked weakness without congestive failure is seen in some cases of acute coronary thrombosis.

It is of primary importance to look upon the left and right portions of the heart separately for, although we generally see the results of failure of both sides, it is often possible to distinguish the phenomena characterizing the failure of each side separately. At times one will observe evidence of pure one-sided failure. The importance of a balance between the two ventricles becomes clear from the following analysis. If, as a result of any cause, the left ventricle expelled one drop of blood less per beat than the right ventricle, within three to four hours about one liter of additional blood would accumulate in the lungs. This would lead to acute pulmonary edema. A condition similar to this occurs in acute left ventricular failure with paroxysmal cardiac dyspnea. On the other hand, if the right ventricle expelled one drop less than the left an equal amount of blood would accumulate on the venous or right side of the circulation, resulting in venous distention, enlarged liver, and, possibly, peripheral edema. However, if both ventricles diminished their output equally, although the circulation would slow up there would be no accumulation on either side, and neither pulmonary congestion nor peripheral edema would result. In other words, although a slight imbalance of the two ventricles may exist for short periods of time, the two ventricles must eventually expel equal amounts of blood if disaster is to be avoided.

The processes involved in the gradual development of congestive heart failure are both numerous and intricate. Let us trace some of the events that occur during the progress of a case of mitral stenosis. As the mitral valve becomes increasingly narrowed the pressure in the left auricle increases. The wall of the left auricle becomes slightly dilated, which has two effects. It tends to make the pressure within its cavity return to normal and, following Starling's "law of the heart," the slight dilatation improves the contraction and compensates for the obstruction of the valve. The circulation is restored to normal but with the result that the left auricle is slightly larger, and eventually the pressure in the auricle and the pulmonary circuit becomes increased. As years go on and the condition progresses the right ventricle feels the burden of the increased pulmonary pressure. The pulmonary second sound increases in intensity. The right ventricle first dilates, thereby increasing its ability to expel blood, and later hypertrophies. It is a matter of general experience that prolonged dilatation precedes and is the stimulus for hypertrophy. In this way the balance of the two sides of the heart is maintained. The equilibrium that now exists in this patient with mitral stenosis is such that, although there is no peripheral congestive failure, there has been a slight increase in the volume of blood in the lungs owing to the prolonged backward pressure behind the stenosed valve. At this stage the patient may be short of breath on effort but shows no rales in the lungs. The vital capacity of the lungs, however, may already have decreased. This measurement often is the first evidence of a diminished cardiac reserve and is the result of a decrease in the total available air space in the lungs. In the early stage, even if the vital capacity is not yet found to be decreased when measured with the patient at rest, it will be found that effort will diminish the vital capacity, whereas the same effort will produce no change in a normal individual.

In following the developments of the above case the progression may take different courses. If the right ventricle has become sufficiently hypertrophied and has not dilated too much, and the mitral obstruction is considerable, increasing breathlessness may result from further engorgement of the pulmonary circuit. In fact, such patients often have attacks of pulmonary edema. At such times, as a result of additional effort or of some nervous mechanism, or for some other ill-defined reason, the right ventricle pumps out more blood than the left and the difference is trapped in the lungs. An adjustment of the circulation occurs as the right side decreases or the left side increases its output. From this one can see how phlebotomy may occasionally be helpful in producing this adjustment. This is the small group of cases with so-called tight mitral stenosis with marked increase in pulmonary pressure, prone to attacks of pulmonary edema but without right-sided failure, who are now being subjected to surgical procedures. This will be further discussed later.

The course of events, however, may be different. The right ventricle may dilate beyond the point of mechanical efficiency. With this there is an increase in the pressure in the right auricle, the venae cavae, and the systemic veins. This increase in the venous pressure (normal values are

40 to 80 mm. of water) is the first evidence of right-sided failure. One of the earliest results of this is engorgement of the liver. Another is the development of pitting edema of the recumbent portions of the body. In some cases, despite the increase in venous pressure, peripheral pitting edema does not occur or is delayed because there are other factors concerned with the production of edema. Among these, one of the most important is the pumping action of muscular contraction of the legs on the venous return. If there has not been enough dyspnea to prevent the patient from walking, the exercise of the legs tends to delay the development of edema. Changes in the walls of the capillaries, the osmotic pressure of the blood, the development of acidosis, and, to a lesser extent, the question of tissue anoxia, which is determined by the volume output of blood, all may have a bearing on the appearance of peripheral edema.

The recent work of Stead and his colleagues has emphasized the importance of forward failure, mainly in the production of edema. According to this concept, in the early stages of heart failure there is a decreased output from the left ventricle. As a result there is a considerably decreased renal flow and retention of sodium. This is interpreted as the primary cause of fluid retention and production of edema. An important point in our new knowledge is that when there is a slight fall in left ventricular output (and even when there is no fall) there may yet be a considerable decrease in renal flow. Different organs partake differently in the changes in blood flow, so that changes in total blood circulation cannot tell us what is happening in any particular organ.

The subject in the above hypothetical case could therefore present himself at one stage as a patient with mitral stenosis complaining of dyspnea on exertion without physical signs of congestion but having a diminished vital capacity of the lungs. At another time this patient might have a good deal of obvious pulmonary congestion with marked breathlessness or he might show considerable venous distention, enlarged liver, with or without pitting edema, and little dyspnea. Finally, all the evidence of failure of both sides of the circulation may be present.

If a hypothetical case had started with hypertension or aortic valvular disease the primary strain would have been on the left ventricle. At first, because of the increased work, the left ventricle would dilate a bit, and thereby compensate to eject the normal amount of blood into the aorta. If it did not do so for any significant length of time, acute pulmonary edema would result. In the course of time the prolonged dilatation and subsequent hypertrophy of the heart progress beyond the point of improved efficiency and the left ventricle fails to propel as much blood as the right ventricle. The result, as in the case of mitral stenosis, is increased pulmonary pressure, congestion of the lungs, and dyspnea. The right ventricle, laboring against a constant increase in pressure in the pulmonary artery, becomes hypertrophied. This accounts for the frequent enlargement of the right ventricle that is found in cases of left ventricular strain. Finally, when the right side is sufficiently embarrassed, peripheral edema, engorged liver, and ascites may develop. Patients who originally had primary left ventricular strain may be seen with various combinations of cardiac failure, some mainly with dyspnea, others with little or no dyspnea and showing for the most part peripheral congestion, and still others with different degrees of both.

There are other effects on the dynamics of the circulation and physiologic functions of the various organs of the body that result from congestive heart failure. The total volume of blood increases. From a normal amount of about 5000 cc. it may increase to 6 or 7 liters or more. This is one of the most constant changes that accompany heart failure. This excess blood is stored throughout the venous side of the circulation, the lungs, and to some extent in the dilated heart. The fact is often overlooked that when a heart is considerably dilated there may be as much as 1 liter or more of blood in excess of normal within its chambers. In such cases there must be a large amount of residual blood in the heart, for no increased amount is expelled with each systole. The total blood volume will always decrease and approach normal with clinical improvement. It has been difficult to explain what happens to the 1 or 2 liters of blood that disappears from the body as congestive failure improves. Recently, however, it has been shown that during congestion there is an increase in red blood cell formation as evidenced by reticulocytosis, and with improvement there is a diminution in blood formation and an increase in blood cell destruction. The latter is indicated by an increase in the icteric index of the blood and a marked increase in the urobilinogen in the stools. The increase in blood volume in congestive failure is so constant that occasionally it may serve as a diagnostic point. I recall an instance in which a man with definite organic valvular disease had a good deal of edema and pulmonary congestion. There was ample evidence that he had nephritis as well. At first the problem was regarded as one of heart failure. It was found, however, that the blood volume was perfectly normal. This and other studies of the dynamics of the circulation all showed that the patient could not have heart failure and that the edema must be due to nephritis. He died shortly thereafter of typical uremia.

Disturbances in the velocity of blood flow are of considerable importance in cardiac patients. In certain hyperdynamic states, such as obtain during fever, exercise, anemia and especially with hyperthyroidism, the rate of blood flow (not to be confused with the heart rate) is increased. Blood moves more rapidly from place to place in the circulation. With congestive failure the blood velocity is slowed up, mainly owing to the increase in the blood volume or circulatory bed. When slowing is considerable there is likely to be pulmonary congestion, but slight slowing can take place in constrictive pericarditis, when the lungs are not congested. One factor that has been neglected as causing a slowing in the velocity of blood flow as usually determined is the volume of the heart itself. There are instances of marked dilatation of the heart, especially of the auricles, when the cavities may contain 2 liters or more of blood.

The circulation time will necessarily be markedly prolonged because of the dilution in this enormous residual pool and the slow movement of blood, even if there is no pulmonary or venous stasis. The methods in common use measure the time it takes for blood to flow from a vein at the elbow to the heart, through the lungs, out of the aorta to the tongue or respiratory center. Normally this requires about fifteen seconds. When delay occurs it takes place for the most part in the lungs or heart. Patients with marked congestion may show an arm-to-tongue time of twenty-five to fifty seconds or more. In fact, if the rate of flow is normal it is unlikely that there is any chronic cardiac congestion of the lungs.

Various methods of measuring the velocity of blood flow are in current use. Sodium dehydrocholate or Decholin (3 to 5 cc. of 20 per cent solution) may be injected into an antecubital vein. Arrival of the drug in the tongue is signaled by the sensation of a bitter taste. Similarly, 2 to 3 gm. of saccharin in a few cc. of sterile water may be injected. The end-point in this case is a sweet taste. Sodium cyanide (0.25 to 0.5 cc. of a 2 per cent aqueous solution) may also be used. The advantage of this method is that the end-point is objective, for the patient will suddenly take deep gasping breaths the moment the drug reaches the carotid sinus. Alpha-lobeline hydrochloride (5 mg.—0.5 cc. of 1 per cent solution intravenously) can be used. The end-point is a sudden cough thought to come from carotid sinus stimulation. Calcium gluconate (2.5 cc. of a 20 per cent solution) may be used, in which case the end-point is a sensation of heat in the tongue or mouth. Caution must be exercised in injecting calcium when the patient has been receiving full doses of digitalis, because of a synergistic action of the two drugs. In all these procedures the patient should be recumbent and relaxed with the arm lying at about the level of the heart. The injection should be rapid and the end-point accurately timed with a stop watch.

The preceding methods measure the time it takes blood to flow from a vein in the arm through the lungs, back to the heart, and out through the aorta. If it is desired to measure the time consumed in the flow of blood through the lungs, the ether method is used. An injection of 0.3 to 0.5 cc. of ether with an equal amount of normal saline is made into the brachial vein. The moment the patient or the observer detects the ether in the breath is the end-point. This time, which normally is about four to eight seconds, subtracted from the arm-to-tongue time, is an indirect measurement of the pulmonary circulation time because most of that delay takes place in the pulmonary vessels.

Measuring the velocity of blood flow is a simple procedure for differentiating many conditions such as emphysema, bronchitis, bronchopneumonia, cancer of the lungs, and aneurysms from heart failure. Not infrequently the condition evidenced by these symptoms, such as dullness, rales, dyspnea, and chest pain, is mistaken for congestive failure. In all of these states the velocity of blood flow is normal or not much changed, whereas if heart failure is present it is slowed. It is evident, therefore, that a prolonged circulation time through the lungs is an indirect indication of failure of the left ventricle. There is one important exception to this general rule. When *acute* pulmonary edema develops in a patient who previously was in fairly normal health, as may happen with acute coronary thrombosis or in a well-compensated hypertensive individual, the velocity of blood flow may be essentially normal. It apparently requires a more chronic state of passive congestion in the lungs, so that pulmonary blood volume is markedly increased, before slowing of the circulation may take place.

An increase in the venous pressure similarly affords an early measure of failure of the right ventricle. This can often be estimated by observing the degree of distention of the cervical veins. Normally these veins are completely collapsed with the patient in the upright or semirecumbent position. The height above the heart to which the distention rises serves as a rough measure of venous pressure. The exact reading can be made directly from the antecubital veins (normally about 40 to 80 mm. of water). In certain cases in which the question of congestive heart failure is in doubt, the determination of the venous pressure may be very helpful. Obviously an enlarged liver or ascites may be due to a malignant growth, alcoholic cirrhosis, inflammatory conditions, or passive congestion. Similarly, edema of the legs may be due to nephritis, varicose veins, or cardiac failure. In all such cases, if the cardiac function is intact, the venous pressure in the arms will be essentially normal.

One of the simplest and most valuable of the measurements that aid in estimating cardiac efficiency is the vital capacity of the lungs. Some of the factors that influence the vital capacity have already been discussed (see Chap. 6). All that is needed to obtain this reading is a spirometer. The apparatus is very simple and inexpensive, and requires no upkeep. The test can be performed in one minute by any physician and will afford valuable information. It has been very much neglected and should be used by all practitioners. Once a diagnosis of heart disease has been made, the vital capacity determinations will be much more valuable in estimating prognosis and in following the progress of a cardiac patient than the more expensive electrocardiograms that are frequently taken. Furthermore, the finding of a normal or supernormal vital capacity practically rules out congestive heart failure. This test is particularly valuable in detecting cases of functional dyspnea, when the readings are so often perfectly normal. Diminution in the breathing space is a very early sign of left ventricular failure. As has been stated, this may precede the appearance of basal rales. The decrease in the vital capacity results mainly from engorgement of the pulmonary vessels, which diminishes the available alveolar spaces, and from a loss of elasticity of the bronchioles. Other factors in some cases are the development of hydrothorax and even the huge size of the heart. The volume of the heart occasionally may be actually 1 or 2 liters greater than normal. It is obvious under such circumstances that, with the thoracic cage remaining unchanged in size, the available space for ventilation must diminish considerably. Normally the average adult having a total breathing space of about 4000 cc. inhales 400 to 500 cc. with each breath and on effort can increase both the rate and the depth of respiration without distress. When the vital capacity is diminished to 2000 cc. he reaches his greatest possible depth of inspiration more readily and will resort to a greater increase in rate of respiration to attain adequate ventilation. Furthermore, with these short and rapid breaths there is an increase in the proportion of the dead space (that upper part of the respiratory tract in which the air is not exposed to the blood for gaseous exchange). In this way a diminished vital capacity is conducive to dyspnea or uncomfortable breathing.

It is also of some interest that pulmonary congestion may set up certain vicious circles which tend to aggravate the very condition that produces them. Bouts of coughing, so common in cardiac failure, tend to increase still further the return flow of blood to the right side of the heart and thereby overburden the pulmonary circuit. The same is true of the act of overventilation or agitated breathing, such as is seen during the period of hyperpnea of Cheyne-Stokes breathing. From this it is clear that whatever tends to quiet cough or vigorous breathing, such as a hypodermic injection of morphine, not only makes the patient more comfortable but actually improves the underlying congestion.

One form of breathlessness common in certain cardiac patients is particularly prone to occur at night. It occurs in varying degrees of severity, from a slight increase in the degree of dyspnea to violent attacks of suffocation. It is often called "paroxysmal nocturnal dyspnea," or "cardiac asthma." It occurs most commonly in association with conditions in which there is a strain on the left ventricle, such as hypertension, aortic valvular disease, and coronary artery disease. It is less frequent in cases of mitral stenosis. The factors that underlie this phenomenon are numerous. When the patient goes to bed there is a slight gradual shift of fluid from the periphery to the pulmonary circuit. Venous return from the legs becomes facilitated, blood volume increases through hemodilution, pressure in the peripheral veins and the right auricle rises, and the right ventricle expels a little more blood than the weakened left ventricle can expel. The metabolic rate of the body also increases slightly as the day progresses. This and the bodily activities during the day tend to produce greater pulmonary congestion. The vital capacity of the lungs which already had been diminished becomes further decreased. Furthermore, sensory perception is obviously diminished during sleep and the reflex stimuli from congested lungs, which are most important in the control of breathing, are less effective than during the waking hours. The result is that a greater degree of pulmonary stasis develops before the reflex stimuli from the lungs are effective in producing exaggerated respirations. Finally the stimulus becomes sufficiently great to arouse the patient from sleep. The respiratory center now responds vigorously. The patient is then found to be breathing laboriously, with evidence of slight or marked pulmonary edema. The cough that frequently accompanies the attack and the vigorous rapid breathing both tend to make the condition worse. The vicious circle may be broken by diminishing the return of venous blood to the right heart, by increasing the output of the left ventricle, or by decreasing the sensitivity of the nervous system. The first is accomplished if the patient assumes the upright position or occasionally if phlebotomy is performed; the second is accomplished by giving digitalis in some cases or by diminishing peripheral resistance, and the last by the use of morphine.

The foregoing discussion explains in general terms the mechanism of nocturnal dyspnea. There are, however, other less important influences involved which may serve as precipitating factors. The act of coughing, a full bladder, abdominal distention, unpleasant dreams, a change in environmental temperature, lowering the head, or a large meal have all been observed to precipitate attacks of paroxysmal dyspnea in cardiac patients. By some methods, probably through nervous reflexes, these factors serve as trigger mechanisms, but they all require a background of pulmonary congestion to be effective in the production of attacks of dyspnea.

Among patients who suffer from breathlessness, especially those with nocturnal dyspnea, and in some who are hardly aware that they have any dyspnea, periodic or Cheyne-Stokes breathing is quite common. Much attention has been given to its explanation but, although some light has been thrown on its mechanism, this peculiar phenomenon still remains obscure. It occurs mainly in patients with left ventricular failure, particularly in older people, and is most marked during, if not entirely confined to, the period of sleep. The breathing waxes and wanes with intervals of apnea varying in length from a few seconds to even a minute. The period of hyperpnea following the apnea may be very violent and awaken the patient in great agitation. In fact, this accounts for many attacks of nocturnal dyspnea.

Apart from the one predominant factor of pulmonary congestion there are other factors that have some bearing on the production of this type of periodic breathing. A diminution in the blood flow to the respiratory center, a decrease in the sensitivity of the respiratory center and of the entire nervous system during sleep, an increase in intracranial pressure, and a diminution in the carbon dioxide content of the blood may all play their respective roles. Once a tendency to periodicity develops it is not difficult to understand why it may continue or become more marked. During the apneic intervals the carbon dioxide level of the blood (which is the main stimulus for respiration) increases, as carbon dioxide is not being expired from the lungs. The oxygen content of the arterial blood is decreasing, as very little oxygen is being absorbed from the lungs. After a sufficient interval has elapsed the stimulus becomes great enough even to arouse the insensitive respiratory center, which responds in an exaggerated fashion. The result is violent hyperpnea which in time gets rid of the accumulated carbon dioxide from the blood through the lungs until the level is again too low to excite the respiratory center and the cycle begins again.

Morphine helps patients with Cheyne-Stokes breathing not by doing away with the periodic breathing, for it may even lengthen the periods of apnea, but by diminishing nervous sensitivity and thereby preventing patients from being aroused by the uncomfortable hyperpnea. Caffeine in large doses, on the other hand, may temporarily eliminate this type of breathing by increasing the sensitivity of the respiratory center. Aminophylline given intravenously in doses of 0.24 to 0.48 gm. ($3\frac{1}{2}$ to 7 grains) has been found very useful. More important are the measures that improve the underlying pulmonary congestion. When cardiac therapy succeeds in producing a diuresis, sometimes even one of slight degree, the condition may be greatly improved. Furthermore, the condition may be greatly helped by having the patient sit up in a chair with the legs hanging down rather than by keeping him in bed. This also tends to diminish the venous return to the right heart.

There are some other sequelae of congestive heart failure apart from those directly related to the dynamics of the circulation. Fever and leukocytosis are commonly seen in conjunction with cardiac congestion. In some instances an intercurrent infection may be the precipitating cause of the heart failure. Frequently, however, congestion itself produces slight fever. When the temperature is over 101° F. it is more likely to be due to some infection like bronchopneumonia, rheumatic fever, or sore throat, or to infarction in some organ, especially the lung. The fact that slight fever (100 to 101° F.) may result from uncomplicated heart failure, although commonly observed in ordinary cardiac patients, is best illustrated in rare cases of paroxysmal tachycardia. Here one may see a patient without organic heart disease suddenly develop a rapid heart rate, and if the attack is prolonged he may gradually show evidence of pulmonary congestion and with it fever and leukocytosis. With disappearance of the congestion the temperature and white blood count return to normal.

Jaundice is another finding in some cases of heart failure. There are three factors involved in the production of this type of jaundice. In the first place, passive congestion of the liver and anoxemia may impair liver function and disturb the excretion of bile through the bile ducts. Secondly, pulmonary infarction is frequently associated with jaundice through the breakdown of red blood cells in the lung. Finally, as congestion improves, there is an increase in blood destruction. The icteric index in some cases may reach levels as high as 20 to 30 or more. As a result of prolonged hepatic congestion, cardiac cirrhosis may also develop. This may produce the picture of portal obstruction added to the already existing cardiac edema. In such cases repeated abdominal paracentesis may be required. Ascites may be quite conspicuous and out of proportion to the other evidences of heart failure. This occurs most frequently in cases of organic tricuspid stenosis and in constrictive pericarditis.

In determining the presence or absence of congestive heart failure, it is helpful to distinguish the objective from the subjective manifestations. Symptoms are more often misleading than signs. Breathlessness may be functional or bronchial in origin. Pain in the chest may be due to spondylitis and not to heart disease. Likewise, the objective signs may also have other causes than the heart. Peripheral edema may be due to varicose veins with the accompanying lymph stasis, rales to pneumonia, and enlarged liver to alcoholic cirrhosis or cancer. It is often much easier to ascertain whether heart disease is present than whether there is heart failure.

In observing and guiding the course of a patient with organic heart disease it is most important to bear in mind the factors that tend to precipitate heart failure. Inasmuch as the underlying original causes, such as rheumatic fever, arteriosclerosis, and hypertension, are difficult to prevent, care must be exercised in protecting cardiac patients against the aggravating or precipitating causes. The most important of these are excessive intake of sodium and infection. The others are for the most part those situations that unduly increase the work of the heart. Excessive physical effort, prolonged emotional strain, obesity, pregnancy, anemia, hyperthyroidism, or any condition that accelerates the heart may be contributing factors. In so far as they can be prevented or remedied, just so far will ultimate heart failure be delayed.

The distinction has already been drawn between congestive heart failure and peripheral circulatory failure. It must also be made clear that both conditions may exist simultaneously. This is particularly true in some cases of acute coronary thrombosis and when organic cardiac patients have intercurrent conditions such as pneumonia or cerebral hemorrhage. When both types of failure coexist, difficulties arise concerning some of the methods of therapy commonly employed. A patient with severe acute coronary thrombosis may have pulmonary edema indicating left ventricular failure, and cold, gray, moist skin with a low blood pressure as a result of peripheral shock. For the former condition phlebotomy might be useful, and for the latter one might reasonably give a transfusion. Likewise, digitalis is beneficial for the former and useless or harmful for the latter. In such cases the physician must weigh the advantages and disadvantages of the treatment in each individual instance.

THE CLINICAL PICTURE OF CONGESTIVE FAILURE

A brief review of the clinical picture of congestive failure may now be presented, even at the risk of some repetition. The type and severity of complaints and the variety of physical findings will depend on the particular case and the stage of the process that has been reached. Symptoms as a rule precede signs. Breathlessness is the most important and generally the earliest evidence of heart failure. As has been discussed previously, it is necessary to rule out other causes, such as those of a functional and pulmonary nature, before regarding breathlessness as due entirely to the heart. In hypertension and aortic and coronary cases, dyspnea may first appear at night, while in other cases it is first noted on effort. Cheyne-Stokes breathing especially during sleep almost always means heart failure. Even before dyspnea occurs most cardiac patients complain of fatigue, "lack of pep," restlessness, insomnia, and nervousness. These general complaints are too common in many other conditions, particularly in neurasthenia, to be very helpful diagnostically.

Edema of the ankles then develops. At first it is transient, disappearing overnight. Later it may persist. When orthopnea does not prevent the patient from assuming the recumbent position at night, edema may spread upward earlier in the progress of the disease and involve the arms and face. The liver becomes engorged and causes pain or discomfort in the upper abdomen, and in the course of time ascites may develop. The amount of urine voided also decreases.

Examination will show various findings in different cases. Basal rales or diminution in respiratory excursion are among the earliest objective evidences of heart failure. Diminution in respiratory excursion is reflected in a diminution of the vital capacity of the lungs. The x-ray may show evidence of pulmonary congestion in the absence of rales. Later free fluid accumulates in the pleural cavities, especially the right. Auscultation of the heart may or may not reveal abnormalities depending on the nature of the lesion. Murmurs, irregularities, and even cardiac enlargement, if present, are not necessarily indicative of heart failure, although they may signify the existence of heart disease. The presence of a diastolic gallop rhythm or pulsus alternans may generally be relied upon as a sign of failure or impending failure.

Cyanosis is apt to appear rather late. In some cases of mitral stenosis and in chronic cor pulmonale, it is often very marked. The cervical veins become distended and may remain so even when the patient is in the semirecumbent position. Gradually, when severe heart failure continues for years, a high degree of cardiac cachexia with marked wasting of tissue takes place. Such patients may show considerable swelling of the lower half of the body, with very thin, emaciated arms and thorax. The urine, which is small in amount, may show albumin and casts, but unlike that seen in chronic nephritis it will be highly colored and of a high specific gravity. An unexpected gain of weight, while the food intake is actually small, often occurs and is due to the retention of fluid. This may take place without obvious edema, for cardiac patients can have as much as 5 liters of excess fluid in the intercellular tissue spaces and yet show no pitting. Slight jaundice, often due to a complicating pulmonary infarction, is not uncommon.

Of greatest importance is the realization that most of the signs and symptoms of heart failure may be simulated in other noncardiac conditions. An enlarged liver may be due to cirrhosis or cancer; pulmonary rales to pneumonia, bronchitis, or tumor; edema of the legs to nephritis, pelvic tumor, varicose veins, or hypoproteinemia; increased venous pressure to superior mediastinal obstruction, and so on. One could further elaborate these similarities. It obviously is necessary to appraise the entire picture most carefully in determining the presence or absence of congestive heart failure.

THE ACTION OF DIGITALIS

There is hardly a drug in medical use that has been studied as extensively as digitalis. Despite the most exhaustive pharmacologic investigations concerning its mode of action, many questions remain unanswered. This discussion will be limited primarily to some of the known effects of digitalis and to the simpler aspects of its clinical indications.

Digitalis in sufficient doses increases the irritability of the heart as indicated by the production of ectopic ventricular beats, first few in number and then in the form of ventricular tachycardia, and finally by the development of fatal ventricular fibrillation. In the experimental animal the latter mechanism is generally the cause of death when lethal doses are given. The therapeutic dose, which averages about 35 to 40 per cent of the lethal dose, causes none of these irregularities except possibly a few extrasystoles.

Digitalis also slows the conduction of impulses. This is especially noticeable in a prolongation of the P-R interval. The effect may be sufficient to result in partial heart block and rarely even in complete heart block.

Most of the slowing that results from digitalis and its allied drugs is produced by its stimulating effect on the vagus nerve. Apparently some of the slowing is extravagal for it is only partly abolished by full doses of atropine. In cases of auricular fibrillation, conspicuous slowing of ventricular rate results. This is brought about mainly by the action of the drug on the junctional conductive tissue. In hearts with a normal regular rhythm, only very slight slowing occurs. This slowing is so slight that it cannot be the cause of such striking improvement as is witnessed in many cases of heart failure with a normal rhythm.

There are other effects on the heart muscle produced by digitalis. Possibly the most important pharmacologic effect of digitalis is that it increases the strength or force of contraction of cardiac muscle. By direct action on heart muscle it lengthens the effective refractory period and slows the rate of propagation of impulses. These effects are counteracted by the indirect action of the drug through the vagus which shortens the refractory period and accelerates the transmission interval. The final effect, therefore, is variable, depending upon which influence predominates. The drug has another direct effect on the ventricular musculature that is shown in a peculiar inversion of the T wave of the electrocardiogram (see Chap. 21). It also causes a slight shortening of the Q-T interval. Animal experimentation has shown that, although therapeutic doses of digitalis produce no pathologic changes in the heart muscle, toxic doses do cause definite necrosis of heart muscle fibers and inflammatory changes and also changes in brain cells. Whether these findings are in any way related to the previously mentioned electrocardiographic evidence of myocardial effects is doubtful.

It has long been known that digitalis diminishes the size of the heart. This has been ascribed to an increase in "tonus" of the heart.

There has been much discussion concerning the action of digitalis on the coronary arteries and coronary blood flow. Most of the evidence points to a constricting action on these vessels due to a vagal effect. It is unlikely, however, that this results in diminished blood flow through the coronary arteries because compensatory effects may result from the accompanying slowing and other actions of the drug.

It is thought that digitalis improves the efficiency of the heart. By this is meant that it enables the heart to do the same work with less expenditure of energy. More knowledge concerning the intimate metabolism of heart muscle is needed. It has been found that with heart failure the potassium and creatine contents of heart muscle are diminished. It is apparent that, when the heart is unduly dilated, a decrease in size brought about by digitalis might well increase the mechanical efficiency of contraction. It can readily be seen that the effect of all these factors on the output of the heart will be variable. The decrease in venous return would tend to diminish and the improvement in cardiac efficiency or capacity would tend to increase the cardiac output. The former effect will predominate in cases in which the heart is normal or essentially normal and there is no abnormal residual blood in the heart, for no matter how efficient the heart may be it cannot pump out more blood than it receives. When there is severe heart failure, however, the decrease in venous return is not a handicap and the improvement of the efficiency of contraction may be sufficient to produce an actual increase in the cardiac output. Direct measurements, in fact, have shown that digitalis actually diminishes the output of the heart in normal individuals and in patients with conditions like pneumonia, in which the heart is regarded as normal. In congestive failure, when the output may be either normal or somewhat diminished, digitalis has been found to produce a variable effect. In many cases there is an increase but in some there is a decrease in the output, depending on which of the two opposite effects predominates.

In the normal heart a small amount of blood still remains within the ventricular cavities after ventricular systole. Emptying of the cavities becomes more complete with effort or when special demands are made. In heart failure there remains a greater amount of residual blood after contraction, and when the need increases the ventricle involved (or both sides) is not able to keep pace and emptying of the chambers becomes even less well performed. Digitalis aids the failing heart in performing this function more adequately.

The beneficial clinical action of digitalis is regarded as limited to the heart. The notable diuretic properties have been thought to be secondary to improvement in cardiac function. Of interest historically is that Withering regarded the primary value of digitalis as a diuretic. Thereafter the cardiotonic action of this drug was regarded as paramount. It was not until twenty-five years ago that interest was redirected to the action of digitalis on the kidney. Gremels showed clearly a chloruretic and diuretic effect of digitalis at a time when there were no detectable changes in the circulatory dynamics of the heart or kidney. His work pointed to a direct action of digitalis on the renal tubules. Confirmation of this concept has currently been obtained by more than one group of investigators. It may be that digitalis interferes with the effects of those adrenal cortical steroids which promote the reabsorption of sodium by the renal tubules. Notwithstanding these direct effects on the kidney, it is still generally thought, and rightly so, that the main diuretic effect following digitalis administration in congestive failure results from the favorable action on the heart.

The main indication for the use of digitalis is congestive heart failure, whether it be left or right ventricular, or both. It does not matter then whether the blood pressure is high or low, whether the heart rate is rapid or slow, or whether the aortic or mitral valve is involved. When there is also a significant pulse deficit, as occurs in cases of auricular fibrillation or auricular flutter, apart from the previously mentioned effects, the drug improves the circulation by eliminating or diminishing the pulse deficit. When there is considerable cardiac hypertrophy, slowing of the rate is more important because a thick musculature needs a longer diastolic rest period for oxygen diffusion. It is open to question whether or not it is desirable to give digitalis continuously to those patients who have no heart failure but who manifest conditions that might lead to failure, such as hypertension with cardiac hypertrophy. If the circulatory dynamics are already normal and the patient has no symptoms it is likely that digitalis in therapeutic doses will upset the patient, and if there is no dilatation of the heart the cardiac output would probably be diminished by the drug rather than increased.

Digitalis is also used for long periods of time, in those patients who recover from heart failure, to maintain the improvement that has been obtained, whenever the underlying condition is chronic and it is feared that heart failure might recur. There are disturbances in cardiac rhythm, not necessarily associated with congestive failure, for which digitalis may be used. Paroxysmal or maintained auricular fibrillation or auricular flutter and instances of paroxysmal auricular tachycardia may often be helped considerably by the judicious use of the drug. The rapid ventricular rate of auricular fibrillation or flutter may be slowed even when there is no heart failure, and especially in the latter condition a normal rhythm is often resumed. When attacks of paroxysmal auricular tachycardia recur frequently, constant administration of digitalis may prevent attacks entirely.

It is important to emphasize that digitalis not only is not indicated but may be harmful in cases of peripheral circulatory failure. In acute infections, surgical shock, heart tamponade from pericardial effusions or constrictive pericarditis, further diminution of cardiac output may result from the drug. There are occasional instances in which the foregoing conditions are associated with true congestive failure and then digitalis may favorably affect the latter to a sufficient degree to be beneficial.

The Treatment of Congestive Heart Failure

Unlike acute infectious diseases or many surgical conditions in which a complete cure is to be expected, the treatment of congestive heart failure is concerned with the amelioration of symptoms. Its purpose is to diminish suffering, to prolong life, and to increase the usefulness of the patient for as long as possible. Although cures are not to be hoped for, except in a small number of cases, because the underlying structural changes in the heart are for the most part irremediable, proper treatment may render individuals more comfortable, may restore some to useful occupation, and occasionally may secure even complete symptomatic recovery. For the most part the best that is accomplished by intelligent care of a patient with chronic cardiac disease is a prolongation of life that compares very favorably with the advantages that are derived from the early diagnosis and treatment of cancer. It is, therefore, with such restricted hopes that we must view this problem.

At the outset, the physician must bear in mind that social and economic factors often enter into consideration in outlining a course of treatment. This is as true of chronic heart disease as it is of many other chronic diseases. A day laborer who suffers from recurrent asthma and hay fever cannot be sent on a sea voyage or to the mountains every so often to rid himself of the offending agents or to avoid exposure to them. On the other hand, patients in a more fortunate economic position often derive considerable benefit from such expensive trips. Similarly, those patients with angina pectoris who are in a position to afford it can go south in the winter and avoid the burden of cold winters and inclement weather. Likewise, the decision whether four or six weeks will be spent in the medical care of an individual case of cardiac failure may depend upon whether the man's job is jeopardized or whether he has sickness insurance, and on other purely nonmedical considerations.

Let us start with an average male of moderate means, 40 years of age, whose occupation is that of bank teller. He has had mitral stenosis for many years and now presents himself in moderate congestive heart failure. There has been increasing dyspnea, some cough, and, finally, peripheral edema. Physical examination shows moderate pitting of the ankles, a slightly engorged and tender liver, rales at the bases of the lungs, and evidence of a slight right hydrothorax. The heart is dilated, the action is absolutely irregular, typical of auricular fibrillation, with a rate of 130, and the murmurs indicate the presence of mitral stenosis. The blood pressure is 150 mm. systolic and 90 mm. diastolic. The Wassermann test is negative, and the other findings are not significant. We may also assume that this patient previously had been receiving inadequate treatment and, in fact, had taken no digitalis whatever.

REST

The first principle in the treatment of such a patient is rest. Some patients, especially men, will rebel at what appears to them as such an extreme measure. They will plead to be permitted to cut down their work, to go into town for only one half a day, or to remain at home resting or "taking it easy." It is best at the outset to explain that more will be accomplished in a shorter time if a strict regimen is carried out. An effective argument is to emphasize that they will start feeling better more quickly and will lose less time from work if they give themselves every advantage for recovery than if they adopt only half-way measures. I have found it helpful to explain that with complete rest, as compared with being merely ambulatory, the average heart saves about 25,000 beats each day and it is this enforced rest to the heart which is so beneficial. The advice "to stay home or in a hospital and rest" often carries with it a grave outlook in the mind of the patient. However, the patient will have a better understanding of its significance and fear it less after a few days when he becomes aware of a distinct improvement. It is desirable to obtain as much mental and physical rest as possible and for this at times it is wise to delay starting the entire course of treatment for a day or two so that the patient may take care of certain matters that would otherwise prey on his mind.

When the patient stays in bed, simple devices should be used to make his bodily position comfortable. The proper number of pillows or a back rest, with supports under the forearms and beneath the knees, will aid considerably and often determine whether a patient will feel relaxed or restless. It will generally be advisable to have him sit in a chair most of the day with the feet hanging down to prevent the shift of fluid from the periphery to the lungs. The use of a commode is often less of a burden than use of a bedpan. During the early days visitors should be restricted, although diversions such as reading the newspapers and listening to the radio may be permitted.

I have become so convinced of the importance of the change in the dynamics of the circulation on assuming the recumbent position, which results in an increase in blood volume and an aggravation of the pulmonary congestion, that I now advise many patients to place wooden blocks under the head posts of their beds. These should be about 8 or 9 inches high and can be used indefinitely. This procedure is not particularly indicated when the main difficulty is hepatic congestion and edema of the legs, or when the element of breathlessness is inconsequential. In some cases, moreover, it is better to have the patient stay in a chair all day. In fact, in recent years I have treated patients with congestive failure more and more by having them stay out of bed, in a chair, most of the day. The bed they use to sleep or rest in has the 9-inch blocks under the head posts so that at no time is the body really horizontal. They then do not need to use the bedpan at all, and many are allowed to take some steps around their room. Patients are happier under this regimen than under the former method of strict bed rest, have fewer complications and, I believe, establish compensation more quickly. (For a more detailed discussion of the "chair" treatment of cardiac patients and its rationale, see page 153.)

DIET

The clinical manifestations of heart failure are, in large measure, the result of congestion due to increase of extracellular fluid brought about by the retention of salt and water by the kidneys. It is now clearly established that the harmful factor is the retention of sodium, not of water. Therapy has therefore become oriented to the restriction of sodium ingestion and the promotion of its loss. In the usual patient with heart failure limiting the intake of sodium to 800 mg. per day (or 2 gm. of sodium chloride) may suffice, in conjunction with other measures already discussed, to eliminate the edema and prevent its re-accumulation. In patients with advanced degrees of decompensation, more rigid restriction of sodium—to a level of 400 mg. daily—may be necessary.

In the average patient being treated in general practice, when it is difficult to achieve sodium restriction, this can be attained by use of a Karell diet, i.e., ingestion of 200 cc. of milk four times a day with as much water as desired. This diet is easily taken and is low in calories, salt, and protein. It often produces a feeling of restfulness and relaxation which improves the general condition, even without any other medication. An inanition diet like this may have beneficial effects because of the same factors that are at work in normal people living on a low caloric intake. It has been found that semistarvation produces a fall in blood pressure, in pulse rate, and in basal metabolic rate. This no doubt may diminish the work of the heart and may thereby improve the circulation when failure is present. The availability of low sodium milk further improves the benefits to be derived from this regimen.

Another method is to permit a general intake of food in small or moderate quantities, but to eliminate the addition of salt in cooking, and its use at the table. Such restriction generally reduces the dietary intake to between 2 and 4 gm. of sodium chloride. This more palatable diet may well be instituted after a preliminary several-day course of the Karell diet. The total caloric intake and the protein content are determined by the degree of weight reduction desired and by the presence of renal impairment. A method of achieving extremely low amounts of dietary sodium has been practiced by Kempner. This diet is limited to rice and fruit, although after some months lean meat may be added. It is thought by most that the merit of the Kempner diet is ascribable to the very low salt content (200 mg. of sodium).

The sodium content of various foods is now well known and physicians should take care that their cardiac patients are not consuming larger quantities of sodium than had been advised. Patients should be cautioned not to use soda bicarbonate or other indigestion preparations that contain sodium. Other drugs, such as sodium salicylate, certain antibiotics, and the like, may also be a source of sodium. Canned foods containing sodium benzoate as a preservative should be excluded. Frozen foods preserved with sodium chloride should be avoided. The palatability of the low sodium diet may be improved for some patients by permitting so-called salt substitutes which do not contain sodium. When this is done, the possibility of excessive potassium intake must be kept in mind, especially in the patient with far-advanced failure.

The appreciation of the role of sodium metabolism in the mechanism of heart failure has been a distinct advance in the treatment of heart disease. It has enabled some patients to weather acute phases of their disability and has considerably prolonged the lives of many who continue to carry on with slight degrees of congestive failure.

SEDATIVES

The care of the patient at night is a most important part of the treatment. If he spends a restless and sleepless night, struggling for air, he will have a poor day following it, but if he obtains a good night's sleep he will more likely show improvement the next day. He is apt to need some sedative at night, and if there has been nocturnal dyspnea it will generally be necessary to use morphine subcutaneously. Although the mildest sedative that is effective should be used, too much time should not be spent experimenting with bromides, phenobarbital, and similar drugs during these early days. The first night a subcutaneous dose of 0.01 to 0.015 gm. of morphine ($\frac{1}{6}$ to $\frac{1}{4}$ grain) is generally advisable. The patient will often tell you that this is the first good night's sleep he has had in weeks. The dose should be diminished so that after three or four days some sedative may be given by mouth and will be found effective. By this time the condition of the circulation would have improved, and comfortable nights might be anticipated by the use of 10 to 15 grains of potassium bromide, $1\frac{1}{2}$ grains of phenobarbital, $1\frac{1}{2}$ grains of Nembutal or 15 grains of chloral hydrate. There is one type of heart failure in which morphine may be harmful and even dangerous. This is advanced cor pulmonale from emphysema, pulmonary fibrosis, or disseminated pulmonary arterial disease. The margin of respiratory function is so slight that further depression by the narcotic may be disastrous. In an occasional patient who, for one reason or another, has not been given digitalis compensation of the circulation will become reestablished, primarily as the result of the proper use of sedatives at night. The care of cardiac patients at night is so important that the intelligence displayed in this regard may be the deciding factor in the recovery of the circulation.

Psychoses are common with severe heart failure, especially in elderly patients and patients who have hypertensive or coronary heart failure. The manifestations are most marked at night and often present a difficult therapeutic problem. The irrational and panicky states in some patients appear to be made worse by narcotics. If the underlying cardiac therapy proves successful and congestive failure improves or disappears, the mental state almost always clears. It may be necessary to try omitting all sedation for a while or to discontinue morphine and give large doses of paraldehyde or chloral to obtain some rest. One must be ready to change from one course of treatment to another with the hope that the heart itself will eventually improve sufficiently that no sedation will be necessary. In some of these cases I am inclined to give intramuscular injections of vitamin B complex daily on the suspicion that avitaminosis, which is not rare in patients with severe cardiac disease, may be playing a role. In other instances getting the patient out of bed and placing him in a chair has seemed to clear the mental state.

CARE OF BOWELS

Vigorous catharsis was formerly employed as a means of ridding a patient of edema. This practice, fortunately, has been discarded to a large extent. I have rarely seen any good come of it. In fact, during the first days of the treatment outlined here, while a patient is receiving very little solid food, it does not matter if there is no bowel movement for two or three days, provided there is no abdominal distention or discomfort. Thereafter a bowel movement every day or two, either occurring naturally or as a result of a mild cathartic or enema, is all that is necessary. Purgation is too exhausting and alters the edematous state too little to warrant its use.

DIGITALIS

Digitalis is the most important drug in the treatment of congestive heart failure. Although it was first introduced into medical practice nearly 175 years ago and its action has been studied in human beings and in animals by a good many students, the intricacies of its effects have not altogether been disentangled. Its indications and limitations have also been matters of heated controversies. Despite this, our knowledge concerning its proper use is gradually becoming more firmly established and greater accuracy now exists concerning what may or may not be expected from it. Not so long ago it was taught that digitalis was contraindicated in aortic valvular disease, in febrile conditions, and in hypertension. As to the latter, it was feared that the blood pressure would be further elevated by digitalis. That fear no longer exists. In fact, when hypertension is present with cardiac failure the blood pressure generally falls during digitalis administration if the congestion disappears, and when it does not fall the outlook is not so favorable. The view that prevails among most authorities is that digitalis is of use in any condition associated with congestive heart failure. In acute coronary thrombosis there is some doubt as to its possible beneficial or harmful effects. Its use is certainly indicated in patients with dyspnea and with peripheral pitting edema of cardiac origin, no matter what the circumstances may be. There still is some dispute whether it acts beneficially in the presence of a regular heart beat. Many of the English clinicians were of the opinion, and some still are, that its use is limited to auricular fibrillation. In America it is generally accepted that, although the most dramatic responses are seen when auricular fibrillation is present, it has a decidedly beneficial effect even when the rhythm of the heart is regular.

A more detailed discussion of the action of digitalis was taken up at the beginning of this chapter.

In using digitalis at the present time the physician is confronted with a great many different names and types of preparations. Over forty years ago pharmacologic studies showed that many of the preparations that were customarily used were below standard potency. In fact, some were found to be almost inert. The present situation is quite different. Now they are practically all satisfactory and carefully standardized by the manufacturer. The physician should choose a preparation that is not expensive for it may need to be used for a long time. He should not be misled into believing a special pill or a tincture will not produce nausea. They all can if they are active. Liquid preparations for oral use have largely been discarded. The currently accepted practice is to use pills in one form or another. The old fashioned digitalis leaf containing 0.1 gm. (1 cat unit) is still a satisfactory preparation. The purified glycosides have now gained wide usage. The advantages of these preparations are the constancy of the active principle which is determined by weight and the fact that they are thought to be nearly completely absorbed in the gastrointestinal tract. The preparations of this type are Digitoxin, Digoxin (Lanoxin), Cedilanid (lanatoside C) and acetyl digitoxin.

Opinions still prevail that certain digitalis preparations will be beneficial when others are not. Careful studies, however, have shown that the margin of safety, i.e., the difference between the therapeutic and toxic or lethal dose, is essentially the same for preparations like digitalis, digitoxin, lanatoside C, strophanthin, or ouabain when given intravenously. Confusion has resulted because absorption of these preparations varies considerably when they are given orally. Ouabain, a pure crystalline glucoside obtained from *Strophanthus gratus*, is absorbed very poorly from the gastrointestinal tract but is suitable for intravenous use (0.25 mg. once or twice the first day and once daily thereafter). Strophanthin, a purified mixture of glycosides derived from *Strophanthus kombé*, is similar in its action to ouabain although the dose is about twice as great. Similarly, lanatoside C (*Digitalis lanata*) is useful for parenteral use, the full digitalizing dose intravenously being 1.5 to 2.0 mg. The oral dose, however, is much greater. Six to 8 mg. given in divided doses during two to three days will be adequate, and the daily maintenance dose is about 1.0 mg. (2 tablets of 0.5 mg.). On the other hand, a preparation like digitoxin (a pure active principle of *Digitalis purpurea*) is completely and readily absorbed by the gastrointestinal tract so that the digitalizing dose is practically the same, orally or intravenously, i.e., 1.20 mg. It is of some interest that this dose is only 3 cat units and is equal in potency to 15 cat units of the tincture or the whole leaf when given orally. The reason for this discrepancy is that it is all absorbed, whereas about four fifths of the ordinary digitalis given by mouth is nonabsorbable. When digitoxin is used the full therapeutic dose of 1.20

mg. may be given orally in one dose, and treatment continued with a daily maintenance dose of 0.1 to 0.2 mg.

During the past ten years or so digitoxin has become increasingly popular in this country. It has been used extensively in France for many years. It has the advantage that it is completely and readily absorbed when given orally and that being a pure chemical it does not need to be standardized biologically. Its potency is therefore constant. It also produces much less nausea when therapeutic doses are administered, for the dosage by weight is about one thousandth of that required when digitalis leaves are employed. There is one disadvantage, however. Because early nausea is less likely to occur one may more readily exceed the therapeutic dose and inadvertently produce toxic results. Another preparation that is being used is Digoxin, a pure crystalline substance derived from *Digitalis lanata*. The methods of administration and the mode of action are somewhat like those of digitoxin. The dose, however, is slightly greater, i.e., 1 to 1.5 mg. for a single rapid oral effect and 0.25 to 0.75 mg. as the daily maintenance dose. It is rapidly absorbed and rapidly eliminated. This drug can also be used intravenously in the above doses.

Let us now return to the treatment of the patient mentioned above and let us assume that he had not received any digitalis before. The average adult will require about 2 gm. or 30 grains of digitalis or 20 cc. of tincture of digitalis given over several days. (The dose required in infants and children is apt to be one and one-half to twice as great in proportion to weight as in an adult.) The exact amount will vary, some patients requiring less and some more. This dose can be given quite rapidly, even within twenty-four hours, but it is very rarely advisable to do so for it may turn out that only 1.5 gm. or less was necessary and the remainder of the dose would have proved excessive and would produce toxic manifestations. When the situation is very urgent and an effect is to be produced in hours rather than in days, the intramuscular or intravenous route should be used instead of the oral. There is no single method of dosage that needs to be followed. Much will depend on the condition of the patient and the frequency with which he will be observed by the physician. Generally it is satisfactory to give one fourth of the total dose or 0.5 gm. the first day and a similar amount the second day. One pill (0.1 gm. each) five times a day will accomplish this. On the third day the dose may need to be diminished. If the apex rate, which was 130, has fallen to 100 it may be planned to give 0.1 gm. three times on this day and after two or three days this may be cut down to one pill a day. The hope is to lower the apex rate to 60 or 70 if possible, without producing any ill effects. If this patient is seen only once a day this is best done in the morning, for then one can witness all the good or harm that the previous dosage has produced and one can outline the amount to be taken during the following twelve hours. Finally, the so-called "maintenance dose" of 0.1 gm. daily is kept up. This is approximately the amount that is utilized or eliminated daily.

The course outlined in the preceding paragraph needs to be modified under certain circumstances. If the patient had previously received digitalis it is better to start with smaller amounts. One pill three times a day may then be sufficient. On the other hand, he may be complaining of nausea and vomiting and doubt arises whether he has already received too much digitalis. More often than not these symptoms are due to circulatory failure, generally accompanied by hepatic engorgement, and demand more rather than less digitalis. If auricular fibrillation is present and the heart rate is still rapid, one can feel quite certain that more digitalis is needed. This same conclusion cannot be drawn if the rhythm is regular, for the rate then may remain rapid even after full doses of digitalis are administered. Occasionally the electrocardiograms may be helpful in deciding the question although they are rarely necessary. When nausea and vomiting are present and further digitalis is to be given the tincture can be used rectally. Three or 4 cc. (diluted in 50 to 100 cc. of water) may then be given daily. I have used this method with success and the vomiting has ceased even in patients who were convinced that it was produced by the previous digitalis that had been taken. The dosage for rectal administration is the same as that for oral.

There are rare instances in which it is difficult or even impossible to decide whether a patient is over- or under-digitalized. Even electrocardiograms may not dispel this doubt. The problem becomes critical when an acute cardiac emergency develops, such as the condition precipitated by an attack of rapid heart action. Such spells, in fact, may be due to paroxysmal auricular tachycardia with block which is easily confused with auricular flutter or fibrillation. Frequent extrasystoles with a rapid ventricular rate may be due to excessive digitalis or to myocardial failure itself. The question may then arise, whether to give more digitalis rapidly or to use measures such as administration of potassium or Pronestyl to counteract the toxic effect of digitalis. For this purpose Lown and his co-workers have devised an acetylstrophanthidin test. A dose of 0.15 mg. of this is injected intravenously while continuous electrocardiographic tracings are being recorded. In five to ten minutes a similar quantity is injected. The effect is carefully observed in the electrocardiograms. If the heart slows or the premature beats vanish the patient needed more digitalis. If the condition grows worse the reverse is true and potassium chloride in doses of 3.0 or more (or Pronestyl 0.5 to 1.0 gm. intravenously) might be very helpful. If only 0.3 mg. of acetylstrophanthidin can be administered before toxic effects appear the patient is adequately or excessively digitalized. If therapeutic action follows after either 0.6 or 1.2 mg. of acetylstrophanthidin the patient requires either partial or full doses of digitalis. The effect of acetylstrophanthidin appears within a few minutes and vanishes in about one-half hour. In that way a rapid estimate can be made of the digitalis requirements of the patient. The difficulty is that the procedure carries some risk. Sudden fatalities have occurred. At present it can only be carried out by those very familiar with the details of the test and especially with the electrocardiographic evidence of the arrhythmias involved and the toxic manifestations of digitalis. Properly performed this test has occasionally proved life saving in very critical emergencies when there was no other way to determine whether a patient needed further large doses of digitalis or was already toxic from its overdosage.

When great speed of action is required some form of digitalis should be used intramuscularly or intravenously. Such preparations are put up in ampules and generally contain 0.1 gm. for each 1 or 2 cc. Whereas most physicians are familiar with the proper oral dosage, the situation is quite different with regard to hypodermic use of the drug. In fact the exact dose with the latter method is not so well known. If 2 gm. is a proper digitalizing dose for a patient when given orally, it certainly would be excessive if it were all given intramuscularly or intravenously in one injection. On the other hand, one ampule containing 0.1 gm. is often given hypodermically, especially by surgeons, hoping to give the patient the benefit of digitalis. It is obvious that this dose is practically valueless. The proper amount to obtain an appreciable therapeutic effect is between 0.5 and 1 gm., given either intramuscularly or intravenously. An effect may be expected with the former route in one to two hours and with the latter in fifteen to thirty minutes. The same dangers exist, however, when digitalis is given intravenously as when strophanthin or ouabain is used, for the margin of safety between the minimal toxic and minimal lethal dose is the same for all these preparations. It is of utmost importance that if the patient has recently been taking any appreciable amounts of digitalis, intravenous preparations should be given with great caution and in smaller doses.

The following experience illustrates the occasional instance when rapid digitalization is imperative. Some years ago I was called to see a woman about 40 years of age who was in a moribund state. She had mitral stenosis with a regular rhythm, and had been ambulatory and getting along very well. She had not been taking digitalis. At 9 p.m. that day she was suddenly stricken with palpitation and dyspnea and in a short time acute pulmonary edema developed. When I saw her at 11 p.m. she was unconscious. There were marked cyanosis and stertorous breathing, and the lungs were full of moist rales. The pulse was imperceptible, but the heart rate as counted at the apex was about 190 and the rhythm was absolutely irregular. She had already received strychnine, camphor, and caffeine hypodermically. This was exactly the condition in which digitalis was indicated, but even minutes were precious. I therefore gave her 8 cc. (0.8 gm.) of digitalis intravenously and in about twenty minutes the heart rate fell to 100 although the rhythm remained irregular. The effect was most dramatic; the breathing quieted down, and most of the rales disappeared. A short time later the patient returned to her customary duties and presented the picture of a patient with well-compensated rheumatic mitral stenosis and auricular fibrillation. A similar dramatic result could now be obtained by giving about 1.2 mg. of Cedilanid or 1.0 mg. of Digoxin intravenously.

It is always important to watch for the indications to diminish or to omit digitalis. The first obvious reason for cutting down the dose is if the desired therapeutic effect is produced. In the case of the bank teller (first discussed on page 363), if the heart rate slowed to 70, the dyspnea and edema disappeared, and the patient was subjectively improved, the dose should be reduced to about 0.1 gm. a day. One therefore does not need to push the dosage to obtain toxic effects if the therapeutic result is satisfactory. The second reason for omitting the drug is detection of evidence of intoxication. This may be either subjective or objective. It is curious how patients differ in their reactions to digitalis. Some will quickly develop the subjective symptoms without the customary objective signs of intoxication, and others do just the reverse. Still others on very large doses develop neither.

The most common early evidence of digitalis intoxication is loss of appetite, nausea, and vomiting. There is often a general mean and sickly feeling accompanying the desire to vomit. When this occurs there is no treatment except omission of the drug. However, Thorazine might be tried. Other symptoms that are less common are diarrhea, yellow vision, dizziness, headache, confusion, and even disorientation. The objective evidence of intoxication concerns the findings in the heart. Among these are undue slowing of the rate of the heart, i.e., to less than 50, the development of extrasystoles not previously present, especially in the form of coupled beats, paroxysmal auricular tachycardia with block, and heart block. The most common finding is digitalis coupling. Here every second beat is a ventricular extrasystole. This can easily be recognized if the rhythm of the heart was regular at the start, but can also be detected at the bedside if auricular fibrillation is present. Any of three forms of heart block may result, first degree (delayed conduction time), second degree (partial block), or complete block. The first cannot readily be detected without an electrocardiogram, but the second is easily recognized on auscultation by noting an occasional dropped beat. However, complete heart block brought on by digitalis offers real diagnostic difficulties. The ventricular rate of complete heart block produced by digitalis is not around 30, as it is in Adams-Stokes disease. It is generally 60 or more and may be over 80 and 100. This mechanism is really an idioventricular rhythm in which the pacemaker for the ventricles is in the upper part of the auriculoventricular junctional tissue. This regular rate will also continue to accelerate on increasing doses of digitalis. In animal experiments this is one of the mechanisms by which death from digitalis intoxication occurs, although the more common mechanism is ventricular fibrillation. As a practical matter, the first two types of heart block from digitalis do no harm and, in so far as slowing of the ventricle results, may be beneficial. They serve merely as a signal that further dosage must be given cautiously. Complete block, although rare, is an indication that the drug should be omitted or the dose should be diminished considerably. Inasmuch as it may be difficult to detect this clinically it is well to omit digitalis if the heart, which was previously grossly irregular, becomes regular on digitalis, until the exact mechanism of the heart beat is known. In such a case, either regularization may be due to a resumption of the normal rhythm of the heart or the ventricles may be beating regularly while the auricles are still fibrillating. In the first instance nothing would be lost by omitting digitalis for a few days; in the latter harm might result by continuing its use. Electrocardiograms might be necessary to aid in making some of these unusual decisions. Digitalis also produces changes in the T wave of the electrocardiograms (Chap. 21, Fig. 181), which do not indicate intoxication but which occasionally may help in estimating the amount of the drug that a patient has received.

Apart from digitalis or its allied drugs, like Urginin, there is little else in the form of medication which acts directly on the heart that one can use in the treatment of congestive failure. Strychnine, camphor, and caffeine had a considerable vogue in the past, but there is very little satisfactory evidence to support their use, except that caffeine may serve at times as a respiratory stimulus. Adrenalin and ephedrine are useful in those cases in which the dyspnea or cough is in part due to an asthmatic or emphysematous state. Potassium chloride or phosphate (1.0 to 2.0 gm. three times daily) may be helpful for certain periods of time, to correct a possible deficiency of potassium in the myocardium in cases of heart failure or to counteract any toxic action of digitalis. I recall an elderly man who had nocturnal dyspnea from left ventricular failure. He had been taking 0.1 gm. of digitalis daily but showed a constant digitalis bigeminy. By adding potassium chloride 1.0 gm. four times daily it was possible to give him digitalis 0.1 gm. three times daily for about one week, with striking improvement in his clinical state. Incidentally the ventricular extrasystoles disappeared during this course of treatment. Although many other drugs are often supposed to have beneficial effects on the heart, they prove to be hardly worth the trial.

DIURETICS

Next in importance to digitalis in the treatment of patients with congestive failure is the group of diuretic drugs. Diuretics are best given after complete digitalization has been accomplished, if there still remains evidence of dyspnea or peripheral edema. It must be remembered that patients may have considerable latent edema in the body after all obvious pitting has disappeared. Furthermore, when the patient has been in bed for some time, it is well to look for subcutaneous edema in the sacral region, for fluid may accumulate there when the ankles are entirely free of edema.

The success of the soluble organic mercurials has caused them to monopolize the field of diuretic agents and to replace the many medications which were formerly in vogue, such as theophylline (Theocin), theobromine sodium salicylate (Diuretin), and urea. The use of the mercury diuretics in the treatment of congestive heart failure has been an important factor in the prolongation of life of chronic cardiacs. The preparations in current usage are Mercuhydrin, Thiomerin, Salyrgan and Mercupurin. Each cubic centimeter of these preparations contains about 40 mg. of organic mercury. In addition, except for Thiomerin, they also contain about 50 mg. of theophylline which decreases local irritation, facilitates absorption, and may augment diuretic action. The diuretic potency of these drugs resides in the mercury ion which is believed to interfere with the reabsorption of salt by the distal tubule of the kidney.

The preferred method of administering the mercury diuretics is by intramuscular injection deep in the gluteal region. This site is generally preferable to the deltoid region. Thiomerin has the slight advantage that it may be given subcutaneously, but it is then likely to evoke local reactions. The patient or a member of the family can often be taught to give the injection and thereby obviate the need of so many calls on the part of the physician. Although the intramuscular route is generally the safest, there are times when it may be given intravenously. This is true when there is massive edema or extensive local induration from previous injections, or when there has been no response, possibly due to impaired local absorption. When it is given intravenously, great care must be exercised that no infiltration into the subcutaneous tissues occurs. If even a small amount of drug leaks out of the vein, there is considerable pain and an ugly and stubborn ulcer may occasionally develop and last for many weeks. There is less risk of harmful effects if the diuretic is diluted with 10 cc. of sterile saline when the intravenous route is used. Within a few minutes after the intravenous injection of a mercurial diuretic, various types of cardiac arrhythmia may appear, particularly extrasystoles. These are transient and harmless. On very rare occasions sudden fatalities have occurred, mainly in cases of coronary artery disease.

One would very much welcome a mercury preparation that would serve as an effective diuretic when given orally. There are some available, such as Neohydrin, which are useful in occasional cases. Such tablets contain 10 to 20 mg. of mercury and about 40 mg. of theophylline. The dose is one to three tablets daily. When three tablets are given daily for many weeks or months, renal impairment, gastrointestinal upset, or other untoward effects may at times result. It is safer to advise one or two tablets a day for a long period of time. Mercurials have been used in the form of rectal suppositories, but they too frequently produce local irritation which makes this method impracticable.

The dose of intramuscular mercury will vary from 0.5 to 2.0 cc., and as often happens it may need to be repeated every few days to every few weeks for a long time. Occasionally it may be beneficial to give mercury every day for several days. When the response wanes it may be necessary gradually to increase both the dose and the frequency of administration. I have seen a patient who had about 250 injections at weekly intervals over a course of five years, always obtaining a most satisfactory diuresis of 5000 to 8000 cc. in twenty-four hours. During this time the individual dose was gradually increased from 1 cc. to 4 cc. At no time was there any evidence of renal damage, despite the enormous amounts of mercury that were used.

In some cases the effect of diuretics may be enhanced by the preliminary administration of acidifying salts, such as ammonium chloride. The dose is 1 to 2 gm. (15 to 30 grains) four times a day for two or three days, followed by injection of 1 to 2 cc. of mercurial diuretic. This may be repeated as indicated, often at weekly intervals. In fact, occasionally a diuresis may be produced as a result of ammonium chloride alone. These large doses of ammonium chloride are rather disagreeable, but the annoying taste may be minimized if enteric-coated tablets are used. It should never be given continuously. Prolonged administration of ammonium chloride may be associated with certain harmful effects, occasionally resulting in fatalities. Serious potassium deficits, ammonium intoxication, and hyperchloremic acidosis are some of the harmful sequelae.

Occasionally, stupor and rapid deterioration in a cardiac patient may be the result of hyperchloremic acidosis secondary to ammonium chloride poisoning. Since acidosis may follow doses of four to six grams daily, coma of this etiology should be suspected in all obscure circumstances. The finding of a plasma carbon dioxide content of less than 12–14 milliequivalents per liter in a patient who is known not to have had diabetes or significant renal disease points strongly to hyperchloremic acidosis. Such patients are likely to have a markedly elevated serum chloride level. A high blood urea nitrogen can also be present, but need not indicate a serious state of renal disease, as the chemical abnormalities may be mostly if not entirely reversible. Treatment consists of administration of large amounts of isotonic sodium lactate or bicarbonate intravenously (usually 1000–3000 cc. in the first 24 hours will be necessary). Should any evidence of pulmonary edema appear the customary measures to counteract this complication need to be employed.

Apart from the above dangers, the very purpose of increasing diuretic responsiveness to mercury is defeated when ammonium chloride is continuously ingested. Within 48 hours after such a chloride load renal compensation ensues with tubular production of ammonium ion.

Aminophylline is a useful adjunct in producing or increasing the diuretic response when the mercurials alone are ineffective. The aminophylline is given intravenously in a dose of 0.5 gm., preferably one to two hours after the intramuscular injection of mercury. It may also be given in the form of a rectal suppository or a solution administered rectally one to three times during the day the patient receives mercury. The object of this is to increase glomerular filtration. When the glomerular filtration rate is markedly reduced, as in advanced cardiac decompensation, the ionic load presented to the renal tubule is much less than the capacity for reabsorption. In such circumstances the tubules are still able to reabsorb the small amount of sodium even after mercurial effects have been produced. It is well to have the patient remain recumbent in bed during the day when mercury is injected intramuscularly, to enhance the diuretic effect.

Notwithstanding the beneficial effects of mercurials, it is well to be aware of the occasional untoward features of mercury administration. Allergic reactions are uncommon, and include chilliness, fever, vomiting, and cutaneous eruptions. Changing to a different mercurial preparation may circumvent this difficulty. Muscle cramps in the legs are quite common, especially after a brisk diuresis. The cause of this is still puzzling. The measures that have been used to combat this include administration of quinine, calcium salts, or potassium salts, but most effective is the reduction of the dose of mercury. Prostration, weakness, fall in blood pressure, hemoconcentration, and thrombosis at times develop. It is reasonable to encourage a liberal intake of fluid during the day of an expected diuresis, especially in the hot weather. Mercury-induced diuresis may provoke digitalis intoxication. Formerly this was thought to be due to the mobilization of digitalis-laden edema fluid which on recirculating produced additional digitalis effect on the heart. The postmercurial redigitalization is now thought to be the result of the potassium loss occurring during the diuresis. Such evidence of digitalis intoxication may be prevented by the judicious prophylactic use of potassium salts.

Ordinarily 75 to 85 per cent of the organic mercury is excreted in 24 hours if it induces a diuresis. When no diuretic effect occurs and repeated doses are given, considerable mercury may be retained in the body. This *can* result in mercurialism with stomatitis, excessive salivation, metallic taste in the mouth, gastrointestinal cramps and diarrhea, and renal impairment with oliguria, hematuria, and azotemia. These complications are more likely to occur from the prolonged oral rather than parenteral administration. The following experience illustrates this type of problem. The patient became unresponsive to mercurial diuretics. It was suspected that he was possibly suffering from mercury poisoning and had mercury retention in the body. He had developed a very distressing dermatitis exfoliativa of unknown origin. Twelve days after the last injection, determination of mercury in the urine showed that he still was excreting considerable quantities. It was therefore decided that he be given a three-day course of BAL (British anti-Lewisite) treatment. After this, when the urinary mercury had decreased markedly, he again obtained a satisfactory diuresis from the same injection of mercury that previously had been ineffective. Incidentally, the dermatitis remained unaltered by this treatment. The dose of BAL was 1.2 cc. three times daily (0.025 cc. per kilogram of body weight).

Probably the most important complication of the use of mercurial diuretics is the possible derangement of the electrolytes in the body.

The ideal drug for relieving the body of sodium and water would be one that blocks their renal tubular reabsorption, promotes a balanced chloride and bicarbonate diuresis without incurring electrolyte derangements, can be taken orally, is palatable, and does not provoke gastrointestinal upsets or other untoward effects. Such a drug will no doubt become available in the foreseeable future. Various oral preparations are currently in use. None are as effective as the mercurial injections. In addition to the oral mercurials, three other categories of drugs are now available: the carbonic anhydrase inhibitors, the uracil preparations, and the cation exchange resins.

Among the carbonic anhydrase inhibitors Diamox has been found to be the most effective. The normal reabsorption of sodium is due to an exchange of hydrogen ion in the tubular cell for sodium in the tubular urine. This is the mechanism for conservation of the fixed base in the body and occurs through the reabsorption of filtered bicarbonate, the acidification of urinary buffer salts, and the excretion of fixed anion with ammonium ion instead of sodium. The source for the hydrogen ion in the renal tubular cell is carbonic acid, which is formed from CO_2 and water. The rapid and adequate formation of carbonic acid is made possible by the presence of the enzyme carbonic anhydrase in the renal cortex. Inhibition of carbonic anhydrase activity by Diamox therefore interferes with the normal hydrogen-sodium exchange mechanism and promotes excretion of sodium from the body.

Like any of the oral diuretics Diamox, when effective, will diminish the need for intramuscular mercury injection. When it is of value, favorable effects from Diamox will be observed within two or three days; otherwise the drug should be discontinued. It is more likely to promote diuresis in patients with mild decompensation; it has been noted to be particularly helpful in patients with chronic cor pulmonale when the blood CO_2 is elevated. However, it is worth a trial in any stubborn case of congestive failure. It has been advised that Diamox in conjunction with large doses of ammonium chloride will induce hyperchloremic acidosis and restore responsiveness to mercury. The usual dose of Diamox is 0.25 to 0.5 gm. once daily or every other day. Untoward effects are not uncommon or very serious. They consist of paresthesias, drowsiness, headache, gastrointestinal upsets, and electrolyte derangements.

Experience with the uracil preparations, namely Mictine and Rolicton, has been too limited to permit final judgment as to their value as diuretics. It would appear that they are effective to a certain extent, and that they do not give rise to serious side-effects. The dose for Mictine is 2 to 4 tablets daily (0.4 to 0.8 gm.) for three consecutive days each week with meals. Gastrointestinal upsets are common, but are less troublesome with Rolicton. The dose of the latter is 1 tablet (0.4 gm.) three to four times daily.

Another method of dealing with the sodium problem is to eliminate it from the gastrointestinal tract where sodium is present in great abundance. For this purpose the cation exchange resins may be employed, as was initially suggested by Dock. These resins are synthetic insoluble macromolecular compounds that contain numerous basic or acidic groupings which undergo ionization when placed in solution and exchange hydrogen ion for other cations present in aqueous medium. When given

orally they liberate hydrogen and bind sodium from the intestinal contents. Since they are not absorbed the bound sodium is eliminated in the
feces. The one I have used is Carbo-resin. Each gram is capable of ab-
stracting about 1 milliequivalent (23 milligrams) of intestinal sodium if
the patient is ingesting 1.5 grams of sodium in the diet. The dose of
Carbo-resin is 15 grams three times daily. The total value of the resins
has not been great because of the difficulties encountered in their use.
They may produce gastrointestinal symptoms, particularly abdominal
distress and constipation. They can result in dangerous losses of other
cations, such as potassium and calcium.

When a cardiac patient in congestive failure becomes refractory to
the above methods of therapy and particularly when he no longer obtains a diuretic response from mercury injection, it is imperative to
review the electrolyte situation. The most common derangement is an
abnormally low blood chloride level. When the chloride concentration
is reduced, the blood CO_2 rises and the urea nitrogen may increase. At
this point mercury injections may be ineffective and make the condition
worse. When mercurial unresponsiveness develops the chloride concentration ranges usually from 80 to 90 milliequivalents per liter. Occasionally the mercurials are without effect when the chloride level is only
slightly decreased. I have observed mercurial fastness when the chloride
was only 98 milliequivalents, only to obtain a sizable diuresis when the
concentration was raised just above 100. When hypochloremia is present,
mercury should be discontinued and ammonium chloride should be administered orally. Rarely it may be necessary to give ammonium chloride
intravenously to restore normal electrolyte balance. It may be given intravenously as a 2 per cent solution to be injected not faster than 100
cc. per hour. As much as 10 grams may be required before the refractoriness to mercury is abolished. The chloride may be given as hydro-
chloric acid; 20 cc. of a 10 per cent solution is diluted to a volume of
1000 cc. and taken with a straw. This provides about 50 milliequivalents
of chloride.

The development of unresponsiveness to mercury may be due not
only to a low serum chloride but also to a low serum sodium concentration. Reduction in serum sodium may occur after a low sodium diet
and mercurial therapy. But it must be realized that it may develop
with little or no treatment. When a patient who has been responding to
diuretics develops weakness, lassitude, and drowsiness, and the blood
chemistry reveals azotemia, hypochloremia, acidosis, and a low sodium,
he may be suffering from depletion hyponatremia, the result of an intensive diuretic program. Intravenous administration of hypertonic
saline solution may abolish the symptoms and correct the electrolyte
derangement. There is another type of hyponatremic syndrome encountered in patients with decompensation which develops gradually and is
generally devoid of any specific symptomatology. The lowered sodium
concentration is believed to be due to dilution and to represent excessive
antidiuretic hormone activity and abnormalities in the volume-regulating

centers in response to severe cardiac failure. The urgent need is not alteration in the electrolyte concentration, but improvement in myocardial function. Dilution hyponatremia occurs without the bodily loss of sodium and is a manifestation of a critical state of decompensation. Attempts to raise the serum sodium level only further compromise the precarious state of compensation. Occasionally it is hard to determine whether hyponatremia is the result of depletion or of dilution. In such cases the slow administration of 5 per cent saline in divided doses of 50 cc. and elevation of the serum sodium level by 5 to 10 milliequivalents may significantly improve the depleted patient and not prove unduly harmful to those with dilution hyponatremia. Fluid should be sharply restricted on the day when the hypertonic saline is administered.

One specific difficulty arising from diuretic therapy in congestive heart failure and requiring additional discussion is disturbance in potassium metabolism. During the chronic progressive stages of congestive heart failure there is often a slow loss of body potassium. Normally deficits are readily replaced by the potassium in the diet. However, when the food intake is curtailed, either because of lack of appetite or by the dietary restrictions outlined by the physician, deficits of potassium may then be incurred. When, in addition, an active diuretic program is carried out, further loss of potassium occurs, resulting in substantial deficits. The patient maintained on rigid salt restriction is the most likely candidate for such depletion. When sodium is in short supply, the distal tubule of the kidney exchanges potassium and hydrogen for the filtered sodium, thereby conserving this cation. The serum level of potassium often does not reflect bodily deficits. In the majority of such cases the serum potassium concentration is normal, although the cells are depleted. The metabolism of potassium has special pertinence to the problem of digitalis administration. In the presence of potassium deficit the myocardium is more sensitive to the toxic properties of digitalis. Even small maintenance doses of digitalis may precipitate serious arrhythmia after potassium has been lost from the body.

Potassium replacement is not a simple matter. The patient with advanced congestive heart failure in whom this problem arises handles potassium poorly; he neither stores it well nor excretes it well. He therefore is prone to serious potassium intoxication when additional amounts are given. Nevertheless, it is well to administer 3.0 to 5.0 gm. of potassium chloride the day before and the day of mercury therapy, when there is some suspicion of potassium deficit. Electrocardiograms are helpful in appraising the effect of potassium and may be particularly valuable in detecting the early evidence of potassium intoxication.

In general the various diuretics have added considerably to the treatment of patients with congestive heart failure. When properly administered it may be expected that beneficial effects will result if the function of the kidneys is good. At times it is no simple matter to anticipate without elaborate functional tests whether the kidney function is adequate or not. Albumin and casts in the urine may result from passive congestion of otherwise fairly healthy kidneys, as well as from true nephritis. In general practice, when it is not easy to perform chemical analysis of the blood, the absence of any anemia and the presence of a high specific gravity of the urine points to a satisfactory functional state of the kidneys even when albumin and casts are present. Only occasionally will it be necessary to determine the blood urea nitrogen or nonprotein nitrogen, or to perform the phthalein test or a concentration test to ascertain more accurately the state of the kidneys. Even when it is found that the kidneys are slightly or moderately impaired, if there is congestive heart failure and edema persists despite digitalis and rest, diuretics may be used. Although the results will not be so beneficial as when the kidneys are normal, such patients may yet do better following the use of mercurial diuretics than without their use.

Cardiac cachexia and inanition are not infrequent results of long-standing chronic heart failure and with this there may be an element of edema, purely as a result of the low protein content of the blood, just as occurs in nephrosis. In fact, on occasions, because of the presence of considerable edema and certain other findings, a patient may be regarded as having heart failure when the edema is entirely due to nephrosis, nephritis, hypoproteinemia, or some deficiency disease. It is now well known that a fall in the total protein content of the blood serum may produce edema. This is particularly true if the albumin content is markedly diminished, resulting in a reversal in the albumin-globulin ratio. Such changes diminish the osmotic pressure in the blood and permit fluid to move from the blood into the tissue spaces. Such hypoproteinemia may result from prolonged dietary deficiency, especially when the protein intake is restricted, from loss of albumin in urine and also from liver disease. These factors not infrequently are involved in patients with chronic cardiac disease. The diets of these patients are often unwisely restricted by physicians, or the patients do not eat because of persistent anorexia, and the liver is frequently in an unhealthy state from passive congestion. The result is that some cardiac patients have edema not only because of decompensation but because of hypoproteinemia. Examination of the blood must be made in all cases of stubborn edema to establish the correct diagnosis. In some cases the edema will not be controlled until special efforts, such as the institution of a high protein diet or infusions of blood or, preferably, plasma, are made. When intravenous injections are difficult or impossible, infusions of blood or albumin may be given intrasternally, an 18-gauge needle being used and the injection being given in the midline.

Occasionally one observes patients in whom adequate response is obtained from the use of mercurial diuretics but who steadily lose ground. As they become edema-free their general condition grows worse. Some seem to grow apathetic, drowsy, and weak. Although this complication has not been thoroughly studied it may be that when it occurs there is an increase in the renal insufficiency and dehydration of the tissues. If this is so, some of the harmful effects might be obviated by increasing the amount of fluid in the diet. When the kidneys are impaired in function and unable to concentrate well it requires a larger volume of fluid intake and of urine output to insure the necessary elimination of waste products. In fact, the prevailing custom of marked restriction in the intake of fluids for patients with congestive heart failure needs some revision because of this.

Fever is common with congestive failure and is an added burden on the heart. Whenever this might be due to an infection responsive to specific therapy, such as penicillin or sulfonamides, appropriate measures must be carried out. Occasionally it will be advisable to use a nonspecific antipyretic, such as aminopyrine (0.2 to 0.3 gm.), for short periods of time, to diminish the work of the heart.

Since Dicumarol has come to be used so generally in thrombophlebitis and acute coronary thrombosis, it also has been given to groups of patients with congestive heart failure. Studies, using the alternate case method of control, have shown that those receiving Dicumarol during their hospital stay had a much lower mortality. This was due to a marked decrease in thrombo-embolic phenomena in those receiving anticoagulant therapy. Therefore, whenever feasible it would be advisable to give Dicumarol while treating patients for congestive heart failure. Similarly it has been my custom to apply elastic stockings to the lower legs in cardiacs under active treatment, to help diminish the likelihood of thrombophlebitis of the legs.

MECHANICAL METHODS OF TREATMENT

The importance of posture in the care of some cardiac patients has already been discussed. Often patients who are put to bed lose their peripheral edema; pitting of the ankles may disappear but congestion of the lungs gets worse. Even fatal pulmonary edema may result. Placing such patients in a chair with the feet down may reverse this process or may have prevented it if employed from the start. Furthermore, nine-inch blocks under the head posts of the bed can minimize the deleterious effects of the recumbent posture.

In cases of acute pulmonary congestion in which circumstances might indicate the need of phlebotomy, tourniquets may be applied to the four extremities. Pressure should be about 40 to 50 mm. of mercury, or enough to prevent return flow of venous blood and yet to permit free forward arterial flow. This traps the blood in the periphery and pressure may be maintained for a half hour to several hours using the following method. Tourniquets are applied on three of the four extremities and every fifteen minutes one is released and applied on the limb that had been free. In this way each extremity has a rest period every forty-five minutes.

Alcohol vapor inhalations have also been recommended for acute pulmonary edema by Luisada. Oxygen is bubbled through 70 per cent alcohol instead of water for this purpose.

Edematous fluid in the limbs can at times be removed by mechanical means. Southey-Leech tubes may be inserted subcutaneously under aseptic precautions into the swollen feet or hands. In this way several hundred cubic centimeters or more of fluid may be lost daily and the edema thereby diminished. I once saw a patient who lost over 15 liters of fluid in three days by this method, and another who lost 20 liters in 52 hours. Some of these patients became responsive to mercury after drainage by the use of Southey-Leech tubes, with further improvement, whereas they had been refractory to mercury before. Penicillin should be given during this treatment to prevent local infection.

There remain several other procedures that are helpful in the treatment of patients with congestive heart failure. It is not uncommon to forget that a diuresis may occur and the urine remain in the bladder. This is particularly to be watched for in elderly male patients. I recall the humiliation I experienced in finding 1500 cc. of urine in the bladder when the postmortem examination was performed in a patient I had treated for heart failure. The retention of urine in the bladder results primarily from prostatic obstruction. Although patient and physician may have been aware of this prostatic difficulty before, at times the first significant evidence of it may occur during the bed treatment for cardiac failure. It is obvious that the temporary remedy for this is catheterization.

A more common complication is hydrothorax. Most patients with advanced heart failure have some free fluid in the pleural cavities. When the amount is small, i.e., 100 to 200 cc., it is not detectable, nor is it of any advantage to remove it mechanically. However, when there is over 500 cc., or especially 1000 cc. or more, considerable respiratory and general relief can be obtained by a thoracentesis. The bases of the lungs, especially on the right, should always be carefully examined in all cases. Dullness or flatness on percussion, diminished breath sounds, and decreased tactile fremitus with or without rales are the findings that help in detecting free fluid at the bases of the lungs. Tapping should be performed if it is expected to obtain more than 500 cc. of fluid. There is no advantage in withdrawing the very last amounts, and the needle should be removed when the fluid begins to come with difficulty or when an uncomfortable cough is produced. It is always best to use a dull needle so that unnecessary scratching or bleeding of the pleurae will not take place.

Abdominal paracentesis should also be employed when there is significant ascites. Here also small amounts of fluid are better left undisturbed. Tapping is indicated if the amount that might be obtained is more than 2000 cc. The removal of smaller amounts does not seem to improve the condition sufficiently to make the procedure worth while. Furthermore, small amounts either in the abdominal or in the pleural cavities can readily disappear in the course of the routine treatment for heart failure, whereas the mechanical removal of larger quantities may expedite recovery. When there is marked ascites, mercurial diuretics may be ineffective until the abdominal fluid is removed by tapping. It would appear that the pressure of the fluid on the renal vessels prevented the mercury from producing its customary effect.

Oxygen therapy may help patients with congestive failure. This is of particular value for brief periods of time during cardiac emergencies when there is severe breathlessness and pulmonary congestion. Use of a positive-pressure oxygen mask may be very beneficial in some cases of acute pulmonary edema. Oxygen therapy is obviously not a procedure that is applicable in most cases of chronic failure which continues for months. However, I observed a middle-aged woman, who had advanced irreversible congestive failure with striking cyanosis, dyspnea, and a very large liver, carry on her work as a school teacher for a few years. Apart from the customary cardiac medication she spent about two hours each day inhaling oxygen through a mask. She was convinced that the oxygen enabled her to carry on.

Finally, a word must be said about phlebotomy. As we all know, bloodletting is an old method of treatment that was in vogue for centuries and used in all sorts of diseases. Much of this practice has been discarded, and I am of the opinion that at present its application in the treatment of congestive heart failure has not been sufficiently utilized. In many of these patients, if not in all, the total volume of blood is increased. The various organs, especially the lungs and the liver, are markedly engorged. The pressure in the venous side of the circulation is increased, as is manifested by prominent distended veins in the neck and an increase in the venous pressure readings taken directly from peripheral veins. There is both experimental and clinical evidence that after a phlebotomy the state of the circulation can be improved in some cases. Venesection in severe hypertensive heart failure has been found to produce a fall in venous pressure and an increase in cardiac output, both favorable effects. Some observations made years ago showed that the removal of 500 cc. of blood from one arm improved the flow of blood in the other arm. I have witnessed a decided decrease in the size of the liver and a prompt disappearance of pain and tenderness in that region directly after the removal of 700 cc. of blood in a patient with mitral stenosis and auricular fibrillation. What is much more striking is the effect of phlebotomy in some moribund patients. The following experience illustrates very graphically some of the results that may occasionally be obtained by this neglected method of treatment. I was once called to see a woman about 73 years of age who had asthmatic bronchitis, hypertension, and myocardial failure. All the customary treatment had been employed, and when I arrived the patient was moribund, unconsciousness having gradually developed that day. In fact, the breathing was such as is witnessed in patients only a few minutes before they die. The chin dropped with each breath, and there were tracheal rattles. There was marked cyanosis and pulmonary edema. The situation was so desperate that I did not even sterilize the needle that was used to puncture the vein. About 600 cc. of blood was removed in twelve minutes, and just as the procedure was completed the patient became conscious. In two weeks she was out of bed and the recovery enabled her to live in comparative comfort for another eighteen months. In a second instance of this sort an elderly man who had been in a coma immediately regained consciousness after a phlebotomy of 550 cc. of blood. Here the children made the simple request that they wished to speak to their father once more. He remained mentally clear that day, then relapsed into a coma and died the following day. In these two and other similar cases the effect must have been a specific result of the bleeding because all other methods of treatment had failed and the improvement occurred literally minutes after the operation was started. The amount of blood to be removed may be gauged by the level of venous pressure. This should not be reduced below normal.

The exact indications for phlebotomy are not clearly defined. Beneficial results are not always obtainable even when the conditions appear to be similar. The following conditions seem to be those in which bleeding may be helpful: engorged or tender liver, distention of the veins of the neck, cyanosis, and pulmonary edema. When the blood pressure is still elevated under the above circumstances greater improvement may be expected from bleeding than if the blood pressure is low. In fact, when a state of shock is present, as in acute coronary thrombosis, it may even be harmful. If the onset of hepatic engorgement has been recent and acute, as occurs shortly after the development of auricular fibrillation, a definite diminution in the size of the liver may result from bleeding. When the liver has remained congested and enlarged for months or years, the secondary cirrhotic changes that take place prevent such a decrease from occurring after bleeding.

A phlebotomy should be carried out very rapidly. As large a needle as possible should be used and the entire amount of blood (400 to 700 cc., depending on the size of the patient) ought to be withdrawn in about ten minutes. The exact mechanism of the improvement that occurs is not clear. Whether it takes place because of a diminution of the work of the heart by decreasing the volume of blood or by increasing the "tonus" of the heart, and thereby its contraction, are matters that need not be taken up here. In so far as it may be due to the latter it becomes desirable for the venous blood to be removed rapidly so that the dilated right side of the heart may decrease in size and regain a better tone before further blood returns from the periphery to redilate these chambers. That this mechanism cannot be the sole one involved is illustrated by the beneficial results that occur from bleeding when acute pulmonary edema takes place in a patient with hypertension and sudden left ventricular failure. Here there is no engorgement of the liver or appreciable venous engorgement. This beneficial effect is probably the result of decreasing the return flow to the right ventricle and, therefore, the output to the lungs. This enables a normal balance between the two ventricles to be established. There obviously remain some important questions concerning this matter that need investigation in order that we may have more accurate indications and contraindications for the use of this valuable method of treatment.

After several weeks of rest treatment, a patient such as we have described may be permitted to increase his activities. At first he may be permitted to walk about in his room. He then is gradually given greater liberties, and finally starts going up stairs and out of doors. When it is planned for him to return to his duties, it is well to have him begin by working only half a day. Some restrictions in his activities must be enforced, as it is apparent that his circulation was not sufficient for the former expenditure of energy. A conference between the physician and the patient and his family will help in ascertaining what part of his work should be curtailed, what entirely given up, and what should be retained. It is wiser to have him continue on only one half the previous amount of work with its decreased income than to try to carry on full duties, knowing that in a short while he will again be bedridden. Medical judgment tempered by good common sense is necessary in giving this advice.

In this connection, there are individuals who are incapacitated permanently and they cannot get to work or return home because of the difficulty with street cars, subways, etc. They are well enough to do their sedentary job if that were all they had to do. They should be advised to use taxis to and from work. This may cost $10 to $15 weekly but will enable some to remain self-supporting and not become a charge on their family or on society. I have had several very advanced cardiacs carry on in this fashion for many years, with great satisfaction to all concerned, after they had been made miserable and unhappy by being prohibited from doing any remunerative work. It has been impressive that some of these very sick cardiacs seemed better rather than worse for returning to work. Physicians should pay more attention to this point of view.

QUINIDINE

In the preceding discussion of the treatment of patients with congestive heart failure no mention was made of the use of quinidine. This brings up a controversial subject and merits a separate analysis. Quinidine was first proposed as a drug that would change auricular fibrillation to a normal rhythm. It was accidentally discovered by Wenckebach who was told by one of his patients with auricular fibrillation that he could make his heart beat regularly by taking quinine. It was later learned that quinidine was more effective in producing this change. This was hailed as a great discovery because auricular fibrillation, once established or continuing for a week or more, was practically always expected to persist indefinitely. In fact it used to be called the perpetual arrhythmia. Furthermore, it was also known that heart failure was often precipitated by and dated its onset from the change of the mechanism of the heart beat to auricular fibrillation. It seemed reasonable, therefore, to hope that any drug which could keep the heart regular would be of great benefit. The early reports concerning its use were very optimistic, but, as with many other therapeutic procedures, unfavorable aspects and limitations of its use gradually appeared and now it is known that the former enthusiasm was not altogether warranted. However, there still remains a distinct field for its administration.

In a sense, quinidine is a cardiac poison when given in sufficient doses. It impairs the conduction of impulses, lengthens the Q-R-S and Q-T intervals of the electrocardiograms, produces slight notching of the T wave, slows the auricular rate in auricular flutter or fibrillation, may evoke ventricular premature beats and rarely even ventricular tachycardia. It also can produce standstill or inhibition of the auricles and theoretically may have a similar effect on the ventricles. The maximum effect in human beings occurs two to three hours after oral administration and parallels the degree of concentration of the drug in the blood stream. There is only a slight amount of the drug in the blood at the end of twelve hours and only a trace after twenty-four hours. The larger the oral dose, the higher the blood concentration. There are some unexplained incompatibilities in the effects of quinidine. I have seen cases of auricular fibrillation that have reverted to normal rhythm only four or six or more hours after the last dose. Regularization must have taken place some time after the peak of blood concentration of the drug. Furthermore, it is puzzling that quinidine can inhibit extrasystoles, tachycardia, and fibrillation of the ventricle and yet at times it produces these very same irregularities.

The pharmacologic action upon which the action of quinidine depends in changing an irregular beat into a regular one consists essentially of two factors. It lengthens the refractory period of heart muscle and it also slows the speed of the cardiac impulse. It will be recalled that auricular flutter and fibrillation are due to a circus movement of an impulse in the auricles. This impulse keeps traveling around the venae cavae at a very rapid rate (300 to 600), always finding cardiac tissue ahead of it that has already recovered from the refractoriness following the previous impulse and thereby permitting a continuous circus motion to persist indefinitely. If the refractory period of the muscle could be lengthened, the impulse might find tissue still refractory and would stop. The circus might be broken up in this way and this would permit the normal pacemaker with its slow inherent rate, which has been held in abeyance by the rapid rate of the circus, to start functioning. On the other hand, if the rate at which the impulse travels around the circus is slowed or the path it takes is lengthened, it affords a longer time for the cardiac tissue to recover from its refractoriness and this would allow the circus wave to continue, thereby tending to perpetuate the circus. One effect of quinidine (lengthening of the refractory period) would tend to break up auricular fibrillation or flutter and the other (slowing of the impulse) would tend to perpetuate it. When the former predominates a regular rhythm is restored and when the latter effect predominates the arrhythmia persists. This explains the variable results obtained from the use of quinidine.

Let us consider what might be expected from restoring a regular rhythm when auricular fibrillation is present. In estimating the results of therapy both subjective sensations and objective changes must be carefully differentiated. Many patients will say they feel much better after regularization, when on close analysis it will be found that they no longer are annoyed by palpitation. The irregular heart beat is easily felt and causes not only discomfort but some apprehension. They feel the heart less or not at all when it beats regularly, and believe that there must be great improvement because they know that a normal heart should beat regularly. This does not necessarily mean that the heart is more efficient. The best indication that the circulatory state is actually improved is the degree of dyspnea or the objective signs of congestive heart failure. Patients with auricular fibrillation who have improved after quinidine may owe their recovery to the rest in bed and digitalis that was given during the period of observation. To differentiate clearly the effects that are solely the result of quinidine, one should employ all the other therapeutic measures available for a few weeks and then, when the patient is in as good condition as possible, measure what further improvement may follow regularization. When this is done the results will not always be favorable.

Some years ago I undertook a study of this sort. Inasmuch as dyspnea is the outstanding evidence of congestive failure and the vital capacity of the lungs is the best index of the degree of dyspnea, careful measurements of the vital capacity were made. The vital capacity would increase as the condition improved following bed rest and digitalis therapy. The heart rate would slow as was to be expected. After the condition was stabilized quinidine was given. When the rhythm became regular, the vital capacity of the lungs showed no constant alteration—it was slightly less, the same, or slightly greater. This meant that breathlessness was not materially improved by regularization of the heart, if the rate previously could be adequately slowed by digitalis. A heart that is beating irregularly at a rate of 60 to 70 can be about as efficient as if it were beating regularly at a rate of 70 to 80. In fact, a slow irregular rate may maintain a better circulation than a rapid regular one. It was occasionally found that, in the presence of stubborn congestive heart failure when the regular rate was 100 or more, improvement might first become manifest only after auricular fibrillation developed. What would happen was that digitalis that was given failed to slow the regular rhythm and when auricular fibrillation began the drug slowed the ventricular rate to 60 or 70 and congestion began to clear. In this sense the irregularity at times is an advantage.

There are, however, some definite advantages of a normal rhythm over auricular fibrillation. The formation of mural thrombi in the auricles with the possible development of emboli is much more likely when fibrillation is present. Also, although the heart rate may be kept slow with digitalis when it is irregular, it accelerates less on effort when regular. As a result of this factor it may well be that when there is no more breathlessness *at rest* with the heart fibrillating than while regular, there will be more dyspnea *on effort* if the rhythm is irregular. To these factors may be added the subjective relief of palpitation.

Taking everything into consideration, it is more desirable that the heart should beat regularly than irregularly. Quinidine sulfate would, therefore, be a very useful drug if this change could be accomplished without risk. However, there are dangers in its use. Rarely it causes sudden and unexpected death and it may result in the production of emboli. The exact cause of death is not clearly understood. It may result from an embolus but it would not be sudden under these circumstances. I have had three unexpected fatalities in which postmortem examinations failed to show either emboli or mural thrombi. A direct toxic effect on the heart may possibly account for some fatalities, as it is known that quinidine can inhibit the propagation of impulses. Inhibition of auricular beats with temporary disappearance of the P waves has been observed following quinidine. If the same type of effect is produced in the ventricles it would cause sudden arrest of the heart. It is also possible that at times quinidine may produce ventricular tachycardia or ventricular fibrillation. In the latter event sudden death would result. Another cause of death is respiratory failure. In cats this, rather than heart failure, is the primary cause of death from toxic doses of quinidine. In fact, when respiration has ceased and the heart is still beating, recovery can result if artificial respiration is instituted and caffeine is administered intravenously even after a lethal dose of quinidine is given to the animal. These experiments showed that the respiratory mechanism can fail while the heart is still viable, and if respirations can be stimulated or maintained during the critical period for a long enough time recovery may take place. Such observations have a direct clinical application, for it follows that caffeine in large doses and artificial respiration may prove effective in tiding over some patients that manifest toxic action from quinidine.

During the early years following the introduction of quinidine it was advised that, in order to avoid unfavorable effects, patients with auricular fibrillation to be given this drug should be selected according to certain definite criteria. It was thought that the most suitable were those in whom there was no great amount of enlargement of the heart, the irregularity was of short duration, and there was no significant heart failure. In other words, those with the least cardiac disability were regarded as the most likely to be benefited. Unfortunately one of the most disastrous results in my own experience occurred when all these favorable factors were present. This woman, about 35 years old, had a well-compensated mitral stenosis and had been able to work steadily. When the patient was first seen her heart was regular and three weeks later auricular fibrillation was found. She came into the hospital for a tonsillectomy and it was decided that the heart should be regularized before the operation. She was in very good condition and, after a preliminary course of digitalis, quinidine was given. The first day two doses of 0.2 gm. (3 grains) were administered. The second day the patient received 0.3 gm. (5 grains) three times. That evening the heart was regular, but there quickly developed marked breathlessness and the patient died in several hours. I thought she had a pulmonary embolism from a thrombus in the right auricle. Postmortem examination showed mitral stenosis and neither pulmonary infarct nor intramural cardiac thrombosis. It was after this experience that the animal experiments on the mechanism of death from quinidine were carried out. In retrospect it seems highly probable that this patient died of respiratory paralysis and that the same procedure that enabled the animals to survive (i.e., artificial respiration and caffeine) might have saved her life.

Apart from the fatalities due to either cardiac or respiratory effects, emboli may become dislodged as the auricles stop fibrillating and start contracting regularly. There is no known method of predicting in which case auricular thrombi are present and whether emboli will occur. When they do take place, embolic phenomena will develop within a few hours or days after the transition to a normal mechanism. The emboli are more often arterial than pulmonary and may affect almost any part of the body. Hemiplegia is the most common disabling complication. Although such emboli occur in patients with auricular fibrillation who do not receive quinidine, they are much more common during this treatment and must then be regarded as the direct result of quinidine administration.

Another limitation in the use of quinidine when organic heart disease (especially mitral stenosis) is present is that, once a normal rhythm is established, in many cases after a short time there is reversion to the auricular fibrillation that existed before. The regular rhythm is often maintained only for a few days or weeks and then the entire process of regularization needs to be repeated. In many, it appears to be impossible or too difficult to keep the heart beating regularly. Finally in only about 50 to 75 per cent of the cases will quinidine be effective in restoring the heart to a normal rhythm.

Notwithstanding the hazards and limitations of quinidine it occupies an important place in therapy. There are occasional instances in which it alone has been responsible for restoring compensation and one might even say in saving life. The pros and cons must be weighed carefully and, with increasing experience, a proper selection of those cases in which its use is justifiable will result. In the first place, from a review of my own experience and that of others, it seems to be safe and effective when given to that group of fibrillators, by no means small, who have no organic heart disease. There is a considerable number who have this arrhythmia without other evidence of heart disease. Here it may be expected that practically 100 per cent of the patients will promptly revert to a normal rhythm with only beneficial results. In one such patient who had documented auricular fibrillation for seventeen years, regularization was obtained which has been maintained for at least three years. In this case the doses of quinidine had to be gradually increased during the few days of treatment until a single dose of 2.0 gm. was reached. Furthermore, it is effective in the small number who continue to show auricular fibrillation two weeks or so after a subtotal thyroidectomy for hyperthyroidism when the basal metabolic rate has returned to normal. It is useless to give quinidine before operation in such cases or even after operation if the basal metabolic rate has not been effectively lowered by the surgical procedure. It is best to wait about two to three weeks after the operation, because in many cases spontaneous change to a regular beat will take place during this time. In fact, if the change does not take place, careful search for an undetected mitral stenosis should be made.

The main problem concerns the use of quinidine when mitral stenosis or hypertensive or myocardial disease is present. These patients comprise the group in which fatalities and emboli occur. At the outset it must be appreciated that we have no certain method of avoiding these accidents. The very early cases cannot be regarded as free from hazard, nor can the advanced cases be given up as hopeless. There are some general principles that may guide us in these decisions. All the disastrous results in my own experience have occurred in patients with mitral stenosis. Although serious complications have been reported in nonvalvular cases, they are not so numerous. I therefore have greater hesitancy in advising it in the former group. When a patient can be restored to a favorable state of compensation on digitalis and the ordinary methods of treatment, it is doubtful whether quinidine should be used. This is particularly true if mitral stenosis is present and the ventricular rate can be kept around 70. On the other hand, if the patient is doing poorly and it seems certain that he will not become ambulatory, one would be justified in hazarding a course of quinidine. Occasionally in cases in which there was apparently no hope, improvement has occurred. Furthermore, when palpitation from the rapid irregular beat is a major and disturbing complaint the drug may be tried. In some cases it is evident that as long as the heart was beating regularly the patient was in comparatively good health and incapacitation dated from the onset of fibrillation. When this disability has been present only a short while, one might risk quinidine therapy in the hope of preventing the slow downhill course that often follows the development of auricular fibrillation.

Since the advent of mitral valvuloplasty the question of quinidine therapy has taken on a new light. One might think that, following a satisfactory enlargement of the valve orifice with a decrease in the pressure and possibly in the size of the left auricle, a regular rhythm might be restored more readily and might be maintained for a longer time. The hopes have not altogether been realized. If auricular fibrillation first developed postoperatively, quinidine has generally been worth while. In cases of long-standing fibrillation the results have been disappointing.

However, occasionally regularization could be obtained some months after the operation when significant improvement in the state of the circulation had already taken place.

Whenever it is decided to use quinidine for persistent auricular fibrillation, the patient should be treated in a hospital unless circumstances do not permit it. The advantage of hospitalization is that changes in the mechanism of the beat may be more readily followed if electrocardiograms can be made whenever needed. Ordinary methods of treatment including digitalis should be employed until as much improvement as possible is thereby obtained. A maintenance dose of digitalis is continued during the period of quinidine treatment. The question of anticoagulant treatment before, during, and after quinidine therapy deserves some mention. The purpose of this would be to prevent emboli from possible auricular mural thrombi. There is no controlled information in this regard. It would take a very large series of cases to supply adequate data, as the complications that might be prevented are rare without anticoagulant therapy; nor is it known how long such treatment would be needed before quinidine is started.

The exact amounts of quinidine that are employed and the speed with which the dose will be increased will vary with the urgency of the circumstances and somewhat with the custom of the physician. The following is a routine course from which one can make individual variations as occasions arise. The first day 0.2 gm. is given at 10 a.m., 0.4 gm. at 2 p.m. and 0.6 gm. at 6 p.m. The dose is increased by 0.2 gm. each time, continuing the following days at the same hours of the day. The patient is examined just before each dose to see if reversion has taken place. If auricular fibrillation persists the dose is increased. If regularization occurs a maintenance dose of 0.2 to 0.3 gm. three times daily is continued for two to three weeks. This dose is then decreased to 0.2 gm. twice daily. Whether quinidine therapy should eventually be discontinued or maintained and at what dosage can only be determined by trial and error and by experience in a given type of patient. In cases of mitral stenosis the maintenance dose should be continued indefinitely unless untoward effects are produced and in some cases it will have to be as much as 0.3 gm. three or four times daily. Another program of quinidine therapy is to quickly increase the dose to 0.4 or 0.6 gm. and then give that dose every two hours until regularization or toxic effects occur. I have preferred the first of these two methods, giving the drug three or four times daily and increasing the dose each time.

The response of different cases varies considerably. In some patients small doses suffice; in others single doses as large as 1.0 or 1.5 gm. will be necessary for reversion. Once the rhythm is regular, if doses larger than 0.3 gm. three times daily are necessary to maintain a regular rhythm, it generally will be better to discontinue quinidine therapy entirely and accept the fibrillation as permanent. I recall an instance in which 0.8 gm. three or four times a day was necessary to restore the heart to a normal rhythm and that same daily dose to prevent a return of the arrhythmia. This was continued for months and enabled the patient to work, whereas otherwise he would have been bedridden with congestive failure.

During the early days when increasing doses of quinidine are given the ventricular rate often rises while the rate of impulse formation in the auricles slows. The acceleration of the ventricles is undesirable and palpitation becomes more uncomfortable. This temporary aggravation of the condition is to be expected but must not be allowed to last too long. In several days it must be determined whether the rhythm will revert to normal or not. The drug should be omitted if any untoward toxic effects, especially syncope or marked acceleration in rate, develop. When it is found that regularization does not occur, quinidine should be stopped entirely. It should not be given in small doses, like digitalis, for long periods of time, because it will fail to restore a regular beat and only make it more difficult for the digitalis, which the patient is receiving, to keep the ventricular rate slow. In other words, quinidine is given to make the heart regular or to keep it so, but it should not be continued for any length of time if auricular fibrillation persists.

There are occasional instances in which noncardiac toxic reactions to even small doses of quinidine occur. These may consist of a skin rash or fever. It is worth while to try to obviate such apparently allergic responses by the simultaneous administration of some antihistamine preparation, such as Benadryl 0.4 gm. four times daily. In one such instance of sensitivity it was possible to start with a small dose of 0.01 gm. and gradually increase the dose, so that the necessary amount of quinidine which previously produced a fever was tolerated and regularization was effected.

There is some reason to believe that quinidine might be useful in the prevention of auricular fibrillation in those prone to develop this irregularity. One might expect that the hazards of its use would be avoided or at least diminished if it were given to some patients before fibrillation develops. The difficulty is that there is no known method of predicting when this irregularity will occur and so one can rarely be convinced that the treatment is accomplishing its purpose. Nevertheless, I occasionally advise patients with well-marked mitral stenosis who are well compensated to take 0.2 gm. of quinidine sulfate two or three times a day indefinitely in the hope that this distressing type of irregularity may be prevented.

Quinidine has other uses than in the treatment of permanent auricular fibrillation. It has been valuable in various forms of paroxysmal rapid heart action in preventing recurrences. For this purpose it needs to be taken daily for long periods of time. It is very effective in controlling ventricular tachycardia and often inhibits the occurrence of extrasystoles of various forms. These therapeutic problems have been taken up previously in other chapters and need not be considered here. Suffice it to recall that it has an important place in the treatment of many arrhythmias.

When cortisone therapy was first introduced it was heralded as having remarkably beneficial effects on rheumatoid arthritis. With increasing experience its usefulness has broadened to encompass a great variety of conditions. In fact, adrenal steroids are being used in many different conditions, especially if they are serious and there is no other available and effective method of treatment. As a result of this attitude, and with the discovery of adrenal steroids that have less of the salt-retaining action, they are now being tried in some serious cardiac states. I have had a few amazing experiences that bear on this point. One elderly patient with calcific aortic stenosis who had been in and out of severe congestive failure finally reached a most critical state. His blood pressure was very low, the skin was clammy, and it did not appear that he would survive another twenty-four hours. He was then given 100 mg. hydrocortisone intravenously in 500 cc. of 5 per cent dextrose in water, over a period of six hours. The following day he was a new man. The skin was dry, his mind was alert, and his appetite returned; from then on his progress was favorable so that he again became ambulatory. Another patient was a man of 60 years who had had previous attacks of coronary thrombosis. He gradually grew weak, had marked anorexia and some dyspnea, but had no chest pain. Extreme asthenia with a cool moist cyanotic skin and a blood pressure of 90/70 were the outstanding features. The day after administration of 200 mg. of hydrocortisone intravenously there was an extraordinary change for the better. For the first time during his hospital stay he actually asked for food and had a sense of well-being.

The mechanism of these results is not at all clear. But the favorable effects in some of these cases were so striking and so prompt that they could not have been due to chance. The problem certainly deserves further investigation. At present, if such therapy is to be tried, it seems preferable to use preparations like Meticorten orally 10 mg. three times a day for a few days then gradually reducing the dose. This will have little sodium-retaining action. When the situation is very critical and even hours are precious, the intravenous route would be indicated. The patients who appear to be helped are those with marked asthenia in a state of semi-shock.

SURGICAL PROCEDURES

The inadequacy of medical treatment for patients with chronic heart disease, just as in other fields of medicine, has impelled the profession to seek further aid from surgery. The heart has been the last important organ to enter the scope of therapeutic surgery. It is evident that operative work on the human heart will necessarily be difficult. The circulation cannot be arrested for more than a brief time without sacrificing the life of the body even if the heart beat can be restored. The brain in particular does not withstand anoxia for more than several minutes. Until a satisfactory artificial circulation could be developed that would nourish the body, especially the brain and heart, any lengthy operative procedures on the inside of the heart would be difficult or impossible. This is just as important as an apparatus for artificial respiration was for the development of pulmonary surgery. Despite these handicaps, heroic attempts now and then were made to explore this new field. Accidental wounds of the heart have been successfully sutured. Considerable progress in pericardial surgery has been made (Chap. 5). Indirect methods of beneficially affecting the heart have been applied by altering the nervous system. Cervical sympathectomy, dorsal ganglionectomy, and paravertebral alcohol injections of the dorsal rami and ganglia have been employed with some success in the treatment of angina pectoris (Chap. 6). Daring attempts at incising and enlarging the orifice of a stenosed mitral valve were made as far back as 1923. These early ventures proved too hazardous and it was only after a lapse of 25 years that the operation was revived, and now thousands of patients are being operated on successfully.

A simple operation has been tried on rare occasions to give relief, when there is marked enlargement of the heart, i.e., decompression of the chest. Surgeons have occasionally done this in the belief that pericardial adhesions were present, only to find subsequently that the pericardium was normal. Despite this mistaken diagnosis, clinical improvement has been noted in some such cases. I had one patient in whom the removal of a generous portion of several ribs overlying the precordium was of considerable benefit. This patient was about 25 years old and had mitral stenosis, auricular fibrillation, and marked cardiac enlargement. The circulation was maintained in a fair state of compensation by the constant use of digitalis. I had followed this case for many years. The patient finally developed dysphagia which resulted from pressure of the enlarged left auricle on the esophagus. This was purely a mechanical difficulty and did not respond to ordinary methods of treatment. The dysphagia was promptly cured by removing, under local anesthesia, portions of ribs overlying the precordium. Not only was the patient able to swallow normally after this operation, but palpitation, which had been very annoying before, was much improved. She then did not feel the rapid irregular heart beat because it was no longer pounding against bony ribs but rather on a soft cushion of muscles and subcutaneous tissue. Even the ventricular rapidity seemed to be better controlled by digitalis than formerly. The patient lived for about nine years after the operation. Such decompression of the chest may be indicated whenever an enlarged heart is producing distressing symptoms as a result of pressure. This may involve not only the esophagus but also the left bronchus, causing harassing cough. Enlargement of the left auricle and of the pulmonary artery may also produce hoarseness or aphonia as a result of paralysis of the left vocal cord caused by pressure on the left recurrent laryngeal nerve. Similar operative procedures that decompress the chest may possibly prove useful in such conditions.

The hopelessness of many cases of advanced cardiac disease was responsible for the development of another surgical procedure, complete thyroidectomy. Its application in the treatment of patients with angina pectoris has already been discussed (Chap. 6). It also was performed for intractable congestive heart failure, due either to valvular or to myocardial disease. The following discussion is taken up mainly to throw light on the theoretical background of the possible value of lowering the basal metabolism in cases of intractable heart disease, not to support the advantages of this operation. In fact, total thyroidectomy has now become practically obsolete, but radioactive iodine therapy, a simple non-surgical method of accomplishing similar results, has come into use. It was known that when the basal metabolic rate is elevated as in hyperthyroidism, and there is congestive heart failure, a subtotal thyroidectomy with a subsequent fall in the metabolic rate caused the heart failure to disappear. It was also known that in myxedema associated with a sluggish circulation, congestive heart failure was very rare. It was, therefore, theoretically assumed that by producing myxedema in a patient without hyperthyroidism who has heart failure the demand on the heart might thereby be lessened to meet the supply. However, it was overlooked that, in the production of myxedema, not only is the demand diminished by lowering the metabolic rate, but the supply is also depressed, for the volume output of the heart is diminished and the velocity of blood flow is slowed in spontaneous and artificial myxedema. If the circulation is improved by this procedure, therefore other factors must be at work. The inherent metabolism of the heart may be altered so that it does its necessary work more efficiently and with less proportionate expenditure of energy. Another possibility is that with a partial myxedema, the heart is less sensitive to certain reflexes or internal hormones such as epinephrine. Finally, a most important factor is the size of the heart. A certain amount of dilatation of the heart may be beneficial, but excessive dilatation impairs the efficiency of the circulation. In congestive heart failure the heart is already dilated to a greater or lesser extent. When myxedema is produced, there is a tendency for further dilation to occur. May not improvement depend on this unpredictable factor, i.e., whether the further dilation of the heart is excessive or not? At any rate, the pathologic physiology of this problem is still unsettled.

The clinical results of complete thyroidectomy were variable. In those suffering from extremely advanced lesions, if improvement occurred, it often did not last long enough to warrant the operation. On the other hand, the operation did not seem justified if the disease was only slight or moderate or if the disability was not great, because of the handicaps attending partial myxedema. There remained a small group of cardiac patients, neither too sick nor too well, who seemed suitable for this operation. There is no doubt that some of the patients who had complete thyroidectomy were improved as far as their symptoms of heart failure were concerned, but it was hoped that a simpler method might be devised to obtain similar results without producing the ill effects that follow the removal of an important vital organ. At present I do not advise total thyroidectomy in chronic cardiac disease.

Nonsurgical methods of decreasing thyroid function and producing a partial myxedema are now being employed. The first consists of administering large doses of propylthiouracil to patients with intractable congestive failure or angina who have a normal thyroid gland. This may need to be continued for several months or more before a lowering of the metabolism occurs. The doses required are likely to be large—100 to 200 mg. three times daily. The second method is the use of radioactive iodine. This is much simpler and is being tried in many medical centers. The reports of Blumgart indicate that the results are fairly satisfactory in the majority of cases of angina but less so in those suffering from congestive failure. The doses of radioactive iodine employed have varied from a total of about 20 to 100 millicuries given in interrupted amounts at varying intervals. No injury to other organs has been observed, although in about one half of the cases a mild sore throat and cough have occurred which disappeared in a week or so. The cholesterol was found to rise before the basal metabolism fell. The results of these two types of treatment need to be observed more extensively and for a longer time before final judgment as to their value can be determined.

From my own experience it would seem that radioactive iodine therapy has some value in a small selected group of patients with intractable anginal pain who appear to be in fairly good health when they are free from pain. The patients should be told beforehand that they will have certain symptoms of hypothyroidism, such as dry skin, sensitivity to cold, and some general sluggishness. When the pain itself is a very distressing factor and relief to a greater or lesser extent is obtained from the treatment, the end-result is still beneficial.

Another surgical procedure that is being employed for hypertension and to some extent for hypertensive heart failure is sympathectomy. Various types of operations are being tried, but it appears that the dorsolumbar sympathectomy of Smithwick is at present most promising. More extensive division of the sympathetic nervous system, including all the dorsal and lumbar branches, may prove to be more effective. Many successful results have been obtained, even when myocardial involvement was present as shown by the presence of gallop rhythm and markedly abnormal electrocardiograms. This approach to the problem of hypertension and its complications deserves our most careful interest and attention.

One peculiar, although rare, form of congestive heart failure responds most dramatically to surgical treatment, i.e., the type following *arteriovenous aneurysm or fistula*. As a result of trauma or, less frequently, following an infection, a communication may become established between an artery and an adjacent vein. Blood is then shunted through the circulation and the work of the heart becomes definitely increased. In the course of time dilatation of the heart, murmurs, and congestive failure are apt to develop if the blood vessels involved are of significant size. The diagnosis is easily made by the history and the findings of a continuous murmur and thrill at the site of the aneurysm, with accentuation during systole. Furthermore, compressing the fistula produces an immediate and characteristic slowing of the heart rate. The surgical obliteration of the communication between the artery and vein can result in a complete disappearance of all subjective and objective evidence of cardiac failure.

An arteriovenous fistula occasionally is discovered in the lungs. Auscultation reveals a continuous murmur which resembles the murmur of patent ductus arteriosus. At times the two conditions may be confused, although an x-ray finding of a shadow in the lung ought to be diagnostic. Apart from the auscultatory findings there may be cyanosis, clubbing, and polycythemia. This condition is curable by surgery.

The various shunting operations to relieve pressure in the pulmonary circulation in cases of mitral stenosis have now been replaced by the direct attack on the obstructing valve. There still may be a rare instance of refractory and severe left ventricular failure with paroxysmal dyspnea, especially in cases of hypertensive heart disease, in which ligation of the inferior vena cava might be beneficial. I have had one such experience in which the result was remarkable and followed immediately after the operation.

The Surgical Treatment of Valvular Disease

GENERAL REVIEW

Cardiac surgery has made tremendous strides during the past decade or two. The first successful operation for mitral stenosis was reported in 1923 by Cutler and Levine. Because the next three cases ended in operative deaths I became discouraged. Shortly thereafter further surgery of the mitral valve was discontinued. About 25 years later Harken and Bailey revived the problem, and now operations of this kind are being performed all over the world. The original attempts were unsuccessful partly because the approach was through the left ventricle rather than the left auricle and because other aids to surgery were not then available. The development of blood banks, antibiotics, and improved methods of anesthesia has now made possible the survival of patients who formerly would have succumbed. Even before this, Gross had already opened the field of surgery for congenital heart disease when in 1938 he performed the first successful operation for patent ductus arteriosus. Rapid advances followed. Blalock and Taussig introduced the surgical approach for tetralogy of Fallot. Potts added a new technique which widened the usefulness of such surgical treatment. Brock then began to operate on the stenosed pulmonary valve directly through the right ventricle. In the meantime Crafoord and Gross simultaneously succeeded in relieving coarctation of the aorta. During the past few years cardiac surgery has continued to progress as a result of the introduction of hypothermia and extracorporeal methods of maintaining the circulation. Operations can now be performed that were technically impossible only a few years ago and much more is to be expected in the near future.

MITRAL STENOSIS

The most common valvular condition at present that is amenable to surgery is mitral stenosis. Here the problem is mechanical to a large extent, if not entirely. The selection of cases is most important. A correct diagnosis is obviously a primary requisite. It is now necessary to try to estimate the degree of constriction of the valve. Normally the size of the opening is 4 to 6 sq.cm. Cardiac reserve is such that patients suffer very little handicap until the valve is less than 2 sq.cm. in area. In fact, many patients do tolerably well until the area has decreased to 1.5 sq.cm. or less. The greater the constriction the greater the improvement to be expected from surgery, other factors being the same. A second consideration is the amount of accompanying mitral insufficiency. Inasmuch as the present operations for mitral regurgitation are not very satisfactory the physician should try to select cases that have pure mitral stenosis—and there are many of them—or that have only a slight degree of mitral insufficiency.

It is of interest that a high degree of stenosis cannot simultaneously exist with a high degree of regurgitation. Anatomically it would seem that when the mitral opening is very small there would be little chance for any considerable reflux. Physiologically it would be impossible with each systole for much blood to return to the left auricle and, at the same time, for an adequate amount to go through the aorta, if the mitral valve is markedly narrowed, for the constriction itself decreases the amount of blood that can reach the left ventricle with each cardiac cycle. In other words when there is a high degree of stenosis the regurgitation can only be slight, and when there is a high degree of insufficiency the stenosis can only be slight. The same considerations apply to the other valves of the heart. A third factor is the state of the myocardium. In most cases this can be regarded as essentially normal. In some it will be clear that coronary artery disease is also present. In others there will be evidence of significant myocarditis. Obviously if valves other than the mitral valve are involved the situation is different. These other complications may be expected to persist even after a successful mitral valvuloplasty.

In the selection of cases for surgery let us first consider pure mitral stenosis. As in all decisions concerning surgery, the risk involved must be weighed against the possible improvement. As the operative risk has diminished, the range of appropriate cases has broadened. At present the operative mortality in favorable cases is not more than 1 per cent. After the diagnosis is made the decision as to surgery will depend on the degree of disability and its rate of progression. If the patient is doing well or has only minor symptoms, is able to do his work, even if he cannot perform violent or extreme effort, and the condition is stationary, surgery is not indicated. At the present time it does not seem wise to advise operation as a prophylactic measure. Many patients with mitral stenosis continue in good health for a great many years. I have under observation a woman 50 years old who is quite well, is working every day to help support her family, and is on no cardiac medication. She first showed definite evidence of mitral stenosis thirty-five years before. Another man, 71 years old, was still working as a janitor, and walking a great deal in his work, twenty-one years after he first showed definite evidence of mitral stenosis and auricular fibrillation. The signs had not changed all those years. There are many such cases that either progress very slowly or remain stationary for very long periods of time.

The inference to be drawn is that detection of progression of the cardiac status is very important. While following a case of mitral stenosis it is necessary to watch for evidence of deterioration. Is dyspnea increasing, is the heart becoming larger, are objective signs of congestion appearing? These and other findings guide us in determining whether the condition is deteriorating or not. If the original condition appears satisfactory and no new developments appear from year to year, one is justified in delaying surgery.

It must be appreciated that when pursuing this conservative course one is taking a calculated risk. The one dangerous unpredictable complication is a cerebral embolus. This may come out of a clear sky when the patient is otherwise doing quite well. Although many such cerebral accidents are transient, without any serious ultimate handicap, some are followed by permanent paralysis of major importance. Although there is evidence that surgery diminishes the likelihood of subsequent emboli in cases of mitral stenosis, there is also the slight possibility of the operation itself resulting in a cerebral embolism. Where all factors are considered it still seems unwise at present to operate on a patient with well-compensated mitral stenosis, who is doing very well and shows no evidence of progression.

The ideal case for surgery is a patient with a definite diastolic or presystolic rumble at the apex, no apical systolic murmur or only a very faint one, an accentuated first sound, a definite opening snap, a reduplicated and accentuated pulmonary second sound, a normal sinus rhythm, an enlarged pulmonary artery, a prominent left auricle without much general cardiac enlargement on x-ray examination, and evidence of right ventricular hypertrophy in the electrocardiograms, with no evidence of left ventricular hypertrophy. When these signs are present and the patient has significant symptoms, surgery is clearly indicated. The symptoms may be increasing breathlessness on effort, recurrent attacks of acute pulmonary edema, bouts of hemoptysis, transient spells of auricular fibrillation, or a past history of some embolic phenomenon. The ideal case described above often proves to have a so-called *tight mitral stenosis*, measuring not more than 1.0 sq.cm. and sometimes even less than 0.5 sq.cm. It must not be expected that all these findings will be present. The heart may be moderately enlarged or auricular fibrillation may have appeared and become permanent. With every evidence of a more advanced state of the lesion the operative risk increases somewhat, but so also does the urgency of surgery.

Numerous exceptions are encountered in this work. I recall a 25-

year-old woman who showed an extremely loud apical systolic murmur (grade V). There was only a very faint or questionable murmur in presystole. Because of other features in this case, operation was performed, and the surgeon found an extremely narrow mitral valve (0.4 sq.cm.) and no detectable regurgitant jet. The explanation of this loud systolic murmur remained obscure.

A difficult problem confronting the physician is the estimation of how much stenosis and how much insufficiency may be present in a given case of rheumatic mitral valvular disease. Patients with marked mitral insufficiency may have a patulous valve with a large orifice resembling a wide-open diaphragmatic shutter of a camera. Such patients can still have a loud (grade III to V) apical diastolic murmur and thrill. They have very little mechanical stenosis of the valve and would only be suitable for surgery when operative measures for mitral insufficiency have been perfected. When there is doubt as to the degree of constriction and this knowledge is important, the gradient of diastolic pressure between the left auricle and left ventricle can be determined. This is done by inserting a catheter through a needle into the left auricle by an approach either through the trachea or from the back. The greater the gradient, the greater the degree of stenosis. This procedure and information obtained from pulmonary wedge pressure determinations may be necessary in order to obtain the answer to some of these questions.

Starting with the ideal case of mitral stenosis with no objective evidence of congestive failure, the next group is one in which there has been edema of the ankles, hepatic engorgement, persistent basal rales or hydrothorax, increased venous pressure, or permanent auricular fibrillation. When one or more of these complications have been present but the condition responds satisfactorily to medical treatment good results may yet be expected. The operative risk is greater in these cases, but in general will be about 2 to 3 per cent. However, when the condition is further advanced and congestive failure is entirely or partially irreversible, the risk mounts to as much as 10 to 30 per cent. There are obviously all gradations in operative risk from very slight to very great, depending on numerous factors. The presence of calcification of the valve, increasing age, the male sex, previous embolism, persistent auricular fibrillation, moderate or marked cardiac enlargement, evidence of significant myocardial involvement (abnormal ventricular complexes) all increase the gravity of the situation to a greater or lesser degree. That does not mean that patients in whom these conditions prevail are not suitable for surgery, but rather that these factors must be weighed in making a decision and in estimating the degree of expected postoperative improvement.

When faced with a patient belonging to the third group, i.e., one with refractory and gross congestive failure, the question of surgery is a difficult one. The decision will often depend on the attitude the patient takes toward his disability and his life. There is no fixed rule to follow.

I have had some most grateful patients who were operated on after some years of increasing disability which finally led to a bed and chair existence. Even on the day of operation such patients still showed marked enlargement of the liver, hydrothorax, and auricular fibrillation. I recall one patient of this type, a middle-aged woman who had such a satisfactory recovery that nine months after surgery she exclaimed that she had been able to dance with her husband for the first time in nine years. She has also maintained this improvement for about four years. Others, however, do not survive the operation and some who do survive are not sufficiently helped to have made the operation worth while. These factors are difficult to appraise and must be decided upon individually. At present we have no clear formulas to guide us.

There are a few contraindications for surgery. Certain acute illnesses, such as bacterial endocarditis, active rheumatic fever, and acute myocardial infarction, would obviously force postponement of the operation. One would hesitate to advise surgery for a patient who is unstable or unsound mentally. In this condition cardiac surgery is a double-edged sword. On rare occasions it may precipitate a severe psychosis, and in other instances the postoperative improvement may favorably alter the mental state.

It is not the purpose here to discuss the surgical technique of mitral valvuloplasty. Suffice it to say that the procedure is fast becoming safer. There still is the occasional risk that operative manipulations may dislodge an embolus from a left auricular thrombus. The serious ones are those that go to the brain. This operative complication, although uncommon, is mainly but not entirely confined to patients who have auricular fibrillation. Another hazard is sudden arrest of the heart or ventricular fibrillation. Despite all these possibilities it is surprising how much surgical trauma the heart can stand and how well even some very sick cardiac patients may do.

If a patient with mitral stenosis or any other cardiac condition develops auricular fibrillation postoperatively, it is desirable to try to restore a normal sinus rhythm. At first, adequate digitalis is given to slow the ventricular rate and then quinidine is administered, following the technique discussed earlier in this chapter. In the majority of cases quinidine will be effective. If auricular fibrillation persists a second course of therapy may be given later. On the other hand, if auricular fibrillation was already present and persistent before operation, it is not advisable to try to obtain reversion preoperatively. In this event it is preferable, although generally disappointing, to try quinidine about two weeks after the operation, or even a few months later. This whole matter is a difficult one, and at present different men hold different views as to the advisability of trying to restore a normal sinus rhythm in such cases. It may still be worth while to try quinidine several months after a successful mitral valvuloplasty, at a time when improvement of the circulation has already become manifest.

Follow-up Study.   In about 10 to 20 per cent of the cases a so-called postoperative syndrome develops a few weeks to a few months after the operation. This is thought by some to be a reactivation of rheumatic activity and by others it is looked upon as a direct late result of trauma of the operation and the presence of fluid or irritation of the pleura and pericardium. It consists of a febrile illness lasting one to two weeks, a temperature rise to 101 to 103° with precordial or pleural pain and grippe-like sensations resembling a virus infection or mild pneumonia with or without limb pains. There are no fatalities from this complication.

The clinical results of mitral valvuloplasty have been most satisfactory. One might have thought that if a fibrosed or calcified valve measuring 0.5 sq.cm. were enlarged by fracture or cutting to 3.5 sq.cm., the same process that originally caused the constriction would start operating all over again. If this were true the operation merely sets the clock back and the condition would only recur. In the five or more years that cases have been observed many patients have not shown recurrences. Some have had a secondary operation, and a few examined at autopsy one or more years after operation have shown what might be interpreted as recurrences of mitral stenosis. The objection raised to this interpretation is that the original operation was not adequate and failed to accomplish the desired result. It is claimed that if the surgeon succeeds in freeing the leaflets properly and attains an opening that is approximately normal, stenosis will not recur. How true this will prove to be only future study will show. The natural course of mitral stenosis is so gradual and may be so slow in its evolution that it will take many years before this question will be answered with any certainty.

From a clinical point of view the majority of cases (75 per cent or more) that survive operation show either marked or sufficient improvement to have made the surgery worth while. The degree of improvement will vary in different cases. In a sense one might say that this improvement is just as great when a patient who has been confined to a bed and chair existence is enabled to walk in the street and drive his car, as when a patient who formerly became short of breath on stair climbing but not on walking is enabled to hurry, make many flights of stairs, and carry on essentially normal duties. Many patients are rehabilitated economically. The mothers are enabled to carry on housework and bring up their children or go through pregnancy safely. Others return to occupations they previously had to give up.

The general improvement in the efficiency of the circulation continues during the postoperative months while the left ventricle is gradually adjusting itself to the increased work that it is permitted to do. It appears that the tendency for arterial emboli has been sharply decreased as a result of the operation, as they have been found to be extremely rare during the years that many of these cases have been followed by Ellis and Harken. In this regard it must be appreciated that in the natural history of mitral stenosis arterial emboli, especially cerebral emboli, become much less frequent years after the onset of auricular fibrillation. Inasmuch as most patients with peripheral emboli have had persistent auricular fibrillation and the patients who had mural thrombi and therefore were prone to have emboli might have had emboli preoperatively, it is not surprising that this complication is much rarer after operation. Despite this criticism the difference seems greater than might be expected. There no doubt is less stagnation in the auricles, the speed of blood flow is increased, and the auricular appendage, which is the most common site of the thrombus, has been removed. All of these factors would tend to decrease embolic phenomena.

During the early postoperative months the patient continues on a more or less strict medical regimen for congestive failure. How vigorously this is carried out will vary in different cases. Low-salt diet, digitalis, and mercury diuretics with or without added ammonium chloride may all be necessary. It is advisable that the patient take penicillin (200,000 units by mouth once or twice daily) to help prevent streptococcus infections and recurrent rheumatic fever. Physical activities should be slowly and gradually increased. At appropriate intervals some of the medical measures or restrictions can be diminished. Simple intelligent guidance, including instructions in breathing exercises, and an optimistic attitude on the part of the patient will enable him to make steady progress.

MITRAL INSUFFICIENCY

Surgery for mitral insufficiency at present is not satisfactory and must be regarded as still in the experimental stage. Various procedures are being tried with varying success. Such patients generally have marked cardiac enlargement, particularly of the left auricle. They also show evidence of left ventricular enlargement on x-ray or electrocardiographic examination. In this regard the electrocardiogram has been much more reliable in detecting ventricular hypertrophy than the x-ray. The left auricle is likely to show active systolic expansion on fluoroscopy. Auscultation is likely to reveal a systolic murmur of grade III intensity or louder. When the mitral valve is both stenosed and incompetent the extent of improvement following operation will depend mainly on the degree of stenosis present that can be relieved. If this is great, the expected improvement will be great. It is of interest that a proper operation for mitral stenosis generally does not produce insufficiency of the valve and may in fact lessen it.

AORTIC STENOSIS

The results of the surgical treatment of aortic stenosis as yet have not been altogether satisfactory. The immediate operative mortality has been considerable. In those who have survived surgery the results, although occasionally excellent, have often been disappointing. The early operative approach through the left ventricle has presently given way to the transaortic approach. Optimistic reports are now coming out from some clinics. It is therefore well to remain hopeful that before long eth operation will have a wider appeal.

AORTIC INSUFFICIENCY

At present the only operation that has had any success is the insertion of the Hufnagel valve into the thoracic aorta. This prevents reflux of blood from below the point of insertion so that the upper part of the body still shows some, but diminished, evidence of aortic regurgitation whereas the lower part does not. The clinical results in many patients are quite satisfactory. The operative risk is still appreciable (about 20 per cent) but probably will decrease as a result of improved technique and more favorable selection of patients. Both congestive symptoms and anginal pain have disappeared postoperatively. Among the serious complications of this operation are sudden death, cardiac arrhythmias during the early days, and distal emboli during the later days. The artificial valve produces, with each heart beat, a clicking sound which is audible to the patient and to those near him. It eventually does not disturb him; in fact he knows that he will remain alive only as long as he can hear it. No doubt new techniques will be devised that will be more effective. Already Sarnoff has performed some successful ingenious experiments on dogs, shunting the blood flow from the left ventricle directly to the aorta, by-passing the aortic valve.

TRICUSPID STENOSIS AND COMBINED LESIONS

The accurate diagnosis of tricuspid stenosis is still difficult but is being made with greater frequency. It always accompanies mitral stenosis and generally aortic stenosis is present as well. Operations occasionally are performed for tricuspid stenosis, but this should be done after the mitral operation. In rare instances more than one valve has been explored at the same operation.

Since surgery for valvular disease has been introduced a new diagnostic challenge has arisen. Formerly it was a common experience for a physician to make a diagnosis of "combined aortic and mitral disease." Now it is necessary, whenever possible, to appraise the relative role played by each valvular lesion in any particular case and even to try to estimate the degree of stenosis or insufficiency that is present. Greater accuracy is now demanded in the diagnosis of the actual anatomical abnormality that the surgeon may find. Although our knowledge in this regard is increasing rapidly, there still are occasions when the situation will remain obscure and exploratory operations will be necessary. This is permissible when the operative risk is not great, and is similar to surgical practices in other parts of the body. Preoperative determination of the differences in pressure on each side of a valve (the pressure gradient) affords a good guide as to the degree of obstruction. The study of the form of the arterial pulse wave and the measurement of the speed of upstroke of this wave will also help in estimating the degree of aortic stenosis. Such studies and others that will become available will no doubt aid in the selection of appropriate cases for surgery.

CHAPTER 21

Clinical Electrocardiography

By HAROLD D. LEVINE, M.D.

The Normal Electrocardiogram

Normally the impulse that initiates the heart beat arises at the sino-auricular node of Keith-Flack, a club-shaped structure consisting of specialized tissue measuring about 1.5 cm. in its greatest length and located high in the right atrium near the orifice of the superior vena cava. This tissue is different in structure from the rest of the cardiac musculature and is rich in nerve fibers and ganglion cells. Although there is reason to believe that rhythmic electrical activity must exist within this structure, thus far conclusive evidence for electrical activity within the node has not been demonstrated. While it has been possible to record electrical activity of a distinctive form in isolated Purkinje tissue, there is, so far as we know, no representation of sinus activity in the normal electrocardiogram. The wave of excitation emerges from the sino-auricular node into the auricular muscle proper. Hence the node is called the pacemaker of the heart. Since there is no specialized conduction path in the auricles, the impulse is then conducted radially over the auricles in much the same manner as a ripple spreads over the surface of a pond when a pebble is dropped into it. Because of the thinness of the auricular walls the epicardial surface is activated simultaneously with the underlying endocardial surface. This wave spreads over the auricles, depolarizing first the greater part of the right atrium, then the greater part of the left atrium. At or shortly before the height of the P wave the right atrium has been activated; the left atrium is activated during the second half of the P wave. The impulse is conducted over the auricles at a fairly rapid rate, in the neighborhood of 1000 mm. per second. The wave of depolarization is followed by a wave of repolarization (the so-called auricular T wave), but this is ordinarily swallowed up in the succeeding ventricular complex of the normal electrocardiogram.

When the first half or so of the P wave has been inscribed and the right auricle activated, the wave of excitation is picked up by the junctional tissue between the auricles and ventricles. This structure is called the auriculoventricular node of Tawara, which continues as the auriculoventricular bundle of His. This junctional tissue also has a

405

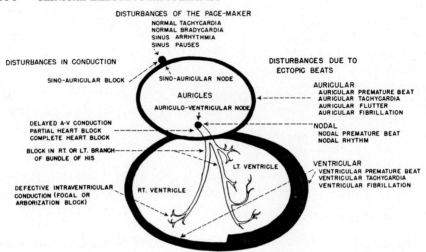

FIG. 1.   *Common Types of Disturbances in Mechanism of the Heart Beat.*

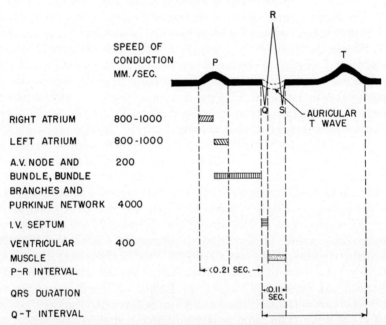

FIG. 2.   *Impulse Conduction in the Heart.*   Speed of conduction in various parts of the heart and its representation in the normal electrocardiogram.

specialized structure like the sino-auricular node. The auriculoventricular node is an ovoid structure located beneath the right atrial endocardium just below the orifice of the coronary sinus. Here the impulse is conducted much more slowly, about 200 mm. per second. It picks up speed as it continues into the auriculoventricular bundle but it is still conducted at a relatively slow rate. The bundle runs forward for a short distance on the crest of the muscular portion of the interventricular septum at its junction with the membranous septum ("undefended space"), then divides into a right and left branch. The impulse travels even faster in the bundle branches which course down on each side of the interventricular septum. The right branch becomes a part of the anterior papillary muscle of the right ventricle and does not branch again until the apical extremity of that muscle is reached (see Fig. 1). The left branch, on the other hand, in most if not all individuals, begins to branch shortly after it has become the left main stem. These specialized conduction paths continue with finer and finer arborizations (Purkinje fibers) and spread throughout the two ventricles, being particularly abundant on the endocardial surface of the ventricles. All of the electrical events described so far, activation of the auricular musculature, the auriculoventricular node, the auriculoventricular bundle, the bundle branches, and the Purkinje network, are included in that part of the normal electrocardiogram from the beginning of the P wave to the beginning of the ventricular complex (Fig. 2). However, the spread of the impulse through the main bundle branches and the subendocardial Purkinje network is so rapid that these events have virtually no duration and are not represented in the normal electrocardiogram.

Probably because of the earlier arborization of the left bundle branch, the left side of the septum, for a brief instant, is activated earlier than the right. But the left side of the septum would probably get this "head start" in being activated even if the left branch did not branch earlier than the right, since the area of distribution of the left branch on the left face of the septum is more widespread than that of the right branch on the right surface. Spread of the impulse in the muscular septum and the free walls of the ventricles is much slower, 400 mm. per second, than spread in the Purkinje tissue, which has been measured at 4000 mm. per second. The spread of the impulse is in the direction from the apex toward the base of the ventricles on the endocardial aspects of their free walls and approximately at right angles to the endocardium from the subendocardial network to the epicardium. Because of the rapidity of subendocardial activation this process is almost synchronous throughout the ventricles. As a result both ventricles are stimulated to contract almost simultaneously. Actually, since the right ventricle is thinner than the left, the impulse has a shorter distance to travel and emerges upon the epicardial surface of the right ventricle earlier than upon the epicardial surface of the left ventricle. Coincident with the latter part of septal activation the free wall of the right ventricle close to the septum is activated. Furthermore, the thinner apical poles are activated earlier than the thicker bases of the ventricles.

ELECTRICAL ACTIVATION OF THE VENTRICLES

It will be helpful at this point to consider certain theoretical aspects of the electrical activation, first of a muscle strip, then of the human ventricles. If a simple muscle strip (Fig. 3) is stimulated at point A an electrical impulse spreads from point A along the strip toward

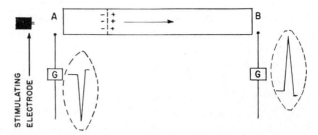

FIG. 3.   *Potential Variations and Electrographic Representation.*   Showing potential variations at each end of a simple muscle strip stimulated at one end. If positivity is indicated by an upward deflection, the recording electrode away from which the impulse moves records a downward deflection, while that toward which the impulse moves records an upward deflection.

point B. The impulse can be regarded as a wave front with positive charges in advance and negative charges in the wake of this advancing wave of depolarization. A recording electrode is coupled through a galvanometer to a remote point of negligible potential. The galvanometer is so arranged that a positive potential at point A is recorded at the galvanometer as an upward deflection and a negative potential at point A as a downward deflection. Since point A is in the negative field of the advancing wave during the passage of the impulse, a downward deflection is recorded at A. If a similar arrangement is set up at point B, an upward deflection is recorded at point B, since B is in the positive field of the advancing wave. It may be concluded, then, that with such an arrangement an impulse moving *from* a point is recorded at that point as a downward deflection and an impulse moving *toward* a point is recorded at that point as an upward deflection. By convention, the connections to the galvanometer in human electrocardiography are identical with those given above, and the same considerations apply.

From present knowledge let us now consider (Fig. 4) the potential variations occurring from moment to moment during ventricular activation at two points in relation to the heart, one (point A) in relation to the epicardial surface of the right ventricle, and the other (point B) in relation to the epicardial surface of the left ventricle. An electrode at point A, facing the right ventricle, being in the positive field of the initial unopposed wave moving across the septum, records a small upward deflection (Fig. 4, *1*). Additional coalescent wave fronts now form on the left side of the septum and, at the same time, presumably at the apex of the right ventricle near the base of its anterior papillary muscle. The electrode is now in relation to a large cone (for although we have represented these electrical events upon the plane of the page they must be thought of in relation to all heart muscle in its three dimensions) of positivity from the spread of the impulse from the left side of the septum, a cone of negativity from the spread of the impulse on the right side of the septum, and a cone of either positivity or negativity from activation of the apical part of the free wall of the right ventricle, de-

pending upon its orientation with regard to the electrode. If the cones
of positivity predominate there is a further increment (Fig. 4, 2) in
positivity at electrode A. At the next instant (Fig. 4, 3) the free walls
of the right and left ventricles are being activated. The much larger
negative fields due to left ventricular activation more than overbalance
the small positive field due to right ventricular activation. Hence the
electrode now shows a change in polarity with consequent reversal in the
direction of the deflection recorded there. Since the area of negativity
facing the electrode becomes still greater the deflection becomes still
more negative (Fig. 4, 4). As the cone of negativity has now reached

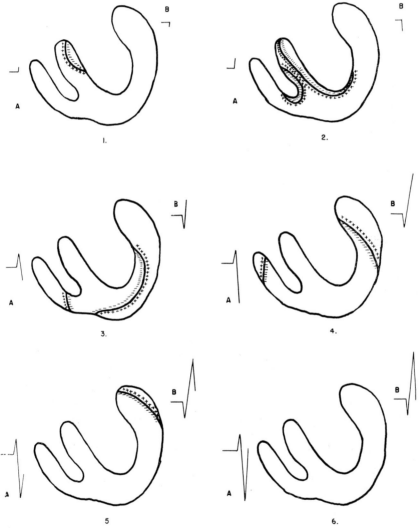

FIG. 4.   *Ventricular Depolarization*.   Schematic representation of current concept of the moment-to-moment manner of depolarization of the ventricles. (After
Ashman.)

its maximum and is now decreasing, the deflection has reached its nadir and moves again toward the baseline (Fig. 4, 5). Finally with total depolarization of the heart the tracing has returned to the isoelectric line. Accordingly the initial ventricular complex as recorded over the right ventricle consists of a small upward R wave followed by a large downward S wave deflection. To indicate the relative size of these deflections this may be designated an rS wave. These considerations are true whether the electrode is in contact with the right ventricular wall (direct lead) or with the precordium overlying the right ventricle (semidirect lead).

An electrode facing the left ventricle at point B, recording the same electrical events, being in the negative field of the initial unopposed activation of the septum from its left to its right side, records an initial downward deflection (Fig. 4, 1). At the next instant electrode B is in relation to the larger and nearer field of negativity due to further activation from the left to the right side of the septum, probably overbalancing the smaller and more distant field of positivity emerging from the region of the apex of the right ventricle; a further increment in the initial downward deflection may thus be inscribed. For the next few moments depolarization of the free wall of the left ventricle brings a much larger area of positivity into relation with the electrode than the area of negativity produced there by depolarization of the smaller and more distant free wall of the right ventricle. Hence the deflection now moves upward. When the area of positivity reaches its maximum the upward deflection reaches its apex. As the area of positivity in relation to the electrode now recedes the deflection moves toward the isoelectric line, and when the ventricle is fully depolarized the deflection has returned to the isoelectric line. Thus in a general way an electrode facing the left ventricle records as the initial ventricular complex a small downward deflection (Q wave) followed by a large upward deflection (R wave). To indicate the relative size of these deflections we may designate this as a qR wave. With some qualification these considerations apply equally to an electrode applied directly to the left ventricular surface (direct lead) and to one on the overlying precordium (semidirect lead). The more directly the electrode faces the left side of the septum, the more prominent should the initial downward deflection appear. Whatever part of the body faces the left side of the septum should show this initial downward deflection followed by a large upward deflection. It should be clear, then, that the normal Q wave is produced by septal activation; it is referred to as a "septal Q wave" and is a normal finding of no pathologic significance.

It is possible that the sequence of septal and free-wall activation is much more complex than has been indicated above. It is likely, for example, that there is more than one wave of activation across the septum. And longitudinal, in contrast to tangential, spread of the impulse may be more important than has been suggested. In essence, however, this simplified conception seems accurate enough for all practical purposes.

PRECORDIAL LEADS

Although some of the pioneer studies in electrocardiography were carried out with chest leads, interest in these leads was abandoned early in favor of study of the electrical events reflected in the frontal plane of the body and recorded in the conventional limb leads. However, in the course of some twenty years certain limitations in the conventional limb leads with regard to the diagnosis of anterior myocardial infarction and certain practical and theoretical developments with regard to the recognition of bundle branch block prompted a renewed interest in these chest or precordial leads. At first a bipolar technique similar to that used for the limb leads was employed; the polarity was such that relative positivity at the precordium was represented by a downward deflection of the tracing and relative negativity by an upward deflection. Later this convention was reversed so that the tracings would be comparable with those obtained in the three conventional leads. It was felt or hoped that the potential of the limb with which the precordial point was paired had an electrical potential which was negligible with reference to the electrical contribution of the precordial point. Actual experience, however, showed that the contribution of the limb potential to the chest lead, whether it was a CF (chest–left leg) lead, CL (chest–left arm) lead, CR (chest–right arm) lead or CB (chest–back, usually over the right shoulder) lead, was by no means always negligible. The reason for this is twofold: (1) Although there is a logarithmic falling off of the recorded cardiac potentials from the heart to the more remote portions of the trunk, which functions as a volume conductor, the limbs act rather as linear conductors and there is therefore no further drop in potential from groin to toes or from axillae to finger tips. (2) The heart, as will become clearer presently, may be so oriented as to have a considerable electrical effect at the limb paired with the precordial point. Only if the heart happens to be so positioned that a mixture of right and left ventricular potentials, mutually extinguishing one another, is reflected to an extremity, would that extremity show a really negligible potential. Therefore none of the limbs can be depended upon to be truly "indifferent." All workers in the field have therefore agreed upon the desirability of an arrangement one of whose poles records the potentials of a precordial point and the other whose potential is zero; this would be a unipolar chest lead. Although opinion is still not unanimous on just how such a unipolar chest lead should be recorded, most of the objections to the Wilson unipolar chest lead have now been met. This consists of two loops, an exploring loop which is attached to the positive pole of the galvanometer, and a central terminal loop which is connected to the negative pole of the galvanometer. The central terminal in turn is connected to each of the three extremities, right arm, left arm, and left leg, through a 5000 ohm resistance. Accepting the validity of the Einthoven triangle hypothesis, to be described more fully below, the potential at the central terminal must be the average of the potentials at the three extremities (Fig. 5). If, for example, at one instant during the electrical

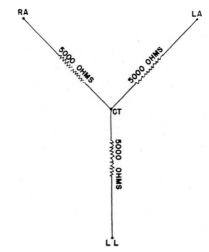

FIG. 5.   *The Central Terminal of Wilson.*

Let VR represent the voltage at RA (right arm),

VL represent the voltage at LA (left arm),

VF represent the voltage at LL (left leg),

and VT represent the voltage at CT (central terminal).

But, by Ohm's law, EMF (voltage in each part of the circuit) =

Current (in same part of circuit) × Resistance (in same part of circuit).

Then VR − VT = Current (RA − CT) × a constant,

and   VL − VT = Current (LA − CT) × a constant,

and   VF − VT = Current (LL − CT) × a constant.

Adding these three equations:

VR + VL + VF − 3 VT = [Current (RA − CT) +

Current (LA − CT) + Current (LL − CT)] × a constant.

But, according to Kirchoff's first law, the algebraic sum of the currents meeting at any point in any network of wires is zero.

∴ VR + VL + VF − 3 VT = 0 × a constant = 0

∴ VR + VL + VF = 3 VT

And VT $= \dfrac{VR + VL + VF}{3}$

Or, stated differently: The potential at the central terminal is the average of the potential at the three extremities.

activation of the ventricles the potential at one of these extremities increases, that at the other two extremities automatically decreases so that the average at the three extremities and, therefore, the potential at the central terminal do not change. Thus a reference point with a nonfluctuating potential is obtained. Actual measurements of the potential at this central terminal show it to be very close to zero, with minimal and unimportant fluctuations from moment to moment during the cardiac cycle, and to show less fluctuation than any single point in the body, no matter how remote from the heart.

Although at first the potentials of only one and later two precordial points were recorded, the desirability, in certain conditions, of recording the potential at several precordial points is now universally recognized.

Precordial leads are of value, frequently decisive, in the study of myocardial infarction, bundle branch block, and ventricular hypertrophy. In most instances a decision regarding any of these three conditions can be made from the study of two or three precordial points, but there are certain instances when decisive changes will be present at only one of six precordial points. This point might be skipped when the potentials of only two or three fixed points are recorded; hence the frequent need for multiple precordial leads. Experience has shown that in those cases in which precordial exploration is necessary the potentials of six precordial points should be taken. These are:

  Point 1. At the fourth intercostal space just to the right of the sternum.
  Point 2. At the fourth intercostal space just to the left of the sternum.
  Point 3. At a point midway between points 2 and 4.
  Point 4. At the fifth intercostal space in the left midclavicular line.
  Point 5. At the same horizontal level as point 4 in the left anterior axillary line.
  Point 6. At the same horizontal level as point 4 in the left midaxillary line.

When these points are paired with the central terminal of Wilson they are called leads V_1, V_2, V_3, V_4, V_5, and V_6, respectively. At times it is necessary to record additional leads to the right of V_1 or to the left of V_6, or cephalad to V_4, V_5, and V_6. This will be discussed later.

EXTREMITY LEADS

In his classical studies of the electrocardiogram Einthoven conceived of the heart as being in the center of an equilateral triangle whose apices are the right shoulder, left shoulder, and left groin, the heart being quite distant from these apices and these apices being distant from one another. He assumed also that conduction of an electrical impulse in the tissues of the body from the heart to the extremities is uniform. This is the Einthoven hypothesis. It is to be distinguished from the Einthoven equation. The latter is a necessary consequence of the arrangement of the electrocardiogram and merely states that at any instant the magnitude and sign of the QRS complex (or the P wave or the T wave) in Lead II must be equal to the algebraic sum of the magnitudes of the QRS complex (or P wave or T wave) as inscribed at the same moment in Leads I and III. It is a valuable fact, often enabling one to detect improper application of the electrodes. However, there has been some disagreement regarding the validity of the Einthoven hypothesis. The points of attachment of the extremities to the trunk do not exactly form an equilateral triangle. The heart is not precisely in the center of a triangle formed by the extremities; in general it is closer to the left shoulder than to the right shoulder or left groin. Conduction is not uniform through muscle, lung, liver, or bone. In spite of these objections, however, the hypothesis is close enough to the facts to have been of inestimable value in the study of the electrocardiogram during the past quarter of a century. Practically all studies have shown that, although there may be some argument about the details, in a general way the Einthoven hypothesis may be accepted as valid and workable.

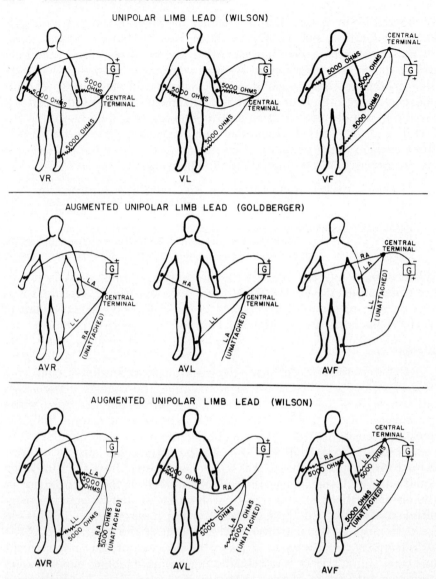

FIG. 6.   *Methods of Recording Unipolar and Augmented Unipolar Extremity Leads.*

The conventional leads described above, being bipolar leads, represent the combined potentials of two of the three points at the apices of the Einthoven triangle. Thus a downward deflection in Lead III might be the result of a downward deflection at the left leg or of an upward deflection at the left shoulder, since an upward deflection at the left shoulder is routed through the galvanometer so that it becomes a downward deflection in writing Lead III. As will become apparent, it is frequently desirable to break down the composite potential of Lead III into its constituent parts. This can be done by the use of formulas or, much more readily, graphically, and strikingly, by the use of unipolar extremity leads. These are similar in theory and practice to the unipolar chest leads described above. By coupling the central terminal of theoretically zero potential through the galvanometer, in turn, to each of the three extremities—right arm, left arm, and left leg, it is possible to record virtually the potential at each of these points and thus to obtain, in relatively pure form, as it were, the potential at the apices rather than along the sides of the Einthoven triangle. These are called unipolar limb leads and are designated VR (right arm), VL (left arm), and VF (left leg or foot). As worked out by Wilson (Fig. 6), a 5000 ohm resistance was included between the central terminal and each of these three extremities to swamp out local differences in resistance between skin and electrode at each of the three limbs. In order to increase the magnitude of the unipolar potentials recorded at the limbs, Goldberger did two things. (1) Contending that little or no difference is produced in the resulting tracings, whether or not resistances are included in the circuit, he eliminated the resistances in the portion of the circuit between the central terminal and the electrodes. (2) Since the potential at the extremity being investigated was routed to *each* pole of the galvanometer and thus, to a certain extent, was pitted against itself, he detached the wire of the combined portion of the central terminal from the extremity being studied. Reference to Figure 6 shows the Goldberger modification more clearly. Thus he obtained "augmented" unipolar limb leads, designated aVR, aVL, and aVF. It is to be noted that, in dropping the central attachment to one of the limbs, the record obtained was no longer strictly unipolar. It can be shown, however, that when a similar arrangement is used at each of the extremities this discrepancy is neutralized. Wilson accepted the second change but retained the 5000 ohm resistances. There is still some controversy as to whether these unipolar limb leads should be recorded at all, whether these unipolar limb leads should be "augmented," and whether resistors should be retained. It is our impression that unipolar limb leads are very helpful in certain cases. A study of the literature would seem to indicate, moreover, that less error is introduced into the method if the resistors are retained. Accordingly the tracings reproduced in this book and labeled aVR, aVL, and aVF are Wilson augmented unipolar limb leads.

ELECTRICAL POSITION OF THE HEART

The heart does not occupy a fixed position in the thoracic cage but may vary in position from individual to individual, and from time to time in the same individual. It is known that, by and large, the trunk of the body acts as a volume conductor, but the extremities function as linear conductors, recording the potentials at their respective points of attachment. Since these points of attachment are invariable, errors due to slight variations in the point of attachment of the electrode on the limb are obviated, a distinct advantage thus being obtained by the use of the extremities for recording the cardiac potentials. In essence, then.

the cardiac potentials recorded at a point may vary (1) with variation in the position of the heart in relation to a fixed electrode, (2) with variation in the position of the electrode in relation to a fixed position of the heart, or (3) with a combination of the two. By the use of extremity leads the factor of variation in the position of the electrode is eliminated, enabling us to study variations in the position of the heart.

The vantage points used for this purpose are the right arm at its attachment to the right shoulder, the left arm at its attachment to the left shoulder, and either the right, or, as is the custom, the left leg at its attachment to the trunk. Because of its pericardial reflections the heart is relatively fixed at its base but enjoys a greater degree of mobility at its apex. The right shoulder faces the base and cavitary aspect of the heart and hence records a predominantly downward deflection (which may be preceded or followed by a small upward deflection depending respectively upon whether a small part of the right or left ventricular potentials are reflected there). The potentials of the left shoulder and leg, on the other hand, show much greater variations. From the latter one may draw certain inferences regarding the electrical position of the heart. Assuming normal activation of the heart we may designate as an *intermediate electrical position* (Fig. 7) one in which the left ventricular potentials are transmitted approximately equally to the left shoulder and left leg. A *horizontal electrical position* (Fig. 8) is one in which the heart has rotated on its anteroposterior axis so that the left ventricular potentials are transmitted to the left shoulder while right ventricular potentials are reflected to the left leg. A *vertical electrical position* (Fig. 9) is one in which the heart has rotated in the opposite direction on its anteroposterior axis so that left ventricular potentials are transmitted to the left leg while right ventricular potentials are reflected to the left shoulder. One can, with Wilson, conceive also of a semivertical or a semihorizontal position. In the *semihorizontal electrical position* (Fig. 10) the rotation of the heart is incomplete so that, whereas left ventricular potentials are transmitted to the left shoulder, the heart has not developed the extreme degree of rotation characteristic of the truly horizontal heart, and a mixture of right and left ventricular potentials is reflected to the left leg, one virtually extinguishing the other, so that the QRS complex recorded at the left leg possesses a low electromotive force. In the *semivertical electrical position* (Fig. 11), whereas left ventricular potentials are transmitted to the left leg, the left shoulder similarly receives a mixture of left and right ventricular potentials, again mutually extinguishing one another, and resulting in a QRS complex of low electromotive force at the left shoulder. Comparison of the unipolar limb and chest leads in the following manner enables one to identify the various positions of the heart:

Vertical position: Lead VL resembles Leads V_1 and V_2; Lead VF resembles Leads V_5 and V_6.

Semivertical position: Lead VF resembles Leads V_5 and V_6; QRS complex of Lead VL is small.

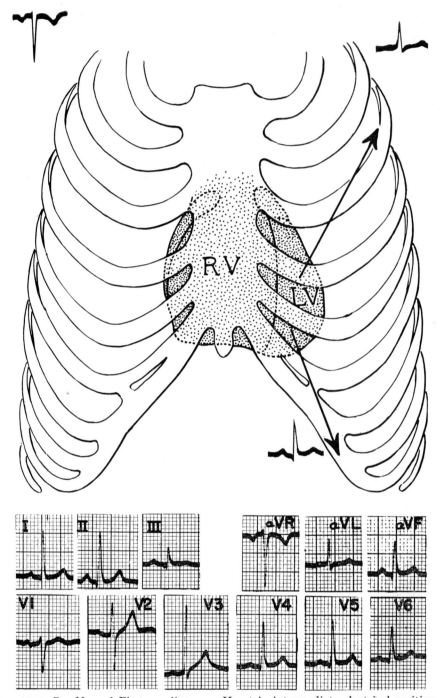

FIG. 7. *Normal Electrocardiogram.* Heart in intermediate electrical position. The left ventricle is so situated that its potentials are reflected equally to the left shoulder and left leg. Hence both Leads aVL and aVF resemble Leads V_5 and V_6. *It is to be emphasized that, although anatomic sketches are here used to illustrate the various positions of the heart, this is merely a graphic method of demonstrating how rotation of the heart can alter its electrical projections with regard to the extremities. These should therefore be conceived of as electrical positions which may or may not correspond to anatomic positions.*

417

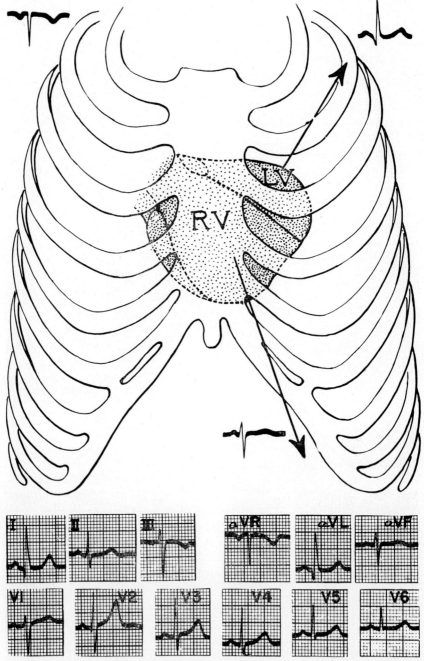

FIG. 8. *Normal Electrocardiogram.* Heart in horizontal electrical position. The heart has rotated in a counterclockwise direction on its anteroposterior and longitudinal axes. This swings the left ventricle into relation with the left shoulder and the right ventricle, through the diaphragm, into relation with the left leg. Hence Lead aVL resembles Leads V_5 and V_6, and Lead aVF resembles Lead V_1. Left axis deviation here is a positional change and is not due to left ventricular hypertrophy. The transitional zone lies between Leads V_1 and V_2.

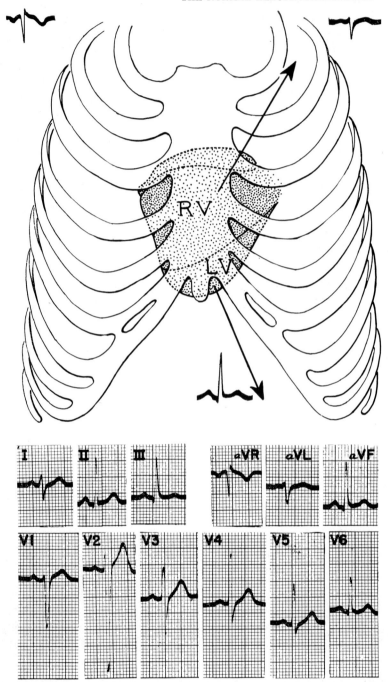

FIG. 9.   *Normal Electrocardiogram.* Heart in vertical electrical position. The heart has rotated in a clockwise direction on its anteroposterior and longitudinal axes. This swings the right ventricle into relation with the left shoulder and the left ventricle, through the left leaf of the diaphragm, into relation with the left leg. Hence Lead aVL resembles Leads V_1 and V_2, and Lead aVF resembles Leads V_5 and V_6. Right axis deviation here is a positional change and is not due to right ventricular hypertrophy. The transitional zone is at Lead V_3.

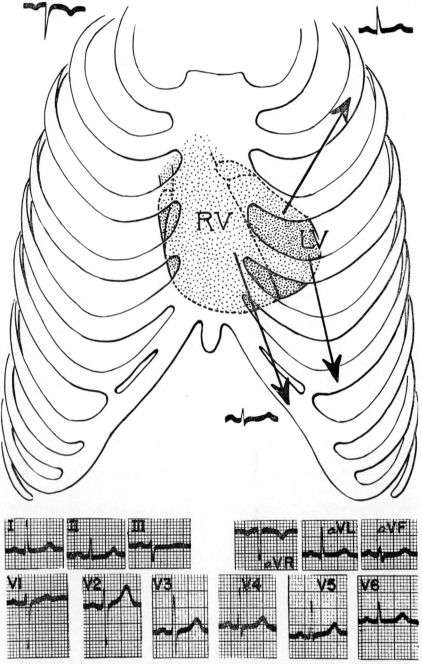

FIG. 10. *Normal Electrocardiogram.* Heart in semihorizontal electrical position. The heart has rotated so that the left ventricle is still in close relationship to the left shoulder, but counterclockwise rotation of the right ventricle is incomplete so that the left ventricle still has some electrical effect upon the left leg. The left leg receives a mixture of left and right ventricular potentials with decrease in the resultant left leg potentials. Hence, while Lead aVL resembles Leads V_5 and V_6, the QRS complex in Lead aVF has a low voltage.

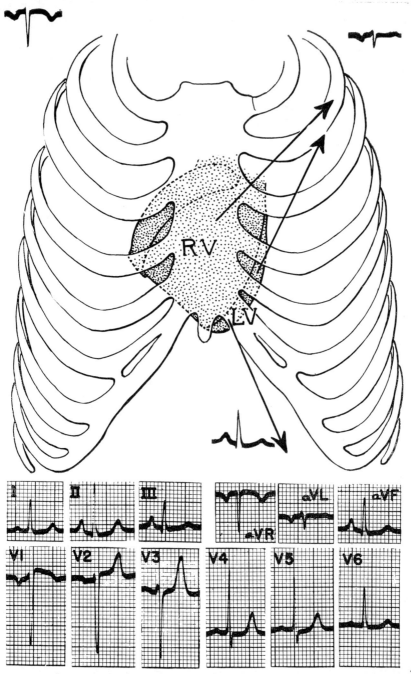

FIG. 11. *Normal Electrocardiogram.*   Heart in semivertical electrical position. The heart has rotated so that the left ventricle is still in relation to the left leg but clockwise rotation of the right ventricle is incomplete so that the left shoulder receives a mixture of right and left ventricular potentials with resultant decrease in left shoulder potentials. Hence, while Lead aVF still resembles Leads V_5 and V_6, the QRS complex in Lead aVL has a low voltage. The transitional zone lies between Leads V_3 and V_4. Many combinations of axial rotations are possible; in the examples given here clockwise rotation on an anteroposterior axis has been combined with clockwise rotation on the longitudinal axis (as viewed from the apex of the heart), and counterclockwise rotation upon the anteroposterior axis has been combined with counterclockwise rotation upon the longitudinal axis.

Intermediate position: Leads VL and VF are similar and resemble Leads V$_5$ and V$_6$.

Semihorizontal position: Lead VL resembles Leads V$_5$ and V$_6$; QRS complex of Lead VF is small.

Horizontal position: Lead VL resembles Leads V$_5$ and V$_6$; Lead VF resembles Leads V$_1$ and V$_2$.

Indeterminate position: No relation demonstrable between the unipolar limb and precordial leads.

Although roentgen examination usually shows that the anatomic position of the heart corresponds to the electrical position of the heart determined in this way, there may be some exceptions to this. Provided these positions be regarded as electrical, these discrepancies need not concern us here. The important point is that attention to the electrical position of the heart often enables us to detect from the electrocardiogram changes in its appearance which are referable, not to disease of the heart, but to changes in its electrical position.

THE CONVENTIONAL LIMB LEADS

Einthoven, impressed with the relatively fixed position of the extremities with relation to the heart, focused the attention of workers in the field upon the use of the limb leads derived from the three points of the triangle formed by the right and left shoulder and the left leg. Thus for some twenty-five or thirty years electrocardiography was dominated by Einthoven's three extremity leads. Lead I he designated as the potential difference between the right and left shoulder, and is recorded by routing the left arm potentials through the string galvanometer so that a positive potential at the left shoulder is written upward, while the right arm potentials are so routed that a positive potential at the right arm is written downward. Thus Lead I is a bipolar lead, and the composite result of the potentials at the right and left shoulder, the left shoulder contributing to Lead I with unchanged polarity while the polarity of the right shoulder potentials is reversed in Lead I. Similarly Lead II records the difference in potential between the right arm and left leg recorded simultaneously, the right arm potentials entering in a negative and the left leg potentials in a positive way into the resultant potentials. Lead III is the composite effect of the potentials at the left arm and left leg, the left arm potentials being routed to the negative and the left leg potentials to the positive pole of the galvanometer. Most of our knowledge of cardiac arrhythmias, conduction disturbances, and abnormalities of the auricular and ventricular complexes was worked out with these bipolar limb leads. However, the limitation of the method with regard to certain cases of myocardial infarction and bundle branch block later redirected attention to the study of the precordial leads. Somewhat later the desirability was appreciated of breaking down the precordial and conventional extremity leads into their constituent parts, and thus led to the development of unipolar lead electrocardiography. Although it is possible that the use of unipolar limb leads may eventually supplant conventional leads, several factors, including current usage of the latter and inadequate experience with the normal variations in the former, compel the retention of the conventional leads at least for the present. Accordingly a description of the normal variations in the three conventional limb leads is warranted.

When the electrocardiogram of a normal individual is taken a series of waves is recorded. They have been arbitrarily called P, Q, R, S, and T waves (Fig. 12). These electrical complexes differ in form in the various leads. The P wave represents the electrical disturbances that take place in the auricles. The first half or so of the P wave represents right auricular activation, the second half left auricular activation. Because of the situation of the auriculoventricular node in the inferior portion of the right atrium, the impulse enters the auriculoventricular node at or shortly before the peak of the P wave. The P wave as well as the other important waves are apt to be most prominent in Lead II. All of the other waves are due to ventricular activity and can be divided into

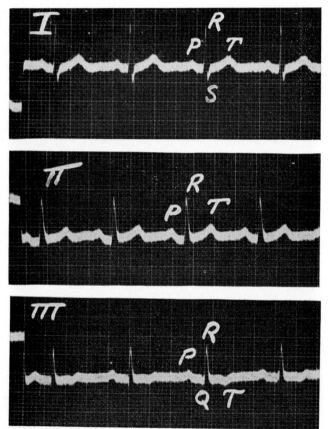

FIG. 12. *Normal Mechanism.* The three curves show the three conventional leads. At the beginning of each tracing the standardization is photographed (1 centimeter = 1 millivolt). P represents auricular depolarization. QRS is the initial (depolarization) and T the final (repolarization) ventricular complex. The time is indicated in 1/25 and 1/5 seconds. Note that T₃ may be flat normally.

two portions, the initial deflections (QRS) and the terminal deflection (T). The first downward wave, if followed by an upward deflection, is called a Q wave. The first upward wave, whether preceded by a downward one or not, is called an R wave. A wave that is directed downward which follows an R wave is called an S wave. When there is a second upward deflection after an S wave, it is called R′ and similarly a second downward deflection after R′ would be S′. If there is only one deflection and it is downward it may be called QS. There is some controversy about the proper terminology of the initial deflections but the above nomenclature has the sanction of present usage. After the QRS complex there follows a brief isoelectric line which gradually blends into a smooth rounded T wave. Occasionally there may be, after the T, a small U wave which has an obscure origin. In potassium depletion a U wave may make its first appearance or, if present previously, it may increase in height or duration or both, generally at the expense of the T wave.

The P wave normally is upright and measures about 0.5 to 2.5 mm. in height. The P-Q or P-R interval which measures the time it takes an impulse to go from auricles to ventricles (conduction time) varies from 0.12 to 0.20 second. An interval greater than 0.20 second is regarded as pathologic. Most of this delay takes place at the auriculoventricular node and bundle of His. The normal P-R interval decreases with increasing heart rates and is shorter in children than in adults. In children under 6 years the range is 0.13 to 0.17 second, and for those between 7 and 13 years it is 0.14 to 0.18 second for rates of 130 to 70, respectively. Table 1, from Alimurung and Massell, shows the maximal P-R intervals at different age levels and varying heart rates. Normally Q and S waves

TABLE 1.   Maximal P-R intervals in seconds at different age levels and varying heart rates.

AGE	RATE					
	<71	71–90	91–110	111–130	131–150	>150
< 1 month			.11	.11	.11	.11
1– 9 months			.14	.13	.12	.11
10–24 months			.15	.14	.14	.10
3– 5 years		.16	.16	.16	.13	
6–13 years	.18	.18	.16	.16		

may or may not be present. When the heart is rotated on its longitudinal axis in a counterclockwise direction as viewed from the apex, a Q wave is present in Lead I and an S wave in Lead III. On the other hand, when the heart is rotated on its longitudinal axis in a clockwise direction as viewed from the apex, the S wave is present in Lead I, the Q wave in Lead III. The R wave varies in height from about 5 to 15 mm. The T normally is upright in Leads I and II, and may be upright or inverted in Lead III. Its amplitude will range from 1 or 2 mm. to 4 or 5 mm. The duration of the QRS is an important part of the study of a tracing.

Normally it will be found to be between 0.04 and 0.08 second. When it reaches 0.1 second it is regarded as delayed. The duration of the Q-T interval, which is an accurate measurement of the length of ventricular electrical systole, is about 0.4 second, but will vary with the cardiac rate.

The QRS complex really measures the time it takes the impulse to spread throughout the two ventricles and reflects the integrity of the two branches of the bundle of His. The thickness of ventricular muscle will affect this time to only a slight extent. The T wave or terminal portion of the ventricular complex may be regarded as due to the process opposite to that producing the QRS. The latter is the advance of the electrical or physicochemical process, the former is the retreat.

Normally the P, R, and T waves, which are regarded as the more constant deflections, should be greatest in Lead II and the sum of the height of the waves in Leads I and III should equal that in Lead II. Because of the great variations in the character of these complexes in normal individuals, a considerable experience is required to become familiar with the normal and caution must be exercised before slight alterations are regarded as significant.

It has been suggested that during the last two months of pregnancy electrocardiographic evidence of the fetal heart can be obtained by taking a lead from the left arm and right leg of the mother. Very minute waves may be seen regularly interspersed among the mother's electrocardiographic tracings. Insertion of electrodes into the rectum or vagina of the pregnant woman may enable one to obtain larger electrocardiograms of the fetal heart.

The Normal Precordial Electrocardiogram

We have seen that it does not matter whether an electrode is applied an inch higher or lower on one of the limbs, since the limbs function as linear conductors. However, in taking leads from the chest, moving the electrode 1 inch over the precordium produces profound alterations in the tracings. This introduces some confusion in comparing precordial tracings obtained in the same patient at different times. The position of the heart may change with relation to the six designated precordial points. Furthermore, the precordial electrode may not be applied to exactly the same point on the chest wall at each recording. By taking the entire panorama of six precordial leads it is possible, often at a glance, to eliminate changes which are due to either of these changes, i.e., change in the position of the heart itself, or a change in the position of the electrode. Herein lies one of the most important reasons for recording six rather than one, two, or three precordial leads.

It is to be remembered that each precordial lead records the potential not only of the part of the heart immediately underneath the electrode but also, to varying degrees, that of more remote parts of the heart. If the heart is close to the chest wall the effect of the adjacent part of the heart upon the electrode will be relatively greater than the effect upon this electrode of more remote parts of the heart. Conversely, if the heart is deep in the chest and relatively distant from the precordium, there will be a greater relative effect of the more remote portions of the heart upon the electrode. In the latter instance, the changes from V_1 to V_6 will proceed more gradually because at each precordial position a fusion of the potential of many parts of the heart is produced. On the other hand, when the heart lies closer to the chest wall, abrupt changes may be detected from one position to the next. Ordinarily the spectrum of changes consists of a progressive change from right to left ventricular potentials; however, if the heart happens to show extreme rotation, Lead V_1 need not show characteristic right ventricular potentials or Lead V_6 need not show characteristic left ventricular potentials. For example, if the heart rotates clockwise on its longitudinal axis (as viewed from the apex) and the apex is also displaced posteriorly, Lead V_6 may still show the rS pattern characteristic of right ventricular potentials (Fig. 179). In that event it would be necessary to take additional leads to the left of Lead V_6 at V_7 (same horizontal level in the posterior axillary line) or at V_8 (same horizontal level over the scapula), or cephalad to these positions in the third or fourth interspace in order to record true left ventricular potentials. On the other hand, the heart may be rotated counterclockwise on its longitudinal axis so that Lead V_1 records left rather than right ventricular potentials. In such a case (Fig. 26), it has been recent practice to take additional leads to the right of Lead V_1 at positions having a relation to the right anterior chest similar to that which Leads V_3 and V_4 have to the left anterior chest. These are designated Leads V_{3R} and V_{4R}, or $V_{3'}$ and $V_{4'}$. These leads should become routine when rheumatic or congenital heart disease is suspected.

Ordinarily Lead V_1 may or may not show an R wave. Absence of an R wave at this location may therefore be a normal variation, and may be assumed to result from the relationship of the electrode to the right ventricular cavity with septal activation proceeding tangentially with relation to the electrode. When an R wave is present it is probably due mainly to septal activation. The S wave is generally quite large. The T wave at this location may be inverted, isoelectric, or upright.

At position V_2 an R wave is usually recorded. If there was an R wave at V_1, it is slightly taller at V_2 than at V_1. The greater size of the R wave is probably related to the closer relationship of the electrode with the septum and the fact that it now faces the septum more directly. The S wave is as a rule somewhat deeper at V_2 than at V_1; this is probably due to closer proximity of V_2 to the heart in most cases. If the heart were strongly rotated counterclockwise on its longitudinal axis the S wave would be larger at V_1 than at V_2 because V_2 would be closer to the left ventricle and to the larger R type of potential. The T wave in adults is generally upright from V_2 to V_6. In children, young women, and, as has been reported, in Negroes, the T wave may be inverted in

V_2, V_3, or even V_4. The exact frequency of this finding in the normal adult population has not been established.

The R wave in Lead V_3 is still taller; by the time this point has been reached it generally measures 2 mm. or more. Failure of the R wave to increase as the electrode moves toward the left is an abnormal finding. This may result from anteroseptal scarring from an old myocardial infarct, with resultant failure of the subjacent muscle to be activated. Even more suggestive of scarring would be a decrease in the magnitude of R once it has appeared at Lead V_1 or V_2. In other words, the R wave should normally show a progressive increase from Lead V_1 to V_4. If it fails to increase or, more strikingly, if it decreases, there may be an infarct of the myocardium in this region. This change may also occur with left ventricular enlargement, particularly if associated with incomplete left bundle branch block. The R wave fails to increase in left bundle branch block because in that disturbance the septum is activated from its right to its left side. The wave which would proceed early from left to right fails to appear and thus fails to antagonize the downward impulse recorded at the right precordium corresponding to activation of the septum from its right side.

Coincident with increase in the height of the R wave in Lead V_3 the S wave decreases. In some cases, especially when the heart is in a vertical position, the R wave in Lead V_3 may actually be larger than the S wave in the same lead, but there is considerable variation from heart to heart in the point at which R first exceeds S.

Usually at Lead V_4 the R wave is much taller and the S wave much smaller. The R wave here is due to activation of the anterior or anterolateral wall of the left ventricle. If the apex is well anterior the S wave may now be quite small or even absent. If the apex is displaced posteriorly the R wave may be smaller and the S wave still relatively prominent. The presence of an S wave signifies that more of the left ventricle (its posterolateral aspect normally) is activated after the muscle near the electrode. If no S wave is inscribed one may conclude that the electrode is in relation to the last part of the left ventricle to be activated.

Because of the intervention of relatively poorly conducting lung tissue between the lateral aspect of the heart and the precordium, the magnitude of all deflections may fall off in Leads V_5 and V_6. In fact, miniature tracings maintaining the same type of relationship between Q and R are not at all uncommon in Lead V_6. In many cases, especially if the heart is in a horizontal position, the R and T waves may be as large in V_6 as in V_4, or even larger. The important point, however, is that whereas a decrease in the height of the R wave from Lead V_1 to V_4 is abnormal, a falling off of the R wave from Lead V_4 to V_6 need not be.

A Q wave is not normally seen in Leads V_1 to V_3. As the electrode moves to the left and faces more and more directly into the left side of the septum, a Q wave appears and becomes more prominent in relation to the R wave. The exact point at which this Q wave is first encountered in going toward the left of the precordium varies, of course, with the position of the septum. It generally does not become well marked until Lead V_5 or V_6 has been reached, and may not be recorded at all in the usual six chest leads. This Q wave is thin, rarely lasting longer than 0.02 second, and, even when most prominent in comparison with the R wave in the same lead, never measures more than a small fraction of that R wave. This Q wave, as we have seen, is a normal finding due to septal activation and has no pathologic significance.

The tracings obtained in Leads V_{3R} and V_{4R}, properly applied, look like that of Lead V_1 in miniature. Their important feature is a QS deflection or an S wave which is deeper than the R wave.

THE "INTRINSICOID DEFLECTION"

If a third recording electrode is placed about halfway along the experimental muscle strip shown in Figure 3, a biphasic $(+-)$ deflection is there recorded as the wave of excitation travels along the muscle strip. This is due to the fact that this new point functions in two ways, first as electrode B or a point toward which the impulse travels, then as electrode A or a point away from which the impulse moves. Hence an initial upward and a final downward deflection are inscribed. The moment when the impulse has arrived at or near the muscle beneath the electrode is signaled by the sudden change in the direction of the impulse and is customarily measured at the beginning of this "intrinsic deflection." Although for some time a similar terminology has been used with regard to points over the precordium, it should be clear that in this situation the electrodes and the muscle being activated are relatively remote from one another. The final downward deflection there has less magnitude and may appear less rapid than directly over the epicardium. Furthermore, the electrode is not arranged parallel to the line of activation of the ventricles. Rather, in a general way, the impulse, moving from endocardium to epicardium, approaches the electrode, then emerges upon the epicardial surface of the ventricles. In terms of the bipole theory the beginning of the final rapid downward deflection coincides with the moment when the largest field of positivity is oriented toward the electrode. As the field of positivity begins to decrease the deflection recedes toward the isoelectric line. This does not necessarily mean that the impulse emerges on the epicardium beneath the electrode at that moment. Actually, this is more apt to occur sometime on the downstroke of the rapid deflection. The term "intrinsic deflection," then, is a concept useful in the experimental study of muscle activation, while the term "intrinsicoid deflection" has been proposed as a more appropriate term for the clinical appraisal of electrical activation of portions of the intact heart.

Whatever its mechanism, the measurement of the time of this deflection over the precordium has proved of considerable value in the study of the normal or hypertrophied heart or, more particularly, the heart with bundle branch block. As a matter of convenience this may be measured from the beginning of the QRS complex to the apex or starting-off point of the rapid downward deflection (ordinarily the beginning of the RS wave); if there is more than one rapid downward deflection the final one should be taken as the intrinsicoid deflection. To be quite accurate, this deflection would have to be measured from the beginning of the earliest Q wave in a simultaneously recorded conventional limb lead; however, since simultaneous leads are not taken in ordinary clinical electrocardiography, the deflection is measured, as accurately as possible, from the beginning of the QRS complex in the same lead.

Because the right ventricle is normally thinner than the left, the impulse activating its wall has a shorter distance to travel than has an impulse activating the left ventricle. Accordingly the intrinsicoid deflection, which we have seen gives a measure of the time of activation of the ventricle, is inscribed earlier over the right than over the left ventricle. Ordinarily the difference between right and left ventricular activation does not exceed 0.02 to 0.025 second. In left ventricular hypertrophy the difference may approach or exceed 0.045 second. This delay parallels the increase in the voltage of the R wave over the left ventricle but it is to be noted that ventricular thickness is not the only factor affecting the voltage of the R wave. The proximity of the ventricle to the chest wall and probably certain chemical changes at the boundary of the heart muscle cells are two other factors to be considered. In right ventricular hypertrophy, apparently depending upon its degree, the difference between the intrinsicoid deflection over the right and left ventricles may be decreased or, perhaps more often, the intrinsicoid deflection may be inscribed later over the right than over the left ventricle. In left bundle branch block the delay in activation of the left ventricle is extreme. In complete or incomplete right bundle branch block the reversal in the normal relationships of right and left ventricular activation is invariable.

THE "TRANSITIONAL ZONE"

The point or area over the precordium at which the form of the ventricular complex changes from that characteristic of the right ventricular potentials in the heart to that characteristic of the left ventricular potentials in the same heart is referred to as the "transitional zone." It is to be emphasized here that, although reference is made to right and left ventricular potentials, what is actually meant is the potentials recorded, respectively, over the right and the left precordium. Each precordial point records the totality of the electrical activation of the heart. One ventricle influences the potential recorded at that point more or less than the other ventricle does, depending on its relative nearness to that point and on the depth of the heart in the chest cavity. Bearing this qualification in mind it may be said that if the heart lies close to the chest wall the transition may be an abrupt one, changing from a right to a left ventricular potential from one of the usual precordial points to the next. If, on the other hand, the heart lies deep in the chest, the change may be smoother and slower, showing a gradual evolution from right to left ventricular potentials over two, three, or more precordial points. The change is more readily determined if the direction of the transitional zone is at right angles to the line of the usual six precordial points, and it is less readily determined if the transitional zone and this line lie parallel to each other. The change may be from the rS complex of the right ventricle to the qR complex of the left ventricle. Very often, however, notching of the QRS complex is noted at the transitional area, an initial R wave corresponding in time to the R wave of one ventricle and a secondary R wave to that of the other ventricle (Fig. 26). This type of notching is a normal variant and is not to be confused with that due to complete or incomplete bundle branch block or to focal block. One cannot be sure of block of either of these types unless the electrode lies clearly in relationship either with the right or the left ventricle. In deciding whether one has recorded true right and left ventricular potentials, it is essential to demonstrate that the "transitional zone" has been crossed, either with the use of the usual six precordial leads, or, if necessary, with additional leads to the right or left of these. As a corollary to this fact, the position of the "transitional zone" is of some value in determining rotation of the heart on its own longitudinal axis. A pronounced shift of the transitional zone to the left may be an important clue to, and in rare cases the sole electrocardiographic evidence of, acute cor pulmonale. When the transitional zone is in relationship with either the left shoulder (aVL) or the left leg (aVF), bizarre notched, low voltage complexes are apt to be reflected to either location. This constitutes one of the criteria for the designation of a semivertical heart in the former instance or of a semihorizontal heart in the latter. If the voltages are small (less than 3 or 4 mm.) at either of these points, analysis of the relative duration and amplitude of the individual components of these deflections is likely to prove misleading in the study of myocardial infarction. Furthermore, one must distinguish between the transitional zone demarcating left and right ventricular potentials and that demarcating infarcted and uninfarcted muscle. This problem is more fully considered in the discussion of myocardial infarction.

The Vectorcardiogram

If Lead I of the electrocardiogram is recorded simultaneously with Lead II or III it will be observed that the apex of the R wave in one lead is not inscribed at the same instant as the apex of the R wave in the other leads. The R wave is clearly "out of phase" in the three limb leads. This results from the fact that the electrical axis of ventricular depolarization changes from instant to instant. In Figure 13 the R wave of Lead I corresponds to an S wave in Lead III. There is obviously left axis deviation, but the leftward "mean electrical axis" just described is an oversimplification. The "vector" as represented in the frontal plane of the three conventional leads does not extend in only one direction

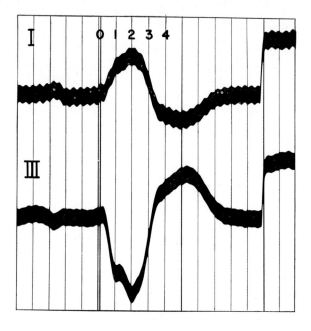

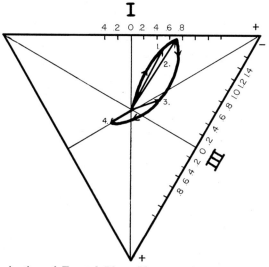

FIG. 13. *Derivation of Frontal Plane Vectorcardiogram.* Leads I and III are recorded simultaneously. At instant zero both baselines are at the isoelectric line. At instant 1 the Lead I trace deviates 5 mm. above the isoelectric line, the Lead III trace 1 cm. below. These two points are marked off on the appropriate sides of the Einthoven triangle. The intersection of their perpendiculars (point 1 on the lower graph) indicates the direction and size of the vector at the first instant. At the moment of the next vertical time mark (instant 2) Lead I shows an upward movement measuring plus 7 mm., Lead III a downward movement of 13 mm. The perpendiculars to these points meet at point 2 in the graph, indicating the instantaneous vector at that moment. Similarly instant 3, with a value of plus 4 mm. in Lead I and minus 3 mm. in Lead III, and instant 4, with a value of minus 3 mm. in Lead I and plus 4 mm. in Lead III, give rise respectively to instantaneous vectors 3 and 4. Clearly the direction and magnitude of the vector as seen in this plane are changing from instant to instant. In this example the deflections do not finish at the zero point; the loop is "open." The leftward "mean electrical axis" is the synthesis of a series of instantaneous electrical axes. A smooth curve (loop) connecting these instantaneous vectors produces a frontal plane monocardiogram or vectorcardiogram.

but proceeds rather through an arc with changing size and direction from moment to moment. The plotting of successive electrical axes is demonstrated in this figure. Thus the electrical activation of the ventricles shows sequential changes in size and direction. Connecting these successive instantaneous vectors produces a "loop" or "vectorcardiogram" as reflected to the frontal plane of the body. This, in turn, is a mere projection of the spatial vectorcardiogram existing tridimensionally in the chest.

This explains why a dynamic sequence of changes is recorded. The same information can also be recorded directly from the body without calculation by plotting Lead I (horizontal deflecting plates) against Lead aVF (vertical deflecting plates) on a cathode ray oscilloscope. The stream of electrons from the cathode of the oscilloscope passes between the paired horizontal and vertical plates and is deflected in a horizontal or vertical direction, respectively, in proportion to the electromotive force of Lead I and Lead aVF. Upon the luminous screen of the oscilloscope there results a series of loops—a very small rounded P loop, a large ellipsoid QRS loop, and a rounded T loop. These may be observed with the naked eye or photographed, during a single cardiac cycle, for further study. This then is the frontal plane vectorcardiogram.

To complete the spatial vectorcardiogram an anteroposterior component is necessary. This may be plotted against Lead I or any other lead whose axis is more or less parallel to Lead I to present a horizontal (transverse) plane vectorcardiogram. Similarly the anteroposterior axis may be plotted against any lead with a vertical axis, such as Lead aVF, to record a sagittal plane vectorcardiogram. There is as yet no universal agreement on the best method of recording a spatial vectorcardiogram—a tetrahedron, a cube, a double cube, or, as more recently suggested, various multiple pole electrodes. Nevertheless all methods give loops that are quite similar in most instances. While it is recognized that any technique that is employed at present may eventually be supplanted by another, the cubic system of Grishman and Scherlis has arbitrarily been chosen. According to this method the electrical forces produced in the heart and reflected through the torso are recorded by means of three bipolar orthogonal (mutually perpendicular) chest leads.

The following exposition attempts a presentation of the general theoretical concepts underlying vectorcardiography. For technical details the reader is referred to the texts of Grishman and Scherlis or Burch. As derived from the cubic arrangement, the normal vectorcardiogram has the following characteristics: In the horizontal plane (H) the loop (Figs. 14 and 15), as viewed from the head of the patient, begins anteriorly and toward the patient's right, then swings counterclockwise and completes an ellipsoid course, terminating at the starting point. In the sagittal plane (S) the loop, as viewed from the patient's right side, starts anteriorly, rotates clockwise as it moves caudally, and then arches posteriorly to return to the null point. In each of these planes, although there is some anterior salience, the bulk of the loop lies posterior to the frontal plane in adults. In the frontal plane (*F*) the loop in general occupies the quadrant between 0 and 90 degrees. When it lies between 0 and 30 degrees it generally takes a counterclockwise course as viewed from the front of the patient. When it lies between 60 and 90 degrees it takes a clockwise course. When it lies between 30 and 60 degrees it may take either a clockwise or a counterclockwise direction. Individual loops need not adhere rigidly to the description just given, for there may be a certain degree of overlap. In this plane the loop may be "open" or it may assume a slender "figure-of-eight" pattern.

The true spatial vector loop has a smooth, full, rounded course and, as reconstructed in three-dimensional space from these projections, its trajectory has a distinct tendency to fall in or near a single plane. The speed of movement of the loop is judged by the distance between individual interrupting time markings. When the loop is moving rapidly the time markers are further apart and appear as streaks; when it is moving slowly they lie close together and appear as closely bunched dots. The direction of the loop is indicated by the use of the "tear-drop" technique. In the illustrations used in this text, the narrowed end of the tear drop points in the direction toward which the loop is moving. The dots are normally bunched more closely together at the origin and

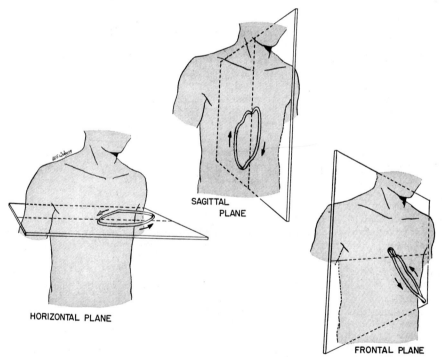

FIG. 14.   *Projections of Spatial Vectorcardiogram upon the Three Planes of the Torso.* The vector normally starts anteriorly and rightward in the horizontal and sagittal planes and has moderate anterior salience but its bulk lies posterior to the null point. The loops shown here were drawn from those actually recorded with the cathode ray oscilloscope (Fig. 15).

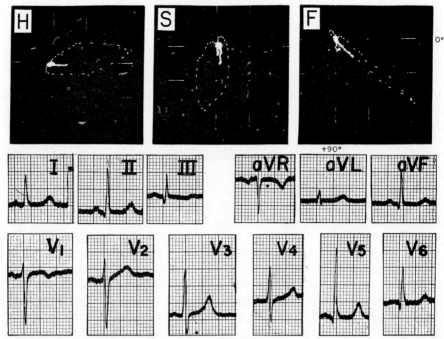

FIG. 15.   *Normal Vectorcardiogram with Electrocardiogram Recorded Same Day.*
In the horizontal plane loops (*H*) illustrated in this book the top of the figure corresponds to the back of the patient's chest and the bottom of the figure to the front
of the chest, the right of the figure to the patient's left side and the left of the figure
to the patient's right side. In the sagittal plane loops (*S*) throughout, the top of the
figure corresponds to the patient's head, the bottom of the figure to the patient's
feet. The right of the figure corresponds to the front of the patient's chest, and the
left of the figure to the back of the chest. In the frontal plane loops (*F*) illustrated
the top of the figure corresponds to the patient's head, the bottom of the figure to
the patient's feet, the left side of the figure to the patient's right side, and the right
side of the figure to the patient's left side. In the horizontal plane (*H*) the loop starts
in an anterior and rightward direction then swings counterclockwise. The greater
part of the loop lies posterior to the null point. In the sagittal plane the loop starts
superiorly or anteriorly and rotates clockwise to finish at the null point. In the frontal
plane (*F*) the loop is generally located in the lower left quadrant, generally rotating
clockwise when located between plus 60 and 90 degrees (more vertical) and generally
counterclockwise when located between zero and plus 30 degrees (more horizontal).
Theoretically and ideally the electrocardiographic appearance of the extremity leads
(I, II, III, aVR, aVL, and aVF) can be predicted from the frontal plane vectorcardiogram, that of the precordial leads (V₁ to V₆) from the horizontal plane vectorcardiogram, and the configuration of the esophageal leads from the sagittal plane vectorcardiogram, and vice versa, but this is not always precisely true. The narrowed end
of the tear drops making up the loop points in the direction toward which the
loop is moving.

termination of the loop, with a lesser tendency to slowing at the point
of maximum deflection.

Since voltage is a very important ingredient in the vectorcardiographic diagnosis of ventricular hypertrophy, the standardization of the
loop in terms of its amplification or attenuation is of considerable impor-

tance. In adults maximum QRS potential difference values greater than about 1.0 mv. are usually associated with left ventricular hypertrophy. With the electrode system described most normal adults achieve maximum spatial QRS potential differences of 0.5 to 1.0 mv.

Ventricular Hypertrophy

The height of the complexes in the three conventional leads is determined in part by the electrical axis of the heart. Ordinarily R waves are highest in Lead II and the sum of the R waves in Leads I and III is approximately equal to that in Lead II. Since the three conventional leads represent the sides of the Einthoven triangle the magnitude of the QRS complex in two of the three conventional leads represents the projection of a "mean electrical axis of the heart" upon these sides of the Einthoven triangle. From the magnitude of these deflections we can calculate the direction and magnitude of the mean electrical axis which must produce them. We arrive then at a vector quantity which has magnitude and direction. Although authorities have set somewhat different limits to the range of normality for this vector, most observers agree that the range from 0 to 90 degrees should be considered normal (Fig. 16). All hearts with axes to the left of 0 degrees or thereabout are considered to show left axis deviation and all those to the right of 90 degrees to show right axis deviation (Fig. 17). Generally when the highest upward deflection (R wave) occurs in Lead I and the lowest downward deflection (S wave) in Lead III it denotes left axis deviation. If the changes are reversed and the lowest downward wave is in Lead I and the highest upward deflection is in Lead III, right axis deviation is indicated. In a majority of cases leftward deviation of the axis is associated with left ventricular hypertrophy, and rightward deviation of the axis with right ventricular hypertrophy. However, as was appreciated early in the development of electrocardiography by Einthoven himself, the electrical axis might lie outside of the so-called normal range in the absence of organic heart disease as a result of abnormal positions of the heart, being pushed to either one side of the chest or the other by fluid in the pleura, by a high diaphragm, or by a malformation of the thoracic cage. In rare cases left ventricular hypertrophy has even been found at postmortem examination in individuals whose electrocardiograms showed right axis deviation during life. Left axis deviation moreover can often be made to disappear by having the patient take a deep breath (Fig. 18). With the descent of the diaphragm the deep S in Lead III may diminish in size and even give way to an upright R wave. It may be concluded, then, that a statement regarding the mean electrical axis must be considered inconclusive evidence for ventricular hypertrophy. Therefore, since the mean electrical axis is not decisive, its calculation is not recommended as a routine in clinical electrocardiography. Recognizing this limitation, however, it seems worth while to report left or right axis deviation when the electrocardiogram is otherwise normal.

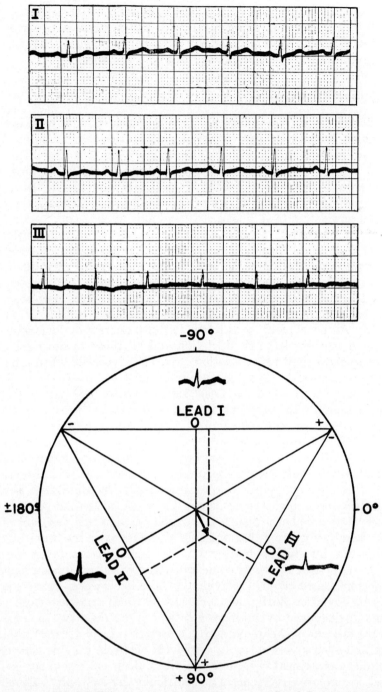

FIG. 16.   *Normal Electrical Axis.* The R wave in Lead I measures 4 millimeters, the S wave 1 millimeter. The net deflection in Lead I is plus 3 millimeters.
The R wave in Lead III measures 4.5 millimeters. Perpendiculars dropped from the
positive side of the Lead I side of the Einthoven triangle and from the positive side
of the Lead III side of the Einthoven triangle meet at the tip of the arrow. This
point is within the normal range of electrical axes (zero to plus 90 degrees).

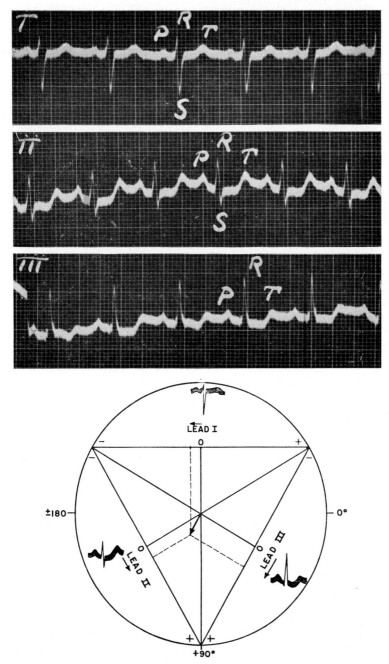

FIG. 17.   *Right Axis Deviation.*   Note that the highest upward wave (R) of the initial ventricular deflection is in Lead III and the lowest downward wave (S) is in Lead I. The projection of the QRS complex is on the negative half of the Lead I side of the Einthoven triangle and on the positive half of the Lead III side. Perpendiculars to these projections intersect in the left lower quadrant of the triangle between plus 90 and plus 180 degrees. This corresponds to right axis deviation. This patient had mitral stenosis.

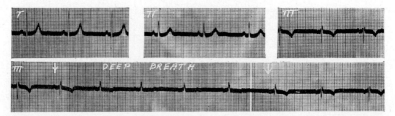

FIG. 18.   *Effect of Deep Breath on Left Axis Deviation.*   The patient was a woman 45 years old, with a normal heart. Note disappearance of S_3 and disappearance of inverted T_3 with deep inspiration.

By use of unipolar extremity and chest leads, however, it is possible readily to separate the effects of the position of the heart from those due to ventricular hypertrophy. In most cases the electrical position of the heart can easily be determined by comparison of the potentials at the left shoulder and leg and those at V_1 and V_2 and at V_5 and V_6 in the manner previously described. In general, hearts in a horizontal or semihorizontal position show left axis deviation and hearts in a vertical or semivertical position show right axis deviation.

LEFT VENTRICULAR HYPERTROPHY

In classic left ventricular hypertrophy the R waves are characteristically very tall over the left ventricle (usually in Leads V_5 and V_6); a small, narrow Q wave is present in one or more of these leads, especially in one facing directly upon the left side of the septum; the RS-T segment is depressed and the T wave inverted in all or some of the leads in which tall R waves are inscribed (Figs. 19 to 22, and 24). As pointed out above it may be necessary to record additional leads to the left of Lead V_6 in order to record true left ventricular potentials. Corresponding to these changes over the left ventricle smaller R waves, deeper S waves, reciprocal elevation of the RS-T segment, and upright T waves may develop over the right ventricle (Leads V_1 and V_2), but these changes are not always present.

If the left ventricle is in relation to the left shoulder, similar potentials will be manifested at Lead aVL and, since Lead aVL contributes to Lead I in a positive way, in Lead I as well. In fact at times, when true left ventricular potentials are not transmitted to the usual precordial points, the diagnosis of left ventricular hypertrophy may be made on the basis of these changes at the left shoulder. The duration of the QRS complex, which should be measured in the conventional leads, is apt to be increased to 0.09–0.11 second. A duration of 0.12 second or more is more likely to be due to a delay or block in one of the branches of the bundle of His. Corresponding to the slight prolongation of the QRS complex there is a greater than normal delay in the timing of the intrinsicoid deflection over the left ventricle, the latter being inscribed 0.04 to 0.05 second later over the left than over the right ventricle. The increased height and delayed peak of the R wave are due to the greater thickness of the left ventricle, the impulse reaching the surface of the left ventricle after a greater than normal delay. It must be remembered, however, as mentioned above, that the voltage of the R wave is a function of other factors than ventricular thickness. The proximity of the heart to the precordial electrode, certain chemical changes such as

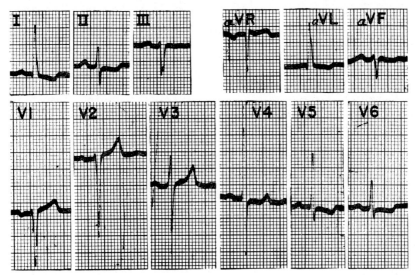

FIG. 19.   *Left Ventricular Hypertrophy.*   Heart in horizontal electrical position. Left axis deviation. Tall R waves in Leads V_4 and V_5, depressed RS-T segments and inverted T waves in Leads V_5 and V_6 indicate left ventricular hypertrophy. Since Lead aVL resembles Leads V_5 and V_6 while Lead aVF resembles Leads V_1 and V_2, the heart is in the horizontal electrical position.

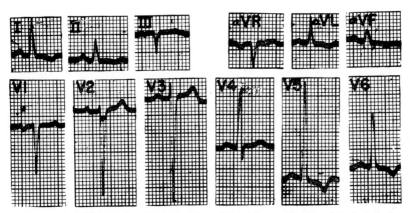

FIG. 20.   *Left Ventricular Hypertrophy.*   Heart in semihorizontal electrical position. The deep S waves in Leads V_2 and V_3, tall R waves in Leads V_4 to V_6, and depressed RS-T segments and inverted T waves in Leads V_5 and V_6 establish the diagnosis of left ventricular hypertrophy. The intrinsicoid deflection in Lead V_6 is measured at 0.04 second. The ventricular complex in Lead aVL resembles those in Leads V_5 and V_6, while QRS in Lead aVF is of low voltage, indicating a semihorizontal electrical position of the heart.

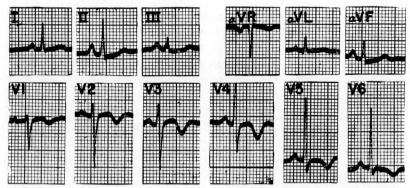

FIG. 21.   *Left Ventricular Hypertrophy.*   Heart in intermediate electrical position. Superimposed T wave changes. The patient was a 63-year-old woman with long-standing hypertension, who was admitted because of recent angina pectoris. The tall R waves and inverted T waves over the left ventricle indicate left ventricular hypertrophy. The QRS complexes in Leads aVL and aVF resemble those in Leads V_5 and V_6. The heart is therefore in the intermediate electrical position. With left ventricular hypertrophy one would expect upright T waves in Leads V_1 to V_3 reciprocal to the inverted T waves in Leads V_4 to V_6. The fact that the T wave in Leads V_1 to V_3 is inverted instead suggested anterior myocardial ischemia or infarction. Subsequent electrocardiographic observation (see Fig. 170) showed waxing of these T wave changes, confirming this impression.

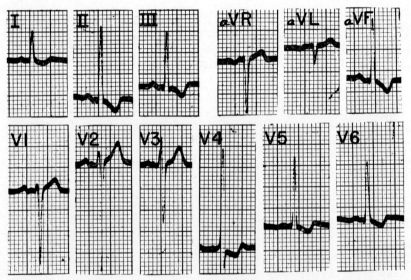

FIG. 22.   *Left Ventricular Hypertrophy.*   Heart in semivertical electrical position. The electrical axis is "normal." Tall R waves, depressed RS-T segments, and inverted T waves in Leads V_4 to V_6 indicate left ventricular hypertrophy. Note reciprocal elevation of RS-T segments in Leads V_1 to V_3, a common accompanying finding not diagnostic of anterior myocardial infarction. Lead aVF resembles Leads V_4 to V_6, while Lead aVL shows a low voltage QRS complex. This places the heart in a semivertical electrical position. Unless the precordial leads were examined one could readily mistake this for right ventricular hypertrophy.

the serum potassium level, and perhaps the state of cardiac compensation also have their effect upon R wave voltage.

The vectorcardiogram in left ventricular hypertrophy (Fig. 23) resembles the normal vectorcardiogram in that the time markings are dashes rather than dots in at least two of the three planes (no significant conduction delay, but often with some slowing in the outgoing limb), in that its initial portion swings anteriorly (as seen in the horizontal and sagittal planes) and to the right (as seen in the horizontal and frontal planes), and in that the loop pursues a counterclockwise course as observed in the horizontal and frontal planes. The initial rightward and anterior course accounts for the small R wave which may be seen in the right precordial leads of the electrocardiogram and for the small Q wave over the left precordium. The loop in left ventricular hypertrophy differs from the normal loop in that it is generally directed in a more posterior direction, namely between −30 and −50 degrees in the horizontal and between −120 and −170 degrees in the sagittal plane. It is this slanting off of the loop posteriorly which accounts for the low to absent R waves over the right precordium in the electrocardiogram

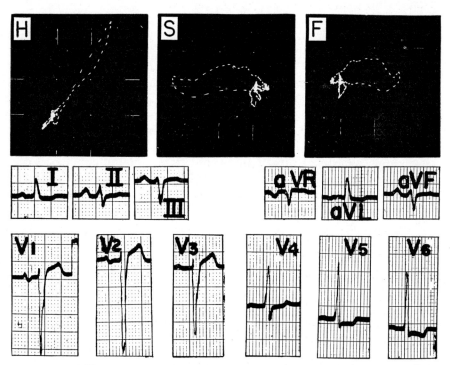

FIG. 23.   *Vectorcardiogram and Electrocardiogram in Left Ventricular Hypertrophy.*   Standardization 6 cm. deflection per millivolt. The loop has an abnormal posterior position in the horizontal and sagittal planes accounting for the lack of a respectable R wave in Lead V₃. In this particular instance the loop shows a figure-of-eight configuration in the horizontal plane. Since the loop starts slightly anteriorly and to the right in this plane it is likely that a small Q wave would be recorded if tracings were recorded further to the left of Lead V₆.

of many individuals with left ventricular hypertrophy. The vectorcardiogram in left ventricular hypertrophy also differs from the normal vectorcardiogram in the greater amplitude of the loop. Because of its large voltage it is generally necessary to cut down considerably in its amplitude in order to accommodate the entire loop in the usual vectorcardiographic field. The QRS loop may not be "closed" prior to the beginning of the T loop. This corresponds to the RS-T shift characteristic of the electrocardiogram of left ventricular hypertrophy. Finally, the principal T wave axis, as observed in at least two planes, lies almost as much as 180 degrees from the principal QRS axis. This in general corresponds to the T wave inversion observed in the electrocardiogram. It should be clear therefore that the vectorcardiographic and electrocardiographic criteria for left ventricular hypertrophy are identical. These consist of changes in the voltage of QRS, occasionally in delay in the ventricular activation time (delayed "intrinsicoid deflection"), shifts in the RS-T segment, and inversion of the T waves. One may demand that all four categories of change be present or be satisfied with only one, e.g., QRS voltage changes. It does seem, however, that the vectorcardiogram gives a much more satisfactory total picture of the orientation of the electrical events studied. But there are as yet no extensive or thoroughgoing anatomic studies available which would designate one of these techniques as superior to the other in the detection of left ventricular hypertrophy.

Let us now examine the concept of the "intrinsicoid deflection" in terms of the vectorcardiogram. The point of the loop furthest removed from its point of origin would correspond with what has been called the "intrinsicoid deflection." This point, where the direction of the loop changes, need not coincide with a similar farthest point in another plane. This emphasizes the arbitrary nature of this designation and raises considerable doubt about its true meaning. Many loops from patients with indubitable left ventricular hypertrophy reach this apogee without more than normal delay. In fact, electrocardiographic studies have shown that significant delay of the intrinsicoid deflection occurs in only about 30 per cent of cases of left ventricular hypertrophy. We have not insisted, therefore, that there must be a delayed "intrinsicoid deflection" to warrant this diagnosis.

Experience has shown that a diagnosis of left ventricular hypertrophy made upon the basis of the electrocardiographic criteria enumerated above was invariably confirmed at postmortem examination, but the additional presence of right ventricular hypertrophy or old myocardial infarction was usually missed. When the autopsy material was considered from the opposite point of view, examining the electrocardiographic findings of all individuals showing left ventricular hypertrophy at autopsy, it was found that two thirds of them showed characteristic electrocardiographic changes of the type described above. Abnormal nonspecific changes were recorded in the electrocardiograms of the remaining one third, but a few showed bundle branch block, and in rare

instances normal electrocardiograms were recorded. In an attempt to
make a correct anatomic diagnosis in some of the cases that would
otherwise be missed the inclination in many quarters has been to broaden
the criteria upon which the diagnosis may be hazarded. Thus some
authorities feel that if the QRS complex measures 0.09 second in duration, if the R waves are exceptionally tall and wide in some of the conventional leads or in Leads V_4 through V_6, if the S waves are exceptionally wide and deep over the right ventricle or in all of the conventional
leads, even if accompanying RS-T segment and T wave changes are
absent, or if certain prescribed combinations of these findings are present,
the diagnosis of left ventricular hypertrophy may be ventured.* However, experience has shown that, while the number of positive diagnoses
is thus increased, the number of false positives is also increased. A state-

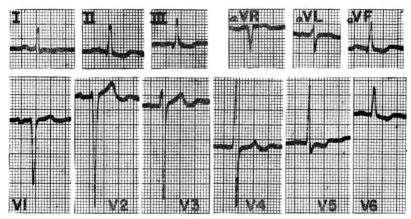

FIG. 24.   *Left Ventricular Hypertrophy.*   Heart in vertical electrical position.
Normal electrical axis. The totality of changes in Leads V_4 to V_6, namely tall R
waves in Leads V_4 and V_5, and depressed RS-T segments and inverted T waves in
Leads V_5 and V_6, indicate left ventricular hypertrophy. Note that deep S waves,
elevated RS-T segments, and upright T waves in Leads V_1 to V_3 mirror the changes
in the left ventricle. In doubtful cases many authorities take these changes into consideration in making the diagnosis of left ventricular hypertrophy. It should be remembered that depth of S waves or height of R waves may be functions of the proximity of the heart to the precordium as well as of ventricular thickness. The identity
of Lead aVF with Lead V_6 and the resemblance of Lead aVL to Lead V_1 would place
this heart in a vertical electrical position. The mere existence of left ventricular
hypertrophy in a heart which is in the vertical position, as illustrated here, raises
the question of combined ventricular hypertrophy.

---

* The following is a partial list of various empirical criteria which have been
proposed for the diagnosis of left ventricular hypertrophy:

R_1 plus S_3 > 25 mm.

R_{aVL} > 11 mm., 12 mm., or 13 mm.

R_{aVF} > 19 mm. or 20 mm.

S_{aVR} > 14 mm.

R_{V_5} or R_{V_6} = 24 mm. or 26 mm. R_{V_5}
= 33 mm. or more.

S_{V_1} plus R_{V_5} or R_{V_6} > 35 mm.

S_{V_1} = 24 mm. or more.

R_{V_6} > R_{V_5} with no S in either V_6 or V_5.

T_{aVL} < 10% R_{aVL} when R = 10 mm.
or more.

R:T ratio V_5 or V_6 = 10 or more.

Delayed intrinsicoid deflection V_5 or V_6
(0.05 sec. or more).

Upright T_{aVR}.

ment that these secondary criteria are suggestive of or consistent with left ventricular hypertrophy would perhaps be the wiser policy.

A straightening and lengthening of the S-T segment, while the T wave remains normal or slightly decreased in amplitude and the Q-T interval remains within normal limits, may serve as a clue to early or incipient left ventricular hypertrophy.

THE VENTRICULAR GRADIENT, PRIMARY AND SECONDARY T WAVE CHANGES

At this point a theoretical digression into the concept of the ventricular gradient will be most helpful. If an ideal cell or muscle strip of the type described in Figure 3, possessing uniform physiologic properties, is stimulated, a wave of depolarization sweeps over this cell or muscle strip from the point of stimulation. If an electrode toward which this impulse moves is connected to the positive pole of a galvanometer and through the galvanometer to another electrode of negligible potential, the movement of the impulse toward the electrode will be recorded at the galvanometer as an upward deflection. This deflection has *large magnitude* and *short duration*. The identity of this deflection with the QRS complex of the electrocardiogram will be apparent. Now, after a pause, the local changes in permeability at the surface of the cell or fiber tend to disappear; the original dielectric effect at the surface is then restored in the same order in which it disappeared. This change occurs much more slowly and the magnitude of the changes reappearing at the cell from moment to moment is much smaller than during the original process of depolarization. The restoration process is referred to as repolarization. Since the electrical changes at the cell surface are now opposite in direction to those which developed during electrical activation of the cell or fiber, the deflection recorded at the galvanometer during this restitution process will have an opposite direction to those initially inscribed. The repolarization process ideally then is one of *lesser magnitude, greater duration*, and *opposite sign* to the depolarization process. Its resemblance to an inverted T wave of the electrocardiogram will be obvious. Since the cell is assumed to be of uniform physiologic properties the area enclosed above this wave must equal that enclosed under the R wave. If the area above this T wave does not exactly equal that under the R wave, or, in other words, if the sum total of the area under the QRS complex and that above the T wave (due regard being had for the signs of these deflections) does not equal zero, then the cell or fiber is not of uniform physiologic properties. This, in a nutshell, is the concept of the ventricular gradient. The existence of a gradient, or difference, indicates local differences in the properties of the cell or fiber. These differences can be the result of differences in the process of depolarization or of repolarization. The latter, however, is much more easily affected than the former by such physical or chemical changes as local cooling, local anoxia, and local intoxication. Only a much more severe grade of injury is capable of altering the depolarization process. This corresponds to the clinical fact that the T wave is much more labile and easily altered than is the QRS complex. The change in the repolarization process is manifested by a greater slowing or delay in the time of recovery in one part of the cell or fiber than in another. Worded differently, there is a local increase in the duration of electrical systole. In the ideal cell or fiber described above, the T wave has an opposite direction to the QRS complex. Physiologists have long been puzzled by the fact that in the human heart the T wave normally has the same direction as the T wave in Leads I and II and those taken over the left ventricle. This must be explained by assuming that in man the physiologic properties of the normal ventricle are not uniform and that there are local differences in the duration of electrical systole. In other words, there is normally a gradient in the human heart.

It will be obvious on the basis of the ventricular gradient concept that T waves may be considered in relation to the QRS complexes preceding them. If the gradient is zero, the area of the T wave may be explained as a necessary consequence of the area of the QRS complex, and the process of repolarization is entirely accounted for by the process of depolarization. In this case the T wave may be considered "secondary" to the QRS complex. Thus if the ventricle is merely activated in a different direction without changing its physiologic characteristics, as in ventricular premature beats or in experimental bundle branch block, secondary T wave changes develop; the gradient is the same in the regular as in the premature or in the aberrant beats. If, on the other hand, the area of the T wave cannot be explained as a necessary consequence of the area of the QRS complex a gradient exists and the T wave shows "primary" changes. Primary T wave changes may be seen in myocardial ischemia, as the result of local chilling of the heart by drinking ice water, in inflammatory diseases of the myocardium, in trichinosis, and in such toxic conditions as diphtheria or emetine poisoning. It is the purpose of the determination of the ventricular gradient to separate these primary T wave changes from the less significant secondary T wave changes.

No attempt will be made here to describe in detail the method of measuring the ventricular gradient. Suffice it to say it consists of measuring the difference of the area of the QRS complex and of the T wave as projected in the frontal plane of the body by appropriate measurements in two of the three conventional leads, preferably recorded simultaneously. Until such time as an accurate practical clinical method of determining the ventricular gradient is available it may be adequate in most cases to judge by inspection and from experience whether the RS-T and T wave changes may or may not be accounted for as consequences secondary to the QRS changes.

"LEFT VENTRICULAR STRAIN"

We have been impressed with the variability of the appearance of the electrocardiograms in hospitalized patients with left ventricular hypertrophy. On one day the R waves might be tall and the corresponding

T waves rather small, on another day there might be characteristic RS-T and T wave changes in addition to tall R waves, on another normal sized R waves with inverted T waves, and, on still another, normal complexes. Of course this does not imply that anatomic hypertrophy was present at one time and not at another. For a variety of reasons, among them this observation that factors other than hypertrophy may affect the resultant electrocardiogram, the designation of "left ventricular strain" has come into rather widespread use, but the exact meaning of the term has varied from one authority to another. The term "ventricular strain" was originally proposed by Barnes in a purely descriptive way at a time when only the three conventional limb leads were being used. He pointed out that in such conditions as hypertensive heart disease and aortic insufficiency, in which the left ventricle bears the brunt of an increased cardiac load, the R wave is tall, the RS-T segment depressed, and the T wave inverted in Lead I while the S wave is deep, the RS-T segment elevated, and the T wave upright in Lead III. Contrariwise he noted that in such conditions as chronic cor pulmonale and certain forms of congenital heart disease, where the right ventricle is overloaded, the S wave is deep, the RS-T segment elevated, and the T wave upright in Lead I, while the R wave is tall, the RS-T segment depressed, and the T wave inverted in Lead III. Since that time there have been many different variations on this original theme. Some consider "strain" to represent the response of a ventricle to a stress, sometimes chemical, sometimes mechanical, and sometimes positional. However, there are certain unwarranted implications in the use of such a term. It might be considered that the hearts of patients with the so-called "left ventricular strain pattern" are near the breaking point, yet experience has shown that this "strain pattern" may persist for twenty or thirty years or even longer. Furthermore, as a matter of experience, the progress of electrocardiography has been impeded in the past because mechanical implications have been drawn from electrical changes; witness the confusion of the T wave with mechanical diastole which persisted for a number of years. It must be conceded that this same criticism can with equal justification be made against the term "left ventricular hypertrophy." It has even been suggested that left ventricular hypertrophy and left ventricular strain are two different concepts and that, whereas hypertrophy produces only high voltage QRS complexes, strain produces only changes in the RS-T segment and the T waves. The validity of this distinction is open to question, but it is possible that this concept may offer a logical approach to the problem of hypertrophy versus strain. It is possible that the determination of the ventricular gradient in these cases might clarify the findings. Thus, if there is no gradient the T wave changes must be secondary and it would not be necessary to assume additional myocardial changes. If, on the other hand, there is a gradient, the T wave changes must be primary and it would be necessary to assume the operation of additional factors, such as myocardial ischemia. One might then conceive of left ventricular hypertrophy with secondary T wave changes and left ventricular hypertrophy with primary T wave changes.

RIGHT VENTRICULAR HYPERTROPHY

In right ventricular hypertrophy (Figs. 25 to 28) leads obtained over the right ventricle (ordinarily V_1 or V_1 and V_2, sometimes V_{3R} or V_{4R}) show an unusually tall R wave which exceeds the S wave in one or more of these same leads. There may or may not be depressed RS-T segments or inverted T waves in these leads. The duration of the QRS complex in the conventional leads is usually normal but may be prolonged to 0.10 second. There is apt to be right axis deviation associated with a vertical position of the heart but this is not invariable. The intrinsicoid deflection is generally delayed over the right ventricle; much more often than not the intrinsicoid deflection is actually inscribed later over the right than over the left ventricle. As the electrode moves further to the left over the precordium the R wave may remain of approximately uniform height or may decrease. In making the decision whether right ventricular hypertrophy is present it is important to be certain that the electrode is to the right of the transitional zone. If, as rarely happens, there is strong counterclockwise rotation of the heart on its longitudinal axis (as viewed from the apex), *left* ventricular potentials may be recorded at positions V_1 and V_2. In such cases R waves which are taller than those usually recorded at these points may be recorded at V_1 and V_2. A smooth unbroken progression in the height of the R wave from V_1 to V_4 can be detected, and at the extreme right position the R wave still exceeds the S wave in magnitude. In such cases it is important to

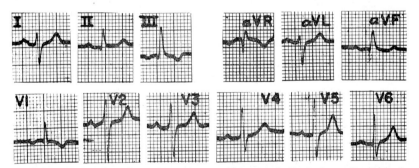

FIG. 25.   *Right Ventricular Hypertrophy; Right Axis Deviation.*   Lead V_1 shows a minute Q wave, a tall R wave, a small S wave, a minimally depressed RS-T segment, and an inverted T wave. In Lead V_2 there is recorded a large S wave exceeding the R wave in magnitude. In Lead V_3 the R and S waves are about equal. As the electrode now moves toward Lead V_5 the R wave increases and the S wave decreases. It is obvious that Lead V_1 is to the right of the transitional zone. Using the criteria enumerated in the text, the position of the heart is generally indeterminate in right ventricular hypertrophy. The patient was a 20-year-old girl in whom a murmur was heard during infancy. At age 10 she had an attack of scarlet fever. Examination during a heart survey when these tracings were taken showed a systolic thrill to the left of the sternum, a harsh grade III systolic murmur in the first and second left interspaces, and a grade II high-pitched systolic murmur at the cardiac apex.

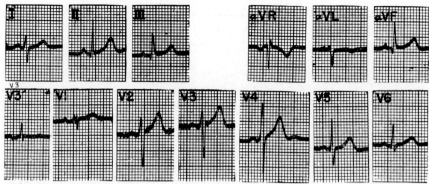

FIG. 26. *Right Ventricular Hypertrophy.* Right ventricular potentials not recorded in usual six precordial leads. The diagnosis of right ventricular hypertrophy is not justified on the basis of changes in Leads V_1 through V_6 but the RR' complex in Lead V_1 suggests that the latter is in relation to the transitional zone and that right ventricular potentials have not yet been recorded. This prompted the recording of an additional lead further to the right at the midclavicular line (Lead V_{3R} or $V_{3'}$); this lead shows a tall R wave and an inconspicuous S wave. This is convincing evidence for right ventricular hypertrophy, assuming accurate placement of the electrode at $V_{3'}$ (V_{3R}).

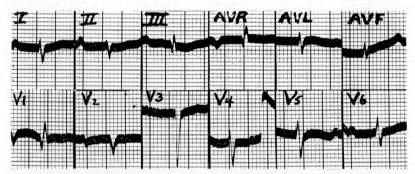

FIG. 27. *Right Ventricular Hypertrophy Simulating Old Anteroseptal Myccardial Infarction ("Chronic Cor Pulmonale").* The patient was a 33-year-old man with lifelong bronchial asthma who developed "right-sided" congestive heart failure. The tracings show low voltage in the conventional leads and a broad Q wave and relatively prominent R wave in Lead V_1. First degree heart block is present. The R wave is absent in Lead V_2 and "embryonic" in Lead V_3. The Q wave in Leads V_1 and V_2 might mislead the electrocardiographer into the diagnosis of anteroseptal infarction, but in right ventricular hypertrophy a Q wave may be present over the right ventricle and the R wave may decrease as the transitional zone is approached. Postmortem examination showed a thick right ventricle (0.7 cm.), pulmonary emphysema, peripheral congestion but no myocardial infarct.

take additional leads to the right of V_1 to record true right ventricular potentials. The change in position from the left ventricle to a hypertrophied right ventricle may be signaled in an electrode moving from the left to the right precordium by an increase in the height of the R wave after it has decreased or by a changing relationship between the R and S complexes in the leads concerned: as the electrode moves toward the right the ratio of the R to the S wave first decreases; after it crosses the septum onto a hypertrophied right ventricle the R wave again becomes taller than the S wave (Fig. 26). A considerable number of patients with right ventricular hypertrophy show a small initial downward deflection which we arbitrarily call a Q wave. This change, in association with an R wave which decreases as the electrode moves from the right to the left precordium, could easily mislead the electrocardiographer into making the diagnosis of anterior myocardial infarction (Fig. 27). If this lead showing the initial downward deflection is recorded simultaneously with other leads it can be shown that this deflection does not correspond to the very beginning of ventricular activation. It probably is actually an S wave preceded by an isoelectric R wave which is not recorded in that particular lead. The force responsible for this "Q wave" is probably developed in the apical pole of the right ventricle, the endocardial aspect of which is faced by the electrode. It is important, then, to avoid the diagnosis of anterior myocardial infarction in association with right ventricular hypertrophy on the basis of an initial downward deflection.

In our experience the diagnosis of right ventricular hypertrophy made on the above criteria has invariably been substantiated at autopsy. In fact, right ventricular hypertrophy is generally apt to be detected by electrocardiography before roentgen ray evidence for right ventricular hypertrophy is present. There are a few cases of right ventricular hypertrophy, as verified at postmortem examination, in which the above described electrocardiographic findings were not present during life. Some

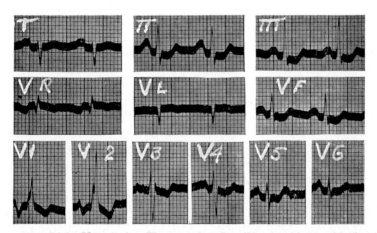

FIG. 28. *Right Ventricular Hypertrophy, Possibly Combined with Incomplete Right Bundle Branch Block; Mitral Stenosis; Right Axis Deviation.* The upper set shows the three standard leads with right axis deviation. The middle set shows the three (unaugmented) unipolar limb leads. The lowest set shows the six unipolar chest leads. The heart is in a semivertical position because Lead VF resembles Leads V_5 and V_6, and the QRS complex of Lead VL is small. There are RR' complexes in Leads V_1 and V_2. The R' waves are tall and broad; the T waves are inverted in Leads V_1 and V_2, and R' decreases from Lead V_2 to V_5. The intrinsicoid deflection is later over the right than over the left ventricle. The patient was a thin woman, 36 years of age, with definite signs of mitral stenosis.

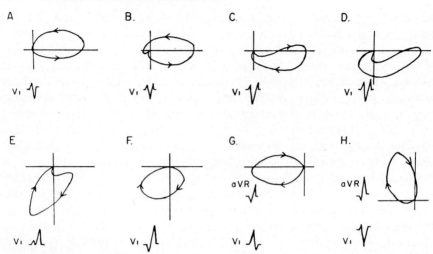

FIG. 29.   *Panorama of Horizontal Plane Loops in Right Ventricular Hypertrophy.*
Associated right precordial lead is shown with each figure. *A*, normal horizontal plane
loop for comparison. *B*, slight fullness of anterior salience. In *B* through *E*, rSr′,
rSR′, or rR′ complexes are inscribed in this plane in the absence of complete or incomplete right bundle branch block. *C*, clockwise rotation of horizontal plane loop with
very little posterior development. *D*, same with minimal posterior development.
E, predominant anterior and rightward development of loop preceded by small initial
counterclockwise segment. *F*, clockwise rotation of loop toward right precordium
only. *G*, same toward both right precordium and right shoulder. *H*, same toward
right shoulder, not toward right precordium.

of these show right bundle branch block. It has been suggested that in
right bundle branch block the presence of a very tall R′ over the right
ventricle might be a clue to the additional presence of right ventricular
hypertrophy. However, tracings of this sort have been induced by catheterization of the right ventricle in a subject with a normal heart, and
in another patient with the same type of electrocardiogram the right
ventricle was of normal thickness at autopsy. This finding of a prominent
R′ in right bundle branch block, then, is not conclusive evidence for
right ventricular hypertrophy. Finally, the empirical observation should
be mentioned that *persistent* incomplete right bundle branch block may
be considered presumptive evidence of right ventricular hypertrophy.
The significance of this observation has not yet been clarified.

The existence of right ventricular hypertrophy is usually seen most
readily in the *horizontal plane vectorcardiogram.* There is no single pathognomonic vectorcardiographic appearance characterizing this condition.
Instead, there is observed a spectrum of changes apparently proportional
to the grade of severity of ventricular enlargement. As observed in the
horizontal plane, the loop ordinarily begins in a normal anterior and
rightward direction (Fig. 29, *B, C, D, E, G, H*), but in many it may
move immediately leftward (Fig. 29, *F*). Which of these two possible
initial movements the loop takes determines whether the electrocardiogram inscribes an initial R or Q wave over the right precordium. The

loop then swings to a greater or lesser degree counterclockwise and to the left; in general, the more pronounced the hypertrophy, the less pronounced the leftward counterclockwise swing. In most cases, instead of continuing to arch in a counterclockwise direction, the loop now reverses its field (Fig. 29, D, E). Its returning loop turns slightly or far anterior to the outgoing loop and continues with unabated speed in a clockwise direction to return to the null point. In some cases, apparently with only slight degrees of hypertrophy, the loop continues its original counterclockwise rotation but fails to show any significant posterior development; in such cases the anterior and rightward "electrical pull" of the hypertrophied right ventricle simply has the effect of causing the returning loop to pass anterior rather than posterior to the null point before returning to the point of origin (Fig. 29, C). With severe right ventricular hypertrophy, the loop may start immediately in a clockwise anterior direction (Fig. 29, F, G, H, and Fig. 30). With extreme hypertrophy the loop may rotate, principally or entirely, superiorly toward the right

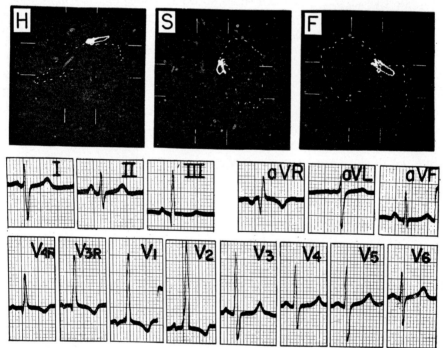

FIG. 30.   *Vectorcardiogram and Electrocardiogram in Right Ventricular Hypertrophy.* In the horizontal plane (H) of the vectorcardiogram the loop pursues a large clockwise rather than the normal counterclockwise course. In the sagittal plane (S) the loop starts in a normal clockwise direction but soon changes to a counterclockwise course. The entire loop is anterior to the plane of the null point. In the frontal plane (F) the loop is fanned out and takes a clockwise direction. The abnormal rightward and anterior development of the loop accounts for the large R waves in Leads aVR and V_{4R} through V_4, the deep S waves in Leads aVL, I, and V_3 through V_6. The Q waves over the right precordium result from the initial clockwise rotation of the loop in the horizontal plane.

shoulder (Fig. 29, G, H). In these instances tall R waves are recorded in Lead aVR. Some of these patients show prominent R waves over the right precordium (Fig. 29, G, Fig. 30). In rare instances, however, these prominent R waves are recorded only in Lead aVR while prominent S waves are recorded over the entire precordium, including Leads V_{3R} and V_{4R} (Fig. 29, H); in this latter circumstance the vectorcardiogram shows right ventricular hypertrophy whereas the electrocardiogram, as judged by the usual criteria, does not. In these instances tall R waves in Lead aVR or deep S waves in Leads V_5 and V_6 may furnish a clue to the diagnosis. In uncomplicated right ventricular hypertrophy there is no terminal slowing of the QRS loop. This point presumably distinguishes pure right ventricular hypertrophy from complete or incomplete right bundle branch block. Pronounced terminal slowing of a horizontal plane loop otherwise corresponding to right ventricular hypertrophy warrants the additional assumption of right bundle branch block, complete or incomplete.

In the *sagittal plane* the loop shows varying degrees of anterior development. The vectorcardiogram may vary all the way from one showing an entirely normal clockwise course with merely a rather full anterior salience, to one which, starting a clockwise course, reverses its direction at varying points from its origin and continues in a counterclockwise arc to return unslowed to the null point (Fig. 30). In some cases the loop takes such a counterclockwise course from its very origin. In the *frontal plane* the loop is generally full and rounded and runs a clockwise course. However, in those cases with a superior and rightward orientation of the vectorcardiogram the frontal plane loop may rotate in either a clockwise or a counterclockwise direction.

rSr' complexes may be inscribed over the right precordium in the absence of right ventricular hypertrophy. Such complexes may be recorded with a normal loop or with right bundle branch block as well. This differentiation can most easily be made with the help of the vectorcardiogram. In the normal heart the loop pursues a counterclockwise course in the horizontal plane; there is generally no terminal slowing, but in young individuals there may be slight to moderate slowing in a terminal rightward appendage. In right bundle branch block, complete or incomplete, the terminal slowing usually produces an appendage which is larger and directed more anteriorly. In right ventricular hypertrophy the loop is generally full anteriorly and in most cases sooner or later assumes a clockwise course as observed in the horizontal plane. In any of these three conditions the electrocardiographic appearance may be similar. Incomplete right bundle branch block is most often confused with mild right ventricular hypertrophy, not with the severe variety.

COMBINED VENTRICULAR HYPERTROPHY

In most cases of combined ventricular hypertrophy the electrocardiogram shows only the features characteristic of left ventricular hypertrophy. In rare instances, however, it is possible to detect electrocardiographic evidence of enlargement of both the right and left ventricles in the same patient (Fig. 31). In these cases the tall R wave decreases as the transitional zone is approached, then reappears or increases after the transitional zone has been crossed. In many such cases it may be extremely difficult to decide whether one is tapping the potentials of only one ventricle or of both. The remaining cases of proven combined ventricular hypertrophy are apt to show nonspecific abnormal electrocardiograms, right bundle branch block, or evidences of such complicating diseases as myocardial infarction. It seems, then, that combined ventricular hypertrophy is rarely detectable in the electrocardiogram but that the accuracy of this diagnosis is improved if one records with certainty both right and left ventricular potentials.

The mere demonstration of evidence for left ventricular hypertrophy in a heart which lies in a vertical electrical position suggests the existence of combined ventricular hypertrophy. All other factors being equal, one would expect that enlargement of the left ventricle should rotate the heart into a horizontal electrical position. The detection, instead, of an electrically vertical heart therefore suggests the operation of factors having the effect of overbalancing this tendency. The most common of these is probably right ventricular hypertrophy. This is what might be called "vectorcardiographic reasoning." As might be anticipated, this type of analysis is more rewarding than the electrocardiographic approach in the diagnosis of combined ventricular hypertrophy. Two

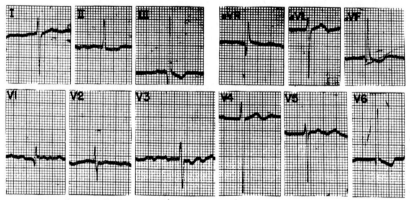

FIG. 31. *Combined Ventricular Hypertrophy*. The patient was a 50-year-old woman with rheumatic heart disease, mitral stenosis, aortic insufficiency, auricular fibrillation, and congestive heart failure. Lead V_1 showed a Q wave followed by an R wave which was larger than the Q wave. An S wave appeared in Lead V_2 and, as the electrode was moved to Lead V_5, increased progressively in relation to the R wave. In Lead V_6 a tall R wave and an inverted T wave indicate left ventricular hypertrophy. The transitional zone was located between Leads V_5 and V_6. On this basis the diagnosis of combined ventricular hypertrophy was made on repeated occasions. At postmortem examination there was hypertrophy of both ventricles, especially the left. Combined ventricular hypertrophy generally cannot be diagnosed electrocardiographically, the tracings usually showing left ventricular hypertrophy alone.

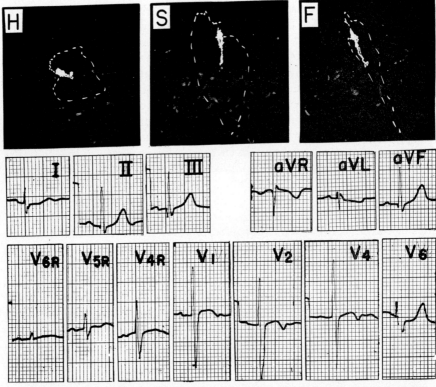

FIG. 32. *Combined Ventricular Hypertrophy.* "Pie-plate" horizontal plane loop in combined ventricular hypertrophy shown with electrocardiogram recorded immediately after vectorcardiogram. An electrical "tug-of-war" between the enlarged right and left ventricles produces an anteroposterior dimension of the horizontal plane loop which is greater than its lateral dimension. The R wave decreases from Lead V_1 to Lead V_2 then increases from V_2 to V_6. This patient had an interventricular septal defect.

distinctive horizontal plane loops are quite suggestive of combined ventricular hypertrophy. One is the *"pie-plate"* pattern; the loop in the horizontal plane has a rather full anterior salience and rotates counterclockwise with an approximately equal posterior development. The anteroposterior dimension of this loop is larger than its lateral measurement (Fig. 32). This loop might be thought of as expressing the early strong anterior "pull" of the hypertrophied right ventricle and the late posterior pull of the hypertrophied left ventricle. This type corresponds to the "Katz-Wachtel" phenomenon of clinical electrocardiography with very large deflections in the precordial leads. A similar balance between the two enlarged ventricles is occasionally expressed in a *thin horizontal plane loop.* This loop is of large amplitude and moves leftward but generally does not point as far posteriorly as the loop of left ventricular hypertrophy. Its greatest long dimension is at least six times that of its maximal breadth (Fig. 33).

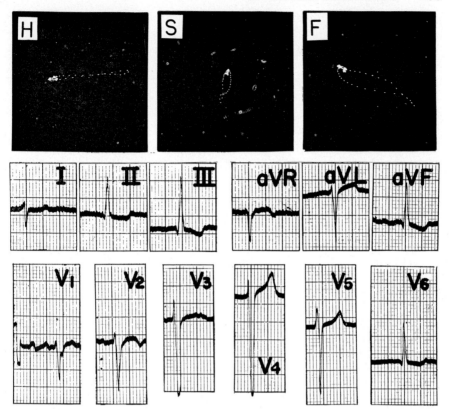

FIG. 33.   *Combined Ventricular Hypertrophy.*   "Thin horizontal plane" loop of combined ventricular hypertrophy and associated electrocardiogram. There are large QRS complexes in the mid-precordial zone between Leads V_2 and V_6 but there is no empirical electrocardiographic evidence for ventricular hypertrophy. The heart is in a vertical electrical position. The greatest length of the needle-shaped horizontal plane is at least six times its greatest width. The patient had rheumatic mitral regurgitation and auricular fibrillation.

CLINICAL IMPLICATIONS OF THE ELECTROCARDIOGRAM IN VENTRICULAR HYPERTROPHY

At birth the right ventricle is larger than the left, and only after several months is the reversed relationship established. On the other hand, during the normal aging process the left ventricle often becomes slightly enlarged even when, from a practical point of view, it is to be regarded as normal. In old age, furthermore, as a result of the increased tortuosity of the aorta, the base of the heart is apt to be pushed down and the apex up so that the heart comes to lie in a more horizontal position. A heart must not be diagnosed as abnormal simply on the basis of axis deviation to the right or left. There are occasions, however, when the electrocardiographic finding of enlargement of one ventricle or the other aids considerably in the differential diagnosis. I recall seeing a war veteran who was supposed to have aortic valvular disease because there were a systolic and diastolic murmur and a systolic thrill at the base of the heart. The electrocardiogram showed right ventricular hypertrophy. This led to an entirely different interpretation, because, if hypertrophy develops in aortic valvular disease, it is expected to involve the left rather than the right ventricle. More careful examination, including x-ray of the heart, showed that the condition was some form of congenital heart disease, which is often associated with right ventricular hypertrophy. Similarly, an elderly woman had congestive heart failure, hypertension, and auricular fibrillation. The diagnosis was nonvalvular heart disease because no diastolic murmur was heard. The electrocardiograms showed well-marked right ventricular hypertrophy. This threw some doubt on the diagnosis because left ventricular hypertrophy should have been found with a senile heart and hypertension. Mitral stenosis was suspected despite the absence of a diastolic murmur, for this could account for the right ventricular enlargement. An x-ray showed a prominent left auricle and later, on postmortem examination, a fish-mouth mitral stenosis was found.

Axis deviation or ventricular hypertrophy does not always develop according to expectations. Disease of the aortic valve and hypertension should produce their effects on the left ventricle by increasing its work. Similarly mitral stenosis, congenital disease of the pulmonary valve, or pure emphysema should increase the burden on the right ventricle by increasing the pressure in the pulmonary system. Although these predicted results generally occur, there are some exceptions that are difficult to explain. Before the role of the position of the heart in producing axis deviation was clearly appreciated, axis deviation and ventricular hypertrophy were often confused. This probably explains many of the discrepancies of the past. Even when this possible source of error is eliminated, there are still some cases in which the increased load is borne by the left ventricle and in which prolonged passive congestion in the lungs with increased pulmonary pressure results in hypertrophy of the right ventricle. The whole heart in this way may be involved in the burden that one might have thought would be limited to one chamber. Such data can, at times, be useful in directing attention to conditions that might otherwise be overlooked. It is particularly helpful in appraising valvular conditions, especially when more than one valve is involved. Let us assume that a patient has an obvious aortic valvular lesion and shows combined ventricular hypertrophy by electrocardiographic examination. This would lead one to suspect the additional diagnosis of mitral stenosis. Evidence of right ventricular hypertrophy in the precordial leads is much more likely to develop in congenital heart disease than in mitral stenosis. Its frequent absence in mitral stenosis may be due to the relatively slight degree of right ventricular hypertrophy or to overbalance by simultaneous left ventricular hypertrophy.

Bundle Branch Block

An impulse may start in the normal sino-auricular node, travel across the auricles, continue down the auriculoventricular node and bundle of His, and yet be blocked in the right or left main branch of the bundle. If the block occurs in the left branch, the impulse descends the right branch normally and reaches the left ventricle in roundabout fashion, probably through the interventricular septum. Generally conduction across the septum consumes about 0.04 second. The reverse process occurs if the right branch is blocked. The ventricles continue to contract regularly so that there is no arrhythmia in the ordinary sense. There is a slight delay, however, in the activation of one ventricle with respect to the other. Thus in right bundle block the left ventricle is activated slightly before the right, a reversal of the normal relationship. In left bundle branch block, on the other hand, the delay in the electrical activation of the left ventricle is even longer than that occurring in the normally activated heart. The ventricular complexes will necessarily be abnormal because of the circuitous route taken by the impulse. In fact, they will resemble a series of ventricular premature beats arising from the unblocked ventricle, or the curves seen in ventricular tachycardia. The QRS complex is characteristically broadened, coarsely notched, and frequently of considerable amplitude, and the RS-T segment is apt to be depressed and the T wave to continue in the opposite direction to the main initial deflection. In pure experimental bundle branch block and in many clinical instances of bundle branch block measurement of the ventricular gradient shows that these RS-T and T wave changes are "secondary" and thus represent changes in the repolarization process contingent upon changes in the depolarization process and are not to be

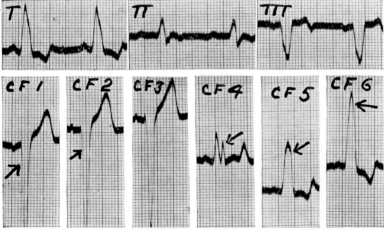

FIG. 34.   *Left Bundle Branch Block.*   The upper set of tracings shows the three standard leads. Note that the QRS complex measures 0.15 second and there is no S_1. The lower set shows the six precordial (bipolar) leads from the chest and left leg, CF_1 to CF_6. Note that the sharp downward stroke or intrinsicoid deflection (see arrow) comes early over the right ventricle (CF_1, CF_2, and CF_3) and very late over the left ventricle (CF_4, CF_5, and CF_6). The latter QRS complexes often show coarse splitting of the waves, as in CF_4. These curves denote delay or block in the left ventricle. The patient was a 53-year-old man who had had a coronary thrombosis two years before.

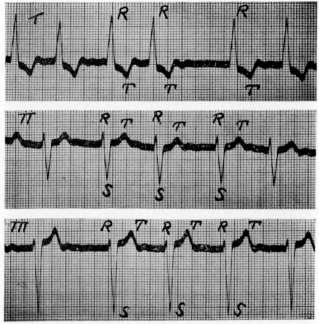

FIG. 35. *Left Bundle Branch Block, with Auricular Fibrillation.* Note the prominent, broad and coarsely notched QRS complexes with oppositely directed T waves. These changes are presumptive evidence of left bundle branch block but require confirmation by the detection of late intrinsicoid deflections over the left ventricle. In this case the rhythm is irregular because of coexisting auricular fibrillation. The patient had hypertensive heart disease and chronic nephritis.

construed as evidence of an altered physiologic state of the myocardium. This point is more fully discussed above in the section on ventricular hypertrophy.

When the broadest QRS deflection is upward in Lead I and downward in Lead III the curves represent *classical left bundle branch block* (Figs. 34, 35, 36, and 41), and when it is downward in Lead I and upward in Lead III it is *classical right bundle branch block* (Figs. 37, 38, and 42). Lead I is generally more helpful than the other two standard leads in determining whether the block is in the right or left branch. If there is a prominent S wave in Lead I, the block is probably on the right side; if there is a prominent R wave and no S wave in Lead I, it is probably on the left. If the QRS complex, measured in the conventional leads, lasts 0.12 second or longer, and late intrinsicoid deflections are inscribed over the left ventricle, then left bundle branch block is present. When we say "late intrinsicoid deflection," we mean that this deflection is the last part of the QRS complex to be written. In such cases the QRS complex over the left ventricle tends to have a flat or turret top. If these criteria are used, many instances of intraventricular block which do not have the classical appearance in the conventional leads will be classified as bundle branch block. In some instances a tracing which

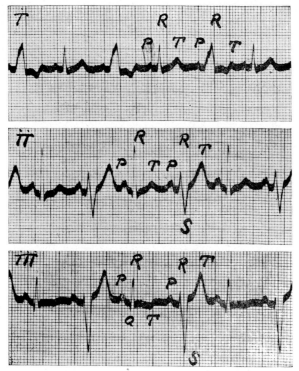

FIG. 36. *Partial (2:1) Left Bundle Branch Block.*   Note that every other ventricular complex has the form similar to Figure 35. The other beats are normal. This indicates that every second beat fails to be conducted down the left branch of the bundle of His. This patient has hypertensive heart disease. Since, in contradistinction to the situation in auriculoventricular block, the conduction tissue distal to the block is usually stimulated by way of the septum with each impulse, this is a very rare phenomenon.

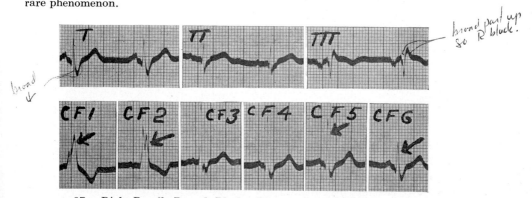

FIG. 37. *Right Bundle Branch Block.*   The upper set of tracings shows three standard leads. Note that S_1 is broad and QRS = 0.13 second. The lower set shows the six bipolar precordial leads from the chest and left leg, CF_1 through CF_6. Note that the last sharp, downward stroke of the R wave or intrinsicoid deflection (see arrow) comes late in the QRS cycle in CF_1 and CF_2 (over the right ventricle) and comes early in CF_5 and CF_6 (over the left ventricle). This denotes that the block or delay is in the right ventricle. The patient was a woman, 48 years of age, with rheumatic aortic stenosis.

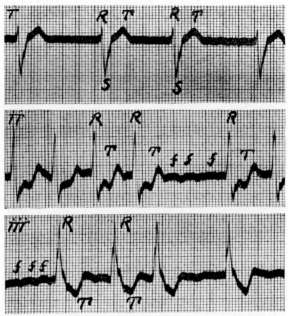

FIG. 38.   *Right Bundle Branch Block, with Auricular Fibrillation.*   Note that the general characteristics of the ventricular complexes (QRS-T) are the same as those in Figures 34, 35, and 36, but that the main deflections are opposite, going downward in Lead I and upward in Lead III. These curves are presumptive evidence of block in the right branch of the bundle of His but should be substantiated by precordial leads showing late intrinsicoid deflections over the right ventricle. In this case the rhythm is irregular due to coexisting auricular fibrillation (f-f-f). At the time these tracings were recorded the patient was 72 years of age, had had such curves for at least eight years, and showed evidence of well-compensated aortic and mitral stenosis and hypertension. He had formerly had frequent attacks of Adams-Stokes syncope.

looks like right bundle branch block in the limb leads shows late intrinsicoid deflections over the left rather than the right precordium. These are probably examples of left bundle branch block with an unusual or extreme electrical position of the heart. It has been the experience of Wolff that the opposite contingency, namely, tracings in which the limb leads look like left bundle branch block but in which the chest leads show late intrinsicoid deflections over the right precordium, are probably examples of true left bundle branch block associated with extensive myocardial infarction. Here the left bundle is blocked but there is little or no remaining excitable left ventricular myocardium to conduct the impulse to the left precordium; by default the right precordium receives the impulse. Figures 39 and 162 are probable examples of this phenomenon.

Unless the situation is complicated by coincident septal infarction a Q wave does not appear over the blocked ventricle. Consideration of the mode of activation of the septum in bundle branch block will make it clear why this is true. In left bundle branch block the impulse which should travel down the left bundle branch is blocked, therefore the left side of the septum does not get its usual head start in being activated. Instead, the right side of the septum is activated first and the impulse travels from the right to the left side of the septum. Since the impulse moves toward rather than away from the left ventricular cavity, the cavity potential must consist of an initial upward rather than downward deflection. Accordingly those parts of the body which face the left side of the septum no longer record an initial downward deflection or Q wave. This change is illustrated in Figure 40, obtained from a patient with acute posterior myocardial infarction. A well-marked Q wave was recorded over the left ventricle when normal intraventricular conduction was present. However, when the process involved the left bundle branch, prolonging the QRS complex to 0.15 second, the Q wave disappeared at those locations where it had previously been present. Actually about 5 per cent of the patients with left bundle branch block do show Q waves over the left precordium. In rare cases such a Q wave may appear and disappear over the left precordium and in Leads I and aVL as a result of changes in the position of the heart induced by respiration. More often a Q wave over the left precordium compels one to assume infarction of the interventricular septum. The infarct, being electrically inactive, permits the potential of the unblocked cavity (in this case that of the right ventricle), which is initially negative, to be transmitted across to the blocked ventricle, so that a Q wave may be recorded over the blocked ventricle. For similar reasons a Q wave should not be recorded over the right ventricle in right bundle branch block unless septal infarction is present.

It has been suggested that localized subendocardial sclerosis ("periinfarction block") may produce broad QRS complexes (0.11 sec. or

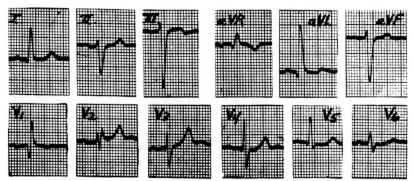

FIG. 39.   *A complicated electrocardiogram* in which the limb leads resemble left bundle branch block, the precordial leads right bundle branch block. The duration of the QRS complex is 0.14 second. There are a small Q wave, a broad, prominent R wave, and no S wave in Lead I. T_1 is not inverted so that the tracing would not be considered a classic example of left bundle branch block. The precordial leads show late intrinsicoid deflections in Leads V_1 and V_2, with R and R' deflections. This is presumably an example of left bundle branch block with extensive myocardial infarction.

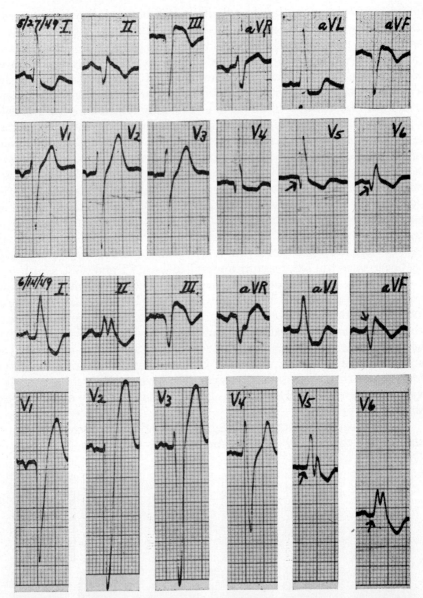

FIG. 40. *Disappearance of Q Wave with Development of Left Bundle Branch Block.*   The initial set of tracings taken early in the course of an acute clinical episode of chest pain shows the characteristic changes of acute posterior, possibly posterolateral, myocardial infarct. Intraventricular block (QRS = 0.11 second) is present. Note the presence of Q waves, indicated by arrows, over the left ventricle, and in Lead aVF. The second set of tracings, recorded eighteen days later, shows the development of left bundle branch block. The QRS complex now measures 0.15 second. Note the late intrinsicoid deflections in Leads V_5 and V_6. Note more particularly the loss of the Q waves in Leads V_5 and V_6 and also in Lead aVF. Septal activation now proceeds from the right to the left side of the septum; accordingly the left ventricular cavity potential now starts with an upward deflection. The decisive evidence of posterior infarction, present in the original tracings, is therefore lacking in the second set. Autopsy showed an acute posterolateral infarct.

longer), an initial Q wave, and late intrinsicoid deflections in leads related to the epicardial aspect of this lesion in the absence of bundle branch block. The resulting electrocardiogram would then resemble that produced by septal infarction in the presence of bundle branch block (Fig. 47). In those cases where RR′ complexes are known to have preceded the development of qRR′ complexes the diagnosis of septal infarction complicating bundle branch block is justified. When the previous electrocardiographic configuration is unknown it seems more reasonable to suggest the alternative explanations of peri-infarction block with subendocardial sclerosis on the one hand and bundle branch block with septal infarction on the other.

At times marked left ventricular hypertrophy may produce waves that resemble those of left bundle branch block, but the former will rarely display a QRS interval as long as 0.12 second, will not show such a tardiness of the intrinsicoid deflection in Leads V_5 and V_6, and may show Q waves in these positions. In considering the time of occurrence of the intrinsicoid deflection, due regard must be had for the thickness of the ventricles. There is some delay because of the hypertrophy itself, but never so much as results from bundle branch block. Although a certain number of patients with ventricular hypertrophy sooner or later develop bundle branch block, practical and theoretical considerations compel us to regard this as a new, emergent, and independent development which is not an integral feature in the course of ventricular hypertrophy. Ventricular hypertrophy and bundle branch block, then, are two unitary concepts. Coincident ventricular hypertrophy and bundle branch block are considered below.

Unless previous electrocardiograms have shown evidence for left ventricular hypertrophy, or subsequent tracings establish this diagnosis, it is generally unjustified to infer the coexistence of left ventricular hypertrophy with left bundle branch block on the basis of tall QRS complexes. The staggered activation of the ventricles in bundle branch block, by throwing the ventricles out of phase, gives the opportunity for the electrical activation of each ventricle to be expressed more or less unopposed and thus may give rise to very large electromotive forces even in the absence of ventricular hypertrophy.

Generally the corroborative evidence for bundle branch block will be found with the usual six precordial leads, but it is necessary to be certain that one has recorded true left or right ventricular potentials, preferably at a point where the final moment of activation of the blocked ventricle is recorded, that is, at a point where an S wave is not inscribed. In order to accomplish this it is occasionally necessary to record additional leads to the right or left of the usual six precordial points. Another note of caution with regard to the diagnosis of bundle branch block is appropriate. Even if all the criteria given above are fulfilled it is still impossible to be certain of the existence of bundle branch block unless these ventricular complexes are actually conducted from the auricles. With complete auriculoventricular block an idioventricular rhythm arising in the opposite bundle branch may produce ventricular complexes identical with those produced in block of the bundle branch on one side. In such cases it is generally wiser to make the noncommittal diagnosis of complete heart block with abnormal ventricular complexes. Unless similar ventricular complexes have been demonstrated previously, or are demonstrated subsequently when all or some of these same ventricular beats have clearly been conducted from the auricles, a definitive diagnosis of concomitant complete heart block and bundle branch block is not warranted. Since it is generally considered that the irregular ventricular beats are actually transmitted from auricles to ventricles in auricular fibrillation, it seems justifiable to diagnose coexistent auricular fibrillation and bundle branch block (Figs. 35 and 38). In occasional cases of this sort, if the ventricular rate is rapid it may be difficult or impossible to differentiate between ventricular tachycardia on the one hand and bundle branch block associated with auricular fibrillation or flutter on the other (Fig. 108).

We have seen that in the normally activated heart septal depolarization proceeds initially from its left to its right side. The impulse produces an upward deflection over the right ventricle. Subsequent activation of the septum from the right to the left side would produce a downward deflection over the right ventricle, but this is antagonized by concomitant and continued activation from the left to the right side of the septum. In left bundle branch block, in which this antagonizing force from the left to the right is lost, the activation from the right to the left is unopposed. This eliminates the tendency of the R wave to increase as the electrode moves over the right ventricle from position V_1 to the transitional zone. As a pure consequence of this abnormal direction of septal activation in left bundle branch block, the R waves are small or absent over the right ventricle. Thus in left bundle branch block the inference of anteroseptal myocardial infarction cannot be made from the presence of small R waves or from the presence of Q waves over the right ventricle. Neither can anterior myocardial infarction be excluded under these conditions. Accordingly, with left bundle branch block one must, from the electrocardiographic standpoint, remain in doubt as to the coexistence of anterior myocardial infarction.

The Vectorcardiogram in Bundle Branch Block. In left bundle branch block the QRS loop is ovoid or round in at least two planes and moves slowly throughout its entire circuit, inscribing closely bunched dots rather than streak-like "tear drops." In the horizontal plane the loop may take off immediately in a leftward and posterior direction and move in a clockwise course; in some cases this plane may show a small initial anterior or rightward and anterior counterclockwise development. In the first instance no R waves are observed in the electrocardiogram over the right precordium; in the second, small R waves may be recorded there (Fig. 41). In the sagittal plane the QRS loop is written in a clockwise direction. The QRS loop does not finish at the null point (Figs. 13 and 41). In other words the loop is "open" at its terminus. And this in turn gives way to a T wave loop which has, in general, an opposite direction in space to the QRS loop.

In right bundle branch block the first and greatest part of the QRS loop is almost identical in all planes with the normal loop of the same individual. The distinguishing feature, however, is the presence in the horizontal plane of a noticeably slow terminal appendage which begins near or behind the null point and extends anteriorly and to the right. It is this finger-like projection which accounts for the broad final R wave over the right precordium and the broad S wave over the left precordium (Fig. 42). The loop may be "open" or "closed," and the T wave loop may lie in space in the same or opposite direction to the QRS loop. The terminal appendage may be quite long, extending far anteriorly and to the right; this circumstance may suggest additional right ventricular hypertrophy. As indicated on page 452, the combination of right

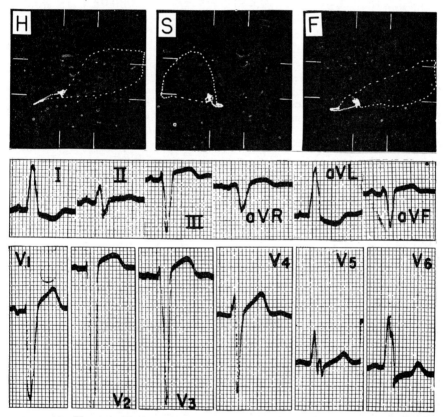

FIG. 41. *Vectorcardiogram and Electrocardiogram in Complete Left Bundle Branch Block.* The time markings are closely approximated throughout their entire sweep. The QRS loop rotates clockwise in the horizontal (*H*) and sagittal (*S*) planes. A small initial rightward and anterior segment in these planes accounts for the small R waves over the right precordium; such an appendage may be absent in left bundle branch block. The QRS loop is fanned out and "open" (RS-T displaced) and opposite in direction to the T loop.

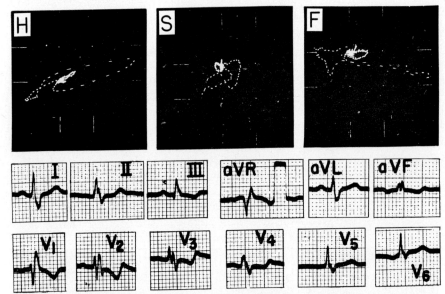

FIG. 42. *Vectorcardiogram and Electrocardiogram in Complete Right Bundle Branch Block.* The earlier portion of the loop in all planes is practically normal. The slowing of the loop is confined to its terminal portion, which extends as a finger-like projection in an anterior and rightward direction. This accounts for the broad R′ wave in Leads V₁, V₂, and aVR, and for the broad S waves in Leads I, aVL, and V₃ through V₆.

ventricular hypertrophy and right bundle branch block may also be suggested by pronounced terminal slowing in a horizontal plane loop whose first portion shows a significant clockwise development and which thus otherwise satisfies the criteria for right ventricular hypertrophy. The vectorcardiogram of pure right bundle branch block is distinguished from that of right ventricular hypertrophy by the terminal slowing of the loop and the counterclockwise rotation of the loop as seen in the horizontal plane. By contrast the vectorcardiogram of right ventricular hypertrophy finishes rapidly; it may start in a counterclockwise direction but finishes in a clockwise direction (Fig. 29).

INCOMPLETE BUNDLE BRANCH BLOCK

There are numerous instances in which there is a delay but no block in one branch or the other, resulting in electrocardiograms resembling those just described, except that the duration of the QRS complex is less than 0.12 second, generally 0.11 or 0.10 second (Figs. 43, 44). Such curves have been recorded in the experimental animal during the subsidence of bundle branch block. If all of the criteria except the duration of the initial ventricular complex are fulfilled the diagnosis of incomplete bundle branch block is warranted. The exact meaning of this finding is still under investigation. Incomplete right bundle branch block may occur as a transient finding in acute myocardial infarction and in acute cor pulmonale, and as a persistent finding in right ventricular hypertrophy. Incomplete right bundle branch block is an almost constant finding in interauricular septal defect. An appreciable number of individuals with hearts normal in all other respects show incomplete right bundle branch block. In making the diagnosis it is important to be certain that the electrode is not higher than the fourth interspace, else the potentials of the pulmonic conus may be recorded. Since the pulmonic conus is one of the last parts of the heart to be activated, an electrode in relation with this structure may show a late intrinsicoid deflection and thus falsely raise the question of incomplete right bundle branch block.

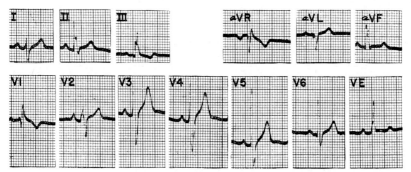

FIG. 43.   *Incomplete Right Bundle Branch Block.*   The patient was a 21-year-old Navy veteran with a record of a dozen Pacific engagements in whom a heart murmur was discovered when he was attempting to re-enlist. Catheterization studies showed the existence of an interauricular septal defect. Note that the duration of the QRS complex is 0.11 second, that an rR' complex is present in Lead V_1, and that a notched R wave is present in Lead V_E, with late intrinsicoid deflections in both of these leads.

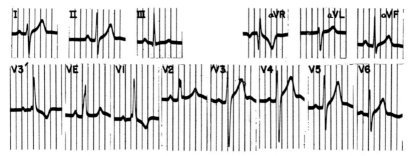

FIG. 44.   *Incomplete Right Bundle Branch Block, with Right Ventricular Hypertrophy.*   The conventional leads show right axis deviation. The zone transitional between right and left ventricular potentials is at Lead V_2. The intrinsicoid deflection is later over the right than over the left ventricle. The presence of an initial R rather than Q wave over the right ventricle is more in accord with incomplete right bundle branch block than right ventricular hypertrophy, but the tallness of R' suggests the additional existence of right ventricular hypertrophy. The patient was a 13-year-old schoolboy with a grade IV systolic murmur and thrill in the third and fourth left intercostal spaces. X-ray examination showed right ventricular hypertrophy and a dilated pulmonary artery. Catheterization studies established the existence of pulmonic stenosis.

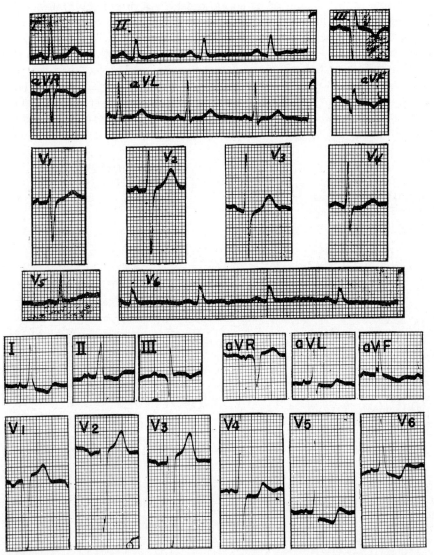

FIG. 45.   *Incomplete Left Bundle Branch Block.*   The upper set of tracings was recorded in a 54-year-old man with a typical attack of acute myocardial infarction. He developed the characteristic changes of an acute posterior lesion associated with a QRS interval of 0.11 second and a late intrinsicoid deflection in Lead V₆. The patient recovered. Note that there is no Q wave in Leads V₄ through V₆ or aVL. The lower set was recorded in a 68-year-old man with hypertensive and rheumatic heart disease. His blood pressure was 220/110. Fluoroscopy showed slight enlargement of the right ventricle and left auricle, and moderate enlargement of the left ventricle. The QRS duration is 0.11 second. The P waves are broad and notched. The voltage of the QRS complexes satisfies the requirements for the diagnosis of left ventricular hypertrophy, but there is no Q wave over the left precordium.

Nor is the significance of incomplete left bundle branch block settled. In all individuals whose electrocardiograms show the characteristic appearance of left ventricular hypertrophy but which lack a Q wave over the left ventricle, the possibility of this condition exists (Fig. 45). As with complete left bundle branch block the abnormal activation of the septum from the right to the left in incomplete left bundle branch block may explain the failure of the R wave to increase over the right ventricle as the electrode moves to the left, which finding may lead to the false inference of anteroseptal infarction. It is the development and recession of incomplete left bundle branch block that is one of a number of factors which may account for the instability of the electrocardiogram of left ventricular hypertrophy (p. 446). The vectorcardiographic features of incomplete right or left bundle branch block are those of the complete varieties.

Bundle branch block is often associated with other types of heart block, such as auriculoventricular or sino-auricular block (Figs. 118, 131). Figure 36 represents a rare instance of 2:1 partial left bundle branch block. At first glance one might interpret this as coupled rhythm due to premature ventricular systoles, but on careful inspection it will be found that auricular and ventricular beats come exactly on time.

CLINICAL IMPLICATIONS OF BUNDLE BRANCH BLOCK

Bundle branch block is fairly common in general practice. Experience with unipolar chest leads has shown that, contrary to previous opinion, block on the right side is much more frequent than block on the left side. Whatever is actually the more frequent, the use of the term "common type" of intraventricular block should be discarded as inexact and equivocal.

Inasmuch as bundle branch block occurs for the most part in patients with regular rhythm it is difficult to recognize this condition without electrocardiograms. Attempts to detect this condition at the bedside or even to verify anatomic interruption of one bundle branch or the other with serial microscopic sections have often been futile. Yet neither failure refutes the incontrovertible electrical evidence of delayed activation of one ventricle or the other. Bundle branch block is a purely electrocardiographic diagnosis. However, it is often possible to suspect its presence. Whenever a diastolic gallop rhythm is heard one should think of the possibility of bundle branch block. Moreover, bundle branch block is often accompanied by a bifurcated or reduplicated apex impulse. Both of these findings need to be looked for carefully and deliberately, for when they are detected bundle branch block is apt to be present. Finally, in such cases pulsus alternans is also very common. In fact, the frequent association of bundle branch block, gallop rhythm, and pulsus alternans should lead one to suspect the presence of the third if the other two are found.

Bundle branch block occurs most frequently in conjunction with hypertensive heart disease, with disease of the coronary arteries, in cases of aortic stenosis, and much less frequently in association with mitral stenosis. It almost always denotes some disease of the myocardium, although in rare instances there is no other clinical evidence that the heart is diseased. The prognosis for patients with left bundle branch block is poor. The average length of life after it is first noted is not more than a few years, but there are patients who carry on fairly satisfactorily for many years. The situation is quite different in right bundle branch block, for here many patients continue in good health for a great many years. In fact, there are instances of this type in which there seems to be very little other evidence of organic disease and the prognosis may be extremely favorable. There is no specific treatment for persons with this disturbance as it does not, by itself, produce any handicap. It merely reflects the condition in the heart muscle, and therapy is directed at the general state of the circulation.

INTRAVENTRICULAR BLOCK

Complete and incomplete bundle branch block are, strictly speaking, special forms of intraventricular block. We have been accustomed, however, to make the diagnosis of intraventricular block by exclusion when bundle branch block cannot be established. Thus if, with a QRS duration of 0.11 second or longer, it is impossible to demonstrate late intrinsicoid deflections over one ventricle or the other, one must, by exclusion, make the noncommittal diagnosis of intraventricular block or defective intraventricular conduction (Fig. 46). Some of these latter hearts will, on further analysis, show localized areas of delayed activation. If the transitional zone can be eliminated as the cause of notching of the QRS complex in one or more precordial leads and if flanking leads show earlier activation, one may be dealing with "focal" or "peri-infarction" block. Occasionally this local area of delayed activation may be restricted to esophageal leads recorded at ventricular levels. This finding probably signifies localized patchy fibrosis, probably involving the subendocardial Purkinje network. The term "arborization block" might be used as the equivalent of focal block, but this should not be confused with the "arborization block" of the older literature. Analysis of many of the tracings showing bizarre, low voltage, prolonged QRS complexes, formerly considered as evidencing "arborization block," would, in the light of the criteria given above, demonstrate many of them to be examples of bundle branch block.

The clinical implications of defective intraventricular conduction are similar to those of bundle branch block. It should be borne in mind that generally a grave condition of the ventricular musculature is indicated and the prognosis should be guarded accordingly. Occasionally, such curves will be found when there is little else to make one suspect heart disease, and in that way they become very helpful diagnostically. In fact, the greatest value of electrocardiography is in the detection of significant abnormalities in the ventricular complexes when the rest of the examination reveals no essential abnormality.

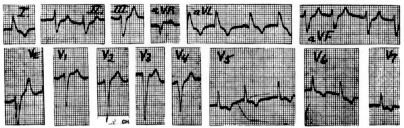

FIG. 46. *Intraventricular Block.*   The QRS complex in the standard leads measures 0.14 second. Although there is a superficial resemblance to left bundle branch block, it will be noted that in Leads I, aVL, and V_5 through V_7 the QRS complex is not flat or turret topped and does not have a true intrinsicoid deflection in the sense of a final rapid downward deflection. The descending limb of the R wave begins relatively early in the QRS complex and shows a smooth, slow, oblique slope. Such curves should be designated intraventricular block. Note also the absence of clearly demonstrable P waves. The patient was a 58-year-old woman admitted for uremia and acidosis. The electrocardiogram suggested potassium intoxication. No postmortem examination was performed.

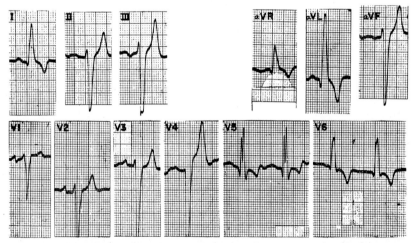

FIG. 47.   *Left Ventricular and Septal Hypertrophy, with "Peri-infarction" Block.* The patient was a 19-year-old man with coarctation of the aorta. The tracings show a QRS interval of 0.16 second, a duration unusual for uncomplicated left ventricular hypertrophy. Late intrinsicoid deflections over the left ventricle and flat-topped R waves in Lead V_6 suggest left bundle branch block. However, deep notching of V_5, of the type seen here, is not usually observed in left bundle branch block and the presence of Q waves in Leads V_5 and V_6 is incompatible with pure left bundle branch block. At postmortem examination the heart was tremendously enlarged (930 gm.), the left ventricle measuring 2.2 cm. in thickness. There was a congenital bicuspid aortic valve. The septum, though strikingly hypertrophied, was the site neither of infarction nor of other disease. There was some scarring in the lateral wall of the left ventricle, most marked subendocardially.

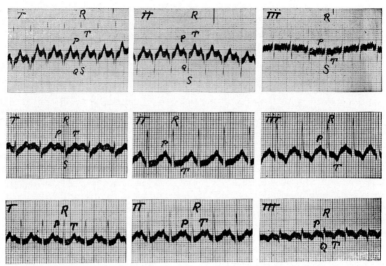

FIG. 48. *Normal Sinus Tachycardia.* Upper tracing is from a boy, aged 9, who had a postscarlatinal tachycardia, rate 143. Middle set is from a youth, aged 18, with neurocirculatory asthenia, rate 146. Note all complexes are normal in sequence but merely come at a rapid rate. The T_2 and T_3 in neurocirculatory asthenia are frequently flat or inverted. Lower set is from a boy, aged 9, with acute rheumatic heart disease, rate 166.

Disturbances of the Pacemaker (Sino-Auricular Node)

NORMAL TACHYCARDIA

It appears that the sino-auricular node has to go through some chemical process in building up material which finally explodes and sends out an impulse. This process normally repeats itself in a fairly orderly fashion at a rate of about 70 per minute. There are numerous common conditions in which the process takes place more rapidly, i.e., exercise, emotion, fever, or hyperthyroidism. Under these circumstances the impulse starts in the normal focus and travels across the heart normally, but the rate at which it is repeated is increased. This is called *normal tachycardia* or *normal sinus tachycardia* (Fig. 48). All the complexes have an essentially normal form and most of the acceleration takes place at the expense of the diastole of the heart (the T-P interval). Such a condition need not indicate disease of the heart. It was doubtful whether any organic heart disease was present in the patient illustrated by the upper curves of Figure 48 and there certainly was no heart disease in the patient from whom the middle tracings were obtained. At times it is very important to distinguish a normal tachycardia from one due to an ectopic rhythm and it may be necessary to produce vagal stimulation, as illustrated in Figures 73, 81, and 124. When a rapid regular rhythm is due to an abnormal mechanism, vagal stimulation either produces no effect, stops the tachycardia, or causes temporary abrupt alterations in the rate, whereas in normal tachycardia the effect is slight or gradual.

There is a tendency for the P-R interval to shorten very slightly in sinus tachycardia. As the rate of impulse discharge accelerates, the site of impulse formation tends to migrate to higher, more cephalad locations in the sino-auricular node. This is manifested in an increased amplitude of the P waves in Leads II and III. Because of the shortening of the P-R interval and the increased amplitude of the P waves, this deflection is generally easily recognized in sinus tachycardia. As we shall see, this contrasts with the puny P wave of paroxysmal auricular tachycardia which tends to be smaller and to be associated with some lengthening of the P-R interval, frequently being lost in the T wave of the preceding ventricular complex.

NORMAL BRADYCARDIA

The vagus and sympathetic control have much to do with the regulation of the rate of impulse formation at the pacemaker. Under certain conditions, either as a result of increased vagal or diminished accelerator tone, the rate of the heart is unusually slow and sluggish, 45 or less (Fig. 49). This occurs in some normal healthy individuals, particularly tall young athletes, with undernutrition, as a result of jaundice, during

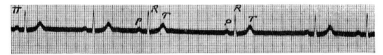

FIG. 49. *Normal Bradycardia*. Rate about 42, from a man, aged 68, who had no symptoms or signs of heart disease. Note that the complexes are normal, the rate is slow, and there is a sinus arrhythmia.

sleep, and after certain infections. The entire mechanism of the beat is normal and, therefore, the electrocardiogram will be normal in every respect except that the diastolic pauses will be great. The condition is called *normal bradycardia*. At times the rate can be below 40 and even 35 with a normal mechanism. At these low levels it must be clearly distinguished from heart block, for with the former the heart is apt to be normal and with the latter the heart is almost always diseased. This distinction can readily be made without special apparatus, for on exercise the rate will gradually rise to a higher level and then return to the original slow rate if the bradycardia is a normal one; when heart block is present the rate will change either slightly or not at all, or sudden interruptions in the length of the heart cycle will be detected. Normal sinus bradycardia is commonly associated with sinus arrhythmia.

SINUS ARRHYTHMIA

There is an irregularity of the heart, called *sinus arrhythmia*, in which gradual acceleration and retardation take place (Fig. 50). It is sometimes called respiratory arrhythmia, because it often is phasic with respiration. The rate speeds up with inspiration and then slows with

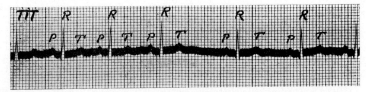

FIG. 50. *Sinus Arrhythmia.*   A woman, aged 38, who had malnutrition but no heart disease. Note gradual increase and decrease of the length of the heart cycles. The changes take place almost entirely in the length of the diastolic pause (T-P interval).

expiration. At times it is independent of breathing. The impulse originates in the normal pacemaker and traverses the heart normally, the gradual changes taking place mainly in the length of diastole. Because it is so common in childhood, it is also called juvenile arrhythmia. When it is marked, or when the changes are abrupt, it may be confused with more serious irregularities, such as auricular fibrillation or heart block. It occurs in many healthy people, in some older individuals with myocardial disease, and after full digitalization. It is apt to disappear entirely if the heart rate is increased artificially by exercise or by diminishing the vagal tone with atropine. The important point is that it must be regarded as an essentially normal phenomenon and does not indicate organic disease. When the heart rate has been rapid and regular for some cause, such as hyperthyroidism or rheumatic carditis, the appearance of sinus arrhythmia is apt to indicate that the condition is progressing favorably and the normal vagal control is returning. In fact, it is rare to find this arrhythmia while active thyrotoxicosis or rheumatic carditis exists. Some instances of sinus arrhythmia are actually examples of sino-auricular block associated with the Wenckebach phenomenon (see page 542).

SINUS PAUSES

The pacemaker of the heart may become inhibited as a result of certain reflex influences and thereby fail to produce impulses for varying lengths of time. Under such circumstances the whole heart fails to contract and, if the pause is sufficiently long, giddiness or actual syncope occurs, presenting clinical features that are similar to those seen in

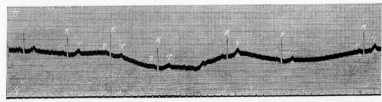

FIG. 51. *Sinus Pauses.*   Note marked irregular slowing of the heart; neither auricle nor ventricle contracts. This resulted from vagus stimulation following gagging (probably a vagovagal reflex). The irregularity of the base line is an artifact and due to movement of the patient. (Author's article in Oxford Loose-Leaf Medicine, vol. II.)

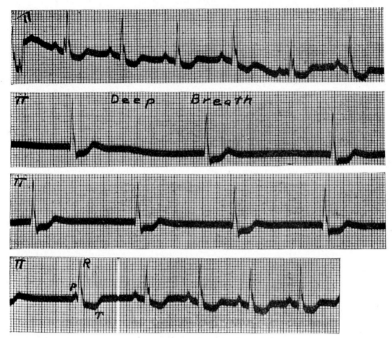

FIG. 52. *Sinus Pauses.* This is a continuous tracing from a man with aortic stenosis and angina pectoris. Note that on taking a deep breath the heart slowed markedly, the P waves disappeared, there was an idioventricular rhythm and a gradual return to normal.

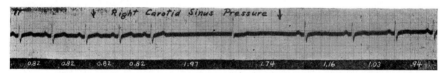

FIG. 53. *Sinus Pauses.* From a man, aged 60, who had syncopal attacks but no heart disease. The right carotid sinus was very sensitive. Note marked slowing of the heart from the carotid sinus reflex.

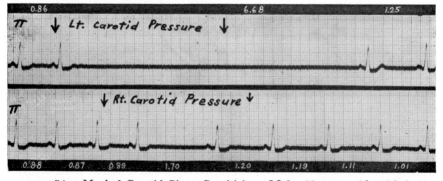

FIG. 54. *Marked Carotid Sinus Sensitivity.* Male, 60 years old, with hypertension, aortic stenosis, and angina pectoris. Note the prolonged asystole of over 6 seconds following left carotid pressure. The effect is less marked on the right.

Adams-Stokes disease. This condition is called *sinus pauses* (Fig. 51). The electrocardiographic complexes are normal in form but there appear long diastolic pauses of varying lengths. This might be regarded as an exaggerated form of sinus arrhythmia. The mechanism of this disturbance depends on a reflex stimulation of the vagus, such as a vagovagal or carotid sinus reflex. Figure 51 is a tracing of a patient who had spells of unconsciousness precipitated by the act of swallowing or gagging and accompanied by a peculiar sensation in the throat. It was found that each time a tongue depressor was applied to the tongue to examine the pharynx an attack occurred, during which the heart stopped for several seconds.

Similar electrocardiograms and syncopal attacks can occur in some individuals with aortic stenosis or in those who have a sensitive carotid sinus. Figure 52 shows the effect of a deep breath in a man with aortic stenosis. The whole heart slowed and the patient grew somewhat faint. Figure 53 shows how readily the heart can be slowed by light pressure over the carotid sinus in some individuals. This man was quite well except that he had frequent spells of unconsciousness which came without warning. He was entirely cured by taking $\frac{3}{8}$ grain (0.025 gm.) of ephedrine sulfate two or three times a day. Another instance of marked carotid sensitivity is shown in Figure 54.

AURICULAR STANDSTILL

On rare occasions electrocardiograms are seen in which the auricular complexes entirely disappear for brief or considerable periods of time. This condition is called auricular standstill, or inhibition of the auricles (Figs. 55 and 56). The ventricular beat is maintained by the idioven-

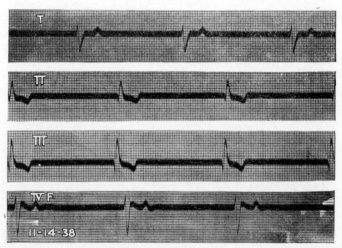

FIG. 55.   *Auricular Standstill.*   Male, 70 years old, who had taken excessive digitalis and developed unconscious spells. Note complete absence of P waves and ventricular rate of 33. Patient made complete recovery, with reappearance of normal P waves.

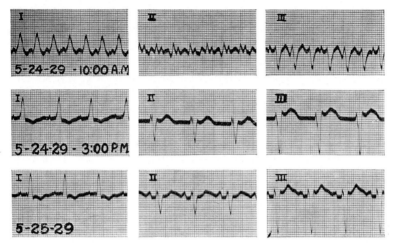

FIG. 56.   *Auricular Standstill Due to Quinidine.*   Upper set of tracings shows paroxysmal ventricular tachycardia with a ventricular rate of 169. Middle set shows auricular standstill in Leads II and III. Lower set shows return of auricular activity. The patient had received a single dose of 1 gm. of quinidine sulfate at 11.30 a.m. on May 24, 1929.

tricular pacemaker. Such curves are occasionally observed during quinidine or digitalis administration and indicate a toxic effect of the drug. Syncopal or Adams-Stokes attacks may occur in patients manifesting this disturbance, and it is imperative that the drug causing the auricular standstill be omitted. Auricular standstill is also apparently a regular feature of the more advanced stages of potassium intoxication.

In deciding whether the auricles are really quiescent electrically, the possibility must be considered that upright or inverted P waves actually coincide with and are obscured by the QRS complexes. If such hidden P waves are upright, the true diagnosis is auriculoventricular dissociation; if inverted, auriculoventricular nodal rhythm with retrograde auricular excitation. To rule out either possibility, special auricular leads or esophageal leads may prove helpful.

Ectopic Rhythms

In the preceding paragraphs we discussed disturbances in the pacemaker of the heart. The second major abnormality in the mechanism of the heart beat is the formation of ectopic rhythms. Impulses can arise in almost any part of the heart: auricles, junctional tissue, or ventricles. When such ectopic beats occur they interfere with the normal sequence of events and produce peculiar and characteristic electrocardiographic changes. The fundamental principle underlying these alterations is that, if an impulse travels an abnormal course through a certain portion of the heart, the electrocardiographic representation of that impulse will be abnormal.

PREMATURE AURICULAR BEATS

Impulses may arise in any portion of the auricular musculature. Ordinarily the tendency for beats to arise in abnormal parts of the heart is held in abeyance, because the pace set by the sino-auricular node is faster and prevents other foci from functioning. Under abnormal conditions ectopic foci are enabled to initiate impulses, and when such isolated beats occur they are called *premature* or *ectopic beats* or *extrasystoles*. On listening over the precordium one hears a regular rhythm (lub-dub, lub-dub) and then suddenly a quick beat followed by a pause, after which the regular sequence is restored. This premature beat may come only at very rare intervals or as frequently as every second or third cycle. Although the beat can be heard over the precordium it may produce such a small pulse wave that it is only barely felt at the wrist or it may be entirely imperceptible. This is so because the heart contracts early in diastole when the volume of blood in the ventricles is quite small.

From an electrocardiographic point of view we must visualize the wave of excitation as arising in some point in the auricle more or less distant from the sino-auricular node. The course through the auricle that this impulse must take will be abnormal. It will travel possibly from left to right rather than from right to left or upward rather than downward. The P wave which represents auricular activity will have to be abnormal in form in one or more leads. How different from the normal P wave it will be will depend on how far away the ectopic focus is from the normal pacemaker. It may, therefore, remain upward or become inverted (Figs. 57, 58, 59). If and when this impulse reaches the sino-auricular node it destroys whatever impulse-forming material has been built up there and the node starts over again in the production of a normal beat. The premature beat is also traveling downward through the auriculoventricular junctional tissue to reach the ventricles. The pathway of this beat through the ventricles therefore should be normal and the QRS-T complex will be of normal form. Generally this is so (Figs. 57 and 59). At times the ventricular complex following a premature auricular beat, however, is abnormal (Fig. 58) and the P-R interval may be delayed. In fact, on rare occasions the beat may be blocked and then it is called a *blocked* or *non-conducted premature auricular beat* (Fig. 204, *D*). This occurs because the beat has come so quickly that the tissue has not recovered completely, and there may be a slight delay in one part or another of the conduction apparatus, distorting the spread of the wave of excitation. The premature and abnormal P wave may need to be sought for carefully. It often is hidden on the previous T wave and is to be detected by a slight alteration in the height or configuration of this T wave (Fig. 57). At other times because the ectopic focus is so near the normal pacemaker the P waves differ only very slightly from the normal ones (Fig. 99, lower curves). The P wave of the premature beat may even be identical with the normal P wave.

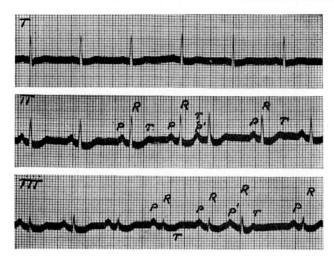

FIG. 57.   *Premature Auricular Beats.*   Note that the irregularity is due to an occasional premature beat (P′) which becomes superimposed on the previous T wave. The ventricular complexes following the premature beats are of normal form (Leads II and III). From a man who had a benign irregularity of the heart.

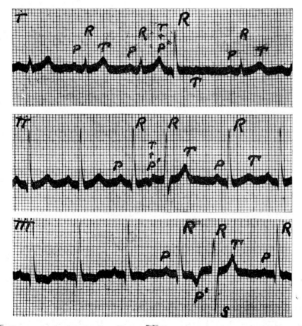

FIG. 58.   *Premature Auricular Beats.*   From a young man with no heart disease. Note that the premature P′ waves fall on the preceding T waves, are inverted in Leads II and III, and are followed by ventricular complexes of abnormal form (aberrant ventricular conduction).

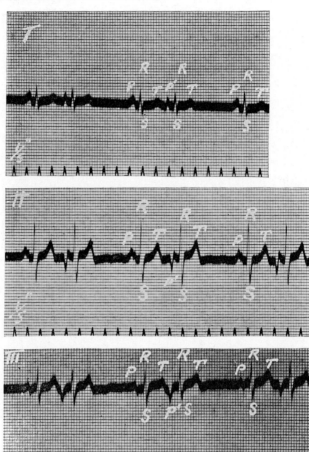

FIG. 59.   *Premature Auricular Beats.*   Note that every second beat is a premature P′ wave which is upright in Lead I but inverted in Leads II and III. This is a
form of coupled rhythm. (Author's article in Oxford Loose-Leaf Medicine, vol. II.)

It may then be difficult to decide whether these premature beats arise
in the atrium proper or in the sino-auricular node. When the pause following such a P wave is equal to the normal P-P interval, it seems more
likely that this beat arises in the sinus node. Occasionally a premature
auricular beat produces no electrical disturbance in one of the leads, but
the finding of a P wave of an abnormal form in one of the other leads
will reveal its abnormal origin.

Premature auricular beats can generally be readily distinguished
from those of ventricular origin. Even when the former are followed by
abnormal ventricular complexes, the QRS waves are not so broad as in
the latter condition. The detection of the preceding abnormal P wave
identifies the beat as auricular.

Finally, the pause after an auricular extrasystole, although longer than the normal cycle, is generally not completely compensatory; i.e., the length of the two cycles including the extrasystole is less than two normal heart cycles, whereas with ventricular extrasystoles it is equal to two normal beats. Occasionally, however, even premature auricular beats are followed by completely compensatory pauses. This may be explained in some cases by the failure of the premature impulse to penetrate the sino-auricular node. The undischarged impulse building up in the node subsequently encounters refractory auricular muscle and is not manifested electrocardiographically. The node then starts anew to build up an impulse which activates auricular muscle, now responsive, on time. The detection of a compensatory pause is not, therefore, a reliable method of differentiating ventricular from auricular premature beats.

Premature auricular beats are fairly common and do not by themselves indicate heart disease. They occur in otherwise well individuals as a purely functional or neurogenic disturbance and need produce no symptoms or disability. When such is the case, the irregularity should not be treated, nor should the patient be restricted in his activities. When these beats produce a good deal of palpitation and are annoying, quinidine or digitalis may be helpful. Occasionally potassium salts (potassium phosphate or chloride, 2 gm. three times a day by mouth) may prove beneficial. Occasionally auricular premature beats result from excessive administration of digitalis, but these are apparently a much less common effect of digitalis overdosage than are ventricular premature beats. Auricular premature beats do occur in patients with organic heart disease, but the diagnosis of structural disease will then have to rest on other evidence. There is some association between this type of extrasystole and auricular disturbances of higher grade, e.g., tachycardia, flutter, and fibrillation. Patients who show the latter irregularities often are found to have premature auricular beats at other times. On following the progress of a case of mitral stenosis this form of extrasystole often occurs for some years preceding the development of auricular fibrillation, and so the detection of the former may lead one to suspect that the latter irregularity will not be long delayed. Likewise, if a patient has paroxysms of some form of rapid heart action, the finding of an occasional auricular extrasystole between attacks helps to throw light on the nature of the paroxysms that have occurred in the past.

PAROXYSMAL AURICULAR TACHYCARDIA

As one continues the consideration of ectopic rhythms in the auricle, a disturbance of somewhat higher degree is paroxysmal auricular tachycardia (Figs. 60 to 69). Here, instead of an occasional impulse arising in some abnormal part of the auricular wall, this focus sends out a series of regular impulses. The pace is then set by this ectopic focus and it may be maintained for variable lengths of time, persisting for hours or days and rarely for weeks. It is argued whether this disturbance is the

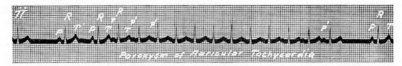

FIG. 60. *Paroxysmal Auricular Tachycardia.* Note the complete cycle of a brief attack of tachycardia, lasting five seconds. P′ is different in form from the normal P wave, but the ventricular complexes are unchanged. The onset and offset are instantaneous, the rhythm is perfectly regular, rate is 158. The patient was a 21-year-old woman without heart disease who complained of palpitation.

result of a circus movement which passes through the sino-auricular or auriculoventricular node or of impulses discharging repetitively from an ectopic auricular focus.

Inasmuch as the origin of the impulse is abnormal, the course it takes through the auricles is abnormal, and in so far as an auricular complex can be identified it will differ from the normal P wave. The course of this wave through the ventricles, however, is normal, and therefore the QRST waves will be the same as when the heart is beating normally. Figure 60 represents a complete brief paroxysm of this type lasting only four to five seconds. It shows that the onset and offset are abrupt and the auricular waves change their form when the paroxysm starts, but that the ventricular complexes remain the same. It is characteristic of this condition that the rhythm is perfectly regular, much more so than in a normally beating heart. It is also peculiar that in most cases the P waves cannot be easily identified, for they probably are fused with the preceding ventricular complex. The result is that one often sees only what appears to be an R and a T wave coming in rapid succession. Even when visible, the P waves are apt to be puny affairs. This contrasts with the P waves of sinus tachycardia, which are generally sharp, clear-cut, and upstanding.

Clinically, this condition is important, because it is common, can cause a good deal of discomfort and concern, and on rare occasions can have serious consequences. It is also important from a practical point of view because it can be readily recognized at the bedside and effectively treated. It occurs for the most part in an individual who has a structurally normal heart. Occasionally it is a complication of organic heart disease and then may produce alarming symptoms. Ordinarily attacks occur without any detectable cause. The patient is apt to blame some particular happening that took place just before the attack, such as a motor ride or eating a certain kind of food. Indigestion or gas is often suspected as being the cause, and yet treatment which is directed at the gastrointestinal tract or the diet will be of no avail. A careful history will frequently bring to light the fact that a certain specific event may act as a trigger in setting off a paroxysm. A sudden turn of the head, or bending over to tie one's shoes, an unexpected emotional upset or a dream all have been known to precipitate such spells. On the other hand, many attacks occur without any obvious cause.

The attack itself is instantaneous in onset and offset (Fig. 60). In most cases the patient is aware of this and will describe it as coming on suddenly, and stopping with a "thump." At times, although the changes are sudden, the sensations will be described as occurring quickly but not abruptly. The patient will complain of palpitation or fluttering

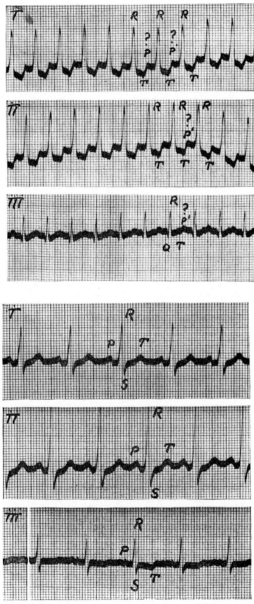

FIG. 61.   *Paroxysmal Auricular Tachycardia.*   Upper three leads show a perfectly regular rate of 172. Auricular complexes (P') probably buried in the previous T waves. Lower three curves on the same patient taken after attack was over show a normal slow rhythm, rate of 83.

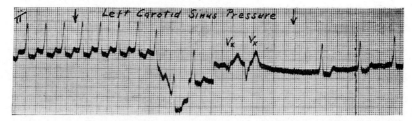

FIG. 62. *Paroxysmal Auricular Tachycardia.* (Same case as Figure 61.) Note the abrupt cessation of the attack caused by pressure over the left carotid sinus. The irregularity of the baseline is due to movements of the patient. Vx indicates ventricular escape beats which are common during the transitions. Patient had hypertension and angina pectoris.

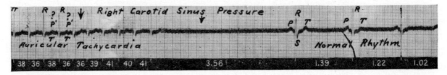

FIG. 63. *Paroxysmal Auricular Tachycardia.* Cessation of attack produced by right carotid sinus pressure. Note long pause followed by resumption of normal rhythm. Rate during attack, 158. P waves during attack not easily identified. Patient had no heart disease.

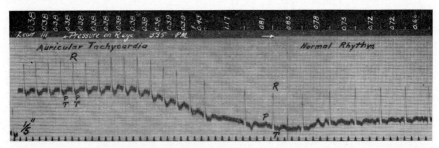

FIG. 64. *Paroxysmal Auricular or Nodal Tachycardia.* Cessation of attack caused by right ocular pressure (oculocardiac reflex). Note sudden transition from regular rhythm with rate of 158 to rate of 80. Numbers above tracing measure the interventricular intervals in hundredths of a second. Note absolute regularity with slight slowing just before the transition. The treatment of auricular and nodal tachycardia is the same. Patient had rheumatic aortic insufficiency. (Author's article in Oxford Loose-Leaf Medicine, vol. II.)

of the heart, become uneasy, nervous, and apprehensive, and want to lie down. Occasionally there is pain over the heart and there may be typical anginal distress even with radiation to the arms. Sometimes nausea and vomiting occur, and with vomiting the attack often ends. This sort of experience convinces the sufferer that it is all due to "indigestion" or to some food that was eaten. After the attack has lasted a variable length of time, it suddenly stops and the patient quickly recovers. Many will feel perfectly well shortly afterward, although a few will be left weak enough to remain in bed a day or so. How distressing the symptoms will be and how severe the evidence of circulatory failure will depend on three factors—the duration of the attack, the rate of the heart during the attack, and the state of the heart before the attack occurred. A normal heart can withstand a rate of over 200 continuously for several days, whereas if mitral stenosis is present evidence of congestive heart failure may develop in hours.

The *clinical diagnosis* of this condition is simple in most cases. It is important to obtain a history or elicit evidence of an abrupt change in rate. The heart rate during an attack of paroxysmal auricular tachycardia ranges from about 150 to 250 per minute, although slower rates may occasionally be found. The rhythm is perfectly regular. By this is meant that contiguous heart cycles will not vary more than 0.01 second in length (Fig. 64). This is very important diagnostically, for the ear is able to detect extremely minor alterations in rhythm. Not only is the heart rapid and regular, but its rate is very fixed for long intervals of time and cannot be altered by simple procedures like breathing or exercise which affect the rate of the normal heart. The rate may change over the course of hours but not during short intervals of time. The bedside application of this peculiarity is to count the rate carefully for sixty seconds by auscultation over the precordium. This should be repeated in several minutes, preferably under different circumstances, after slight exercise or with the patient sitting up rather than lying down. If there is a significant difference in the two rates one can be fairly sure the condition is not paroxysmal auricular tachycardia. With the latter the first count might be 169 and the second 168. If the second count were 174, it would point to a normal sinus tachycardia (Fig. 48). The difference should be no greater than two beats if the count is made carefully. Even this difference is to be accounted for by the difficulty in timing the first and last beats as one follows the second hand of the watch in its complete circuit. One often hears the statement that the rate, though regular, was too rapid to be counted. Although this may be so when the rhythm is irregular, I believe it means careless observation or lack of interest in accurate counting when it refers to a rapid regular rate. I had the opportunity of testing this in a case that showed a heart rate of 250. Three independent observers counted rates of 248, 249, and 250. When the rate is over 200 the actual counting process may be facilitated by tapping on the table with a pencil synchronously with the heart beat and then counting the taps. Emphasis is placed on this because the constancy of the rate can be determined by any physician and helps to distinguish a normal from an abnormal tachycardia.

The various methods that are used to stop an attack also serve as diagnostic procedures, for there is no other type of rapid heart action that can be made to return to a normal rate by such simple means and so quickly. Not only does a normal tachycardia reach its rapid rate gradually, starting from about 70 or 80 and then increasing to 100, 120, and finally 160 or 170, but when it returns to normal it does so gradually. If vagus stimulation is produced by pressure over the carotid sinus or the eyeball during paroxysmal tachycardia, the rate will remain entirely unaltered or it will abruptly fall to normal; i.e., the rate may change from 190 to 80 in one or two beats (Figs. 62, 63, 64, 81). With normal tachycardia, there is apt to be temporary slowing with gradual return to the previous rapid level (Figs. 81, 124). A similar effect is generally obtained if the tachycardia is due to auricular flutter (Fig. 73), and when ventricular tachycardia is the cause of the acceleration vagus stimulation produces no effect whatever. It is evident, therefore, that the diagnosis can generally be made at the bedside and only rarely will electrocardiograms be necessary.

The *treatment* of the condition can be divided into two problems. The first and easier task is to stop the attack. The second and more difficult is to prevent its recurrence. Most attacks will end if left alone and no harm will result. Occasionally severe congestive heart failure or anginal pain may develop and rarely may prove to be fatal. For thirty years one extraordinary patient was followed who had yearly severe attacks, in 1911, 1912, and 1913. During one of these he developed aphasia, which cleared in several months; during another he had a hemiplegia, which disappeared in a few months, leaving only a very slight spasticity; during the third, dry gangrene developed, necessitating amputation of the left arm at the shoulder. The tachycardia in these spells lasted from five to eleven days, without cessation. When the patient was seen during his fourth attack, the heart rate was 250. The blood pressure was about 94 mm. systolic and 88 mm. diastolic. He developed a fever of 101° and an appreciable leukocytosis. He also complained of a constant distressing constricting pain in the chest. There were a few rales at the bases of the lungs. Many of these features resemble those of an acute coronary thrombosis, a condition with which any severe form of paroxysmal rapid heart action can be confused. In fact, the heart was found to have dilated 2.5 centimeters, compared with its size on x-ray examination after the attack was over. Such dilatation is unusual in paroxysmal tachycardia, for in most cases there is very little or no dilatation. It is quite evident that proper treatment was very urgent in the case just cited. At first it was found that carotid sinus pressure was ineffective, but vigorous pressure over the eyeball ended the attack immediately. Subsequent attacks were readily controlled by pressure over the carotid sinus, and the patient was taught how to perform this procedure. For some unknown reason, the attacks gradually became quite rare. The patient remained in excellent health for over twenty years but later developed typical mild anginal pain on effort which was not associated with attacks of tachycardia.

Further illustrations of the urgency of proper treatment are the rare instances in which attacks occur in patients on the operating table during anesthesia. Breathing may cease entirely and the patient may become pulseless. Fatalities may even occur. I have seen several cases in which the condition seemed critical but was readily controlled by simple methods.

The simplest means of stopping an attack is to have the patient hold a deep inspiration as long as he can. He might be advised to make a quick expiratory effort with the glottis closed after a deep breath is taken. Many attacks can be ended quite readily in this way. The patient should be told that, if this fails, he might try to induce vomiting by placing his finger down the pharynx. The act of gagging, retching, or vomiting often ends attacks. This may be brought about by the hypodermic injection of apomorphine. More effective still is 1 to 4 teaspoonfuls of syrup of ipecac. Some patients have learned that lying down or lowering the head may be effective. Often, when the attack continues, morphine is given, and during the subsequent hour or two the heart returns to normal. When this occurs it is difficult to say that the medication causes the attack to end. The most valuable treatment is carotid sinus pressure. This is performed by placing two fingers over the carotid artery just below the jaw, where a slight bulge is felt as the common carotid artery divides, and pressing and massaging the artery against the spine for several seconds. First one side and then the other may be tried, but not both at the same time. This stimulates the vagus nerve reflexly (carotid sinus reflex), although it used to be thought that the vagus nerve which lies just behind the artery in the carotid sheath was stimulated directly. In the majority of cases, when this is properly done, the attack will end instantly. If this fails, ocular pressure may be tried (Fig. 64). One eye at a time should be firmly pressed backward. To be effective the pressure will have to be painful, but this method may succeed when others have failed. It is particularly applicable if the patient is already under an anesthetic, for then the pain will not be felt. In this procedure the reflex goes up the fifth cranial nerve and down the vagus (oculocardiac reflex). There have been rare instances in which carotid sinus pressure has resulted in hemiplegia. I have seen one such case in an elderly man. Very likely when marked cerebral sclerosis is present the fall in blood pressure and cessation of the circulation may result in local cerebral thrombosis. In fact, in extremely rare cases, fatalities have occurred because after a pause in the heart the normal beat was not resumed.

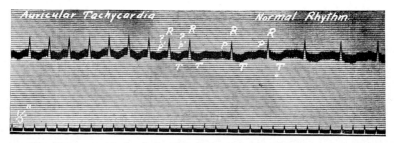

FIG. 65. *Paroxysmal Auricular Tachycardia.* Cessation of attack following 0.3 gm. of quinidine sulfate given intravenously. Abrupt transition occurred about thirty seconds after injection, from rate of 181 to 97. The patient had carcinomatosis but no heart disease. (Author's article in Oxford Loose-Leaf Medicine, vol. II.)

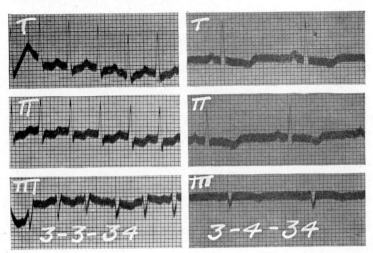

FIG. 66.   *Paroxysmal Auricular Tachycardia, Stopped by Digitalis.*   Tracings on the left show regular rate of 196. Set on the right taken twenty hours later, 1 gm. of digitalis having been given orally, shows normal rate of 69. The patient was a 62-year-old man with bronchopneumonia and a fever of 103° F., who recovered satisfactorily.

Finally, there are drugs that may stop attacks of tachycardia. One of the most successful is Prostigmin given subcutaneously in doses of 0.5 to 2.0 mg. Or, if the patient has received no digitalis in the preceding two weeks, rapid digitalization by the oral (Fig. 66) or by the intravenous route with Digoxin may gradually arrest an attack. The initial dose is 1 mg., followed by 0.25 mg. every two hours until reversion or toxicity develops or a total of 1.5 mg. has been given. An alternative measure would be administration of Cedilanid, 0.8 to 1.2 mg. Neo-Synephrine, 0.5 to 1.0 mg. intravenously, may stop attacks in one or two minutes, but this medication should be avoided in hypertension or coronary artery disease. Mecholyl chloride (acetyl-beta-methylcholine chloride) has been reported as very effective (Fig. 67). The average adult dose is about 20 mg. given subcutaneously. This produces a rather powerful stimulating effect on the vagus apparatus and often aborts an attack in a few minutes. Because of occasional untoward reactions, atropine should always be available for immediate hypodermic use in doses of 1 to 2 mg. Asthmatics or strongly allergic individuals should not be given Mecholyl. The alarming period of asystole which may ensue before the normal pacemaker resumes control of the rhythm makes one hesitate to use this medication.

Quinidine given orally has also had a wide vogue in the treatment of auricular tachycardia. Some rapidly acting preparation should be used since, if successful, its effect is prompt, total, and convincing. If, instead, quinidine is given in progressively increasing doses by mouth, as is often practiced, it is very difficult to be certain whether reversion is spontaneous or quinidine-induced. This point is of more than academic importance, since experience in one attack often determines how subsequent attacks are to be handled. In this sense the treatment of each attack is a titration for future reference. If the condition of the patient has become desperate and all other methods have failed, quinidine may be given by vein in the manner described under paroxysmal rapid heart action (Chap. 13). Instant fatality may follow the intravenous use of quinidine, so it cannot be recommended unless the circumstances warrant the risk. The literature also contains reports of the successful use of magnesium sulfate in the dose of about 2 gm. by vein (Fig. 68), calcium gluconate (10 to 20 cc. of 10 per cent solution given slowly intravenously), Atabrine in doses of 0.1 gm. of a 1 per cent solution by vein or 0.3 gm. in 1 per cent procaine solution intramuscularly, and Pronestyl as described under ventricular tachycardia. It is well worth remembering that if any of these drugs has been ineffective of itself, stimulation of the carotid sinus at the time of the maximum physiological effect of the drug may be followed by reversion. In general it will be found that the paroxysm can be controlled by one or another of the methods described.

The prevention of attacks presents a more difficult problem. If they recur infrequently, once a year or so, it hardly seems wise to institute a course of drug therapy because, not knowing when the attack is due, it will be necessary to keep the patient on the medication all those inter-

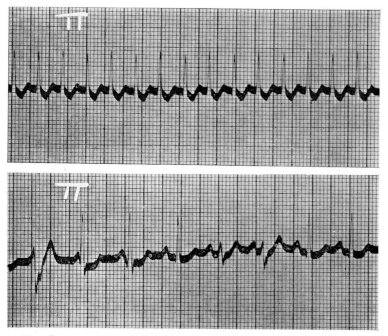

FIG. 67.   *Paroxysmal Auricular Tachycardia, Stopped by Mecholyl.*   Upper tracing shows regular rate of about 225. Lower set taken one minute after 25 mg. of Mecholyl was injected subcutaneously shows slow rate with occasional extrasystoles. The patient was a 36-year-old woman with no organic heart disease. Note electrical alternation of the R waves during tachycardia.

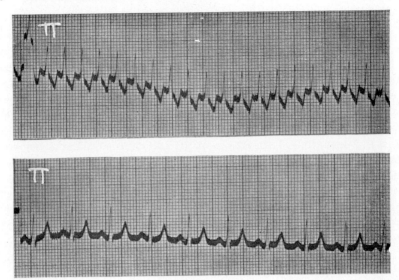

FIG. 68. *Paroxysmal Auricular Tachycardia, Stopped by Magnesium Sulfate.* Upper tracings show regular rate of 257. Lower set was taken two minutes after the intravenous injection of 3 gm. of magnesium sulfate and shows a normal rhythm. The patient was a 68-year-old man with probable spinal cord tumor but no heart disease.

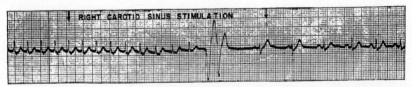

FIG. 69. *Paroxysmal Auricular Tachycardia.* Recording of Lead II showing supraventricular tachycardia with rate of 192. At first sight the small sharp inverted P waves deforming the RS-T segments immediately after the QRS complexes seem to be retrograde from the auriculoventricular node to the auricles. Attention to the last beat in the paroxysm, terminated with carotid sinus stimulation, shows no such inverted P wave following the QRS complex. It is clear, then, that the inverted P waves are not conducted back from the ventricles, but rather are conducted to the ventricles after a prolonged P-R interval. A pair of ectopic ventricular beats interrupt the paroxysm, are followed by a pause, and then the normal sinus rhythm is resumed at a rate of 108.

vening months with the hope of inhibiting this rare spell. It is better to do nothing and then to stop the attack when it occurs. When attacks come frequently the problem is different for they may be very annoying and it is possible to ascertain whether or not drug therapy is effective. Occasionally the constant administration of 0.2 to 0.3 gm. (3 to 5 grains) of quinidine sulfate will prevent attacks. Even more effective is constant complete digitalization. This must be carried out just as it is done in congestive heart failure. One or the other of these methods frequently obviates or at least diminishes the frequency or severity of the attacks.

PAROXYSMAL AURICULAR TACHYCARDIA WITH BLOCK

In classic paroxysmal auricular tachycardia the P-R interval may be in the upper reaches of normal or beyond (first degree auriculoventricular block). There is a distinctive form of paroxysmal auricular tachycardia in which higher degrees of auriculoventricular block (partial or complete) may occur spontaneously (Fig. 70) or be induced deliberately (Figs. 71, B, and 124). Carotid sinus stimulation does not abolish this arrhythmia as it does classic paroxysmal auricular tachycardia (Fig. 81); in this respect paroxysmal auricular tachycardia with block resembles auricular flutter. The auricular rate generally ranges from 150 to 200 but occasionally may reach 250. The auricular rhythm may be perfectly regular or very slightly irregular. The P waves may be taller or lower than normal P waves; they generally are shorter and are upright in the standard leads. An isoelectric baseline separates these distinct upright waves. The slower rate and quiescent baseline generally distinguish this disturbance from auricular flutter, but at times this differentiation cannot be made on purely electrocardiographic lines. Yet it is of the utmost importance that every effort be made to distinguish this arrhythmia from flutter and from classic auricular tachycardia, for it

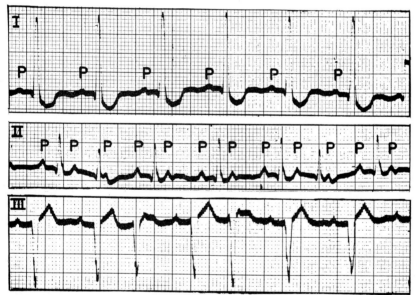

FIG. 70.   *Paroxysmal Auricular Tachycardia with Block.*   Normal sinus rhythm in Lead I with heart rate 89 and P-R interval 0.18 second. In the second strip (Lead II) paroxysmal auricular tachycardia (auricular rate 176) with block (ventricular rate 107) is recorded. Note the isoelectric period between the P waves contrasting with the constantly moving baseline characteristically seen in auricular flutter. The patient was a 63-year-old man with calcific aortic stenosis and aortic insufficiency, angina pectoris, and congestive heart failure, who had been treated with digitoxin, 0.1 to 0.2 mg. daily, over a two-month period, associated with nausea, vomiting, diarrhea, and photophobia. After seven days without digitoxin the abnormal rhythm and the other symptoms disappeared.

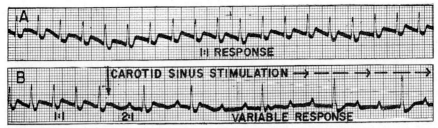

FIG. 71.   *Paroxysmal Auricular Tachycardia, with "Latent" Block.*   In tracing *A* there is a 1:1 response; classic paroxysmal auricular tachycardia appears to be present. In tracing *B* carotid sinus stimulation produces first a 2:1 then a variable ventricular response. The auricular rate is 173, the auricular rhythm slightly irregular. If this were classic paroxysmal auricular tachycardia either carotid pressure would have had no effect at all or it would have abolished the disturbance.

carries with it distinctive therapeutic implications. This is not an extremely rare condition. In fact, because of the widespread familiarity of the medical profession with paroxysmal auricular tachycardia, paroxysmal auricular tachycardia with block may be seen more commonly in hospital practice than classic paroxysmal auricular tachycardia. In about four fifths of the cases it is indicative of digitalis toxicity, the result either of actual overdosage with any of the various digitalis preparations, or of relative overdosage somehow implicated by potassium loss. It generally develops in very sick patients with organic heart disease and advanced congestive heart failure undergoing various forms of depletion therapy (mercurial diuresis, salt restriction, etc.). It is frequently the immediate and unrecognized cause of the death of these individuals. The electrocardiogram merely arouses the suspicion of that variety of paroxysmal auricular tachycardia with block related to digitalis therapy. A definitive clinical diagnosis of that condition must not be made except in the context of a background such as that just described.

Treatment consists of the omission of digitalis and, assuming adequate renal function, the administration of potassium. In the milder cases potassium chloride may be given by mouth in the dose of 5 gm. (67 milliequivalents) in iced orange juice. If this is unsuccessful in aborting the arrhythmia, half this dose may be repeated four hours later. Additional doses may be given if the auricular rate slows or the ventricular rate increases, but careful constant electrocardiographic control is essential to forestall the development of potassium intoxication, especially in very sick or elderly individuals. Patients in severe heart failure or those unable to retain the medication because of vomiting should be given potassium by vein, again with cautious electrocardiographic control. To this end 3 gm. (40 milliequivalents) of potassium chloride is infused slowly by vein in 500 cc. of 5 per cent glucose in water, over the course of an hour. The infusion is stopped immediately reversion occurs. If the auricles slow but reversion has not yet been induced, additional potassium may be given until a normal mechanism is restored. Experience indicates that procaine amide may also be effective in abbreviating this arrhythmia. This may be given orally (1 gm. at once, followed by 0.5 gm. every 3 to 6 hours) or intravenously (50 mg. every 2 minutes, with repetitive observations of blood pressure, the intervals between injections being lengthened if the blood pressure is lowered or the drug discontinued altogether if the pressure continues to fall). Potassium and procaine amide may be given simultaneously if the auricular rate is rapid. In those cases where differentiation between auricular flutter and paroxysmal auricular tachycardia with block is impossible on electro-cardiographic grounds, therapeutic testing with potassium or acetyl-strophanthidin (see p. 370) may enable one to make a clinical differentiation.

In about one-fifth of patients with paroxysmal auricular tachycardia with block the disorder is not due to digitalis and may even be helped by this medication, or by quinidine. These patients frequently have no heart disease whatever and may continue to demonstrate the arrhythmia for long periods of time, even months or years, often with little disability. These cases are not helped by potassium.

AURICULAR FLUTTER

A still higher degree of auricular disturbance is auricular flutter (Figs. 72 to 80). In this condition the auricular rate generally is between 200 and 350, and, except in very rare instances, the ventricles respond to only a fraction of this number, as the junctional tissue cannot conduct impulses so rapidly; i.e., there is in a sense a certain degree of auriculoventricular block. In exceptional cases all auricular beats come through to the ventricles and the heart rate is then very rapid (Figs. 76 and 105). During quinidine therapy the auricular rate may fall to as low as 150. It has been considered that the mechanism of this peculiar abnormality is the development of a circus movement. By this is meant that an impulse gets started and encircles the auricles around the venae cavae and on its return to the original focus finds the tissue out of its refractory state and continues around again and again, always meeting muscle bundles ahead of it that are ready to conduct the impulse. In auricular flutter this pathway is constant and therefore the waves will be regular and constant in form. In auricular fibrillation, to be discussed later, because the rate is more rapid, each impulse finds bits of tissue ahead of it that are still refractory following the previous contraction, so that it has to deviate to one side or another, constantly seeking fibers that will conduct. The result is a sinuous course, and more irregular and more inconstant fibrillary waves occur. Auricular flutter has therefore been regarded as a pure circus motion, whereas auricular fibrillation has been regarded as an impure one. The validity of this concept has long been denied by continental writers. Cinematographic and electrographic studies on experimental flutter in this country by Prinzmetal have cast further doubt on the traditional teaching.

The electrocardiograms of auricular flutter are very peculiar and characteristic. In Lead I the auricular waves are represented by small

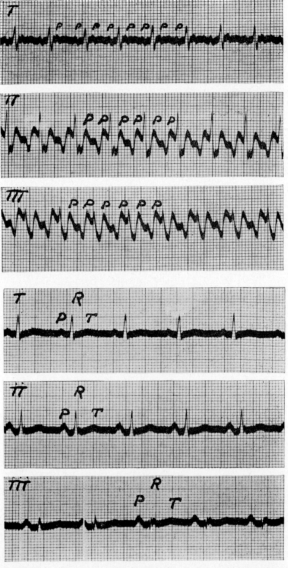

FIG. 72. *Auricular Flutter.* Upper three leads were taken during auricular flutter, lower three were taken four weeks later during normal rhythm. During tachycardia the auricular rate is 278, ventricular 139 (2:1 block). Identity and rapidity of auricular beats are difficult to make out until the ventricles are slowed (see Fig. 73). Note the small P waves in Lead I, prominent triangular P waves in Leads II and III with a sharp upstroke and a coarsely notched downstroke. Normal mechanism was established on quinidine therapy. The patient had no heart disease but complained of syncopal attacks for three years.

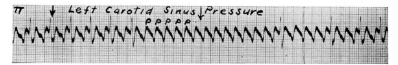

FIG. 73.   *Auricular Flutter.*   Effect of left carotid sinus pressure. (Same case as Fig. 72.) The ventricular rate is temporarily inhibited, permitting the undisturbed rapid auricular mechanism to become clear.

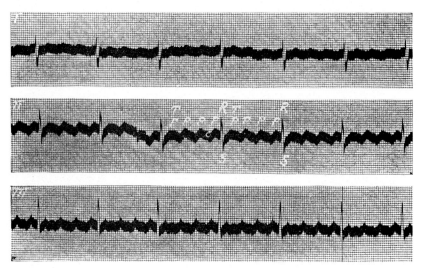

FIG. 74.   *Auricular Flutter.*   The P waves are regular, rate 208; the ventricular complexes are regular, rate 52; there is a 4:1 block. Note triangular form of P waves in Leads II and III. The slow ventricular rate resulted from digitalis. (Author's article in Oxford Loose-Leaf Medicine, vol. II.)

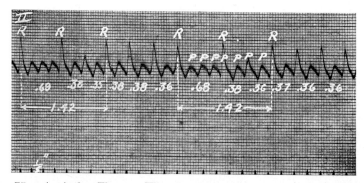

FIG. 75.   *Auricular Flutter.*   The ventricular beats (R) come irregularly, but because of responses to regularly beating auricles (P) there is equal grouping of beats, i.e., not an absolute irregularity. (Author's article in Oxford Loose-Leaf Medicine, vol. II.)

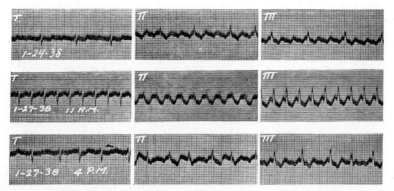

FIG. 76.   *Auricular Flutter.*   Upper curves show mainly a 3:1 block. Middle set shows a 1:1 rhythm. Both auricular and ventricular rates are 191. Lowest set shows a changing degree of block.

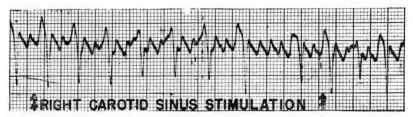

FIG. 77.   *Auricular Flutter, with Extremely Rapid Flutter Rate.*   The patient was a 54-year-old woman who developed auricular flutter with a flutter rate of 440 and a 3:1 response during a thyroid storm. Note slowing on right carotid sinus stimulation, disclosing characteristic sharp ascent and interrupted descent of the flutter waves. Extremely rapid rates in this range are only rarely recorded.

notches (Fig. 72). In Leads II and III the waves have a triangular form. The upstroke is sharp and smooth and the downstroke more prolonged and notched at its midpoint. It seems as if there is a hesitation on the downstroke where the isoelectric line might have occurred. It makes one think that each auricular cycle begins at this point and that the entire complex is diphasic rather than beginning either at the top or bottom of these P waves. The flutter waves are continuous; as one cycle ends the next begins. There is also a similarity between the flutter waves in different patients. In untreated patients there will generally be found a 2:1 heart block, every second beat failing to reach the ventricles. The auricular rate may be 320 and the ventricular 160. It therefore may be difficult to distinguish the auricular waves or count their rate because they become superimposed on the ventricular complexes. With experience one learns to detect flutter from the appearance of the electrocardiograms, but if there is any doubt as to the underlying mechanism, vagal stimulation can help to identify the condition (Figs. 73 and 78). In Figure 72 it may be questioned whether there are one or two auricular complexes between each ventricular beat. However, when the ventricles are inhibited for a short period of time by pressure on the carotid sinus

(Fig. 73) or by digitalis (Figs. 74 and 75), it is then possible to see the flutter waves undisturbed. The true rapid rate easily becomes apparent and is found to be twice the original ventricular rate. The continuous activity of the auricles is also readily visualized from such tracings.

The rhythm of the auricles is strikingly regular. The ventricular rate and rhythm will depend on the degree of heart block. When there

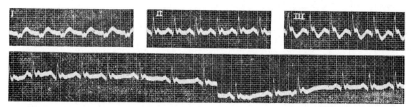

FIG. 78. *Carotid Sinus Stimulation.* Value of carotid sinus stimulation in deciphering an abnormal auricular rhythm. The patient was a 68-year-old man with an acute myocardial infarction. The upper set of electrocardiograms showed a ventricular rate of 136. An upward deflection, particularly well seen in Lead II, was interpreted by one observer as auricular flutter, and by another as paroxysmal auricular tachycardia with block. The lower tracing, after right carotid sinus stimulation, shows that what was thought to be a P wave was actually part of the QRS complex. Precordial leads showed this secondary R wave to be an evidence of right bundle branch block.

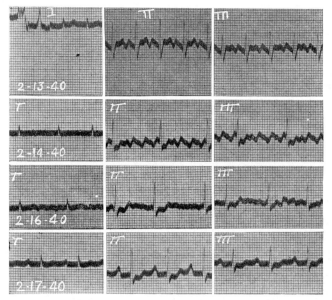

FIG. 79. *Auricular Flutter; Effect of Digitalis.* Upper set of tracings shows auricular flutter with 2:1 rhythm; auricular rate 300, ventricular rate 150. Second set shows flutter with 4:1 rhythm, auricular rate 300, ventricular 75. Third set shows auricular fibrillation with ventricular rate about 75. Lowest set shows normal rhythm rate about 95. The patient received 0.4 gm. digitalis orally on February 13, 1940, and 0.6 gm. on February 14, 1940, then digitalis was omitted. This patient was 63 years old, had mitral stenosis and insufficiency with marked dyspnea and palpitation.

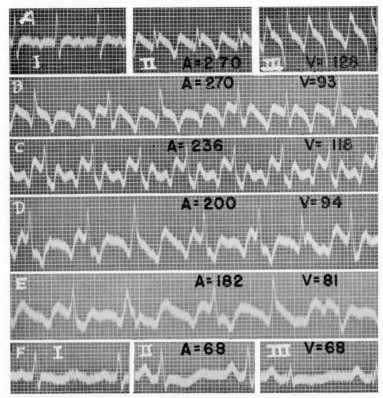

FIG. 80. *Effect of Quinidine.* Effect of quinidine on auricular and ventricular rates in auricular flutter. The patient was a 38-year-old man without evidence of organic heart disease who complained of spells of palpitation for three years, occasionally associated with syncope. *A*, Leads I, II, and III on admission, before quinidine. Auricular flutter with 2:1 response. Auricular rate 270. *B*, second day; on digifolin. Auricular flutter with varying (2:1, 4:1) response. Auricular rate 270. *C*, fourth day, after increasing doses of quinidine (0.5 to 1.5 gm.) for two days. Auricular rate 236; ventricular rate 118. Note that the ventricles have speeded up while the auricles have slowed. This is a frequent finding and apt to be alarming, but the drug should be continued despite this. *D*, fifth day. Auricular rate 200. *E*, seventh day. Auricular rate 182. *F*, tenth day; still on quinidine. Normal sinus rhythm, rate 68. Note slowing of auricular rate from 270 to 182 before reversion to normal rhythm. The "sawtooth" contour is present at rapid and slow flutter rates.

is a 2:1 block, as is commonly the case, the ventricles will necessarily be perfectly regular, contiguous cycles not varying more than 0.01 second in length, just as in paroxysmal auricular tachycardia. We now have four conditions that might account for a rapid regular heart rate; i.e., normal tachycardia, auricular tachycardia, auricular tachycardia with block, and auricular flutter. It often is possible to distinguish these at the bedside. If the regular rate that is counted at the apex is 190 or more, the condition is most likely paroxysmal tachycardia, for a normal tachycardia rarely reaches that high level; the condition is not likely to be auricular flutter, because the auricular rate would have to be 380 which is too fast, or 190, which not only is too slow but would necessi

tate a 1:1 mechanism which occurs but is extremely rare (Fig. 76). I
have only rarely seen instances of flutter with auricular rates of 380
to 440, twice during a thyroid storm (Fig. 77) and once during lobar
pneumonia. It must be remembered that on auscultation only the ventricular beats are heard, as the auricular beats are inaudible. Furthermore, if vagal stimulation produced by breathing, carotid pressure, or
ocular pressure terminates the rapid rate completely, the condition must
be paroxysmal tachycardia, for neither normal tachycardia nor flutter
ever responds in this fashion. If the ventricular rhythm is temporarily
disturbed and slowed, the diagnosis of auricular tachycardia is eliminated, for in the latter the tachycardia either would be unaffected or
would disappear entirely. When the ventricular rate is slowed, therefore,
the condition may still be either flutter, paroxysmal auricular tachycardia with block, or normal acceleration (Figs. 73 and 124). The length
of the heart cycles during these interruptions, the method by which the
rapid rate is resumed, and other factors may then distinguish the one
from the other. During the long pauses, if frequent auricular waves can
be seen in the jugular pulse, auricular flutter or paroxysmal auricular
tachycardia with block is present. Either of these conditions would be
present if the heart rate at any time, even for one cycle, is found suddenly to be halved. Differentiation between the more common flutter
and the less common paroxysmal auricular tachycardia with block would
then depend upon the clinical setting, the auricular rate, and, at this
point, the configuration of the auricular deflections in the electrocardiogram. Figure 81 illustrates the response of various types of rapid heart
action to vagus stimulation produced by carotid sinus pressure. From
such observations one is frequently enabled to distinguish one type from
another by simple bedside examination.

When digitalis is given to a patient with auricular flutter the original
degree of block increases. Instead of every second beat, only every fourth
beat may reach the ventricles (Fig. 74). The ventricular rate will now
necessarily be perfectly regular and slow. If we assume the original
auricular rate to have been 300, and the ventricular 150, the auricular
rate will be the same but the ventricular rate will be 75. When a patient
is seen for the first time under such circumstances, the underlying mechanism can easily be overlooked for one would not suspect that the rhythm
was abnormal with a regular rate of 75. If one thought about the possibility of auricular flutter, one might search for and detect numerous
auricular waves in the jugular veins because the auricles are contracting
constantly. Of greater help than this is to have the patient exercise a
bit. The heart rate may be found to jump suddenly to exactly twice its
former rate for a short time; i.e., the original 2:1 block returns, or an
irregularity will develop that will lead to the proper diagnosis.

A further effect of digitalis is that the ventricular rate may become
irregular. The degree of block then varies. Sometimes every second beat
or every third or fourth beat comes through to the ventricles (Fig. 75).
The irregularity may seem to be gross and resemble the total irregularity

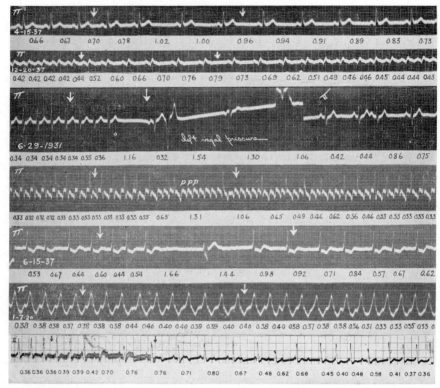

FIG. 81.   *Effect of Vagal Stimulation.*   Arrows in each tracing indicate duration of carotid sinus pressure. Numbers indicate duration in seconds of respective heart beats. First set shows normal gradual slowing in *normal rhythm.* Second set shows gradual slowing with gradual return toward the original rapid rate in *normal tachycardia.* Third set shows instant cessation of an attack of *paroxysmal auricular tachycardia.* Fourth set shows temporary slowing of the ventricles with irregular return to the original rapid rate in *auricular flutter.* Note that the auricular rate remains unaffected. Fifth set shows temporary slowing of the ventricles in *auricular fibrillation,* with return of original grossly irregular rhythm. Sixth set shows no effect in *ventricular tachycardia,* slight irregularities persisting throughout. Last set shows transient slowing with irregular return to original rapid rate in *paroxysmal auricular tachycardia with block.* The effect resembles that in auricular flutter but the auricular rate is 162, the P waves upright, and the baseline isoelectric between the auricular deflections. (The AC interference was introduced by the examiner and could have been avoided by having a dry towel between his fingers and the patient's neck.) These effects characterize each type of mechanism.

of auricular fibrillation. On careful examination, however, it will be found that there still remains a dominant rhythm, as the ventricles respond to regularly beating auricles. Beats will occur in groupings of equal lengths, inasmuch as they correspond to equal numbers of auricular cycles (Fig. 75). This distinguishes it from auricular fibrillation.

Unlike paroxysmal tachycardia, which generally occurs in otherwise normal hearts, auricular flutter is apt to be associated with organic heart disease, either valvular or myocardial, although it can manifest itself as a purely functional disturbance. It may occur in the form of paroxysms lasting hours or days and be transient, but more often once established it is permanent unless the patient is treated. It can persist for many years. It occasionally develops during coronary thrombosis, hyperthyroidism, rheumatic fever, pneumonia, pericarditis or other infections, or as a terminal event in chronic nephritis. In very rare cases flutter can actually be the result of overdosage with digitalis.

The aim in the *treatment* of patients with auricular flutter is to restore the normal rhythm or, if this is impossible, to keep the ventricular rate slow. When digitalis is given, in about one third or a half of the cases the following changes will take place. First the ventricular rate slows, the flutter continuing. Then after several days the mechanism changes to auricular fibrillation. If the digitalis is omitted at this point, a normal mechanism may quickly be re-established (Fig. 79). Often the flutter continues on digitalis therapy with a slow ventricular rate, or the fibrillation that develops persists. It is preferable to have the latter rather than the former condition. Quinidine is also a valuable therapeutic agent in auricular flutter. On increasing doses the auricular rate will actually slow, at times to well under 200, while the effect on the ventricles will vary. The ventricular rate may be slowed or accelerated. With the diminished rate of the auricles a larger proportion of the beats may reach the ventricles (Fig. 80). Finally the circus motion in the auricles may be broken up and a normal mechanism established. At times large doses of quinidine are necessary to accomplish this, even as much as 1.5 or 2 gm. (22 to 30 grains) in a single dose (Fig. 80). It is advisable to try digitalis first, as it is safer, and if it does not accomplish the desired effect it is better to have the patient digitalized before giving quinidine. Patients with auricular flutter receiving drug treatment require careful observation and should be in a hospital, where the condition can be followed with frequent electrocardiographic records.

AURICULAR FIBRILLATION

The highest degree of auricular disturbance is called auricular fibrillation. In this condition the number of auricular impulses is very great, 350 or more. The mechanism has been regarded as due to a circus motion in which the path is impure and irregular. The auricles do not actually contract, but rather remain distended in diastole and show fibrillary twitching. There is no constant pathologic change in the auricles to explain auricular fibrillation and at present it is regarded as a functional derangement accompanying a variety of states. The condition can be easily reproduced in the experimental animal by faradizing the auricles and has been observed repeatedly in the living hearts of patients undergoing cardiac surgery. The number of auricular impulses is so great that only a portion of them can be conducted through the junctional tissue. Therefore, there is always some degree of heart block associated with auricular fibrillation. The ventricular response is grossly irregular, short cycles and longer cycles occurring without rhyme or reason. The

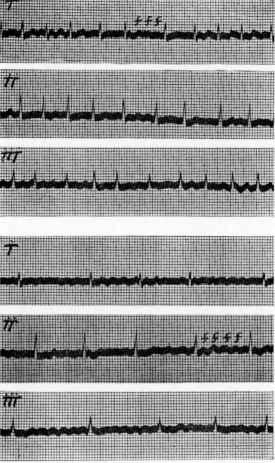

FIG. 82.   *Auricular Fibrillation; Effect of Digitalis.*   The upper three leads were
taken July 9, 1935. Note the gross irregularity of the ventricular beats (rate 147),
the absence of the normal P wave, and the presence of the auricular fibrillary waves
(f-f-f), rate 391. The lower three leads taken July 10, 1935, after 1.5 gm. of digitalis
had been given, show fibrillation continuing but the ventricular rate is now 60 and
still irregular. The patient had mitral stenosis and decompensation.

peripheral pulse is necessarily irregular both in time and in force of contraction. In the past it has been called perpetual arrhythmia, absolute
or total irregularity, and delirium cordis. In more recent years the true
nature of this disorder has been clarified, and the name "auricular
fibrillation" given to it.

It follows from the preceding description that whatever results from
the normal presystolic contraction of the auricles would disappear when
fibrillation develops. In the electrocardiogram the normal P wave will
be absent and instead there will be found irregular rapid fibrillary waves
(f-f-f) for the most part throughout the cardiac cycle, as the auricular
activity is continuous. There will also be a totally irregular ventricular
response (Figs. 82 to 89). Inasmuch as the impulses that succeed in

reaching the ventricles travel down the normal auriculoventricular conduction path, the ventricular complexes are normal in form. These three features of the electrocardiogram, i.e., the absence of the P wave, the presence of fibrillary waves, and the gross irregularity of ventricular beats, make it quite simple to identify auricular fibrillation. Sometimes the fibrillary waves are quite prominent, especially in mitral stenosis, and they may resemble those seen in auricular flutter. It would seem as if the circus motion in places becomes almost perfectly regular. Furthermore, these fibrillary waves may be entirely absent in one or more leads (Fig. 84, Lead III). Occasionally the diastolic interval is perfectly smooth, in which event the diagnosis of auricular fibrillation will rest on the other criteria or on taking esophageal, precordial, or special auricular leads. Finally, under certain circumstances, although the auricles are fibrillating, the ventricles contract regularly (Fig. 89). In some cases, when digitalis is administered, this takes place. It is thought that complete heart block results, and while the auricles continue fibrillating the pace is set for the ventricular rate at the auriculoventricular node or the junctional tissue. When this takes place as a result of digitalis, the regular ventricular rate of complete heart block is not the slow one customarily seen in Adams-Stokes disease. On the contrary, the rate will be 55 to 70 or more, and when the dose is increased it may exceed 100. In fact, if digitalis is continued in large doses, a fatal intoxication may result. The important inference from this is that when a patient with auricular

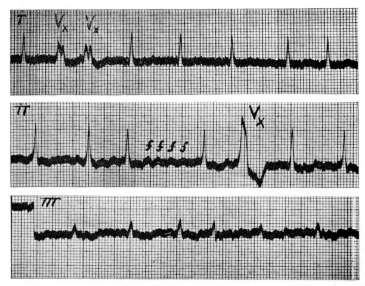

FIG. 83.   *Auricular Fibrillation.*   Note the absolute irregularity of the ventricles, the rapid fibrillation of the auricles (f-f-f), and the absence of normal P waves. The abnormal ventricular beats in Lead I may be paired ventricular premature beats. That in Lead II represents aberrant ventricular conduction (see p. 522). The patient had no heart disease and the rhythm became regular on increasing doses of quinidine.

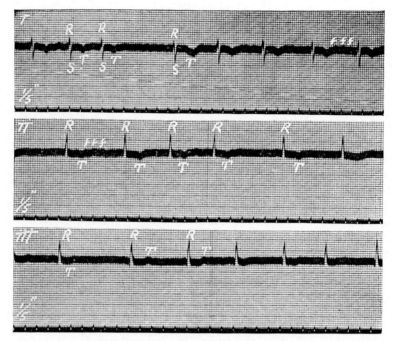

FIG. 84. *Auricular Fibrillation.*   Note the absolute irregularity of the ventricles and the absence of the P waves. The fibrillary waves (f-f-f) are very small in Leads I and II and practically invisible in Lead III. The patient had mitral stenosis and decompensation. (Author's article in Oxford Loose-Leaf Medicine, vol. II.)

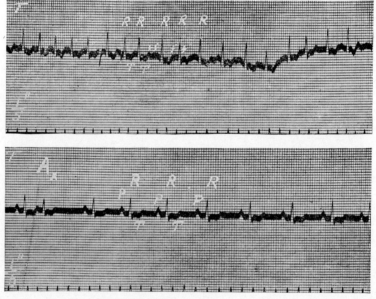

FIG. 85. *Auricular Fibrillation, Paroxysmal.*   The upper tracing shows typical auricular fibrillation with an irregular ventricular rate of 157. The lower tracing, taken a few days later, shows normal auricular contractions (P waves), rate 85. There is one premature auricular beat (Ax). (Author's article in Oxford Loose-Leaf Medicine, vol. II.)

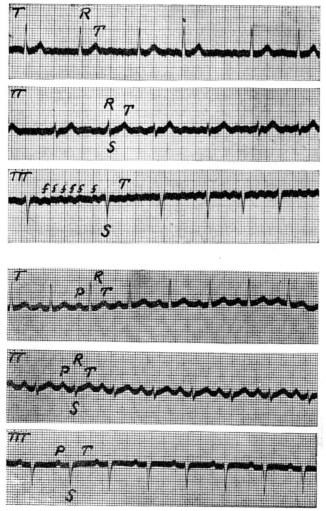

FIG. 86. *Auricular Fibrillation; Effect of Quinidine.* Upper three leads taken
June 19, 1935, show typical auricular fibrillation. Lower three leads taken June 28,
1935, show a normal rhythm. Increasing doses of quinidine sulfate, up to 0.5 gm.,
had been given in the meantime. Contrast this with the effect of digitalis, Figure 82.
This patient had no organic heart disease.

fibrillation develops a regular rhythm while taking digitalis the change
may be due either to a resumption of the normal rhythm or to the
development of this peculiar type of complete heart block. On rare occasions true spontaneous complete heart block with a ventricular rate of
30 may be associated with auricular fibrillation. This subject is further
considered below in the discussion of digitalis toxicity.

From a clinical point of view auricular fibrillation is the most important of all disturbances in the mechanism of the heart beat. It is extremely common, it produces considerable disability if untreated and

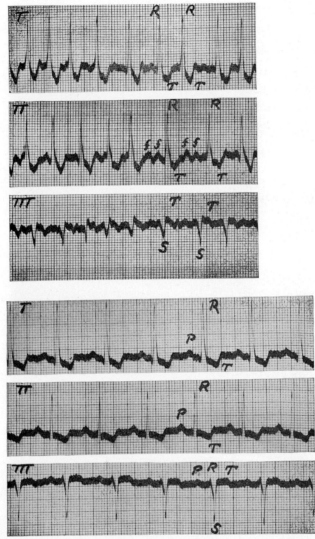

FIG. 87. *Auricular Fibrillation; Effect of Quinidine.* Upper three leads are typical of auricular fibrillation; lower three leads show a normal rhythm. Regularization occurred the morning after three doses of 0.3 gm. of quinidine sulfate were given. The patient was a 25-year-old man with mitral stenosis and aortic insufficiency.

responds very satisfactorily to treatment. It occurs in the transient (Fig. 85) as well as in the permanent form. When paroxysms occur they generally last several hours or a day or so. When the irregularity has lasted for about a week it may be expected to persist indefinitely unless specific measures are taken to restore the normal mechanism. The most common conditions with which it is associated are rheumatic valvular disease with mitral stenosis, hypertensive heart disease, coronary artery disease, and hyperthyroidism. It occasionally develops suddenly during acute infections, such as pneumonia and rheumatic fever. It is common during the early days following an acute coronary thrombosis. Gallstones are not infrequently found in some of the elderly individuals who have the transient form of auricular fibrillation, but whether there is any association between the two conditions is not certain. On rare occasions auricular fibrillation develops as a result of digitalis therapy. Finally, it may be present either as a paroxysmal or as a permanent phenomenon in otherwise healthy individuals. This latter group of patients is an important one, and, curiously, most of its members are males. Paroxysmal auricular fibrillation is more common than is generally supposed. It is particularly characteristic of hyperthyroidism and may be the single clue that leads one to this diagnosis. In fact, it is wise to suspect hyperthyroidism whenever a transient spell of this irregularity occurs.

The bedside recognition of this condition is generally simple. A rapid, apparently grossly irregular heart with an appreciable pulse deficit (the count at the apex being 10 beats or more greater than at the wrist) is due to auricular fibrillation nine times out of ten. The common association of a past history of rheumatic fever or chorea, the presence of mitral stenosis, and auricular fibrillation enables one to predict the presence of the third of these factors if the other two are known to exist. If a patient had rheumatic fever and shows signs of mitral stenosis, then a grossly irregular heart is almost always due to auricular fibrillation. If this irregularity is present and there is a history of rheumatic fever, there probably is mitral stenosis. Finally, if the patient has mitral stenosis and auricular fibrillation, he has been rheumatic whether a positive history can be obtained or not. Exceptions will be found for these generalizations, but it is surprising how frequently they will be valid.

When auricular fibrillation first develops the ventricular rate is quite rapid except in rare instances in which some defect in the junctional tissue already is present. When digitalis is given it slows the ventricular response. Figure 82 shows such an effect, the ventricular rate falling from 147 to about 60 in twenty-four hours after a large dose of digitalis was administered. It must be borne in mind that the fibrillation of the

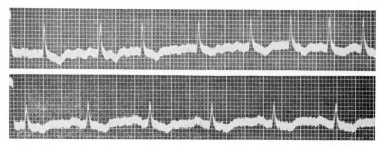

FIG. 88.   *Auricular Fibrillation; Effect of Propylthiouracil.*   Upper curve shows auricular fibrillation in Lead II when patient was thyrotoxic. The lower curve was recorded one month later, when evidence of thyrotoxicosis had disappeared and normal sinus rhythm had been restored following oral administration of propylthiouracil, 200 mg. daily.

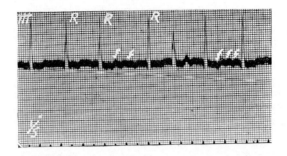

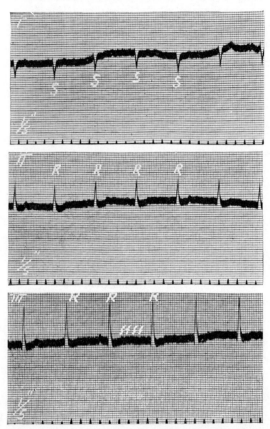

FIG. 89. *Auricular Fibrillation with Regular Ventricular Rhythm.* The upper curve shows the typical gross irregularity. The lower three leads, taken after complete digitalization, show that the fibrillation continues although the ventricles are perfectly regular, i.e., probably complete heart block of the toxic type due to digitalis. (Author's article in Oxford Loose-Leaf Medicine, vol. II.)

auricles persists. Digitalis does not stop the fibrillation; it merely, through its vagal influence on the conduction tissue, prevents many of these rapid beats from reaching the ventricle. Physicians are too inclined to use the expression that "the fibrillation is less," when what is meant is that the ventricles are slower or their contraction is less tumultuous.

The fibrillation of the auricles is either present or absent; from a practical point of view there are no degrees of fibrillation. When the ventricular rate slows, however, the pulse deficit diminishes and may entirely disappear. At this time the bedside rule of thumb is no longer diagnostic. If a physician first sees a patient under these circumstances, the diagnosis is more difficult and must be made on other criteria. Irregularities of the heart beat and of the pulse, though slight, will still be present. The condition may resemble other arrhythmias. Exercise may accelerate the rate and make the more characteristic features return. Rarely will it be necessary to have electrocardiograms before a final decision can be made. There is one additional clinical finding that may help to distinguish fibrillation from a very irregular rhythm due to numerous extrasystoles. In both conditions cycles of short, long, or medium duration may occur at various times. In irregular rhythm due to extrasystoles, it will be found that with extrasystoles all the long pauses are preceded by quick beats because they are compensatory. The same auscultatory phenomenon is present with auricular fibrillation. However, if one listens long enough and hears a sudden pause not preceded by a quick beat, this points to auricular fibrillation. (See the fifth heart cycle in Lead II, Fig. 84). In other words, a sudden lengthening of the heart cycle after a beat of normal length is more characteristic of auricular fibrillation than is a sudden shortening of the cycle.

The customary *treatment* for patients with auricular fibrillation is digitalis. The purpose is to slow the ventricular rate and, if this slowing does not result from adequate dosage, one may rightly suspect that the drug is not sufficiently potent or that the patient has hyperthyroidism. Ordinarily the slowing is marked, and the specific effect of the drug can be compared to the action of quinine in malaria. Furthermore, no similar slowing of a normal tachycardia can be expected from digitalis. This explains why some cardiac patients improve after fibrillation develops, for the digitalis that had been given previously without effect only then begins to slow the rate.

Quinidine, on the other hand, is used at times to treat patients with auricular fibrillation (Chaps. 13, 20). The purpose here is to restore the heart to a regular rhythm (Figs. 86, 87). In terms of the circus rhythm hypothesis it does so by lengthening the refractory period of the auricular musculature so that when the wave completes its circuit it finds the tissue ahead of it still refractory and the circus ends, permitting the normal pacemaker to send out its impulse and re-establish ascendency over the beat of the heart. The reason that quinidine does not always break up fibrillation is that it also slows the speed of the impulse, which would tend to perpetuate the circus motion by allowing sufficient time for tissue to recover from its refractoriness. When the first effect predominates, fibrillation ceases; when the latter predominates, it continues. Quinidine is particularly useful in restoring normal rhythm if there is no organic heart disease and in a few other selected cases of auricular fibrillation.

ECTOPIC AURICULOVENTRICULAR (NODAL) BEATS

Abnormal beats may arise in the auriculoventricular node or in the bundle of His. The pacemaker in the junctional tissue may control the rhythm of the heart for long periods of time (Figs. 90, 91), or only isolated beats may arise (Fig. 93). The impulse will travel down the ventricles through normal pathways, and therefore the ventricular complexes will be normal. It reaches the auricles, however, in a reversed direction, and so will produce abnormal P waves. The contraction of the auricle may take place shortly before or after that of the ventricle, depending on which receives the impulse first.

It has been assumed that if the focus is near the top of the auricular end of the node, the impulse will reach the auricles quickly, but the P-R interval will be shorter than normal. If the focus is lower in the node, the impulse may be conducted into the auricles and ventricles at the same time, and the P and R waves may coincide. In this instance the P wave is hidden in the QRS complex. If the focus is still lower in the node, the ventricles will respond before the auricles, and an R-P interval rather than a P-R interval results (Fig. 91). But a designation of "high," "mid," or "low" nodal rhythm on this basis is subject to some uncertainty since one cannot be sure that the rate of conduction is uniform throughout the auriculoventricular node and bundle. In fact, as has already been mentioned, there is physiological evidence that the speed of conduction picks up as the impulse descends the node, and it is not known whether local changes in conduction velocity may occur under pathological circumstances. At times within the same tracing varying positions of the P wave will be found, sometimes before or after or even simultaneously with the R wave. At other times the origin of the beat may vary in different parts of the sino-auricular node and also in the auriculoventricular node, or one node may compete with the other in controlling the beat. This condition is called a wandering pacemaker and will display different shapes of P waves (Fig. 92). The normal beat from the sino-auricular node may produce auricular contraction before a nodal impulse reaches the auricles. In this case the regular sequence of the P waves remains undisturbed despite occurrence of the premature nodal beat (Fig. 93). The auriculoventricular node often escapes whenever there is a long pause of the normal pacemaker, because it has its own irritability and rhythmicity which is then permitted to manifest itself.

Nodal rhythms have no great clinical significance and cannot be identified without graphic methods. They may occur during anesthesia, deep breathing, or vagal stimulation, and can be produced by certain drugs. There are no practical diagnostic, prognostic, or therapeutic problems involved in this type of irregularity.

Although nodal beats cannot be accurately identified without graphic methods, when a series of such beats arise and the relation of auricular and ventricular systole keeps changing, one may suspect the

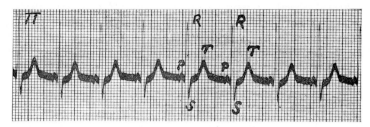

FIG. 90. *Nodal Rhythm.* Note that the P waves have a peculiar form and that the P-R interval is very short (0.06 second). The ventricular complexes are normal. This patient had acute rheumatic carditis.

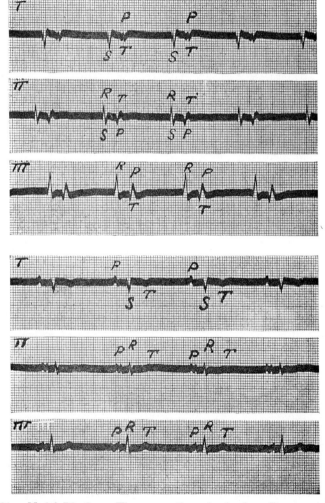

FIG. 91. *Nodal Rhythm.* The upper three leads show P waves of a peculiar form coming at a constant interval after the R waves (R-P interval of 0.23 second). The lower three leads show a return to the normal rhythm with a P-R interval of 0.22 second. The patient had alcoholic cirrhosis of liver.

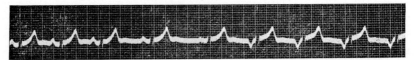

FIG. 92. *Wandering Pacemaker*. The first four beats arise in the sino-auricular node, the last four in the auriculoventricular node. The intervening (fifth) beat shows a flat P wave representing composite activation of the auricles from both the sino-auricular and the auriculoventricular node, so that the upper part of the auricles is stimulated from the sino-auricular node and the lower part of the auricles from the auriculoventricular node. This, then, is a combination or fusion auricular complex. This sequence depicting migration of the pacemaker from one node to the other is one form of wandering pacemaker. The pacemaker may also wander from the upper to the middle or to the lower part of the sino-auricular node, or to the auriculoventricular node.

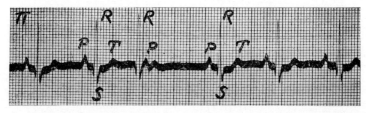

FIG. 93. *Premature Nodal Beat*. Note that the premature beat which arises in the auriculoventricular node produces a ventricular complex of normal form. The auricular rhythm is undisturbed as the P wave comes exactly on time. There was no heart disease here.

presence of this type of arrhythmia by detecting a changing quality or intensity of the first heart sound. This alteration is the result of the differences in the position of the auriculoventricular valves at the moment ventricular systole occurs. A similar mechanism accounts for variations in the quality of the first heart sound in other arrhythmias, for this sound is mainly, if not entirely, due to the snap of the auriculoventricular valves. At times the appearance of extraordinarily large pulse waves in the neck veins may furnish a clue to the presence of a "mid" or "low" nodal rhythm. This can be attributed to contraction of the right auricle against a closed or closing tricuspid valve. Similar pulsations may also be observed with ventricular premature beats.

PAROXYSMAL NODAL TACHYCARDIA

One would presuppose that a paroxysm of tachycardia might arise from the auriculoventricular node or junctional tissue just as it does from the auricles or ventricles. It is difficult to be certain of this, for when such a tachycardia displays abnormal P waves it cannot be determined whether such waves are the result of impulses arising in the auricles, in which event it really indicates paroxysmal auricular tachycardia, or whether they come from the auriculoventricular node. It is almost impossible to identify which ventricular complex is related to the

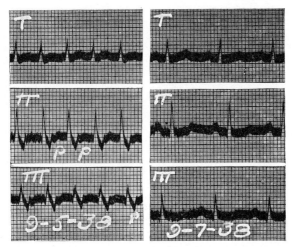

FIG. 94.   *Paroxysmal Nodal Tachycardia (Probable).*   The first set shows regular rate of 201. Note that P waves seem to occur at the R-T junction. The second set shows normal slow rhythm. Some of these attacks were stopped by carotid sinus pressure. The patient was a 54-year-old man with tubercular constrictive pericarditis and obliterative pleuritis.

particular P wave (Fig. 94). In Figure 69, although at first sight this was regarded as paroxysmal nodal tachycardia, attention to the last beat in the paroxysm shows that the final ventricular beat in the paroxysm does not show an inverted P wave immediately after the QRS complex. It is thus apparent that the inverted P waves following each of the other QRS complexes in the paroxysm is not retrograde from the ventricles but rather is conducted after a long P-R interval (0.24 second) to the ventricles as the succeeding QRS complex. From a clinical point of view whatever has been said about paroxysmal auricular tachycardia applies to the condition that might be called "paroxysmal nodal tachycardia."

ECTOPIC VENTRICULAR BEATS

Premature beats arising in some ectopic focus in the ventricle are extremely common (Figs. 95 to 102). This arrhythmia is generally the cause of what the physician calls an "intermittent pulse." This latter expression should be given up because intermittence of the peripheral pulse can be due to a variety of disturbances of the heart beat, which can be properly diagnosed on auscultation of the heart. In this condition the heart is beating regularly, when suddenly a quick beat is heard, followed by a pause. The premature beat may occur so early in the previous diastole that the pressure and volume of blood in the ventricles often are not great enough to produce a pulse at the wrist (Fig. 100) and occasionally may not even open the aortic valves. In the latter event only one heart sound may be heard over the precordium for that particular beat. I have even observed instances of the occurrence, while electrocardiograms were being taken, of ventricular premature beats

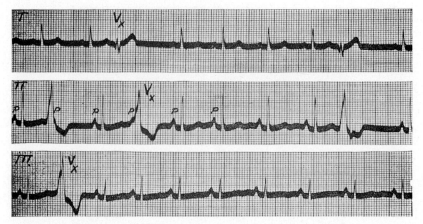

FIG. 95.   *Premature Ventricular Beats, Probably Arising from Left Ventricle.*   The normal rhythm is occasionally interrupted by ventricular complexes having a decidedly abnormal form (V_x). Note that the regularity of the auricular beats (P) is not interrupted although some are buried with the extrasystole. The patient had neurocirculatory asthenia.

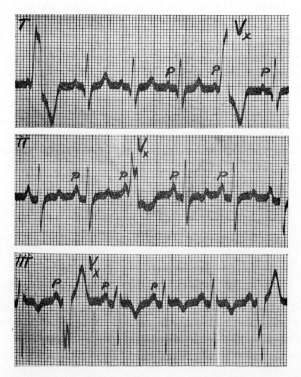

FIG. 96.   *Premature Ventricular Beats, Probably Arising from Right Ventricle.* Note the premature beats with abnormal ventricular complexes (V_x). They are only very slightly premature so that they actually follow the P wave. This patient had congenital heart disease.

which were entirely inaudible during auscultation that was performed simultaneously.

The spread of the impulse from the ectopic focus through the ventricle is abnormal and so the ventricular complex will be bizarre (Figs. 95 to 102). The direction the waves will take will depend on whether the impulse arises in the left or right ventricle and in the basal or apical

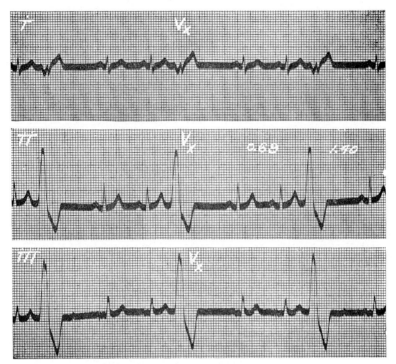

FIG. 97. *Premature Ventricular Beats; Trigeminy.* Note the typical ventricular extrasystoles (V$_x$) coming regularly after two normal beats. This patient had no organic heart disease. The length of normal cycle is 0.69 second. The length of the two beats including the premature beat is just twice that of the normal beat, 1.40 seconds. Therefore the pause is completely compensatory.

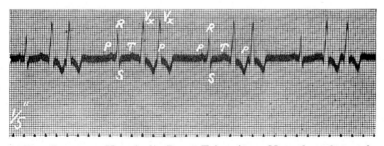

FIG. 98. *Premature Ventricular Beats; Trigeminy.* Note that after each norma beat there are two consecutive premature beats (V$_x$) followed by a compensatory pause. The auricles (P) continue regularly. The patient had rheumatic valvular disease. (Author's article in Oxford Loose-Leaf Medicine, vol. II.)

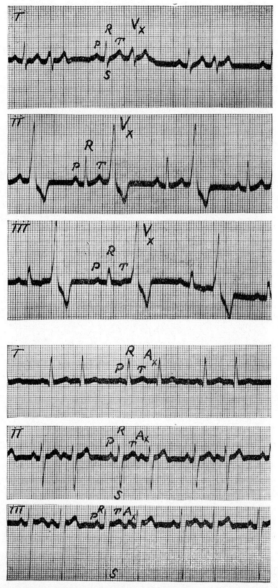

FIG. 99. *Premature Ventricular Beats; Bigeminy.* The upper three leads show a ventricular premature beat (V_x), occurring after each normal beat, and the lower show an auricular premature beat (A_x), producing in each case a coupled rhythm. Note the abnormal form of the ventricular complexes above and the normal ventricular complexes below with auricular waves of abnormal form. Organic heart disease was not present in either case.

region. In general the complexes are broad and coarsely notched, and the T waves extend in the opposite direction to the main initial ventricular deflections. Inasmuch as the ventricle contracts prematurely, the normal auricular beat coming down about the same time finds the ventricle refractory so that it cannot respond again. There follows then a pause until the next normal auricular beat. This pause is completely compensatory, for the rhythm of the pacemaker is not disturbed and the duration of the two beats including the premature beat is equal to two normal heart cycles (Fig. 97, Lead II). The P wave is often lost in the ventricular complex (Fig. 97) or may appear before or after the QRS waves (Figs. 95 and 96).

These beats may occur so very rarely that the physician is unable to detect them at the time of his examination, or they may be frequent. They may come every second beat (bigeminy) (Fig. 99) or every third beat (trigeminy) (Fig. 97). Auricular and ventricular premature beats are only two of a number of possible causes of a bigeminal rhythm. Although ventricular premature beats are far and away the most common explanation for a coupled rhythm, it is generally wise to record an electrocardiogram when this is first detected to rule out other mechanisms.

Sometimes ventricular premature beats come in succession, so that there may be a run of two or more, producing curious types of irregularity (Fig. 98). When they arise in different parts of the ventricles they will have various forms (Fig. 102). Such a condition is apt to be associated with digitalis intoxication or serious heart disease. The elucidation of the site of origin of a ventricular premature beat is an interesting academic exercise but of no practical significance. But the mere presence of more than one form of ventricular premature beat is of considerable importance. These have generally been designated as "multifocal" premature beats, but in the presence of auricular fibrillation it is not always certain that they arise from more than one focus. At least under these circumstances the noncommittal label of "multiform" ventricular premature beats is therefore preferable (Fig. 102).

Occasionally ventricular premature beats are interpolated between two normal beats. The heart is beating so slowly and the premature

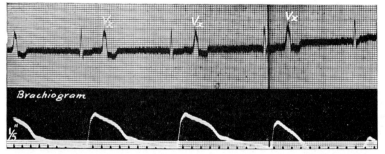

FIG. 100. *Premature Ventricular Beats; Bigeminy; Auricular Fibrillation.* Every second beat is a ventricular extrasystole (V_x). Auricular fibrillation is present but the normal ventricular beats come regularly, i.e., complete heart block. Such curves result from toxic doses of digitalis. Lower tracing is from the brachial artery and shows that the extra beats do not reach the wrist. Apex rate 60, pulse rate 30. (Author's article in Oxford Loose-Leaf Medicine, vol. II.)

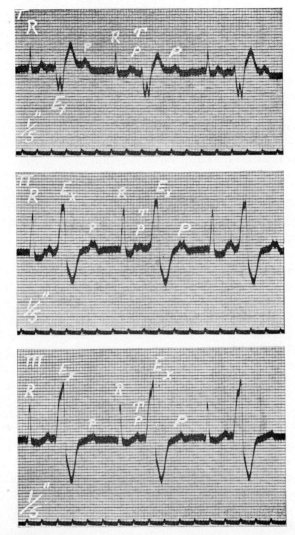

FIG. 101. *Digitalis Coupling.* Every second beat is a ventricular premature
beat with the typical abnormal form. The auriculoventricular conduction time or
P-R interval is markedly delayed, measuring 0.42 second. Both of these effects are
typical of digitalis intoxication. Note the cupped depressed RS-T segments of the
normal complexes, typical of the effect of digitalis. (Author's article in Oxford Loose-
Leaf Medicine, vol. II.)

beat occurs so early in diastole that the next normal auricular impulse
finds the conduction tissue and the ventricles ready to respond (Fig.
103). There is no compensatory pause, and instead one hears three rapid
beats, the second one of which is the premature beat. Another possible
explanation of this mechanism is that the impulse from the ventricles
travels through the junctional tissue to the auricles in a retrograde
fashion and starts a new impulse at the normal pacemaker. Occasionally
the beat following the interpolated ventricular premature beat displays

prolongation of the P-R interval or of the QRS complex (ventricular aberration), and the interval between the beat before and the one after the premature beat may be longer than that between successive regular beats (Fig. 103). These ventricular premature beats which are sandwiched between regular beats are the only truly "extra" systoles. They produce a more rapid rate than is counted when the premature beats are absent. By contrast, ventricular premature beats of the "garden variety," being followed by compensatory pauses, cause no change in the heart rate. Since the term "extrasystoles" may be misleading, it is thus preferable to refer to all varieties as "ventricular premature beats" and to qualify them as "interpolated" when appropriate.

Ventricular premature beats occur very frequently in otherwise normal individuals. They are also common in those having organic heart disease, but the diagnosis of structural disease of the heart will have to rest on other criteria than the irregularity. When they are numerous and

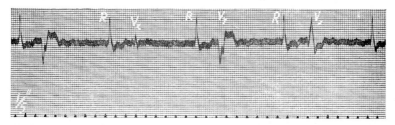

FIG. 102.   *Multiple and Multiform Premature Ventricular Beats.*   Following each normal beat (R) there are ventricular premature beats having varying forms (V_x, V_y, V_z). These beats arise in different foci in the ventricles or have different conduction paths. Such beats serve as a very important clue to digitalis over-dosage but may at times be recorded in other conditions, such as myocardial infarction. (Author's article in Oxford Loose-Leaf Medicine, vol. II.)

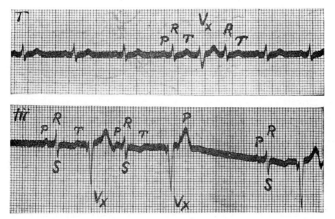

FIG. 103.   *Interpolated Premature Ventricular Beats.*   Upper tracing shows a single ventricular extrasystole (V_x) interpolated between two normal beats. Lower curve shows both an interpolated ventricular extrasystole and an extrasystole followed by the customary compensatory pause. The first patient had no heart disease, the second had angina pectoris.

the patient requires digitalis for heart failure, they indicate a grave outlook, for it is more difficult to administer as large doses of the drug as would otherwise be possible. In fact, digitalis in large doses often produces ventricular premature beats, especially in the form of digitalis coupling (Figs. 100, 101), even if none were present before the drug was used. Coupling may occur whether the rhythm was previously normal, in which case the P-R interval may also be delayed (Fig. 101), or if auricular fibrillation was present (Fig. 100). When this occurs it indicates a toxic effect of digitalis, and the drug must be omitted or the dose should be diminished. Coupling due to premature beats, however, may occur without digitalis and even in the absence of heart disease.

Ordinarily it is not difficult to recognize premature beats at the bedside. When they are numerous they may resemble auricular fibrillation, but they may generally be differentiated by the method discussed in a previous paragraph. It is regarded as impossible to distinguish auricular from ventricular premature beats without graphic methods. One may detect certain features that help to identify the one from the other. If the observer taps with his foot in rhythm with the regular beats, and continues the same pace when the premature beat occurs, the foot will come down synchronously with the following beat if it is a ventricular premature beat. This will generally not be so if it is auricular, because the pause following the premature beat is not completely compensatory. Furthermore, the character of the sounds is different in the two types. An auricular premature beat sounds more like the normal beat, only coming prematurely. A ventricular premature beat has a peculiar clicking sound which is different from the normal first heart sound of the particular patient, because the ventricles are apt to be contracting simultaneously with the auricles or at least in an abnormal relationship to auricular systole. This results in another distinguishing sign that may be elicited. The fact that the auricles contract while the ventricles are in systole makes the auricular impulse in the jugular pulse more prominent and one may see a large "a" wave in the jugular vein. This takes place because the blood from the right auricle is prevented from going into the right ventricle and is forced back through the superior vena cava. However, when it is important to identify the type of premature beat with certainty, graphic methods will be necessary.

The *main symptom* that is produced by ventricular premature beats is palpitation. This will be variously described by different individuals and generally the diagnosis can be made from the history itself. The various expressions used are "skipping of the heart," "a sudden flop or hesitation," "the heart flutters for an instant and then stops," "a thump in the neck or chest," "a sudden sinking or faint sensation, or a wave," and other terms often very graphic in their description. Occasionally a momentary darting pain occurs with each premature beat. In many individuals they produce no symptoms and are only accidentally found on examination. This is more commonly the case in stout patients and in those who are more phlegmatic. It seems that with a thin chest the somatic disturbances within the chest cavity are more readily felt. They are most frequent and most troublesome at rest, especially while a patient is trying to fall asleep, and often are entirely absent during physical activity. This may be due to the fact that, as the heart slows with rest, the diastolic pause lengthens and there is a greater opportunity for a premature beat to arise during longer than during shorter pauses. There are other neurogenic factors that determine the development of these beats at one time or another, apart from the heart rate. There is no doubt that emotional disturbances can be responsible for their presence. The following experience is quite illustrative. This man who had the typical complaint of skipping of his heart did not happen to show any irregularity during my examination. The symptom first began after the death of his child, nine months before. While his electrocardiogram was being taken and the heart was beating regularly, I asked him what illness his child had had, and as he began to speak about his child the extrasystoles appeared. This fits in very well with the physiologic work, showing that there is a center in the hypothalamic region which controls ventricular extrasystoles.

There is another type of ventricular premature beat that develops only on physical effort. In general this is more serious and may even predispose to the development of ventricular tachycardia on effort. Occasionally in certain individuals they are produced by coffee or smoking. More often when this is thought to be cause and effect, carefully controlled observation will show no such relationship. Often no known cause can be detected for their presence.

As to *treatment*, it is best for the physician to regard extrasystoles lightly. The patient should be clearly told that they have no serious significance and do not mean heart disease. Some persons have them all their lives and are not handicapped thereby. Such individuals should not be restricted in their activities unless there is some other reason for such restriction. When extrasystoles produce no symptoms, no medication should be advised. When they are troublesome, quinidine sulfate, 0.2 to 0.3 gm. (3 to 5 grains) two or three times a day, or taken just before they usually occur, may eliminate them entirely. Procaine amide (Pronestyl), 0.25 to 1.0 gm. three or four times daily, may be similarly effective. Occasionally moderate doses of digitalis, curiously enough, also inhibit extrasystoles. Strychnine, 0.001 gm. ($\frac{1}{60}$ grain) three times a day, has also been recommended. In some cases I have found that the extrasystoles disappear when the patient is given 2.0 gm. (30 grains) of potassium phosphate or chloride three times a day. Atropine sulfate may diminish vagal tone and increase the heart rate sufficiently to prevent their development. In general, it may be said that when it is important to eliminate extrasystoles, one or another of the various drugs that are available will prove effective in most cases.

ABERRANT VENTRICULAR CONDUCTION

Ventricular premature beats may be mimicked by supraventricular mechanisms associated with aberrant conduction of the impulse in the ventricles. An important determinant of aberrant ventricular conduction is the chance arrival of the impulse from the auricles in the ventricles in their relative refractory period. If this impulse happens to arrive at the ventricles in their absolute refractory period there is, of course, no ventricular response and no ventricular complex. The refractory period is related to cycle length. When the cardiac rhythm is regular, a slow heart rate is associated with a prolonged refractory period, a rapid heart rate with a shortened refractory period. When the cardiac rhythm is irregular the refractory period of a particular beat is conditioned by the interval immediately preceding that beat. Thus in auricular fibrillation a long pause sets up a prolonged refractory period in the beat following the pause. A supraventricular impulse which happens to filter down from the auricles and arrive at the ventricle during the relative refractory period of this post-pausal beat pursues an abnormal course in the ventricle and results in aberrant ventricular conduction. Thus in auricular fibrillation, if all of the ectopic beats are preceded by "normal" beats which in turn are each preceded by a long pause, or a longer than usual pause, the diagnosis of aberrant ventricular conduction, not ventricular premature beats, is favored (Fig. 104). Certain other features help differentiate aberrant ventricular conduction from ventricular premature beats. In aberrant ventricular conduction the first part of the ventricular complex is generally narrow, the last part broad; most aberrant beats thus resemble right bundle branch block (Fig. 104). This is not true of ventricular premature beats. Aberrant ventricular beats are not followed by compensatory pauses; ventricular premature beats, on the contrary, even in the presence of auricular fibrillation, are apt to be followed by a compensatory, or compensatory-like, pause. Aberrant ven-

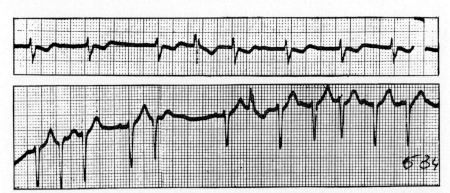

FIG. 104. *Aberrant Ventricular Conduction.* Tracings taken on two patients with auricular fibrillation (Lead V_1 in each case). The abnormal beats follow a ventricular complex which in turn follows a long pause. The abnormal beat has the characteristics of right bundle branch block and is not followed by a "compensatory" pause. Each of the patients benefited from further digitalis therapy.

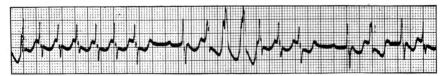

FIG. 105.   *Repetitive Aberrant Ventricular Conduction.*   Tracing made in patient with auricular flutter being treated with quinidine. The first burst of seven beats represents auricular flutter with a 1:1 response. The flutter rate was 207. The following pause and "normal" beat sets up ventricular aberration in the succeeding four beats. The rate during this salvo is identical with that of the underlying flutter. The rapid ventricular rate per se was not the cause of aberration for the two succeeding beats, with unchanged rate, show normal intraventricular conduction. This phenomenon simulates paroxysmal ventricular tachycardia. Quinidine therapy was abandoned at this point, with disappearance of aberration and of the 1:1 response.

tricular beats generally have a random time relationship to the preceding ventricular complex, whereas ventricular premature beats generally follow the preceding complex by a fixed time interval. Frequently, judged by these criteria, all of the ectopic beats fall clearly in one category or the other; the differentiation is then simple. At other times some abnormal beats conform to ventricular premature beats and some to aberrant ventricular conduction. They should be reported as such. It is mandatory, however, so far as possible, to distinguish one from the other, for, to the extent that ventricular premature beats may be an index of digitalis overdosage, this distinction guides subsequent therapy. There is good evidence that aberrant ventricular conduction is not a contraindication to further digitalis therapy; ventricular premature beats, on the other hand, may well be. Furthermore, ventricular aberration, conditioned in the manner described above, may be repetitive. In other words, not one, but a pair or salvo (Fig. 105) of abnormal ventricular beats may occur in succession and suggest the presence or imminence of ventricular tachycardia. Such repetitive beats have been observed in the same strip with isolated aberrant ventricular beats, and all have disappeared on digitalis therapy. The significance of aberrant ventricular conduction, as opposed to ventricular premature beats, in relation to the initiation or continuance of quinidine therapy, has not yet been established.

PAROXYSMAL VENTRICULAR TACHYCARDIA

An ectopic ventricular rhythm of still higher grade is paroxysmal ventricular tachycardia. This may be regarded as a consecutive series of ventricular extrasystoles arising from an ectopic focus in the ventricle. There is much in the nature of this mechanism that resembles a circus motion, and it may eventually be proved to be a disturbance in the ventricles similar to flutter in the auricles. Starting as it does from an abnormal focus in the ventricles, the impulse travels an abnormal course and the resultant ventricular complex will be abnormal (Figs. 106, 107, 109–112). Each individual complex resembles a ventricular extrasystole. The impulse may travel in a retrograde fashion up the junctional tissue

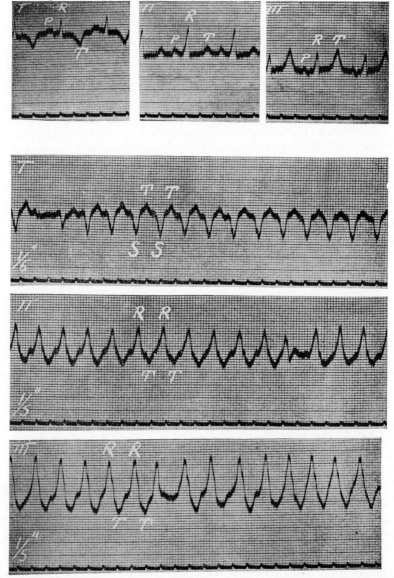

FIG. 106. *Paroxysmal Ventricular Tachycardia.* The upper three leads show
a normal rhythm, rate 89. The lower three leads were taken the next day, during an
attack of tachycardia, rate 172. Note that the form of the ventricular complexes
(RST) changed markedly in the corresponding leads. There are slight irregularities
in the length of the heart cycles during the tachycardia. (Author's article in Oxford
Loose-Leaf Medicine, vol. II.)

and produce auricular contractions. Because the rate is rapid, there may
be a retrograde block so that only every other ventricular impulse
reaches the auricles. At other times the auricles contract independently
and follow their own pacemaker in the sino-auricular node. It is often

impossible to identify the P waves because they are buried in the QRS-T complexes.

It may be difficult to distinguish ventricular tachycardia from a rapid auricular rate with a block in one or the other bundle of His (Fig. 108). Both conditions will show similar ventricular complexes. The finding, while the heart is beating slowly, of isolated ventricular extrasystoles which resemble the complexes when the rate is rapid, or the identification of P waves that are not in the normal relationship to the ventricular complexes, will prove that the condition is ventricular tachycardia. Figure 108 is an example of auricular flutter with bundle branch block which at first sight resembled paroxysmal ventricular tachycardia. In this case the differentiation was relatively simple. The problem may be more difficult with auricular fibrillation and a rapid ventricular rate combined with intraventricular block, since the rhythm is irregular in both auricular fibrillation and ventricular tachycardia. In general, it may be said that the irregularity is much more obvious and more easily detected in auricular fibrillation than in ventricular tachycardia. In ventricular tachycardia the irregularity must generally be deliberately sought.

The most reliable method of distinguishing ventricular from supraventricular tachycardia is the demonstration, during a paroxysm with broad QRS complexes, that an impulse which happens to be conducted from the auricles to the ventricles ("ventricular capture") produces a shorter ventricular complex which is the normal or usual complex for

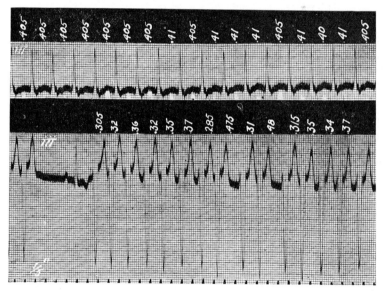

FIG. 107. *Paroxysmal Ventricular Tachycardia.* The upper tracing was made during an attack of auricular tachycardia; the lower one shows the onset of ventricular tachycardia in the same patient. The numbers indicate the length of the heart cycles. Note the absolute regularity of the auricular tachycardia and the distinct irregularity of the ventricular tachycardia.

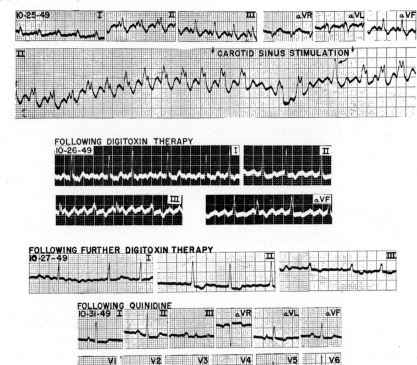

FIG. 108.   *Auricular Flutter with Bundle Branch Block Simulating Paroxysmal Ventricular Tachycardia.*   Initial tracings suggested paroxysmal ventricular tachycardia but the smooth hump between ventricular complexes suggested auricular flutter in the background. Carotid sinus stimulation (Lead II) slowed the ventricular rate, disclosing continuous flutter waves. Following one long pause during induced slowing normal intraventricular conduction (see arrow) was produced, indicating that the intraventricular block was a fatigue phenomenon which would be eliminated on slowing the ventricles. Following digitoxin therapy auricular flutter with slower and varying ventricular response and, as anticipated, normal intraventricular conduction were produced. After further digitoxin therapy auricular fibrillation occurred. Following quinidine therapy normal sinus rhythm with ventricular complexes characteristic of left ventricular hypertrophy was produced.

that lead (Fig. 109). Since the possibility of normal intraventricular conduction is demonstrated in the conducted auricular beat, the abnormal ventricular beats must arise off the beaten path from auricles to ventricles. They could not therefore be interpreted as auricular or nodal in origin with bundle branch block or aberrant ventricular conduction. A similar deduction is warranted if fusion beats interrupt the paroxysm. Here one would argue that a supraventricular beat activates one part of the ventricle while the remainder of the ventricle is activated from the same focus that produces the broad, bizarre complexes characteristic of the remainder of the paroxysm. The blend of the normal and the ectopic beat produces a ventricular complex somewhere intermediate in appearance between the two (Fig. 110).

For some hours or days after any attack of paroxysmal rapid heart action the ventricular complexes may remain distinctly abnormal, showing inverted T waves. These changes may occasionally occur when the heart is structurally normal and therefore cannot necessarily serve as evidence of heart disease. They probably indicate heart muscle fatigue or local relative anoxia of parts of the ventricles, but the curves return to normal eventually. Lack of appreciation of this will lead to incorrect diagnoses of coronary or myocardial disease.

There are numerous important clinical aspects of paroxysmal ventricular tachycardia, and this disturbance needs to be differentiated from other forms of rapid heart action. It can occur as paroxysms or it may

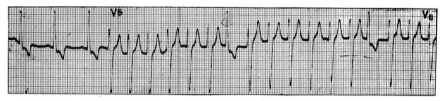

FIG. 109. *"Captured" Beats.* Normal conduction of "captured" beats during paroxysmal ventricular tachycardia. The bout of tachycardia starts as a premature beat following three normal beats which show left ventricular hypertrophy. The seventh and fourteenth beats of the paroxysm occur on time with the other beats of the paroxysm, but are identical with the indigenous beats of the same lead. This indicates that beats conducted from auricles or the auriculoventricular node have a configuration differing from that of beats characterizing the tachycardia. This is strong evidence that the tachycardia arises in the ventricles.

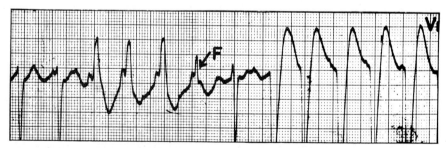

FIG. 110. *Fusion Beat Following Brief Burst of Ventricular Tachycardia.* The strip shows two bouts of ventricular tachycardia with ventricular complexes of one configuration in the first salvo, of an opposite configuration in the second. The first, second, and seventh beats were normal for that lead (Lead V_1). The sixth beat (F) probably represents a synthesis of the normal complex with the ventricular complexes characterizing the first paroxysm and offers conclusive evidence that the latter are genuinely ectopic. The flutter rate was 235, the rate of the ventricular tachycardia 128. When use of quinidine was abandoned the abnormal mechanism disappeared.

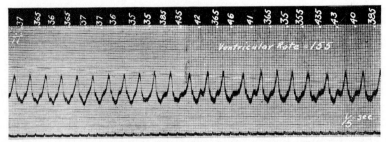

FIG. 111.   *Paroxysmal Ventricular Tachycardia.*   Numbers above indicate the interventricular intervals in hundredths of a second. Note that although the first nine cycles are quite regular, distinct variations in rate occur thereafter.

remain permanent if treatment is not instituted. The rate is apt to be around 160 to 180, and very rarely reaches the high levels of 220 or more that occur in auricular tachycardia. Unlike the latter, it generally accompanies grave heart disease, especially disease of the coronary arteries, but it may be present as a purely functional arrhythmia in an otherwise healthy heart. Furthermore, there are bedside methods that enable one to diagnose this condition. When paroxysmal, the attacks begin and end suddenly (Figs. 107, 109, 110). The rate is rapid, but in most cases slight irregularities can be detected on auscultation, in marked contrast to auricular tachycardia (Fig. 64). Occasionally the rhythm will be perfectly regular, but more often, if one listens long enough, interruptions will be heard. The first nine cycles in Figure 111 are just as regular as the cycles that occur in auricular tachycardia, but thereafter there develop appreciable differences in the length of the cycles that will never be seen in association with the latter condition. Furthermore, on auscultation slight but definite differences in the intensity and quality of the first sound will be heard, which are due to the different relationship between the ventricular and auricular systoles in various cycles. This latter auscultatory finding will not be present either in normal tachycardia or in paroxysmal tachycardia. It also has been pointed out that the auricular pulsations as seen in the jugular vein will be fewer in number than the ventricular rate, and some of these jugular pulsations are particularly conspicuous. Finally, this type of rapid heart action is never influenced by any of the methods used to stimulate the vagus, such as carotid pressure, ocular pressure, or deep breathing.

Therapeutically, the problem of ventricular tachycardia is peculiar. In most cardiac conditions in which there is heart failure digitalis is indicated and a beneficial, or at least not harmful, effect is anticipated. When ventricular tachycardia is present, digitalis not only will fail to improve the situation but may well worsen it. I have seen two instances in which digitalis, on repeated trials, accelerated the ventricular rate while the tachycardia was in progress and aggravated the state of the circulation. Quinidine, on the other hand, is almost a specific drug for this type of tachycardia. In most cases it will restore the normal rhythm.

The amount necessary to accomplish this will vary greatly, from a single dose of 0.3 gm. (5 grains) to as much as 1.5 gm. (22 grains) administered five times a day. Before the heart becomes regularized the ventricular rate will gradually slow (Fig. 112). This slowing enables one to follow the effect of the drug and guide its dosage. On rare occasions even large doses of quinidine will slow the ventricular rate but fail to do away with the abnormal mechanism, the original rapid rate returning as the effect of the drug wears off. On two such occasions 2 mg. ($\frac{1}{30}$ grain) of atropine sulfate, given subcutaneously about one hour after a large oral dose of quinidine, promptly restored the normal rhythm. The pharmacologic action of atropine is to lengthen the refractory period of cardiac muscle. If the condition of the patient seems urgent or deteriorating at the outset, or after oral therapy has already been started, resort may be had to intravenous administration of quinidine. The contents of an ampule of 0.6 gm. of quinidine sulfate or lactate is added to 200 cc. of 5 per cent dextrose solution. This solution is infused slowly by drip under constant electrocardiographic control. The infusion is stopped immediately when reversion to normal rhythm has occurred. If necessary, the quinidine may be injected undiluted in a 10 cc. syringe at the rate of 1 cc. a minute, again with careful electrocardiographic control. In either event one must watch carefully for evidence of respiratory arrest. If this develops the infusion must be halted. Some authorities prefer the intramuscular to the intravenous injection of quinidine. An advantage

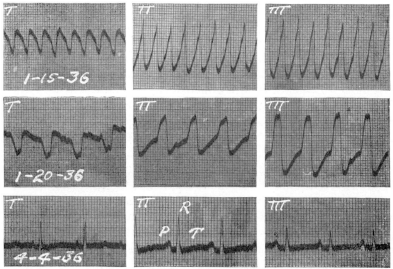

FIG. 112.   *Paroxysmal Ventricular Tachycardia; Effect of Quinidine.*   First set shows ventricular tachycardia, the rate is 247. Second set shows marked slowing of the rate (122) as a result of quinidine, but ventricular tachycardia persists. Lowest set shows normal rhythm. Enormous amounts of quinidine were necessary to produce regularization, single doses being gradually increased from 0.2 gm. to 2.0 gm. The patient was desperately ill with advanced congestive failure, although after recovery there was no evidence of heart disease.

of the latter is the greater ease of maneuverability; the infusion may be discontinued promptly at the earliest indication of toxicity. A disadvantage of the intravenous method is its effect of lowering the blood pressure.

In the last few years procaine amide (Pronestyl) has come into widespread use for ventricular tachycardia. Its effects are similar to those of quinidine, but it may be somewhat less toxic when given by vein. For oral administration the dose is 0.25 to 0.50 gm. every two to four hours until the attack is controlled. For intravenous use the contents of a 10 cc. ampule (100 mg. per cc., or a total of 1 gm.) is injected at a rate no faster than 1 cc. per minute while electrocardiograms are recorded. The injection is discontinued once reversion has occurred. If a single ampule has been ineffective, injection of up to another 1 gm. may yet produce reversion. The decision to employ either of these drugs, quinidine or procaine amide, should never be made lightly. The use of each is subject to certain definite risks. Each, in moderate or large doses, is capable in itself of inducing ectopic rhythms and of prolonging the Q-T and QRS intervals of the electrocardiogram. Some authorities consider the development of pronounced intraventricular block a contraindication to proceeding with quinidine, and, by inference, with procaine amide. In desperate situations, where the gravity of the situation warrants, it may, however, be justified to continue either drug for the arrhythmia may yet be abolished.

It is worth remembering that in some cases 4 to 8 cc. of a 50 per cent solution of magnesium sulfate may produce instant reversion to normal rhythm.

VENTRICULAR FLUTTER(?)

If one continues the sequence of abnormalities of ventricular origin, as was done in the auricles, one should naturally consider ventricular flutter. This generally has been omitted, as no condition has been recognized as ventricular flutter in the electrocardiograms. Figure 113, however, may possibly represent such a condition. These rapid, slightly irregular oscillations were taking place at the very time that very rapid heart beats could be heard. The patient was unconscious. However, she recovered from this attack. Ordinarily one has considered such curves as signifying ventricular fibrillation, but the presence of heart beats and the fact that the circulation was being maintained militate against this diagnosis and denote that the ventricles were actually contracting. Undulations of the baseline producing a continuous sine wave have also been observed in advanced potassium intoxication. This appearance may also be considered an example of ventricular flutter.

VENTRICULAR FIBRILLATION

The final and most extreme disturbance of the ventricles is ventricular fibrillation. With this there are numerous impulses traversing the ventricles so rapidly that coordinated contractions do not occur. When the condition is produced experimentally by faradizing the ventricles, tying the branches of the coronary arteries, or by drugs such as digitalis and epinephrine, fibrillary twitchings will be seen but no mechanical expulsion of blood results. From the point of view of the dynamics of the circulation, the heart suddenly stops. The electrocardiograms that represent this state show very bizarre, rapid and irregular ventricular complexes (Figs. 114, 115). The initial phase of the ventricular waves (QRS) is broadened, and the T waves fuse with them, so that they become indistinguishable. They also vary in height from oscillations of large amplitude to coarse low movements of the base line.

It is extremely rare to find ventricular fibrillation in clinical practice, because in most cases it is the cause of instant death. By mere

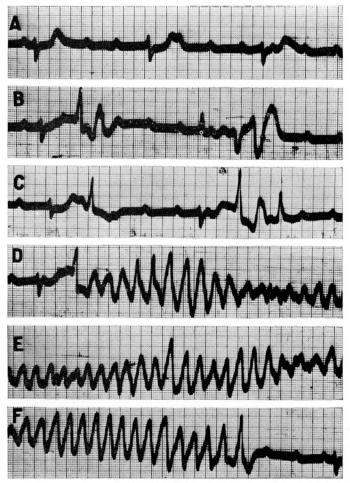

FIG. 113.   *Ventricular Flutter (Possible).*   Strips of a continuous tracing (Lead I) from a woman 59 years old with complete heart block and Adams-Stokes disease. *A* indicates complete block. *B* and *C* show ventricular extrasystoles of different types. *D, E,* and *F* show oscillations that have been interpreted as ventricular fibrillation, but because heart beats were audible throughout this period it is suggested that it be called ventricular flutter. The last complex shows return of complete block

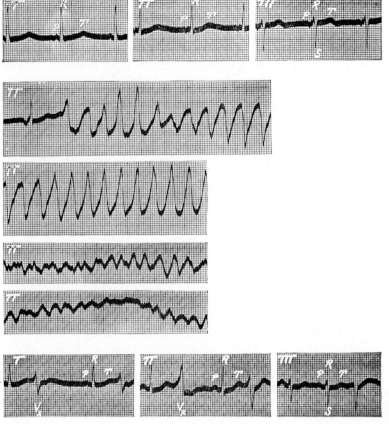

FIG. 114.   *Transient Ventricular Fibrillation.*   The three leads in the upper row show a normal mechanism. The following four curves are portions of a continuous tracing taken during an attack of syncope and are characteristic of ventricular fibrillation. The patient had a convulsion and there was no heart beat or pulse for about one minute. The three leads in the lowest row show a return to a normal beat with occasional ventricular premature beats (V_x). The patient became ambulatory.

chance, examples have been recorded when a patient happened to have an attack while the electrocardiograms were being taken. This was the case in an instance of sudden death from an attack of angina pectoris in which the postmortem examination showed disease of the coronary arteries but no acute thrombosis. This mechanism probably is a common cause of instant death in disease of the coronary arteries and in such events as electrocution. Figure 116 shows the recording made when a patient happened to have an attack while electrocardiograms were being made. This patient had previous angina and had had a recent myocardial infarct. He was doing quite well, but just after the first lead of the electrocardiogram was taken he expired. Leads II and III, taken only a few seconds afterwards, showed that ventricular fibrillation was present.

Occasionally recovery takes place in human beings after ventricular

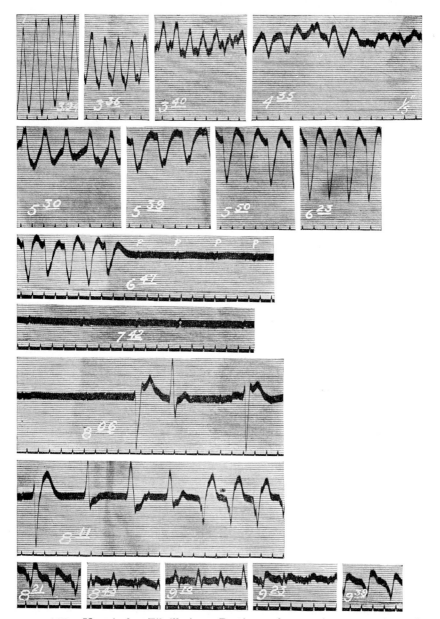

FIG. 115. *Ventricular Fibrillation.* Portions of a continuous tracing taken during an attack of Adams-Stokes syncope lasting five minutes. The numbers indicate minutes and seconds. The patient was unconscious throughout the attack, breathing ceased, and there was no detectable heart beat. Note the early development of ventricular fibrillation with eventual cessation of all electrical activity except for small auricular waves (P). During this time epinephrine was injected directly into the heart and contractions were resumed. The patient recovered and became ambulatory. (Published in "Heart," vol. 12.)

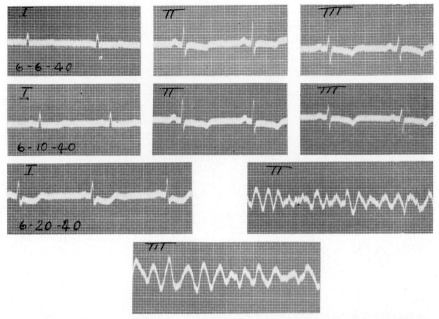

FIG. 116.   *Ventricular Fibrillation (Cause of Sudden Death in Coronary Disease).*
This patient, a man 60 years old, had typical angina for three weeks, with many
attacks daily, promptly relieved by nitroglycerin. On the last day he had a severe
attack, requiring two injections of morphine, and died instantly two hours after onset
of the attack while tracings were being taken. Note the normal rhythm in Lead I of
lowest set and ventricular fibrillation in Leads II and III, taken only a few seconds
later.

fibrillation has set in. Figure 114 shows an example of this sort, in which
repeated attacks of syncope were due to this mechanism and were generally preceded by brief periods of increased numbers of ventricular premature beats and ventricular tachycardia. The number of attacks
seemed to be lessened by constant quinidine administration. Figure 115
shows not only periods of ventricular fibrillation but also complete cessation of all electrical responses in the ventricles, extending over a period
of more than five minutes, with recovery. Whether the epinephrine that
was injected directly into the heart was responsible for the recovery is
not certain. This occurred in a woman about 50 years of age who was
suffering from Adams-Stokes disease with attacks of unconsciousness.

Ventricular fibrillation is one of two possible mechanisms producing
sudden arrest of the heart, such as may occur during surgery. The other
mechanism, ventricular standstill, will be discussed in a later section. In
either case no heart beat is heard and no blood pressure recorded. Irreparable brain damage results from arrested cerebral circulation after
only four minutes of fibrillation or standstill. If at all feasible electrocardiograms should be recorded to define which of these disorders is
present, for the management of one is quite different from that of the
other. If a monitoring cardioscope is available in the operating room, the

diagnosis is at hand. In view of the four-minute deadline it may be justifiable, if an electrocardiograph is not readily available, to perform an immediate thoracotomy and incision of the pericardium. Direct inspection of the ventricles will then establish the diagnosis. Continuous artificial respiration and provision of 100 per cent oxygen is maintained throughout the efforts at resuscitation. Rhythmic compression of the heart at a rate of about 40 times a minute ("cardiac massage") is begun immediately and will maintain an adequate cerebral blood flow. Attempted compression of the heart through the diaphragm when the abdomen is already opened is generally unsuccessful and loses valuable time. If spontaneous recovery does not occur electric defibrillation is attempted. This consists of a high-voltage, single shock, applied directly to the heart through two plates. Applied early enough, this procedure has been followed in a number of cases by resumption of a normal rhythm and the saving of life. Massage should be resumed if electric defibrillation has been ineffective.

In this regard Zoll has devised a new apparatus which can initiate and maintain rhythmic ventricular contractions if there is standstill of the heart, and can defibrillate the heart if ventricular fibrillation is present. This can be accomplished by the application of electrodes to the surface of the thoracic cage and therefore requires no surgical operation. It has already proved successful in a small number of cases.

Disturbances in Conduction

SINO-AURICULAR BLOCK

Having considered the disturbances that may arise in the normal pacemaker of the heart, and then the abnormalities in the origin of impulses (ectopic rhythms), the third main problem involves the abnormalities in the conduction of impulses. The impulse after it is formed in the normal sino-auricular node may be blocked before it reaches the auricular musculature. This is called *sino-auricular block* (Figs. 117, 118). Neither the auricles nor ventricles receive an impulse, and there results the loss of a complete heart cycle. If only one of those normal impulses is blocked, the pause will be approximately equal to two normal heart beats as the pacemaker remains undisturbed. Occasionally this pause will be equal to three or four heart beats, in which event two or three impulses are blocked. Slight differences in measurements will be found because there often is an accompanying sinus arrhythmia that slightly affects the pace. Furthermore, after the pause, the first beat may be an idioventricular beat or nodal escape.

At times, with successive beats there is apparently a progressive delay in the sino-auricular interval leading up to a dropping out of an auricular response. This is a special application of the Wenckebach phenomenon which is described under second-degree auriculoventricular block. The P-P interval shows a progressive shortening before the pause. The P-P interval, including the pause, is shorter than any two con-

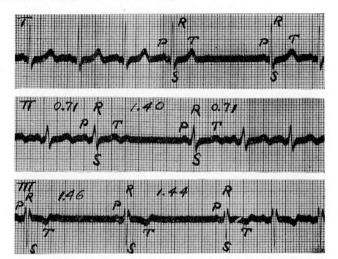

FIG. 117.   *Sino-auricular Block.*   Note that the pauses (1.4 seconds) are equal to twice the length of the normal beat (0.71 second). Neither auricles nor ventricles contract during the pauses as the impulse is blocked at the pacemaker. The patient was a young woman with palpitation but without organic heart disease.

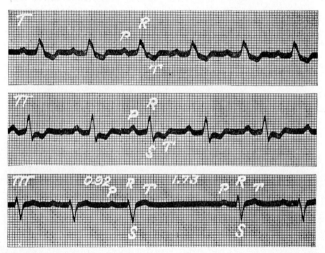

FIG. 118.   *Sino-auricular Block.*   There is a pause in Lead III (1.73 seconds) approximately twice the normal heart cycle (0.92 second). Both auricles and ventricles failed to contract. Curves also show bundle branch block and delayed conduction time (P-R = 0.27 second). The patient had hypertensive heart disease with coronary artery sclerosis.

secutive P-P intervals, and the P-P interval following the pause is longer than that preceding it. One can apply the same reasoning regarding the R waves in Wenckebach-type second degree auriculoventricular block to the P waves in Wenckebach-type sino-auricular block. This arrhythmia is generally interpreted as sinus arrhythmia. This does no particular harm, but a precise understanding of its mechanism explains the abrupt changes in cycle length which occur in this variety of sino-auricular

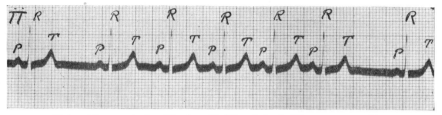

FIG. 119.   *Sino-auricular Block, with Wenckebach Phenomenon.*   Note progressive speeding up of auricles before pause. In this variety the P-P interval after the pause is longer than that preceding it. The abrupt changes in cycle length contrast with the smooth waxing and waning of rate that characterizes sinus arrhythmia. The subject was a 6-year-old boy with a normal heart.

block. In classic sinus arrhythmia, on the other hand, there is rather a smooth progressive waxing and waning of the heart rate.

Sino-auricular block is rare, compared with auriculoventricular block. In general it occurs under the same conditions but has much less practical importance. It can be suspected clinically by detecting a complete loss of a heart cycle on auscultation. Because neither auricles nor ventricles contract during this pause, no auricular or "a" wave will be seen in the jugular pulse. If such a small wave is detected on careful examination of the veins of the neck during the long silent interval, the block is at the auriculoventricular node rather than at the sino-auricular node. Treatment is generally not indicated for patients with this arrhythmia unless it produces syncope, when ephedrine or atropine may prove effective as in the ordinary type of block.

AURICULOVENTRICULAR BLOCK

First Degree Heart Block (Delayed Conduction Time).   The more common type of heart block is that which occurs in the junctional tissue, at the auriculoventricular node or bundle of His. When the defect is slight, impulses are merely delayed in their passage through the main conduction path but eventually reach the ventricles. There really is no blocking of beats, and the heart remains regular. The conduction time (P-R interval), which normally measures about 0.16 second, becomes prolonged, and when it reaches the duration of more than 0.2 second it is arbitrarily regarded as an indication of pathologic change (Figs. 120 to 124). The actual path that the impulse travels is normal and therefore the electrical complexes are all normal in form. The P wave may precede the ventricular complexes sufficiently to fall on the previous T or R wave. Under such circumstances it may become difficult to recognize the P wave and it may confuse the interpretation of the electrocardiograms. At first glance the tracings in Figure 124 as represented by the first three beats could be interpreted as classic paroxysmal tachycardia (rate 162) in which the auricular waves are not visible. Vagal stimulation, however, shows that the P waves are on top of the T waves, and that there is a slightly delayed P-R interval.

In general, auriculoventricular block of all degrees results from three

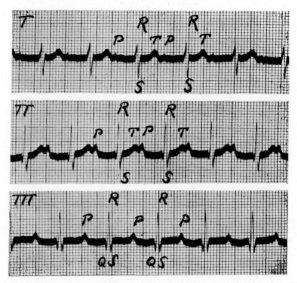

FIG. 120.   *Heart Block, First Degree (Delayed Conduction time).*   The P-R inter-val measures the time it takes for an impulse to go from auricles to ventricles and normally should be between 0.12 and 0.2 second. Here it measures 0.3 second. None of the beats is blocked so that the heart remains regular. The patient was suffering from postscarlatinal rheumatism.

main causes. Digitalis probably is the most common of all. When full doses of this drug are given any degree of heart block may be produced, especially delayed conduction (Figs. 89 and 101). Even sino-auricular block may be caused by digitalis. Heart block rarely occurs during the ordinary infections met with in general practice, such as scarlet fever or mumps. It is more common as a complication of rheumatic fever and diphtheria. When heart block of the higher grade occurs in diphtheria the prognosis is very grave. In rheumatic fever heart block is particu-larly common and often is the only evidence of a rheumatic infection. It can then be interpreted as positive evidence of a rheumatic carditis, and it may be present when there are no rheumatic pains and when the heart itself shows no significant abnormalities on ordinary examination except this electrocardiographic finding. In fact, it is practically the only reliable evidence of an acute myocarditis. Because of the infrequency of heart block in other acute infections, this finding should be sought for and will often serve as a valuable diagnostic aid in identifying many conditions as rheumatic that otherwise would remain obscure. Figure 120 (P-R = 0.3 second) was obtained from a patient who had some vague aches in the legs after scarlet fever and was interpreted as indicative of a smouldering rheumatic fever. Another patient (Fig. 122) merely had a slight "cold" and a questionable murmur in the heart. The markedly delayed conduction (P-R = 0.32 second) meant that the child was suffering from a mild rheumatic fever. More important still was the case illustrated in Figure 123. Here a girl of 13 was spared an unnecessary

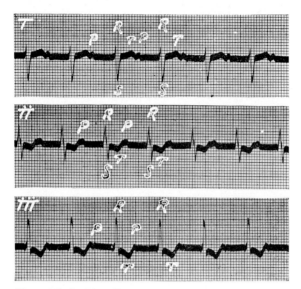

FIG. 121. *Heart Block, First Degree.* The P-R interval is markedly delayed, measuring 0.32 second, but no beats are blocked. The patient had rheumatic mitral stenosis and insufficiency.

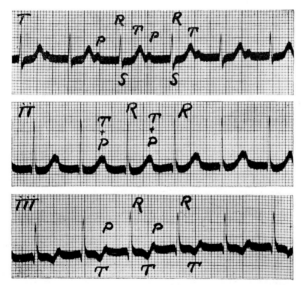

FIG. 122. *Heart Block, First Degree.* The P-R interval is delayed to 0.32 second, but the rhythm remains regular. Note that in Lead II the P wave is practically fused with the preceding T wave. The patient was a boy of 13 who had an apparent "cold," the electrocardiographic changes being the only evidence at the time that the infection was rheumatic.

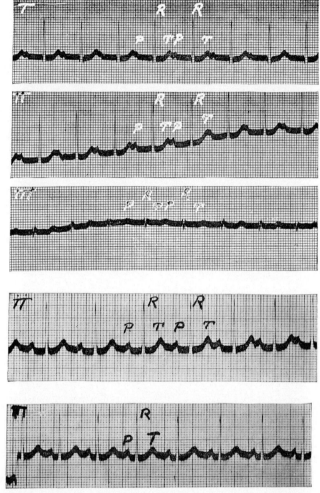

FIG. 123.   *Heart Block, First Degree.*   The upper three leads, taken June 20, 1935, show delayed P-R interval of 0.3 second. The fourth tracing, taken July 5, 1935, shows that the P-R time is much shortened (0.23 second). The lowest curve taken September 5, 1935, shows normal P-R interval (0.16 second). The patient was a girl of 13 with vague abdominal symptoms, who was sent to the surgical service for appendectomy. The electrocardiograms were the main clue that she had rheumatic fever.

operation for appendicitis by the interpretation of the abdominal pain, slight fever, and leukocytosis as rheumatic. The third major cause of conduction defects is chronic organic heart disease, especially coronary artery sclerosis and less frequently rheumatic valvular disease (Fig. 121). Hyperthyroidism and syphilitic disease involving the junctional tissue are also rare causes of heart block. When delayed conduction results from digitalis, it disappears within two or three weeks if the drug is omitted. When rheumatic fever is the cause, it may persist longer but generally clears up entirely (Figs. 123 and 126). However, when it is part of a chronic cardiac problem it remains indefinitely and may become more marked, eventually leading to complete heart block. I once saw a 59-year-old man who had fainting attacks with convulsions due to heart block. On postmortem examination a lesion was found in the upper portion of the interventricular septum resembling Fiedler's myocarditis. There was no evidence of syphilis and no significant coronary artery disease. In another somewhat similar case of Adams-Stokes disease the pathologist described lesions in the interventricular septum that were characteristic of sarcoid.

It must be borne in mind that slight and occasionally marked delay in auriculoventricular conduction may be found in otherwise healthy and normal individuals. During the Second World War a P-R interval of 0.4 second was detected in some healthy Air Corps men while recumbent, which became normal when they sat up. In other instances, second or third degree block was changed to first degree when the subject assumed the upright position.

Although first degree heart block is easily recognized in the electrocardiogram, it is difficult and often impossible to detect clinically. The heart remains regular and the rate is often essentially normal. Unless the possibility is kept in mind, there may be no suspicion that a defect in conduction is present. There are two auscultatory findings that may lead one to the correct diagnosis, i.e., the presence of a gallop rhythm

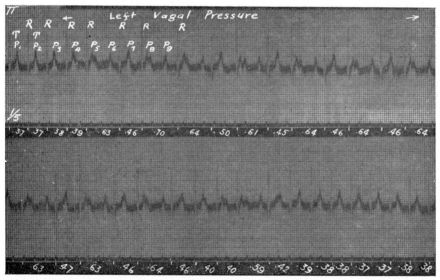

FIG. 124.   *Heart Block, First Degree.*   Effect of vagal stimulation. A continuous tracing at the beginning of which the heart was regular and rapid, rate 162. The auricular waves were obscured and it was thought that classic paroxysmal auricular tachycardia was present. Pressure over the left carotid sinus (indicated by signal above) slowed the ventricles and uncovered normal P waves. Note that P_5 and P_8 are not followed by ventricular complexes. The patient had acute myocarditis following erysipelas. The tracings may be interpreted as showing paroxysmal auricular tachycardia with block. (Author's article in Oxford Loose-Leaf Medicine, vol. II.)

or a decrease in the intensity of the first heart sound. It may be that auricular systole is so far removed from the oncoming ventricular beat that it becomes audible, or auricular contraction produces some other effect on the valves or muscle which results in a sound. This finding should make the examiner particularly suspicious if it occurs during or following an acute infection. Of course gallop rhythm is much more common in other conditions in which the P-R interval is normal. Nevertheless, it may direct attention to an important disturbance that otherwise would be overlooked. Similarly, if the loudness of the first heart sound has been noted to decrease during the days of observation, it may mean that the P-R interval has lengthened.

Second Degree Heart Block (Partial Heart Block).   When the defect in conduction is greater, impulses from auricles to ventricles find it increasingly difficult to pass through the junctional tissue until finally one is blocked. This condition is called *partial heart block* (Figs. 125–128). This may occur once every seven or more beats, or much more frequently, i.e., every second beat (Figs. 126, 127, 128). In fact, more than one beat may be blocked before the next one goes through. These various degrees of partial block will be called 7:6, 2:1, or 3:1, depending on the relation of the P waves to the ventricular complexes. The auricular and ventricular complexes are normal in form for that heart because the path which the impulses take is normal. The P waves may have to be sought for carefully in a preceding T wave. A slight notching or increase in height of the latter may indicate the presence of the former (Fig. 122). The time relation between the two will be abnormal. Figure 125 shows a rapid increase in the P-R interval in the first four cycles, and then the intervals remain the same until a beat is blocked. The increase might have continued but to a slighter degree before the final pause. Because of this diminishing increment in the P-R interval, the heart speeds up before the pause and the shortened P-R interval after the block makes the length of the pause slightly less than two normal heart cycles (Wenckebach phenomenon). Furthermore, the R-R interval following the pause must be longer than that preceding it. These features of the Wenckebach phenomenon as applied to the R-R interval in second degree auriculoventricular block (namely, a progressive shortening of the R-R interval before the pause; a pause which is shorter than any two consecutive R-R cycles; and an R-R interval following the pause which exceeds that preceding the pause) are also observed as part of the structure of the Wenckebach phenomenon seen in one variety of sinoauricular block. In the latter (p. 536 and Fig. 119) the P waves speed up before the pause, the P-P interval including the pause is shorter than any two consecutive P-P cycles, and the P-P interval following the pause is greater than that preceding it.

It is not difficult to recognize partial heart block at the bedside. When only an occasional beat is blocked an essentially regular rhythm will be heard, and then a sudden pause that will be slightly shorter than two normal cycles. A small auricular wave may be observed in the

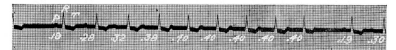

FIG. 125. *Heart Block, Second Degree (Partial Heart Block).* Note that the conduction time (P-R) first rapidly increases and then remains prolonged, and finally a beat is blocked (Wenckebach period), the process repeating itself. The patient had advanced heart failure with hypertension and was on full digitalis dosage when these tracings were taken.

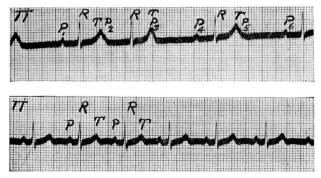

FIG. 126. *Heart Block, Second Degree, with Wenckebach Phenomenon.* The upper tracing was taken June 25, 1929, during acute rheumatic fever; the lower, October 20, 1930, when the patient was well and showed no evidence of heart disease. Note that P_3 and P_5 are not followed by ventricular beats. The lower tracing shows that the heart block has entirely disappeared.

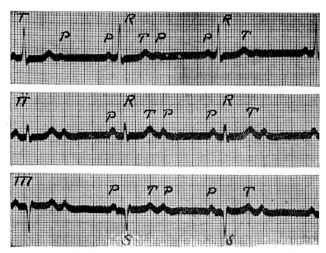

FIG. 127. *Heart Block, Second Degree.* Every other auricular beat (P) is not followed by a ventricular beat; i.e., there is a 2:1 heart block. Auricular rate 86, ventricular rate 43. The patient had hypertension and angina pectoris but no syncope.

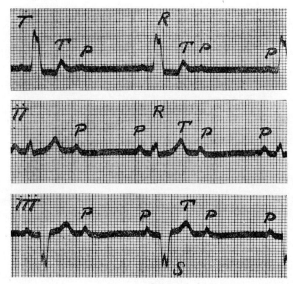

FIG. 128. *Heart Block, Second Degree.* Every other auricular beat (P) is blocked (2:1 heart block). Auricular rate 80, ventricular rate 40. The ventricular complexes (QRS-T) indicate bundle branch block in addition. Note that the P-P interval embracing the ventricular complex is shorter than the clear P-P interval ("ventriculophasic" sinus arrhythmia). The patient had hypertension and fainting attacks.

jugular veins during these pauses. It must be clearly distinguished from premature beats for in both conditions the pulse is intermittent. With the latter an extra clicking beat will be heard in early diastole. On rare occasions I have confused this sound for the faint sound made by auricular systole in partial heart block. When there is a 3:2 block a coupled rhythm results, and this may be misinterpreted as due to some other mechanism. If every second beat is blocked (2:1), a slow regular rate of about 40 is the result. It will need to be distinguished from a normal bradycardia and complete heart block. This often can be done by detecting auricular impulses in the jugular veins and trying to disturb the rate by exercise, breathing, carotid sinus pressure, or drugs such as atropine or amyl nitrite. The effect in normal bradycardia will be most marked and gradual; in complete heart block the rate will be unaffected or only slightly changed, the rhythm remaining regular; with partial block abrupt changes in the length of the heart cycle may result. Atropine or amyl nitrite may lessen the degree of partial block by diminishing vagal tone, and vagal stimulation may increase the block and slow the heart further. Occasionally the reverse occurs, and ventricular rate accelerates with vagal stimulation. In an elderly man with 2:1 partial heart block, carotid sinus stimulation on three different occasions promptly produced a 1:1 rhythm by slowing the auricular rate slightly. There appeared to be a critical level at which all beats could be conducted and above which 2:1 block occurred. This may explain the occasional beneficial

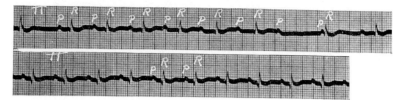

FIG. 129. *Heart Block, Second Degree; Effect of Atropine.* The upper tracing
shows gradual lengthening of P-R interval from 0.21 to 0.32 second and final blocking of a beat. The lower tracing taken five minutes after the intravenous injection
of 1.0 mg. of atropine shows regular rhythm, P-R = 0.17 second.

effects of digitalis on heart block. Careful attention to the physiologic
functions involved and to the exact length of the heart cycles as determined by auscultation will often suffice to differentiate the cause of the
slow heart rate.

Partial heart block generally requires no specific treatment. When
it accompanies rheumatic infections, treatment is directed at the underlying disease. It merely indicates that a longer period of convalescence
is desirable but the prognosis ordinarily is favorable. If it follows digitalis, no harm results. It serves as a warning that the dose of the drug
should be lessened. When it is present with chronic organic heart failure,
one need not be afraid to give digitalis. Specific treatment will be required if syncopal attacks are threatening. This will be discussed under
complete heart block. One might expect that atropine would be of aid
in partial heart block by inhibiting the vagus, and occasionally it is very
effective in eliminating the block entirely and doing away with the accompanying symptoms (Fig. 129).

Third Degree Heart Block (Complete Heart Block). The highest degree of block occurs when the defect is sufficiently great to prevent all
impulses from reaching the ventricles, i.e., complete heart block. In this
case the auricles contract in sequence to their own pacemaker in the
sino-auricular node and the ventricles establish their own rhythm in
sequence to a pacemaker just below the defect, either in the lower
portion of the auriculoventricular node or in the bundle of His (Figs.
130 to 136). Inasmuch as the inherent rhythmicity of the ventricles is
slow, the rate is generally about 30 and regular. The auricles and ventricles contract independently of each other. Sometimes the P wave
precedes the R, at other times it follows it or comes on the T wave.
Occasionally the auricular rate may happen to be just about twice the
ventricular, and an apparent 2:1 heart block will be seen. However, if a
sufficiently long tracing is followed or an attempt made to disturb the
mechanism, a P wave will generally be found to change its relation to
the R wave and actually pass it. The complexes have forms that are
essentially normal for that particular heart as the spread of the excitation wave is normal through auricles and ventricles. The Q-T interval
is apt to be lengthened because of the slow rate and the increased duration of systole. Although the ventricular rhythm is usually regular,

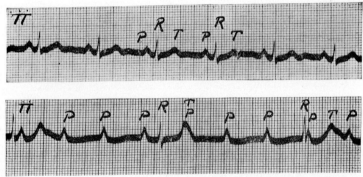

FIG. 130. *Heart Block, Third Degree (Complete Heart Block).* The upper trac-ing, taken September 23, 1931, shows a normal rhythm. The lower tracing, taken May 23, 1933, shows complete block; auricular rate (P) is 103, ventricular (R) is 29. Note the inconstant relationship between P and R waves. The pacemaker of the ventricles is in the auriculoventricular junctional tissue. The patient had angina pectoris and Adams-Stokes disease.

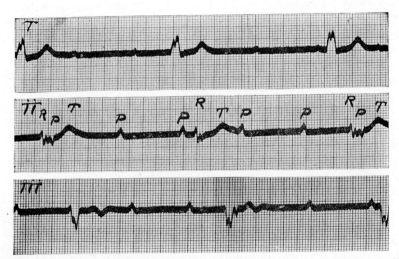

FIG. 131. *Complete Heart Block.* Auricular rate 66, ventricular rate 27. Note that the auricular waves (P) may come just before, during, or after the ventricular complexes (R-T). The patient had rare attacks of Adams-Stokes syncope but was able to do hard work. The ventricular complexes are regular. They could arise in the auriculoventricular node and be blocked in one of the bundle branches, or they could arise as ectopic idioventricular beats in or near the opposite bundle branch. In view of this uncertainty it is safer to refer to them with the noncommittal diagnosis of complete heart block with abnormal ventricular complexes.

slight irregularities may be present. Curiously, the ventricular contrac-tion may disturb the auricular rhythm (Fig. 128), possibly by changes in blood supply, through nervous reflexes, or through the phenomenon of "synchronization." The converse may also occur, and auricular sys-tole disturb the regularity of the ventricles in complete heart block. Oc-casionally this appears to be related to the so-called "supernormal

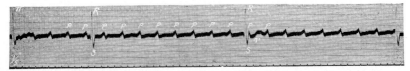

FIG. 134.   *Complete Heart Block.*   The auricles (P) are beating regularly at a rate of 111; the ventricles are contracting slowly and irregularly at a rate of about 16. The two rhythms are independent of each other. (Author's article in Oxford Loose-Leaf Medicine, vol. II.)

are due to further slowing of the ventricles or to complete ventricular standstill. When the rate remains constant, even as low as 30, the efficiency of the circulation may be normal. I have seen many instances in which patients were able to do hard physical work for many years with such slow hearts. Danger arises when the ventricles stop contracting entirely. Such pauses come suddenly, and the symptoms they produce will depend on their length. If the pause lasts several seconds the patients may feel only a faint wave or light-headed sensation like a petit mal. If it lasts a little longer, they faint away for several seconds. If it continues for twenty to sixty seconds they will lose consciousness and have a convulsion, with stertorous breathing. If it lasts a few minutes, breathing ceases and death generally ensues. On very rare occasions the normal beat may be resumed even after the heart has ceased beating for several minutes (Fig. 115). Attacks of syncope may occur at the sudden onset of the complete heart block, before the new ventricular rhythm takes on its function. They may also come at the time of the transition between a partial and complete block or when further depression of the pacemaker occurs and the rate falls below 20 (Fig. 134). When, for some reason, possibly through changes in blood supply or nervous influences, the ventricles, which were contracting regularly at the rate of 30 or 20, suddenly stop entirely syncope will occur. Finally, if an attack of paroxysmal ventricular tachycardia develops in a patient with complete block, it is apt to be followed by complete standstill of the ventricle (Fig. 115). The precarious feature of complete heart block is, therefore, not the slow regular rate of 28 but the temporary complete failure of the idioventricular pacemaker to send out impulses. Similar syncopal attacks may occur even without complete auriculoventricular block if the ventricles fail to contract, as may take place reflexly from a sensitive carotid sinus or in sino-auricular block.

The clinical recognition of complete block is ordinarily a simple matter when the rate is very slow and regular, as there is no other condition in which this occurs. When the rate is between 35 and 50 or more it can be confused with other conditions, especially partial block. The differentiation has already been discussed in the paragraphs on partial heart block. There is one additional sign that is pathognomonic of complete block, i.e., the changing quality and intensity of the first heart sound. On careful auscultation it will be noted that with occasional cycles the first heart sound may become muffled, accentuated, or reduplicated. This results from the changing relationship between the auricular and the ventricular contractions. In some cases the auricular rate is exactly twice the ventricular rate for long periods of time, so that only after prolonged auscultation will this valuable diagnostic sign become apparent (Fig. 135). Furthermore, it is often possible to hear extra-auricular sounds over the precordium during the long pauses, to see extra-auricular waves in the jugular pulse, and even to feel, in the radial pulse synchronously with auricular systole, faint waves which are due to an impact against the aorta. All these latter signs merely indicate that the auricles are contracting more frequently than the ventricles and that there is some degree of block. The changing quality of the first heart sound and other criteria prove that the block is complete.

The clinical conditions in which complete heart block occurs were taken up under partial heart block. In some cases of otherwise inexplicable complete block the conduction defect appears to be related to a severe attack of diphtheria in childhood. In many conditions, once established, complete heart block is apt to be permanent, although occasional reversion to a block of lesser degree or to a normal mechanism occurs. Although mild degrees of heart block are common during the acute stages of rheumatic fever, complete heart block is rare. Furthermore, it is very uncommon to find permanent complete block as a sequel of rheumatic fever unless it develops many years later as an accompaniment of valvular disease.

Although the majority of cases of heart block associated with attacks of Adams-Stokes syncope will show a slow heart and complete block between spells there is a considerable number of patients who have a normal rate and no block except when they are having attacks. It follows, therefore, that finding a normal rhythm in a patient with fainting spells by no means rules out the diagnosis of Adams-Stokes attacks (Fig. 136). In Figure 137 is illustrated an unusual condition in

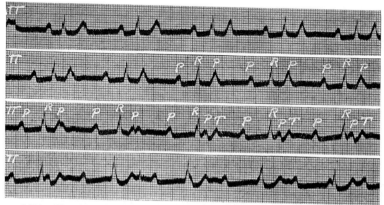

FIG. 135. *Complete Heart Block (False 2:1 Block)*. Continuous tracing shows that, although for a long period (upper two strips) a 2:1 relationship appears to exist, complete block finally develops (lower two strips), with the P waves crossing the R waves.

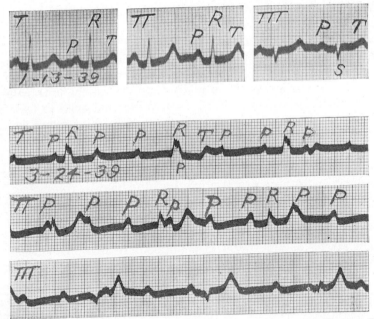

FIG. 136.   *Complete Heart Block (Adams-Stokes Attacks with Normal Rhythm between Spells)*.   The patient was a 60-year-old woman with hypertension and mitral stenosis. At the time the first tracing was taken she already had had frequent attacks of unconsciousness. Two months later she showed typical complete block and syncopal attacks continued.

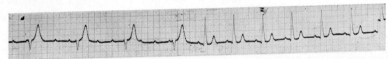

FIG. 137.   *Complete Heart Block Resulting from "Bilateral" Bundle Branch Block*. The patient was a 64-year-old man with Adams-Stokes attacks. The auricular rate remained unchanged throughout the tracing. During the second half of the tracing there was second degree (2:1) auriculoventricular heart block with left bundle branch block, during the first half of the tracing complete heart block with abnormal ventricular complexes resembling block in the opposite bundle branch. The changes can be explained as the result of block in both bundle branches, equivalent to complete heart block, during the first half of the strip, and of disappearance of block in the right branch during the second half.

which complete block is transient, changes to 2:1 block, and may be a manifestation of bilateral bundle branch block.

Therapy in complete heart block is important because it is often effective. Treatment is not directed at the slow steady rate, for this may be productive of no symptoms and may even be a protection to a heart that is threatened with congestive failure. However, the slow rate is no contraindication to the use of digitalis if congestive signs are present. The main concern is the attacks of syncope. When they occur at rare intervals, once every year or more, the problem is difficult, because preventive medication would have to be continued all this time and it might even then be doubtful whether or not the cessation of attacks was due to the drugs. When attacks occur frequently, many times a day, as may happen during acute coronary thrombosis, epinephrine given subcutaneously may be life saving. It may be necessary to give a dose of 0.3 to 0.5 cc. of a 1:1000 solution every two hours for a day or so. The frequency and duration of the treatment will depend on the circumstances. For a period of an hour or more after epinephrine is injected all attacks may cease. The drug increases the irritability of the ventricles and not only prevents the pauses of the ventricles but actually increases their rate in complete heart block.

As an alternative to repetitive subcutaneous injections, the intravenous infusion of epinephrine or isopropylarterenol (Isuprel) may be tried. Four cc. of epinephrine (1:1000) in 1000 cc. of 5 per cent dextrose in water or 1 mg. (five vials) of Isuprel in 250 cc. of dextrose in water is allowed to run in at an initial rate of 15 drops a minute. The rate of flow is increased, depending on the response of the heart rate. The latter should be kept between 35 and 40. Ectopic rhythms can develop with either preparation. In the event of their inception, the infusion should be stopped temporarily and then resumed at a slower rate. After a stable heart rate has been established, an attempt is made to cut down on the rate of the drip and eventually to stop it. There have been recent reports of the successful use of intravenous molar sodium lactate solution in dosage varying from 15 to almost 1000 cc. Finally, the procedure of external electrical stimulation of the heart ("artificial pacemaker") may be used. The important point here is that this method is of value in ventricular standstill, not in ventricular fibrillation.

A considerable number of syncopal attacks in patients with established complete heart block result not from primary ventricular standstill but from an initial period of ventricular tachycardia, perhaps followed by ventricular fibrillation and then standstill (Figs. 113 and 115). Therapy in this group of cases is ill defined. Recent experience indicates that the use of quinidine or Pronestyl is contraindicated. The use of Isuprel, epinephrine, or molar sodium lactate seems more encouraging.

When the condition is chronic and the attacks occur in an otherwise ambulatory patient, Isuprel, 5 to 10 mg. sublingually or orally, or ephedrine sulfate, 0.025 gm. ($\frac{3}{8}$ grain) or even larger doses, administered by mouth two or three times a day may prove effective. Occasionally barium chloride, 0.03 to 0.06 gm. ($\frac{1}{2}$ to 1 grain) three or four times a day, given by mouth, will inhibit all attacks. In stubborn cases a great variety of procedures have been employed, and when an apparently favorable result has been obtained it is difficult to be certain of the efficacy of the agents employed in treatment. Among these are inhalations of 1:100 epinephrine, Benzedrine, propadrine, full doses of atropine, intravenous injections of 50 per cent dextrose, thyroid tablets, Cardiazol, and digitalis or Urginin. It must be remembered that quinidine should be given with caution to patients with disturbances in conduction as it can increase the inhibition of beats.

Congenital Heart Disease

In only one congenital condition, namely, true congenital dextrocardia, is the electrocardiogram absolutely pathognomonic. The electrical axis of the heart lies in the direction opposite to normal, i.e., from left to right. When the three standard leads are taken, therefore, Lead I will be a mirror picture of the normal Lead I. All the waves will be inverted (Fig. 138, upper tracing, and Fig. 139). Lead II will resemble a normal Lead III, and vice versa. Similarly Lead aVR resembles normal Lead aVL and Lead aVL resembles normal Lead aVR. Leads over the left precordium resemble those over the normal right precordium, and vice versa (Fig. 139). If the right and left arm electrodes are reversed, curves of normal appearance will be obtained (Fig. 138, lower tracing). Care must be taken in making the diagnosis of dextrocardia from electrocardiograms, because accidental interchange of the arm electrodes will produce similar curves. This mistake is not at all uncommon.

In three other congenital conditions the electrocardiogram provides decisive evidence of the nature of the defect, if considered in the light of the clinical findings. These are congenital complete heart block, congenital atresia of the tricuspid valve, and congenital origin of the descending branch of the left coronary artery from the pulmonary artery. The electrocardiographic clue to the diagnosis of congenital tricuspid atresia is the presence of left ventricular hypertrophy in a cyanotic infant. In anomalous origin of the left coronary artery from the pulmonary artery, electrocardiographic evidence of anterolateral ischemia has been reported. Apart from these conditions it is a fairly valid general rule that extreme right axis deviation or extreme right ventricular hypertrophy indicates some form of congenital heart disease.

The electrocardiographic examination must be regarded as a very important incident in the work-up of every patient suspected of having a congenital cardiovascular lesion. The electrocardiogram parallels the anatomic and physiologic changes quite closely and records changes if the abnormal flow or the pressure changes are adequate to produce hypertrophy. Thus, in a general way, the electrocardiogram corrects or confirms the roentgenographic and fluoroscopic findings regarding ventricular hypertrophy. Indeed, the electrocardiogram is somewhat more reliable than x-ray examination in the detection of right ventricular hypertrophy. Although the x-ray may detect ventricular enlargement in general, it is relatively inaccurate in telling which ventricle is enlarged. In pulmonic stenosis the electrocardiogram generally shows right ventricular hypertrophy or persistent incomplete right bundle branch block (Fig. 44), but when the degree of stenosis is slight the electrocardiogram may be normal. In atrial septal defect the electrocardiogram generally shows incomplete right bundle branch block (Fig. 43) or right ventricular hypertrophy, or a combination of the two, but here again the tracings may be normal if the defect is small. It is a curious fact that atrial septal defects are more commonly associated with intraventricular block (prolonged QRS complex) and auriculoventricular block (prolonged P-R interval) than are ventricular septal defects. Arrhythmias, including auricular fibrillation, are not uncommonly seen in atrial septal defects.

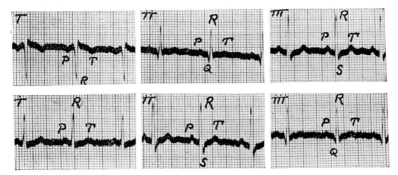

FIG. 138.   *Dextrocardia.*   The upper tracing shows the ordinary three leads in a case of congenital dextrocardia with situs inversus of the abdominal viscera. Note that all the waves (P-R-T) are inverted in Lead I. Leads II and III appear interchanged. The lower curves were obtained on the same patient by placing the right arm electrode on the left arm and *vice versa*. They then appear to be normal curves.

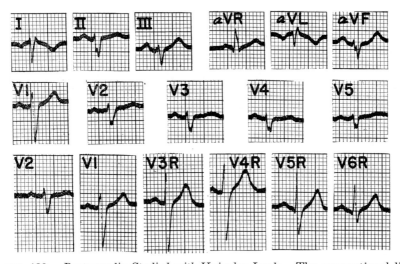

FIG. 139.   *Dextrocardia Studied with Unipolar Leads.*   The conventional limb leads show the same type of change described in Figure 138. Note that Lead aVL here resembles the normal Lead aVR. Lead aVF has a normal relationship to the heart. The second row of tracings shows Leads V_1 to V_5 taken in the usual manner. Note that, instead of increasing as the electrode moves to the left, the R wave actually decreases. By interchanging Leads V_1 and V_2 and continuing over the right side of the chest, representing the true precordium, a series of tracings is obtained comparable to the usual set of precordial leads. Note now that the R wave shows a progressive increase in height to Lead V_{5R}, and therefore that, when rearranged properly, the electrocardiogram has a normal appearance. The patient was a healthy 23-year-old man whose abnormal heart shadow was detected in a mass miniature x-ray survey for tuberculosis.

In the tetralogy of Fallot there is always an extreme degree of right ventricular hypertrophy, and the P waves are apt to be tall and pointed. Right ventricular hypertrophy may also be seen in transposition of the great vessels or in anomalous entrance of the pulmonary veins into the right auricle.

In patent ductus arteriosus, where the greater mechanical burden is borne by the left ventricle, left ventricular hypertrophy may be detected by the electrocardiogram. In many cases, when the defect is small, the electrocardiogram may appear normal. First degree heart block is not uncommon. Coarctation of the aorta and congenital aortic or subaortic stenosis are also apt to be associated with left ventricular hypertrophy (Fig. 47). In ventricular septal defects the forces are generally balanced so that the electrocardiogram is usually normal; occasionally, however, one ventricle appears to be predominantly overburdened so that either right or left ventricular hypertrophy may be recorded. The vectorcardiogram (Fig. 32) frequently shows combined ventricular hypertrophy. Occasionally the defect appears to intercept the auriculoventricular bundle, producing congenital complete heart block, but the latter condition may also occur with an intact septum. Congenital complete heart block may be rather well borne; the heart rate is generally more rapid than that seen with acquired complete heart block.

Changes in Form of the Auricular Complex

The auricular complex (P wave) varies somewhat in form in normal individuals. In general, with faster rates the P wave is taller, and with slower rates it is smaller. This is due to the fact that impulses arise high in the sino-auricular node when the rate is rapid and low in the sino-auricular node when the rate is slow. Generally the P wave shows a much more conspicuous deflection in normal sinus tachycardia than in paroxysmal auricular tachycardia. Occasionally this fact may be helpful in making the difficult differential diagnosis between these two types of tachycardia. Tall, narrow P waves are a regular feature of potassium depletion in the dog and have been recorded in a number of humans exhibiting this derangement. One peculiar type of P wave is present so frequently with mitral stenosis that it is fairly diagnostic. It is prominent, broad, somewhat flat-topped and notched (Figs. 45, lower set, 140, and 141). These characteristics are generally displayed in Leads I and II, and often in Lead III the P wave is inverted. This type of P wave usually denotes an enlargement of the auricles, and as this occurs almost exclusively in mitral stenosis it has important clinical value. When curves are found, such as are represented in Figures 45, 140, and 141, one can be quite certain that mitral stenosis is present. There may be an additional tricuspid stenosis, but this never occurs without the presence of mitral stenosis as well. Occasionally broad notched P waves of the type described above may be observed during acute myocardial

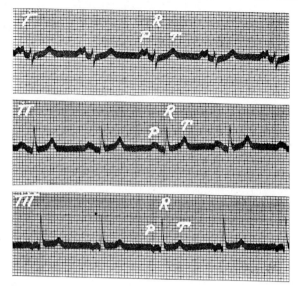

FIG. 140. *Auricular Hypertrophy.* Note that the P waves in Lead I are broad, flat topped, and notched. The patient had well-marked mitral stenosis.

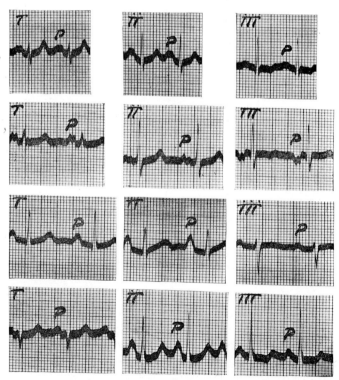

FIG. 141. *Auricular Hypertrophy.* Four sets of curves showing large, broad, and notched P waves. Note that P waves may be most prominent in Lead I or II and may be inverted in Lead III. All four patients had rheumatic mitral stenosis with or without aortic or tricuspid involvement.

infarction. Mitral valve disease may also be associated with broad biphasic P waves over the right precordium. The initial portion of these auricular deflections is upright and the final portion broad and inverted. Such P waves may occur with or without "mitral" P waves in the conventional leads. Notched P waves, generally not so broad as those seen in mitral valve disease, may also be observed in constrictive pericarditis. This may denote auricular scarring, an evidence of involvement of the auricular myocardium in the epicardial process. Deviations of the P-R segment have been described in the auricular infarction which may accompany infarction of the ventricle.

Sharp, narrow, and large P waves may be seen in hyperthyroidism, and it is suspected that tricuspid stenosis may have a prominent P wave that is taller and narrower than those just described for mitral stenosis.

Often, in association with other evidence of right ventricular hypertrophy, the P waves are tall (2.5 mm. or more) and pointed ("gothic" P waves) but not broadened in Leads II and III. These have been referred to as "P pulmonale." Whether this change is due to auricular hypertrophy or simply to a peculiar position of the auricles has not been determined. This change is frequently seen in pulmonary emphysema.

Changes in Form of Ventricular Complexes

There now remains for consideration a heterogeneous group of conditions in which the ventricular complex becomes abnormal, and the clinical significance of such changes. It will be seen that in some conditions the electrocardiographic findings are most important and helpful; in others they may be only suggestive, and frequently the changes may be misleading because they are not sufficiently distinctive.

VENTRICULAR COMPLEXES OF LOW AMPLITUDE

When the height of the R wave or the depth of the S wave is 5 mm. or less in all leads it is regarded as abnormal (Figs. 142, 143). Upward measurements should begin with the top of the isoelectric shadow of the string and downward measurements from the bottom of it. Such low curves may occur with advanced cardiac failure from any cause, either valvular or nonvalvular, with acute coronary occlusion (Fig. 143), anemia, myxedema, Addison's disease, pericardial effusion, or any condition showing considerable edema. They are also frequently present, even without evidence of heart failure, in patients with well-marked emphysema of the lungs. The low complexes are due either to the development of an electromotive force of small potential within the heart or to some electrical effect of the edema of tissues around the heart. The curves may become larger if the edema disappears or the congestive state improves. In myxedema (Fig. 144) not only are the QRS waves diminished, but the T waves are flat. Such curves can return to normal on thyroid therapy. When they are found after a coronary occlusion they are apt to persist indefinitely and be compatible with a satisfactory state of health for years. In general, curves of very low amplitude indicate a fairly grave condition of the heart, but there are exceptions to this rule.

There are tracings that show ventricular complexes of low amplitude which require a different interpretation. They are not apt to be quite so

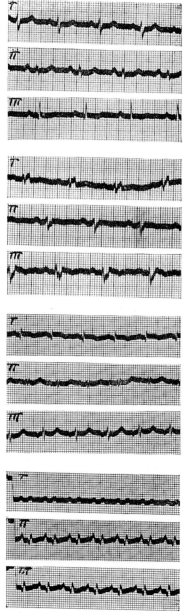

FIG. 142.   *Abnormal Form of Ventricular Complex* (*Low Voltage*).   Four sets of tracings showing QRS complexes of low amplitude in all leads. The lowest curves show the normal standardization. All four patients had serious heart disease of the coronary artery type.

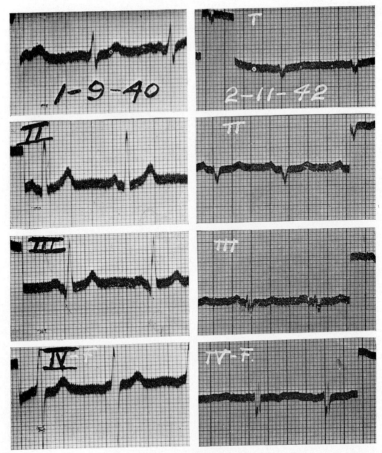

FIG. 143.   *Abnormal Form of Ventricular Complex (Low Voltage)*.   The tracings at the left, taken January 9, 1940, show nothing very abnormal. An attack of acute coronary thrombosis occurred in the summer of 1940. The tracings at the right, taken February 2, 1942, show marked decrease in amplitude of QRS and T waves. The patient had no peripheral edema, although there was a moderate right hydrothorax.

small, although they may be, but they appear otherwise normal. The QRS waves are not notched or spread, and the T waves have a normal configuration. These features distinguish them from the abnormal ones described above. They are found in individuals who are well and show no evidence of organic heart disease. Low voltage in the limb leads is more significant if there is associated low voltage in the precordial leads. It has been shown that in certain cases with low voltage in the limb leads the largest deflections occurred in Lead V_2, whereas normally the largest deflections occur in Lead V_4. This suggests not heart disease but a shift of the mean electrical axis of the heart toward the sagittal plane of the body. It is evident, therefore, that ventricular complexes of low potential must be interpreted with due care and should be considered only in conjunction with other data as indicative of heart disease.

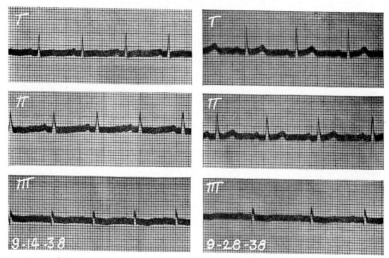

FIG. 144.   *Myxedema.*   The tracings at the left were taken September 14, 1938, when the basal metabolic rate was −35 per cent. The tracings at the right were taken fourteen days later, after thyroid therapy, the basal metabolic rate being −10 per cent. Note the increase in height of T and R waves.

VENTRICULAR COMPLEXES IN CORONARY THROMBOSIS AND MYOCARDIAL INFARCTION

The most important contribution that electrocardiography has made to medicine is in the diagnosis of coronary thrombosis and myocardial infarction. This goes back to the early observations of Pardee when he first called attention to the displacement of the S-T segment in acute myocardial infarction. When the ventricular complexes change after such an attack they do so because of alterations in the musculature supplied by the vessel involved and not because of the thrombosis itself. It would be more proper to designate these abnormalities as indicative of myocardial infarction, which generally results from coronary thrombosis, but which may come from disease of the arteries such as narrowing without thrombosis.

Myocardial injury produces changes in the electrocardiogram which vary with the degree of injury, the size of the area injured, and its location. These changes are of two sorts: (1) changes in the repolarization process (T wave and RS-T segment); and (2) changes in the depolarization process (QRS complex). We have seen that the T wave is the most labile part of the electrocardiogram, changing readily as the result of chemical, mechanical, anoxic, or thermal influences, whereas the QRS complex is relatively fixed and capable of change only by the most severe grades of injury. This corresponds to the clinical fact that changes in the T waves of themselves are to be regarded as nonspecific in their implications, whereas changes in the QRS complex generally correspond to profound muscle damage.

Although animal experiments have shown the earliest electrocardiographic consequences of impairment of the blood supply to the heart to be a sharp inversion of the T waves, this is not ordinarily observed clinically since patients are rarely seen at the very onset of an attack of myocardial infarction.

The T waves may normally be inverted over a small part of the right precordium in men, and over a larger part in women and children. But in general there is a progressive change from inverted to upright T waves as the electrode is moved toward the left. Inversion or notching of the T waves in one or more of the mid-precordial leads while the flanking leads show upright T waves is distinctly abnormal. In rare instances these have been described as a normal variation. Experience at the Peter Bent Brigham Hospital indicates that they are more often a harbinger of anterior wall infarction (Fig. 145). Certainly under suspicious clinical circumstances the detection of this change makes further electrocardiographic observation mandatory. In some of these cases, then, these T wave changes may represent the "ischemic" phase of myocardial infarction in man.

The use of a scatter of precordial leads permits a precise delineation of these changes in anterior wall infarction. It seems reasonable that similar T wave inversions recorded elsewhere, as in Leads II, III, and aVF, may portend infarction in the corresponding regions, but the topography and sequence of the changes are not generally so convincingly demonstrable.

Deeply inverted T waves may appear also at the margins of an infarct later in the course of an acute episode. By and large, however, the earliest changes recorded consist of displacements of the RS-T segments. An electrode overlying a subepicardial or transmural lesion records an upward displacement (elevation) of the RS-T segment, while an electrode overlying the opposite healthy ventricular wall records a reciprocal downward displacement (depression) of the RS-T segment. On the other hand, an electrode overlying an acute infarct which is subendocardial in its location records a depressed RS-T segment while an electrode, such as that at Lead aVR, which faces the ventricular cavity and hence the injured subendocardial layers, records an elevated RS-T segment. This latter is the same sort of change which may readily be induced transiently in certain individuals with angina pectoris. It is difficult to reconcile this clinical phenomenon of easily induced RS-T segment depression with the experimental experience that RS-T segment elevations are recorded in animals only on a more prolonged coronary artery ligation than produced the T wave inversion described above. It is convenient, however, to correlate the three types of electrocardiographic changes with three stages of myocardial impairment, the QRS changes corresponding to myocardial necrosis, the RS-T segment deviations to injury effect, and T wave inversion to myocardial ischemia.

The RS-T segment displacements occurring during an acute myocardial infarction generally last only a few days, gradually returning to the isoelectric line. After a variable interval they are usually accompanied by terminal inversion of the T wave, giving rise to a characteristic appearance in the RS-T segment and T wave variously described as a "coronary T wave," "Pardee T wave," "cove-plane T wave," "round-shouldered T wave," or "upwardly bowed T wave." The Q-T interval in these instances is ordinarily prolonged. The T waves may become very deeply inverted and V-shaped; corresponding to this change the opposite ventricular wall may exhibit very tall pointed T waves. The changes in the T wave generally outlast those in the RS-T segment and may persist for weeks, months, or even years, but they are apt to lose their characteristic shape and the T waves become merely inverted but otherwise are of normal appearance. In time these may become iso-electric or normal upright T waves.

Frequently at the same time, but occasionally at variable intervals after these changes in the repolarization process, changes may also appear in the QRS complex. These changes probably correspond to actual death of parts of the myocardium which are no longer capable of responding to the activating impulse. If the entire thickness of the ventricular wall thus becomes electrically inert, the cavity potentials are transmitted passively through the infarct to an overlying electrode just as they would be through the electrically inactive auriculoventricular valve ring to an electrode (such as an esophageal electrode at auricular levels) facing the ventricular cavity. Since the remaining healthy ventricular myocardium is still activated from endocardium to epicardium, the impulse moves away from the ventricular cavity and a downward deflection is recorded in the cavity. The electrode overlying the transmural infarct therefore picks up the same potential and records a QS deflection. This QS wave ordinarily has considerable duration, 0.03 second or more from onset to nadir, 0.04 second or more in total breadth. If only the inner layers of the myocardium are destroyed and the outer layers are still

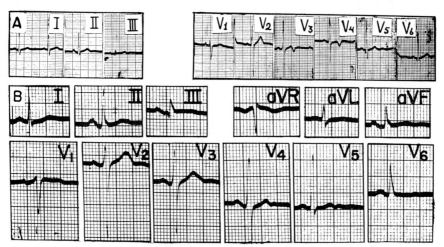

FIG. 145. *"Localized" T-Wave Changes as Expression of Myocardial Ischemia.* The upper strip (*A*) was recorded during the incipiency of an acute transmural myocardial infarction. The lower tracing (*B*) was recorded in a patient suffering with throat discomfort. This change disappeared in two days, but he then showed a positive exercise test for coronary insufficiency.

absolutely or relatively healthy, an overlying electrode records first a
Q wave, corresponding to unopposed activation of the healthy subendocardial muscle of the opposite wall, followed by an R wave corresponding
to activation of the healthy subepicardial muscle under the electrode.
However, this R wave is not so tall as the original R wave recorded over
the same area. Therefore the R wave decreases in height and a Q wave
appears if the infarct is subendocardial, whereas the R wave disappears
to be supplanted by a QS deflection if the infarct is transmural. These
considerations assume the validity of the traditional teaching regarding
the electrical activation of the ventricular wall. The observations underlying this concept have recently been contradicted by Prinzmetal. The
matter will be discussed further under Subendocardial Infarction (p.
586).

Which of the changes described is recorded by an electrode depends
upon its relation to the center or margin of the infarct. Direct leads
record T-wave inversions only at the margins of experimental infarcts.
In clinical myocardial infarction, however, T-wave inversion is apt to
be recorded in the same ventricular complex in which QS deflections are
present; in this case the electrode is a semidirect one and picks up a
mixture of the potentials over the infarct and in its vicinity. If the area
of transmural infarction is small, QRS changes may be missed in the
twelve-lead electrocardiograms now in more general use, or they may be
recorded in only one lead. Here is another reason for taking multiple
leads.

The area over which QRS, RS-T, and T-wave changes develop depends, among other considerations, upon the size of the infarct. QS or
QR waves may be detected over a wide area if the infarct is large.
Although one might expect that the prognosis is worse in larger than
in smaller infarcts, we know of no study which establishes this possibility. The area showing changes in the ventricular complex depends also
upon the orientation of the infarct with relation to the electrodes. From
the characteristic changes developing in certain leads it is possible to
localize an infarct quite accurately. This procedure is described at greater
length below. It must be emphasized, however, that at present localization of infarcts is of more academic than practical interest. Once decisive
evidence of acute myocardial infarction has been obtained, a record of
the sequential changes that subsequently occur is of no clinical value;
it is a matter of little moment if there is a lateral component to an
anterior or posterior myocardial infarct.

As an infarct heals the scar is apt to contract to a smaller and
smaller area. One which produced cavity potentials over perhaps four
of the usual precordial points might then become so small that decisive
changes are now recorded at only one point. If the scar is not located
strategically with relation to these precordial points it may not be
recorded at all.

In contradistinction to the RS-T and T-wave changes which may
be evanescent and disappear entirely with healing of the infarct, the

QRS changes are relatively fixed. Once they appear they are likely to persist, usually for the remainder of the patient's life. On rare occasions Q waves appear and disappear. This is often difficult to explain. By and large the decision regarding *old* myocardial infarction rests upon the detection of characteristic changes in the QRS complexes. The electrocardiographic diagnosis of *acute* myocardial infarction, on the other hand, is made on the basis of characteristic sequential changes in the RS-T, T, and QRS complexes. As indicated below there are some cases of old infarction, especially in association with aneurysm formation, in which the QRS, RS-T, and T-wave changes may remain fixed over months or years. Rarely acute myocardial infarction may be associated with characteristic changes in the RS-T segment and T waves only. If a good clinical history suggestive of an acute episode is obtained, the diagnosis of acute infarction is justified in patients with these electrocardiographic findings. These patients are said generally to do well and on recovery may show no electrocardiographic residue of infarction. Some patients go through an entire clinical episode of acute myocardial infarction without developing corroborative electrocardiographic evidence for the diagnosis. Others will yield decisive or suggestive electrocardiographic findings only after several tracings have been recorded. In one patient electrocardiographic changes did not appear until the third week of a typical clinical episode. Hence, although, as stated above, serial tracings are not helpful once the diagnosis has been established, they are imperative until that diagnosis has been made or another diagnosis has been substituted.

Anterolateral Infarction (Antero-apical Infarction). When an infarct involves both the anterior and lateral aspects of the heart changes of the type described above are generally recorded between Leads V_3 and V_6. A clue to anterolateral infarction is a decrease in the height of the R wave as the electrode is moved to the left of Leads V_1 or V_2, but this is not conclusive. QS deflections corresponding to transmural infarction may be present over one, two, or three positions. At one or more positions to the left of the QS wave, and corresponding to a subendocardial extension of the infarct, QR waves may be recorded (Figs. 146 to 148). RS-T and T-wave changes of the type described above generally occur in association with the QRS changes. The exact leads in which these changes are recorded vary with the position of the heart and of the infarct with relation to the precordial leads and with the precision with which the electrodes are placed at the same precordial positions at each recording of the electrocardiogram.

In these cases the infarct generally extends far enough laterally to be registered at the left shoulder, especially if the heart lies in a horizontal electrical position. Even if the heart is not horizontal the infarct may extend high enough on the lateral surface to be recorded at the left shoulder. Accordingly changes in the ventricular complex are apt to be recorded in Lead aVL as well as in the lateral precordial leads. Since the potentials of Lead aVL are written with unchanged polarity in Lead I, this lead shows prominent Q waves, elevated RS-T segments, and char-

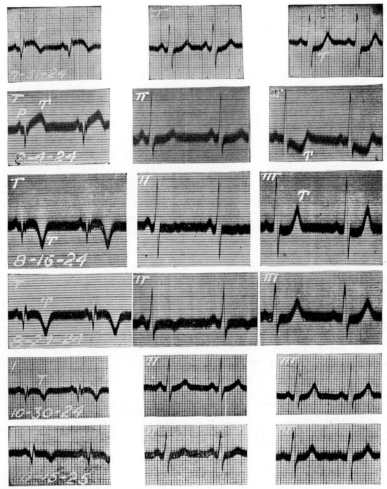

FIG. 146. *Anterolateral Myocardial Infarction.*   A series of tracings following an attack of acute coronary thrombosis which occurred July 20, 1924. Note that the high take-off of the T wave and the subsequent sharp inversion occur in Lead I. Somewhat similar changes but in the opposite direction occur in T_3. Also there is a distinct Q_1 which persists even the following year. These tracings were recorded before the advent of chest leads, but probably would be associated with changes in Lead aVL and in the left lateral chest leads similar to those recorded in Lead I, and therefore probably represent infarction of the anterolateral portion of the left ventricle. (Author's article in Oxford Loose-Leaf Medicine, vol. II.)

acteristic inversion of the T waves. On the other hand, since Lead aVL has a reversed polarity in its contribution to Lead III, Lead III is apt to develop smaller R waves, deeper S waves, depressed RS-T segments, and upright T waves. Thus Leads I and III may have a mirror image relationship as a result simply of the particular galvanometer poles through which left shoulder potentials are routed. Another cause of reciprocal changes in the electrocardiogram is described below under posterior myocardial infarction.

If the infarct is so oriented that only T-wave changes are transmitted to the left shoulder, Lead I will record only an inverted T wave. This T wave might or might not have a so-called "coronary" contour. Thus only dubious evidence for infarction will be present in the standard leads when decisive evidence is recorded in the precordial leads.

Following healing of the infarct the only residuals may be a prominent Q_1 and the presence of decreasing R waves, of absent R waves where R waves are ordinarily recorded, or of QS or QR complexes in the lateral precordium. Generally these changes are much more readily appreciated in the precordial than in the standard or unipolar limb leads.

Anteroseptal Infarction. Here the changes are recorded in the region of the sternum, usually in Lead V_1 through V_4 (Figs. 149 to 153). Changes in Lead V_1 and V_2 are said to be more commonly associated with infarction of the septum, whereas lesions located nearer the apex are likely to be associated with a small R wave in Lead V_1, giving way to QS or QR complexes in Leads V_2 and V_3. A decrease in the size of the R wave as the electrode moves to the left is presumptive but not conclusive

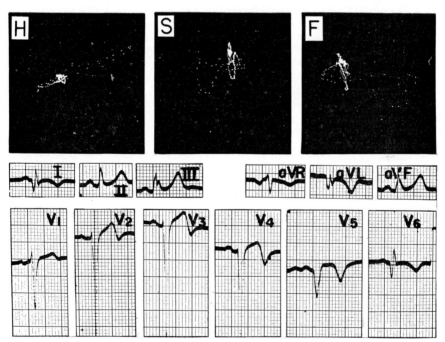

FIG. 147. *Vectorcardiogram and Electrocardiogram in Acute Anterolateral Myocardial Infarction.* In the horizontal and frontal planes there is an extraordinarily large initial anterior and rightward development. This accounts for the large Q waves in Leads I, aVL, V_5, and V_6. The subsequent anterior and leftward salience expected in a normal horizontal plane loop is largely lost. This explains the small and decreasing R waves from Leads V_2 to V_6. In the sagittal plane the loop is twisted. In the frontal plane both the initial and the final appendages seem to come off the null point on a common stalk. This leads to notching of the QRS complex in Leads III and aVF.

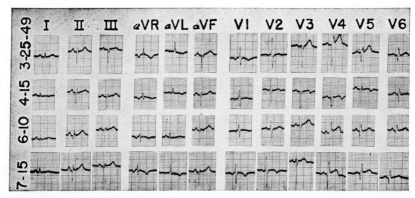

FIG. 148.   *Acute Anterolateral Changes Possibly Superimposed upon an Old Posterolateral Myocardial Infarct(?).*   The patient was a 62-year-old widow, without a previous history of angina pectoris or myocardial infarction, who developed severe crushing midchest pain five days before admission. The initial set of tracings, recorded shortly after admission, showed prominent QS deflections in Leads III and aVF, and broad, prominent Q waves in Leads II and V_4 through V_6. The RS-T segments were elevated in Leads V_4 and V_5 and slightly elevated in Leads III and aVF. These changes indicate myocardial infarction, probably acute. During the first week the patient developed an elevated sedimentation rate and leukocytosis. The second set of tracings, taken three weeks later, show persistence of the QRS changes, return of the displaced RS-T segments toward the isoelectric line, and a terminal dip in the T waves in Leads I and V_2 through V_6. The next two sets of tracings, taken two and three months later, show return to the appearance noted in the original tracings. The patient recovered. In this case the RS-T and T wave changes were most marked anterolaterally while the QRS changes persisted posterolaterally. It is possible that QRS changes were present posterolaterally before the current attack and that the only recent electrocardiographic developments were "ischemic" anterolateral changes. The persistent changes four months after the attack suggest ventricular aneurysm. This series illustrates the occasional difficulty in interpreting tracings when more than one infarct, of varying duration, may be involved.

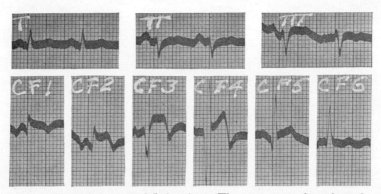

FIG. 149.   *Acute Anteroseptal Infarction.*   The upper set of tracings shows the three standard leads that are not definitely diagnostic of myocardial infarction. The lower set of six bipolar chest leads shows absence of an initial upward deflection in CF_1 through CF_5, and an elevation of RS-T in CF_1 through CF_4, with late inversion of T waves. These are diagnostic of anteroseptal infarction. The patient was a 75-year-old man with a known old gastric ulcer, who developed pain in the xiphoid region which was first misinterpreted as due to a subacute perforation of the stomach. If these changes were static, ventricular aneurysm would be suggested.

evidence of old anteroseptal infarct (Fig. 153). In rare cases elevation of the RS-T segments and inverted T waves may be inscribed at Leads V_1 and V_2 in the absence of more distinctive QRS changes than are ordinarily present in these areas. Fortunately myocardial infarction is not prone to develop in the age and sex groups which may normally show inverted T waves over the right ventricle.

RS-T and T-wave changes may be recorded to the left of Leads V_3 or V_4, but only rarely are diagnostic changes reflected in Lead aVL or Lead I. The reason for this is that, by and large, the electrical forces are oriented in an anteroposterior plane and have little or no projection upon the frontal plane of the body. Infarcts in this location were particularly liable to be missed when only the three conventional leads were

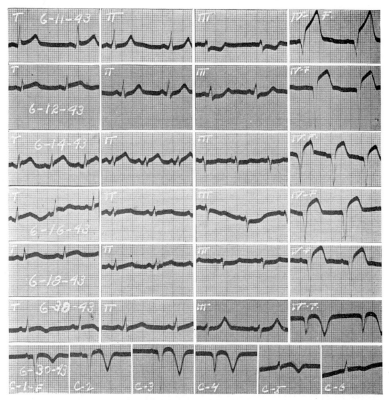

FIG. 150. *Acute Anteroseptal Myocardial Infarction.* This series shows three standard leads and CF_4, the first tracings being taken about four hours after onset. The standard leads go through the customary changes of anterior infarction, i.e., elevation of RS-T_1 and a depressed RS-T_3 becoming a sharply upright T_3. Note that the first set shows a very high take-off of RS-T_{IVF}, which remains elevated for over a week and finally becomes sharply inverted. The R_{IVF} is absent throughout. This is characteristic of anteroseptal myocardial infarction. The lowest set shows the six precordial leads, CF_1 to CF_6. Note that R is absent and T is sharply inverted over the first four positions, indicating a large area of infarction. The patient was a 41-year-old man who recovered and became symptomless.

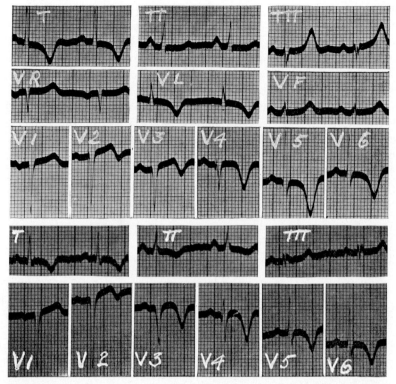

FIG. 151. *Acute Anteroseptal Myocardial Infarction.* The upper three strips, taken October 5, 1941, show the three standard leads, the three unipolar limb leads (VR, VL, and VF), and the six precordial leads (V_1 to V_6). Note the absence of R waves in V_1 to V_3 and the gradual appearance of dipping and inversion of T from V_2 to V_6. The lower two strips, made October 27, 1941, show slight regression of the abnormalities. The patient was a 53-year-old woman who had a coronary thrombosis two months earlier and another twelve hours before the first tracing was made. Recovery was satisfactory.

in use. They can also be missed if one takes only a single precordial lead located to the left of the infarct.

Occasionally it is difficult to decide from leads taken over the right precordium whether old anteroseptal infarction is present. Since the R wave may normally be absent or small in Leads V_1 and V_2, and since R waves may be small or absent over a larger area (V_1 through V_3 or even V_4) in individuals with left ventricular hypertrophy or complete or incomplete left bundle branch block, it may be difficult or impossible to decide whether an old anteroseptal infarct is present. In such cases it may be necessary to report that all of the changes can be accounted for by left ventricular hypertrophy, for example, but that old anteroseptal infarct cannot be excluded.

High Lateral Infarction. Localization of an infarct to the upper left border of the heart, sparing the apex and not detectable with certainty in the usual six precordial leads, is rare. In cases of this sort a clue to the

existence of high lateral infarction may be the presence of a prominent
Q wave followed by an R wave at the left shoulder. Some difficulty is
encountered in evaluating this finding in vertical hearts which may also
show a prominent Q or QS wave at Lead aVL. The finding of an inverted
P wave preceding this QRS complex would be more consistent with a
vertically placed heart, for then auricular as well as ventricular depolarization proceeds away from the left shoulder. One would then have to
conclude that the left shoulder electrode must face the auriculoventricular valve ring through its auricular aspect, and that the Q wave inscribed at the left shoulder lead represents cavity potential transmitted

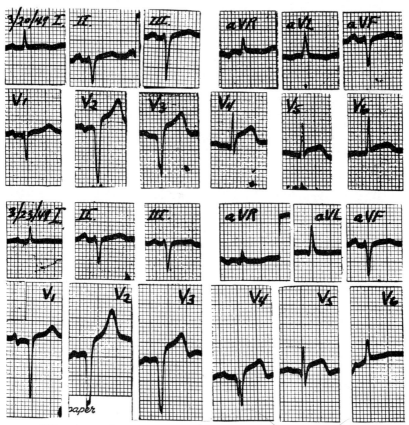

FIG. 152.   *Acute Anteroseptal Myocardial Infarct.*   The upper set of tracings
show the characteristic changes of anteroseptal infarction interpreted as of uncertain
duration. Late inversion of the T waves in Leads V$_3$ to V$_5$ of the lower set of tracings
suggested that the process was acute, and the QR complex in Lead V$_5$ indicated subendocardial extension of the infarct. The patient was a 78-year-old man who had a
typical clinical attack of coronary thrombosis following a fracture of the wrist. He
died five days after the second set of tracings was recorded. Postmortem examination
showed a large anteroseptal infarct extending almost the entire distance from the
apex to the auriculoventricular sulcus with subendocardial hemorrhage, and involving the anterior half of the septum. Popliteal thrombophlebitis and a large pulmonary
embolus to the right lower lobe of the lung were also found.

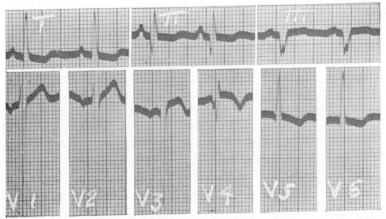

FIG. 153.   *Old Anteroseptal Myocardial Infarction.*   The upper set of tracings shows the three standard leads and the lower the six precordial leads taken February 16, 1943. Note that the R wave gradually decreases in size from V_1 to V_3 so that it is absent at V_3. There are also changes in T in V_4 to V_6. The broad prominent Q wave in Lead II and the notched QS wave in Lead III may be explained by a coexistent old posterior lesion, by anteroposterior (Roesler-Dressler) infarction, or, if the heart were in an extreme vertical position, by transmission of the cavity potentials from the anterior surface of the heart to the left leg. The patient was a 39-year-old man with severe chronic arthritis, who had had an acute coronary thrombosis in April of 1942.

through the valve ring. If, on the other hand, the P wave is upright, auricular depolarization must proceed toward the electrode. Unless the electrode happens to lie in precise relation to the epicardial aspect of the auriculoventricular sulcus, one would be justified in assuming that it overlay the infarcted free wall of the left ventricle, passively transmitting cavity potentials to it. Generally a final decision as to high lateral infarction cannot be made from this finding. However, if additional leads are then taken in the second, third, and fourth interspaces in the midclavicular, and in the anterior and midaxillary lines, one may find unequivocal evidence of infarction in broad prominent Q waves with or without RS-T and T wave changes, distributed over a considerable area. In our experience high lateral infarcts have constituted portions of infarcts already easily detected elsewhere, but they have been reported in the literature as lesions localized to the left upper margin of the heart.

Posterior Myocardial Infarction.   The posterior aspect of the heart lies upon the cupola formed by the left leaf of the diaphragm. The potentials of the posterior wall are transmitted through the diaphragm to the left leg, which is relatively remote from the heart. Lead aVF therefore records the composite potentials of the posterior and, to a lesser extent, of other aspects of the heart. Hence posterior wall infarcts are generally detected in Lead aVF. Lead aVF contributes in a positive way to the potentials of both Leads II and III. Other things being equal, these two standard leads may also detect the changes of posterior wall infarction (Figs. 154 to 157). Until the advent of unipolar lead electrocardiography prominent Q waves, elevated RS-T segments, and inverted T waves in Lead III, and, to a lesser extent, in Lead II as well, have been the evidence upon which the diagnosis has been made. However, Leads II and III are composite leads. A Q wave in Lead III may result from a Q_{aVF}, or from an R_{aVL}. The use of these unipolar limb leads enables one to decide, at a glance, which of these two possibilities explains Q_3 and therefore, in large measure, enables one to decide whether a prominent Q_3 is the result of posterior myocardial infarction or of left ventricular epicardial potentials transmitted to the left shoulder. It is in this differentiation that the unipolar limb leads have their greatest field of usefulness. In the decision of insurability, for example, a prominent Q_3 may be the only residual of a previous posterior infarct. If, with such a finding, a prominent R_{aVL} but no Q_{aVF} (Fig. 27) or an inconspicuous Q_{aVF} are found, one may dismiss the Q_3 as evidence of an old posterior scar. In the same circumstances a broad, prominent Q_{aVF} would be decisive evidence of old posterior wall infarction (Fig. 45). Authorities differ as to just what yardstick should be used to decide whether Q_{aVF} is significant. We have adopted the criteria of Myers, who states that if QRS has a total deflection of 5 mm. or more and the Q wave measures 25 per cent or more of the R wave in that lead and the Q wave measures

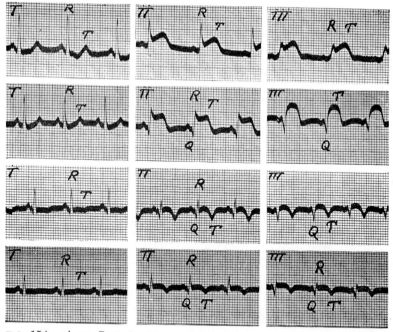

FIG. 154.   *Acute Posterior Myocardial Infarct.*   First set of curves taken four hours after onset of attack, June 14, 1934. Subsequent tracings taken June 20, July 6, and August 17, 1934. Note very high take-off with monophasic action current in Lead III of first set. Note also that Q waves have not yet developed in the first set. The RS-T segment returns subsequently to the isoelectric line, and the T wave inverts. A Q_2 and Q_3 gradually develop and persist.

0.03 second or more from onset to nadir, the unequivocal diagnosis of posterior wall infarction can be made. If only one of these two criteria is present the tracing must be regarded as borderline and consistent with that diagnosis. In our experience, if the Q wave measures 0.04 second from onset to nadir, posterior infarction is probable. It is dangerous to draw conclusions from the form of the QRS complex if the total excursion is less than 5 mm. In that case one may well be dealing with the "transitional zone," recording the composite potentials of both the right and left ventricle. In any case the associated presence of RS-T and T-wave changes enhances the value of changes in the QRS complex which of themselves may be of dubious significance. The important point should be stressed that even with the help offered by Lead aVF it still may be necessary to report equivocal findings. The vast majority of cases showing prominent Q_3 but no significant Q_{aVF} do not have posterior infarction, but we have observed a few exceptional cases in which posterior infarction was present under these circumstances. In these cases, however, the

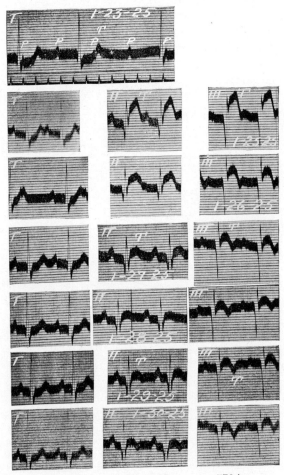

FIG. 155 (A).   (Legend on page 573.)

development of associated RS-T changes generally was sufficient to establish the diagnosis. It is possible that in these cases the patient died before the QRS changes had sufficient time to develop, that the potentials of the infarct were directed at right angles to the frontal plane of the body, or that the infarct was not oriented toward the left leg because of some other peculiarity in the electrical position of the heart. A prominent QS complex in Lead aVF is much more difficult to evaluate. This

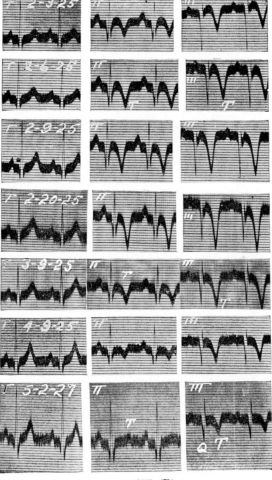

FIG. 155 (B)

FIG. 155. *Acute Posterior Myocardial Infarction.* Attack of coronary thrombosis on January 12, 1925. Note the sequence of changes (*A* and *B*) in the ventricular complexes, beginning with a high take-off of the RS-T segment in Lead III, gradually becoming lower and dipped, and finally marked inversion of T_3. Partial heart block was present in the early days. A prominent Q_2 and Q_3 developed and persisted. Had unipolar limb leads been taken in this case Lead aVF would certainly have recorded the same type of changes as those recorded in Leads II and III. The patient did well for five years after the attack. (Author's article in Oxford Loose-Leaf Medicine, vol. II.)

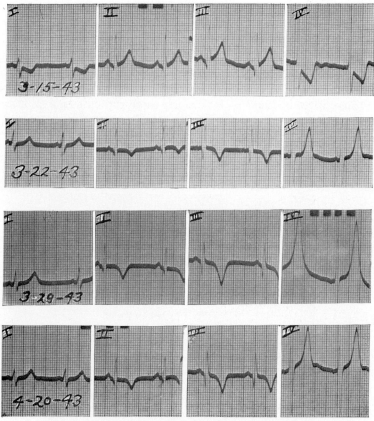

FIG. 156.   *Acute Posterior Myocardial Infarction.*   The first set of tracings was taken six hours after onset of a typical attack of coronary thrombosis. Note depressed RS-T segment in Leads I and IV$_F$, with elevation of RS-T segment in Leads II and III, a distinct Q$_2$ and Q$_3$, and then the gradual development of sharp inversion of T$_2$ and T$_3$ with a marked exaggeration of the upright T wave in Lead IV$_F$. These tracings illustrate the two respects in which the precordial leads may be of possible help in the diagnosis of posterior infarction, namely, depression of the RS-T segment and the development of very tall T waves in one or more precordial leads. These changes may be the earliest clue to that diagnosis. The patient was a 42-year-old man who, while shoveling sand, had severe pain in the chest radiating down both arms. He had slight fever, leukocytosis, and increased sedimentation rate, and the blood cholesterol was 410. Recovery was excellent.

appearance is occasionally seen with left ventricular hypertrophy in the absence of posterior infarction. It has been claimed that this is due to the transmission of cavity potentials to the left leg but just how this can come about is not clear. The point, however, is that a prominent Q$_{aVF}$ is likely to signify posterior infarction only if it is followed by an R wave, however small.

The precordial leads may occasionally be of some help during the acute stage of posterior myocardial infarction. Two types of change, singly or in combination, may be present. These consist of the presence of tall T waves or depressed RS-T segments (Figs. 156 and 157). The former are to be distinguished from the tall, narrower, pointed T waves which occur in potassium poisoning and the latter from the depressed RS-T segments which can develop in subendocardial ischemia or infarction involving the anterior wall of the heart. The described changes in the precordial leads in posterior infarction may actually precede the development of QRS, RS-T, or T-wave changes in Lead aVF, II, or III. They are apt to be very transitory in their appearance. Hence the precordial leads are not of much help in the diagnosis of *old* posterior myocardial infarction.

In the section on anterolateral infarction it was pointed out that reciprocal changes may develop in Leads I and III merely as a consequence of the fact that left shoulder potentials are routed through the electrocardiograph in one direction in writing one of these leads and in

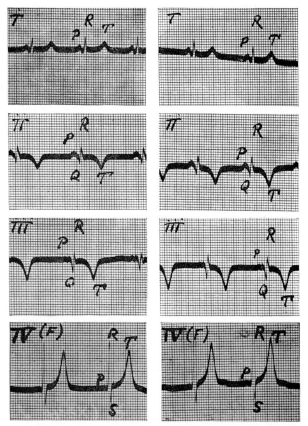

FIG. 157. *Acute Posterior Myocardial Infarction.* The attack occurred June 24, 1934. The first tracing was made July 11, and the second July 18, 1934. Note rounded and dipped T_2 and T_3. Lead IV$_F$ shows a normal R wave and an exaggerated upright T wave. Similar T waves may be observed in potassium intoxication, but the T waves in the limb leads are apt to be pointed and upright in that condition rather than inverted as here.

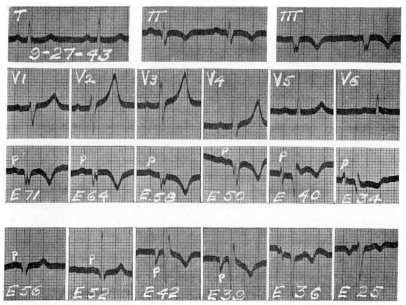

FIG. 158.   *Posterior Infarction.*   The upper set of tracings shows three standard leads suggestive of a posterior infarction. The next set shows the six precordial leads using the central terminal, and gives no positive evidence of infarction. The third set was taken with an electrode in the esophagus at various levels from the external nasal orifice (number of centimeters). Note that at distance E 71 to E 50, when the electrode was adjacent to the left ventricle, there were no R waves and the T waves were inverted. Contrast these with esophageal curves from a normal individual shown in the lowest set (E 56 and E 52). The appearance of sharp P waves marks the presence of the electrode behind the left auricle and only ventricular complexes below this point are significant. The upper three tracings afford positive proof of posterior infarction.

the opposite direction in writing the other. However, reciprocal changes in the electrocardiogram can also develop because one electrode may face one aspect of a current of injury while another electrode faces its opposite aspect. This is the explanation for the reciprocal changes described in the preceding paragraph. In certain cases of acute posterior myocardial infarction the left leg electrode faces the epicardial aspect of the infarct and records an elevation of the RS-T segment, whereas one or more of the precordial leads may face the endocardial aspect of the infarct and therefore record depressed RS-T segments.

It should be obvious that, because of the distance of the left leg or, for that matter, of the groin, from the heart, one lacks in Lead aVF the precise delineation of the presence and extent of a posterior infarct that the multiple precordial leads possess in the detection of anterior infarcts. With the usual precordial leads tapping the potentials approximately over a horizontal plane on the chest one can demarcate anteroseptal, anterolateral, massive anterior, or, with additional leads, high lateral lesions. No such precision is possible with posterior wall infarcts. Esophageal leads recorded at ventricular levels, indicating changes in a more vertical plane in the body, may offer some help in this regard, but the procedure is somewhat annoying and should not be tried if the patient's condition is too critical. In chronic cases in which Lead aVF gives equivocal evidence of posterior infarction our experience has shown that esophageal leads are apt to leave one just about as much in doubt. This deserves further study. Mere repetition of the entire set of tracings, which may happen to change the relationship of the heart to the left leg, is less disturbing, and, in many cases, reveals decisive changes one way or the other. The practice of Goldberger of having the patient take a deep breath during the recording of Lead aVF may accomplish the same purpose. Generally speaking, esophageal leads are much more helpful in the study of electrical activity in the auricles.

Normally, as the electrode rises from the lower esophagus, near the diaphragm, the auricular waves are very inconspicuous until the electrode reaches a point just behind the left auricle. Then very sharp P waves appear (Fig. 158). This makes it very simple to know that the electrode is lower than the auricle and therefore adjacent to the posterior portion of the left ventricle. From this latter position the ventricular complex normally should display a prominent R wave, possibly preceded by a very small Q and followed by an upright T. If the posterior wall is infarcted the ventricular complex will show the same changes that are found with an anterior infarction when the precordial electrode is placed over the precordium, i.e., an absent R, an inverted T (Fig. 158), and possibly a deviation of the S-T segment during the acute stages.

The various grades of auriculoventricular heart block may occur with anterior myocardial infarction but, because the bundle of His and associated tissues are irrigated through the same artery that generally nourishes the posterior aspect of the heart, namely, the right coronary artery, this complication is much more frequent with posterior infarction.

Posterolateral Infarction. If the posterior as well as the lateral aspects of the heart are infarcted, the potential changes produced by the infarct are reflected to Lead V_6 or Leads V_5 and V_6 as well as to Lead aVF. Figures 159 and 160 show electrocardiographic findings in infarcts of this type. Since these leads may be located about 180 degrees around the ventricles from Leads V_1 and V_2, one may find reciprocal changes in the latter leads (Fig. 159). Thus the deep Q waves and elevated RS-T segments of Leads aVF, V_5, and V_6 may be associated with tall R waves and depressed RS-T segments in Leads V_1 and V_2. The development of a tall R wave over the right side of the precordium, resulting from unbalanced forces (the failure of the posterior wall to be normally activated accounting for the release of these R waves), may obscure the previous evidence of old anteroseptal infarction. This phenomenon probably accounts for many of the failures to detect an old infarct in the face of fresh infarction, or to detect multiple old infarcts.

It is important to bear in mind that, in addition to the possibility of posterolateral infarction, changes suggesting coincident posterior and anterior infarction may be produced in two other ways: (1) In the so-

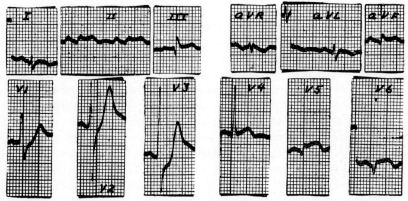

FIG. 159. *Acute Posterolateral Myocardial Infarction.* The tracings show prominent Q waves, elevated RS-T segments, and terminal inversion of T waves in Leads II, III, aVF, V₅, and V₆. Note reciprocal depression of the RS-T segments in Leads V₁ to V₃. The patient was a 62-year-old diabetic who had a typical coronary occlusion two days previously. He died on the morning of admission. Postmortem examination showed a large posterolateral infarct and a thrombus in the circumflex branch of the left coronary artery, which in this case supplied the posterior wall of the heart.

called anteroposterior (Roesler-Dressler) infarct, which involves the interventricular septum and the contiguous portions of the posterior and anterior ventricular walls, deep Q waves, elevated RS-T segments, and T waves may be recorded in Leads aVF, II, III, and in general in one or more of the leads between Lead V₁ and Lead V₄. (2) If the heart is in an extreme vertical position the potentials of the antero-apical portion of the heart may theoretically be transmitted through the diaphragm to the left leg and accordingly to Leads aVF, II, and III. Similar unusual rotations may account for variations in the standard descriptions of the electrocardiographic changes described here. It must be pointed out, however, that it is frequently quite difficult to define the electrical position of infarcted hearts. Infarction may render a considerable part of the ventricles electrically inactive and thus give preponderant electrical weight to the uninfarcted part of the heart, quite independently of the position of the heart. The estimation of the electrical position of the heart depends upon the definition of right and left ventricular potentials and their reflection to the extremities. In infarction, changes from one type of potential to another may be due to a transition not from one ventricle to another but from an infarcted to an uninfarcted area, and in any given case it may be impossible to decide which. With this limitation in mind it is frequently possible to estimate the electrical position of the infarcted heart.

A word of warning about the accuracy of the electrocardiographic diagnosis of myocardial infarction, a warning perhaps not adequately sounded in recent publications. Although it is true that the introduction of multiple chest leads and unipolar limb and chest leads has increased the accuracy of detection and localization of infarcts, its more important contribution has been to a better understanding of the electrophysical principles involved. As was true before the advent of these more elaborate studies, infarction, especially old myocardial scars, can still be missed by the electrocardiogram. Thus, in a recent electrocardiographic-pathologic correlation, although the electrocardiographic diagnosis of acute anterior or posterior myocardial infarction was invariably substantiated at postmortem examination, a small minority of patients with an acute anatomic lesion failed to show diagnostic electrocardiographic evidence for fresh infarction. In those few cases in which the diagnosis was missed the electrocardiogram was abnormal but nonspecific, or the changes of acute infarction were obscured by bundle branch block, left ventricular hypertrophy, or acute infarction elsewhere in the heart. In the cases of healed myocardial infarction, moreover, although the electrocardiographic diagnosis was almost invariably substantiated when made (the single exception showed decreasing R waves in Leads V_1 to V_3, with no scar at autopsy), the greater majority of scars found on the postmortem table were missed electrocardiographically. Here again the electrocardiogram was abnormal but not diagnostic, and the changes were obscured, among other causes, by left ventricular hypertrophy, bundle branch block, or old or recent infarction elsewhere in the heart.

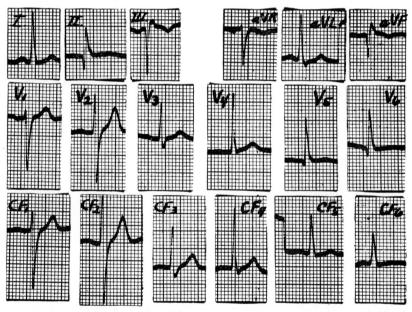

FIG. 160.   *Old Posterolateral Myocardial Infarction.*   The broad prominent Q waves in Leads II and III are associated with a broad prominent Q wave in Lead aVF. This establishes the existence of a posterior infarct. Intraventricular block is also present (QRS = 0.11 second). Note how the Q waves present in Leads V_5 and V_6 are missed in Leads CF_5 and CF_6. This results from the large Q wave in Lead aVF which contributes an R wave to the bipolar CF leads. The patient was a 60-year-old man who had had an acute coronary occlusion one year previously, and later died of a severe viral pneumonia. Postmortem examination showed a large posterolateral scar. In this case the failure to detect the lateral component of the infarct by the CF leads was not important clinically.

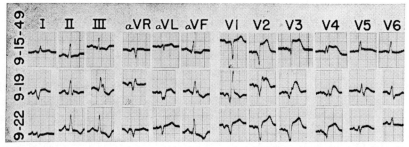

FIG. 161. *Transient Right Bundle Branch Block Complicating Anteroseptal Myocardial Infarction.* The patient was a robust, 54-year-old fireman without previous angina pectoris who was hospitalized because of severe chest pain and shock. Tracings on admission showed elevated RS-T segments in Leads V_1 to V_5. Note "monophasic" action currents in Leads V_2 to V_4. This extreme degree of current of injury is no more ominous than slight but definite RS-T segment elevations. In the second set of tracings the original evidence of acute anteroseptal infarction, i.e., deep Q waves and elevated RS-T segments, is still present despite the supervention of right bundle branch block. Three days later the right bundle branch block disappeared. The patient died on his eleventh hospital day. Postmortem examination showed a massive anteroseptal infarct principally involving the septum. There was also an aneurysm of the apical part of the left ventricle.

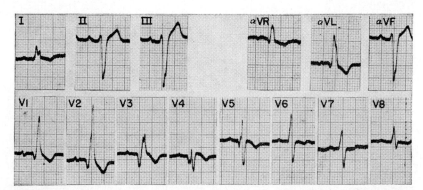

FIG. 162. *Bundle Branch Block with Old Anteroseptal Myocardial Infarction.* QRS duration 0.14 second. Broad Q waves and late intrinsicoid deflections are recorded over the right precordium. These Q waves can be explained by septal infarction, permitting passive transmission of left ventricular potentials to the right side of the precordium. Left ventricular potentials are not recorded until Lead V_8 is reached. Although one might consider this an example of right bundle branch block because of the late intrinsicoid deflections over the right ventricle, vectorcardiographic evidence suggests that this is left bundle branch block with extensive myocardial infarction. The left bundle is blocked but since there is little or no remaining left ventricular myocardium to which the impulse may be conducted, it is conducted, in a delayed timing, to the right precordium by default (Fig. 39). The patient was a 71-year-old man with angina pectoris for twenty-two years and congestive heart failure since a definite episode of myocardial infarction seven years before these tracings were taken.

Myocardial Infarction with Bundle Branch Block. Pure infarction of the right ventricle is almost unknown. When part of the wall of the right ventricle is infarcted anteriorly or posteriorly this is but a small component of an infarct involving largely the contiguous interventricular septum and left ventricle. By and large, then, myocardial infarction is a left ventricular affair. To understand the electrocardiographic changes which occur in myocardial infarction complicated by or complicating bundle branch block, it is important to bear this point in mind.

In right bundle branch block the septum is activated, as normally, from its left to its right side. Therefore the left ventricular cavity potential shows an initial downward deflection; if now the free wall of the left ventricle is infarcted this downward deflection (Q wave) may be transmitted through a transmural infarct to Lead aVF if the infarct happens to be posterior in location, or to the left side of the precordium if the infarct happens to be anterior in location (Figs. 161 to 164). Hence the QRS changes of left ventricular infarction persist with right bundle branch block. Furthermore, since the bundle branch of the ventricle (right) opposite that in which we are interested is the one which is blocked, there is nothing to mask the development of the other electrocardiographic features of left ventricular infarction, namely RS-T segment and T wave changes. Hence the changes of myocardial infarction may be expected to remain in spite of the persistence or inception of right bundle branch block.

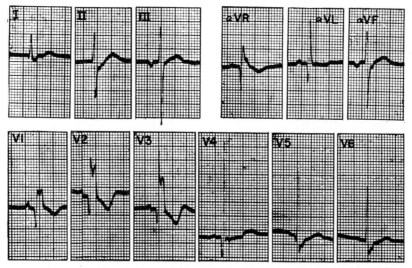

FIG. 163. *Right Bundle Branch Block with Old Anteroseptal Myocardial Infarction.* The duration of the QRS complex is 0.12 second. Late intrinsicoid deflections are recorded over the right ventricle. The Q waves are passively transmitted across the septum from the left ventricle to the right side of the precordium. The patient was an 82-year-old man with a chronic duodenal ulcer. He gave no history suggesting angina pectoris or coronary occlusion, but he showed evidence of cerebral softening and therefore was an unreliable informant. Here the electrocardiogram gave decisive evidence not otherwise obtained.

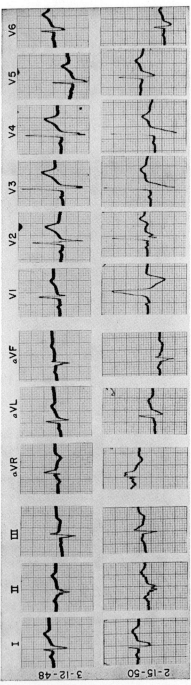

FIG. 164. *Old Posterior Myocardial Infarction, Complicated by Right Bundle Branch Block.*   The initial set of tracings, taken March 12, 1948, shows conclusive evidence of old posterior myocardial infarction (broad prominent Q waves in Leads II, III, and aVF). The QRS duration is 0.10 second. There is right axis deviation but the prominent R in Lead V_1 is not an evidence of right ventricular hypertrophy. It is probably evidence of the posterior infarct. The electrical forces activating the anterior wall of the heart are not antagonized by forces directed posteriorly since the latter are abolished as a result of the infarction. Here the anterior forces are able to express themselves unopposed. In the second set of curves, taken February 15, 1950, the evidence of old posterior myocardial infarction persists despite the development of right bundle branch block. The position of the heart is unchanged. Note how the initial 0.05 or 0.06 second of ventricular activation is the same whether or not right bundle branch block is present. Note the prolongation of the Q-T interval in the second set of curves. This results from staggered activation of the ventricles and not from an inherent change in the ventricular muscle.

When, on the other hand, left bundle branch block is present, the electrocardiogram generally fails to show the evidence of left ventricular infarction. In left bundle branch block septal activation proceeds from its right to its left side. Therefore the left ventricular cavity records an initial upward (R) deflection which is transmitted through a transmural infarct to the left precordium or the left leg, depending on the location of the infarct. The loss of a deep, broad cavity Q wave with the development of left bundle branch block is illustrated in Figure 40. If this patient had been first seen at the time of the second set of tracings the diagnosis

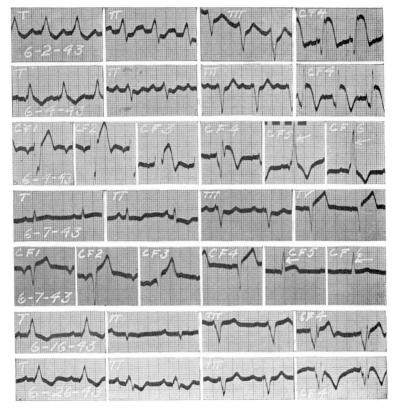

FIG. 165. *Anterior Myocardial Infarction with Transient Left Bundle Branch Block.* The first set of tracings was made a few hours after the onset of an attack of acute coronary thrombosis. Note the left bundle branch block. Lead CF$_4$ is most unusual in that it shows a very high RS-T junction. This is extremely rare in left bundle branch block and is very suggestive of acute anteroseptal infarction. The six precordial leads on June 4, 1943, show a late intrinsicoid deflection (arrow) over the left ventricle, confirming the diagnosis of left bundle branch block. Curves on June 7, 1943, show that the left bundle branch block is gone. Now the intrinsicoid deflection (arrow) is early. The lowest set, June 26, 1943, shows that finally T in Lead CF$_4$ becomes sharply inverted. The patient was a man, 75 years of age, who had an operation for hernia under spinal anesthesia. Preoperative blood pressure was 190 systolic and 110 diastolic, but quickly became imperceptible. One hour after the fall in blood pressure, as operation was completed, pain in the chest was first felt. The patient then ran a typical course of acute coronary thrombosis and recovered satisfactorily.

of posterior myocardial infarction could not have been made on electro-cardiographic grounds. Since, moreover, the left ventricle is the delayed ventricle, the slurred turret-top portion of the ventricular complex gen-erally encroaches upon the area in which RS-T segment elevations may be expected to develop. The RS-T segment depression and T wave inver-sion which are present over the blocked left ventricle may be explained as changes "secondary" to the bundle branch block and to the abnormal direction of activation of the heart. Hence one does not generally get much help from the RS-T segment or T-wave changes in left bundle branch block. If, on the other hand, as rarely happens, the opposite type of RS-T segment deviation, namely elevation, is observed over the blocked left ventricle, one may assume acute infarction (Fig. 165), espe-cially if the degree of elevation recedes while the patient is under obser-vation. Here a series of tracings reveal definite and characteristic changes. The bundle branch block in this case was also transient so that curves could be studied in block and out of block. Both the early and the late abnormalities of muscle injury are apparent. In the vast majority of cases of left bundle branch block and myocardial infarction, however, the electrocardiogram shows the fixed changes of left bundle branch block, and the decision regarding fresh myocardial infarction must rest upon other laboratory or clinical findings.

Septal Infarction and Peri-infarction Block. When the septum is infarcted the lesion is usually the septal component of a lesion of the anterior or posterior wall of the heart. Those involving the posterobasal portion of the septum are more frequently associated with auriculoven-tricular block. With involvement of either the anterior or posterior part of the septum, bundle branch block is quite common (Figs. 162 to 167). In rare cases the infarct may extend through the entire anteroposterior extent of the septum and involve the adjacent portions of the posterior and anterior walls (anteroposterior or Roesler-Dressler infarcts), produc-ing changes in Lead aVF and in some of the precordial leads.

A Q wave is not expected over the right ventricle in uncomplicated right bundle branch block or over the left ventricle in uncomplicated left bundle branch block. The detection of Q waves over a blocked ven-tricle may be interpreted in either of two ways. The first explanation would be the presence of concomitant septal infarction. In right bundle branch block the septum is activated, as normally, from its left to its right side. If the septum is intact an initial upward deflection therefore appears in the right ventricular cavity and is transmitted to the right precordium. If under the same circumstances the septum is infarcted, the left ventricular potentials, including its initial downward deflection, may be transmitted passively through the infarcted septum to the elec-trode over the right ventricle where Q waves are recorded (Figs. 162 and 163). On the other hand, in left bundle branch block the septum is activated from its right to its left side. If the septum is intact an initial upward deflection appears in the left ventricular cavity and is transmitted to the left precordium, where an initial R wave is inscribed.

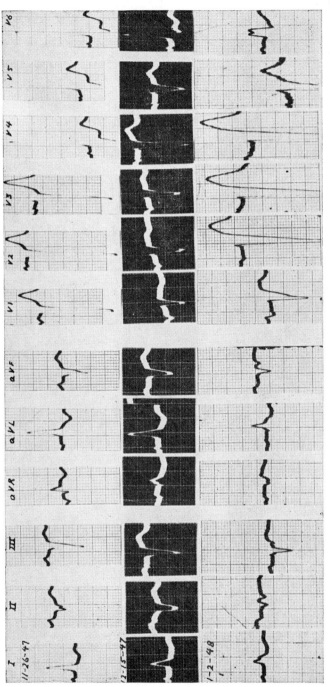

FIG. 166. *Acute Posterior Infarction Complicated by Left Bundle Branch Block and Pulmonary Infarction.* A 65-year-old man with long standing angina pectoris developed constant chest pain lasting one day and followed by congestive heart failure and shock. The initial set of tracings showed prominent QS_3 and QS_{aVF}, in the presence of left ventricular hypertrophy, suggestive but inconclusive evidence of posterior infarction. The pronounced depression of the RS-T segments in Leads V_4 to V_6 is consistent with left ventricular hypertrophy but is possibly a reciprocal change associated with acute posterior infarction. Note that the transitional zone was between V_3 and V_4. The second set of tracings shows a shift of this zone to a location between V_5 and V_6, mildly suggesting right ventricular dilatation and acute cor pulmonale. The final set shows left bundle branch block with late intrinsicoid deflections in Lead V_6. Postmortem examination showed a large acute infarct of the posterior wall of the left ventricle and the posterior aspect of the septum, scattered fibrosis throughout the rest of the myo-cardium, and a small infarct in the lower lobe of the right lung. The QRS complex measured 0.10 second in the initial set, 0.12 in the second and third sets. It is possible that if additional leads had been recorded to the left of V_6 on December 15, 1947, left bundle branch block would have been established at that time.

585

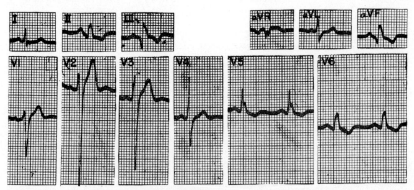

FIG. 167.   *Left Bundle Branch Block with Old Posterior Myocardial Infarction,*
or "Peri-infarction" Block.   The QRS complex measures 0.12 second. A late intrinsicoid deflection and a turret-topped QRS complex in Lead V₆ suggests left bundle
branch block. The broad Q wave in Lead aVF establishes the existence of an old posterior myocardial infarction. The patient was a 65-year-old man who had had an
acute posterior occlusion five months previously. Roentgen ray examination showed
calcification in the descending branch of the left coronary artery.

If, now, the septum is infarcted, the initial downward deflection of the
right ventricular cavity may be transmitted passively through the infarct
to the left ventricular cavity and thence to the left precordium, where a
Q wave is recorded (Fig. 167). An alternative explanation is that of
so-called "peri-infarction block." Left bundle branch block is not present
at all. A Q wave is recorded at an electrode overlying a subendocardial
scar by virtue of activation of the remaining uninfarcted wall away from
the left ventricular cavity. The impulse is delayed from reaching the
epicardium because it must percolate through or around the damaged
tissue. Now on emerging into the healthier subepicardial elements the
impulse approaches the epicardium, and the electrode, rapidly. Thus one
detects intraventricular block (slurring of the QRS complex), preceded
by a Q wave and terminated by a rapid deflection. Except for the initial
Q wave this may resemble bundle branch block. Such an explanation
may be given for the electrocardiogram (Fig. 47) recorded in a patient
with a subendocardial scar of the free wall of a markedly hypertrophied
left ventricle, proved at autopsy. In view of these dual possibilities, how
shall such qRR' complexes be interpreted? In those cases in which the
qRR' complexes are observed to develop sequentially to RR' complexes,
the complicating diagnosis of septal infarction is probable. When, on the
other hand, the previous electrocardiographic configuration is unknown,
it seems more reasonable to give the alternative explanations of peri-
infarction block without bundle branch block versus bundle branch block
with septal infarction.

   Subendocardial Infarction.   Until recently it was commonly held
that as an electrode, insulated except at its tip, is drawn progressively
from the endocardial to the epicardial surface of the free ventricular
wall, there is recorded a smooth build-up in the voltage of the R wave
and decrease in the voltage of the S wave. Thus at the endocardial level

QS waves are recorded; at a point about a fourth of the distance from endocardium to epicardium rS waves are recorded; about midway between endocardium and epicardium equiphasic RS waves are inscribed; at about the three-fourths mark Rs deflections are recorded; and finally, at the epicardium, R waves are registered. Most transmural infarcts are wedge shaped with the broad part of the wedge on the endocardial aspect of the heart. Assuming the validity of the above enumerated considerations one would expect that an electrode overlying the transmural part of an old infarct should record a QS deflection, whereas one in relation to the peripheral portion of this same infarct should record a QR deflection, the Q wave being due to unopposed activation of the opposite ventricular wall, and the R wave to subsequent activation of the relatively healthy subepicardial muscle overlying the infarct. Such changes have indeed been recorded over the margins of transmural infarcts and over old scars which are purely subendocardial. The recent investigations of Prinzmetal, however, seem to show that an electrode such as that described above records QS deflections in the inner three-fourths or so of the ventricular wall. The progressive build-up of R and decrease of S, in this experience, does not begin until the outer shell of the ventricle is reached. If this finding is substantiated, not QR deflections but R waves of smaller amplitude would be expected at an electrode overlying a subendocardial infarct. Brigham Hospital experience with acute subendocardial infarction has been that Q waves are not inscribed. Although other explanations have been offered to explain this fact, it should be acknowledged that it is quite consonant with the findings of Prinzmetal. More extensive experimental and clinicopathological corroboration is awaited.

Acute subendocardial infarcts apparently can produce displacements of the RS-T segment in either direction. An extremely interesting subgroup in this latter category are those cases showing electrocardiographic changes similar to those classically developing during stress tests for

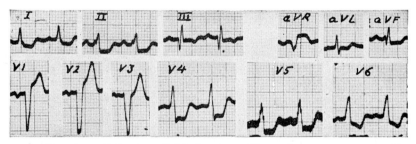

FIG. 168. *Acute Subendocardial Infarction.* The patient was a 53-year-old man with a positive serologic test for syphilis and typical angina pectoris for ten months. Following four days of extreme pain he was admitted in shock. The tracings show depressed RS-T segments in Leads I, II, aVF, and V_4 to V_6, and an elevated RS-T segment in Lead aVR. The R waves are very small in Leads V_1 to V_2. Autopsy showed a fresh circumferential subendocardial infarct and syphilitic disease of the coronary artery orifices and right common carotid artery. Tracings of this type may be recorded as a transient change during angina pectoris.

coronary insufficiency, namely, depressed RS-T segments over the precordium and an elevated RS-T segment in Lead aVR, without concurrent QRS changes (Fig. 168). In some cases of this sort, developing characteristically under circumstances in which there seems to be a total rather than a segmental impairment of the coronary blood flow, postmortem examination may show rimlike subendocardial infarcts involving all or most of the subendocardial muscle. The RS-T segment depressions in the precordial leads and the RS-T segment elevation in Lead aVR, which faces the ventricular cavities, are probably due to the orientation of the injured area toward the endocardium.

Since, as stated above, QRS changes may not develop, it is often impossible from a single tracing to decide if the changes represent subendocardial ischemia or infarction. The persistence of these changes over a number of days, especially if associated with correlative clinical or laboratory findings, would favor the diagnosis of infarction.

The Vectorcardiogram in Myocardial Infarction. The vectorcardiographic loop may be regarded as recording the sum total of the electrical output of all active muscle units of the heart. Each unit makes its contribution to the normal salience of the loop. If a segment of the heart muscle thus becomes electrically inert, two things may happen. If the opposite part of the ventricle, namely, that about 180 degrees around its circumference, is still electrically active, the electrical effect of the damaged portion is now more or less overbalanced, resulting in the loss of a smaller or larger part of the salience of the loop. This displaces the loop away from the area of infarction. From being rounded out it may be flattened (Fig. 147) or it may present a large excavation or bight. Furthermore, the normal loop follows an orbit which lies more or less in a single plane. On meeting an electrically inert island of muscle as it sweeps in its course, the loop in infarction glances in one direction or another out of this plane of predilection. This produces a twisting of the loop. In extreme cases such distortions may give rise to clover-leaf, figure-of-eight, or stalk-like deformities of the loop (Figs. 147 and 169). This may be manifested in electrocardiograms as notching of the QRS complex.

This "biting out" process may result in the loss of the initial rightward and anterior limb in the horizontal plane in anteroseptal infarction, in an abnormally large initial rightward and anterior limb in the same plane in high lateral infarction, in an abnormal superior development of the loop as it is seen in the frontal and sagittal planes in posterior infarction (Fig. 169) or in an abnormal rightward and posterior direction of the mid-portion ("body") of the loop in the horizontal plane in anterolateral infarction. Except in the latter instance these changes involve principally the very earliest part of the vectorcardiogram. This change in the direction of the first 0.03 to 0.04 second of the loop corresponds to the effect of such infarcts in producing abnormal Q waves in the electrocardiogram.

Using such criteria, some observers consider that the vectorcardio-

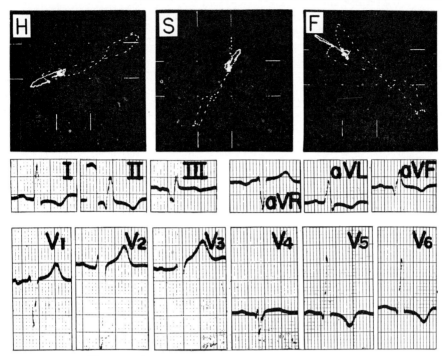

FIG. 169. *Vectorcardiogram and Electrocardiogram in Old Posterior and Anterior Myocardial Infarction.* The loop is figure-of-eight in all three planes. The first half of the loop is markedly slowed. There is no significant anterior salience in the horizontal or sagittal plane. This accounts for the decreasing R waves in Leads V_2 to V_4. There is a large slow cephalad development in the sagittal and frontal planes. This is due to lack of initial inferiorly oriented forces, produces prominent Q waves in Leads II, III, and aVF, and signifies posterior myocardial infarction.

gram is superior to the electrocardiogram in the detection of myocardial infarction. It has been suggested that this is particularly true of the diagnosis of posterior myocardial infarction. If this is substantiated, this technique will be a great boon to electrocardiographer and clinician. The experience of the author in the vectorcardiographic diagnosis of myocardial infarction has not been extensive enough to justify an opinion on its value in this difficult diagnosis.

Acute Myocardial Infarction without QRS Changes. Attention has just been directed to the fact that subendocardial infarction may develop without significant QRS changes. There appears similarly to be a small group of cases of infarction resembling pericarditis in that RS-T and T-wave changes develop without QRS changes, but differing from pericarditis in the degree of these changes. In these cases a diagnosis of myocardial infarction may be justified if there are convincing clinical and laboratory findings sustaining that diagnosis. In the absence of a clear-cut clinical story, and particularly if fever, leukocytosis, and elevated sedimentation rate are lacking, it is probably more accurate to refer to these changes as "ischemic" in nature (Fig. 170). The prognosis

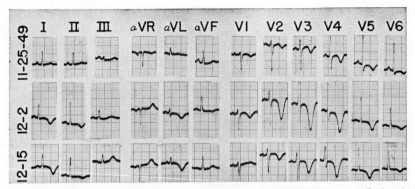

FIG. 170. *Myocardial Infarction in the Absence of QRS Changes ("Ischemic T Waves")*. The patient, a 63-year-old woman, had had repeated episodes of angina pectoris, abating on rest or nitroglycerin, shortly before and during her hospitalization. The initial tracing (see also Fig. 21) showed the characteristic changes of left ventricular hypertrophy, but the T waves over the right ventricle were inverted rather than upright as one would expect them to be in left ventricular hypertrophy. This change suggested anteroseptal myocardial ischemia or infarction. Subsequent tracings showed waxing and waning of the inverted T waves and prolongation of the Q-T interval (K = 0.49), suggesting but not proving anterior myocardial infarction without QRS changes. This patient presented no laboratory evidence confirming infarction, improved, and was discharged. The same changes in association with corroborative clinical and laboratory findings would be acceptable evidence for acute myocardial infarction. Most patients with electrocardiographic changes of this type do well so that anatomic proof of infarction is generally lacking.

appears to be good in either case. Thus far there is a paucity of reports of autopsied cases which showed only RS-T segment and T-wave changes. In some of them intramural infarction may be demonstrated.

Ventricular Aneurysm. RS-T segment displacements developing during acute myocardial infarction are generally short-lived, subsiding within a few days or a fortnight. In some cases, however, these changes persist indefinitely. Since a Q wave is also present and the T wave may show late inversion (Fig. 171), the appearance may be identical with that seen with fresh infarction. Electrocardiograms taken on such individuals seen by a physician for some unrelated or related condition, especially if the latter clinically resembles acute myocardial infarction, can therefore mislead the physician into making the diagnosis of acute infarct. However, under such circumstances, serial tracings will show an appearance which is quite fixed, whereas with acute damage one should find an unstable electrocardiogram. Hence, although the combination of QRS, RS-T, and T-wave changes in a single tracing generally signifies acute infarct, strictly speaking that diagnosis should be made only if sequential electrocardiographic changes are subsequently demonstrated. It has been shown empirically that this finding of fixed QRS, RS-T, and T-wave changes is frequently associated with aneurysm formation in the myocardial scar as demonstrated by fluoroscopic, electrokymographic, or pathologic examination, and therefore may constitute a clue to the existence of that condition. Why aneurysms should produce these

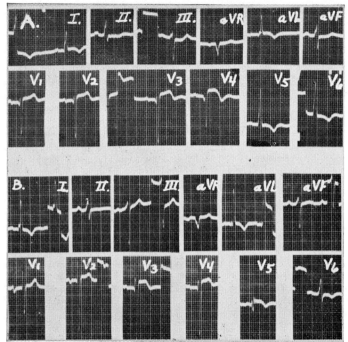

FIG. 171.   *The "Fixed Pattern" of Acute Myocardial Infarction in Ventricular Aneurysm.*   The patient, a 66-year-old man, had an acute myocardial infarction in 1946. The first set of tracings, taken sixteen months later when the patient complained of dyspnea and angina, show deep Q waves, elevated RS-T segments, and terminally inverted T waves in Leads V_2 to V_4. As such, these curves suggested acute myocardial infarction, but there was no clinical or laboratory evidence suggesting this diagnosis. Physical examination showed a systolic precordial bulge and fluoroscopy showed a paradoxical outward thrust with ventricular systole. The second set of tracings was obtained eleven months later when the patient was in congestive failure. They show essentially the same electrocardiographic features again in the absence of clinical or laboratory evidence for fresh infarction. These are two of a long series of tracings showing the same appearance. Right bundle branch block developed by March, 1950. The patient died suddenly one month later. Postmortem examination showed a large aneurysm of the left ventricle which was tremendously hypertrophied.

changes is not clear. It has been suggested that it may be due to transmission to the electrode of the endocardial potentials produced in the hypertrophied ventricular wall opposite the aneurysm, to chronic coronary insufficiency or myocardial ischemia, or to a traumatic pericarditis. The contribution of the muscle fibers remaining in the aneurysmal wall or of changes in the rim of intact muscle at the base of the aneurysmal sac is not known.

'STRESS" TESTS FOR CORONARY INSUFFICIENCY

In numerous instances the physician will be left in doubt as to whether a patient has angina pectoris or not. In fact, the differential diagnosis not infrequently may be between serious coronary artery dis-

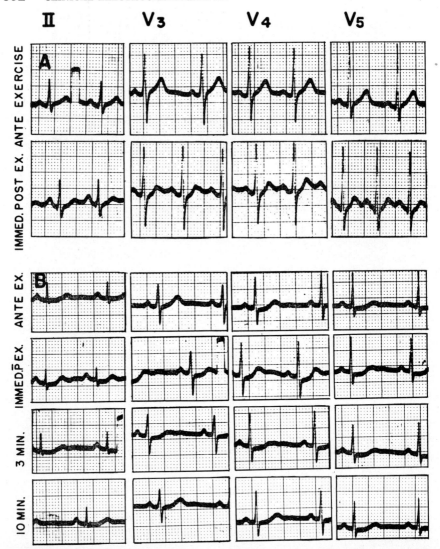

FIG. 172.   *Master "Two-Step" Exercise Test for Coronary Insufficiency.*   Upper set (*A*) shows cardiac acceleration immediately after exercise. At that time the P wave begins on the downstroke of the preceding T wave. Relative to the T-P segment there is apparent RS-T depression, but relative to the P-R segment there is no true RS-T depression. The P-R segment should be used as a baseline. This is a "negative" double Master test in a 38-year-old man with neurocirculatory asthenia. Lower set (*B*) shows a "positive" (abnormal) test in a 55-year-old man, applying for increased insurance coverage, who denied cardiovascular symptoms. Examination was negative except for a gallop rhythm. Following exercise there is definite RS-T segment depression of 1 mm. in Leads V_3 and V_5, 1.5 mm. in Lead V_4. Re-examination of the pre-exercise tracings shows minimal RS-T segment depression which in retrospect must have been due to coronary insufficiency. The test should be carried through ten minutes after the cessation of exercise, for in rare cases abnormal reactions only then become apparent. The use of Leads II and V_3 to V_5 has recently been recommended as being the most informative.

ease and no organic disease of the heart. When the electrocardiogram is normal or equivocal under these circumstances, one is tempted to perform "stress" tests to bring out significant alterations in the tracings. For this purpose two methods are commonly used. The first and simpler one is to take a series of electrocardiograms immediately after a brief effort or "two-step test" and to compare them with the control graphs (Fig. 172). The second method is to take a series of tracings before and for five to fifteen minutes after allowing the patient to inhale 10 per cent oxygen. Characteristic anginal pain may be produced by each of these procedures. From an electrocardiographic point of view the tests are regarded as positive evidence of coronary insufficiency if well-marked deviation (usually depression) of the S-T segment results. There are decided limitations to these tests, as some patients with significant coronary artery disease will show a negative reaction and others with no coronary disease, especially patients who have been taking digitalis or who have rheumatic mitral valve disease, may show suggestive changes. Furthermore, these procedures, like all others in which one tries deliberately to reproduce anginal pain or coronary insufficiency, carry some risk. Rare fatalities or instances of coronary thrombosis with myocardial infarction have occurred. Despite these possibilities, such tests may be indicated on rare occasions.

VENTRICULAR COMPLEXES IN ACUTE COR PULMONALE

Acute overloading of the right ventricle resulting from pulmonary embolism or other causes (e.g., massive collapse of several lobes of the lung) may produce electrocardiographic as well as clinical changes re-

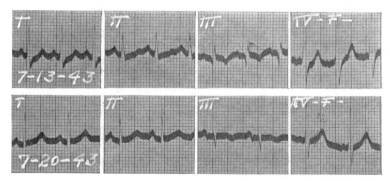

FIG. 173.   *Acute Cor Pulmonale (Pulmonary Embolism)*. The patient, a 42-year-old man, was well except for an inguinal hernia. His heart was normal. Operation was performed on July 1, 1943, under spinal anesthesia. He was doing well when on July 13, 1943, while on a bedpan, he had sudden pain in the left anterior chest, dyspnea, tachycardia, and apprehension. The pulse rate was 140, respiration 28, blood pressure 130 systolic and 80 diastolic. His legs showed nothing abnormal. X-ray showed slightly cloudy left base and elevated left diaphragm. On July 14, 1943, bilateral ligation of the femoral veins was performed. The patient ran a temperature of 101 to 102° F. for five days and recovered. The first tracings show changes indicative of acute cor pulmonale, i.e., an S_1, a Q_3, a depressed S-T_1, an elevated S-T_3, and an inverted T_3. Note the disappearance of these changes in the second tracing.

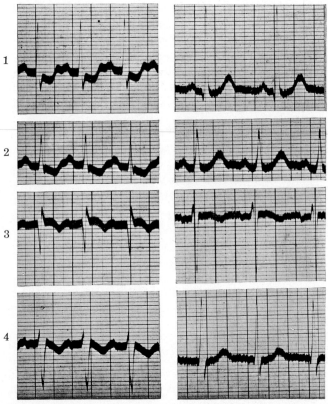

FIG. 174. *Acute Cor Pulmonale (Pulmonary Embolism).* The patient was a 19-year-old woman who had repeated pulmonary emboli post partum several days before the first tracing was made. Note S_1, Q_3, depressed and inverted S-T$_1$, and slightly elevated S-T$_3$. These changes are not present in subsequent tracing. (Courtesy of Dr. Paul D. White.)

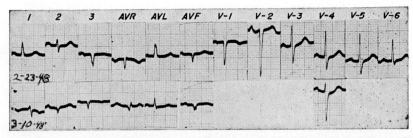

FIG. 175. *Acute Cor Pulmonale, with Leftward Shift of Transitional Zone.* The patient was a 67-year-old woman with carcinoma of the breast. The initial preoperative electrocardiogram shows a prominent QS in Leads III and aVF, strong presumptive evidence of old posterior myocardial infarction. The lower tracing, taken two weeks postoperatively, a few hours after the onset of shock and tachypnea, shows the development of S in Lead I, depression of RS-T in Leads I and aVL, and a persistent QS in Leads III and aVF. The transitional zone which originally lay between V_2 and V_3 now was located to the left of V_4. The patient died eight hours later. Postmortem examination showed emboli in both pulmonary arteries and an old posterior myocardial infarct.

sembling those of acute myocardial infarction. Myocardial infarction, moreover, may be complicated by acute cor pulmonale, and acute cor pulmonale may be complicated by coronary insufficiency. In this difficult differential diagnosis the roentgen ray offers some help, particularly if oblique films are made of the region back of the heart. However, it must be remembered that the roentgen ray diagnosis depends largely upon the demonstration of infarction of pulmonary tissue, whereas the electrocardiographic changes probably depend rather upon the sudden increase in pressure which the right ventricle must support in some of these cases. This may apparently develop as the result of widespread spasm in collateral pulmonary artery branches even if only a small pul-

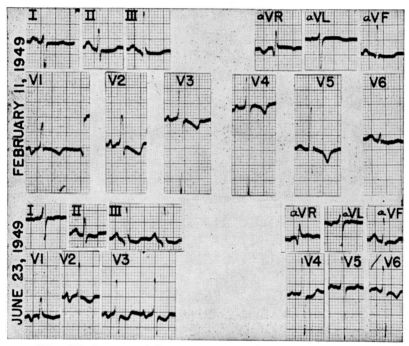

FIG. 176.   *Displacement of Transitional Zone to Left as Clue to Acute Cor Pulmonale.*   The initial set of tracings, made February 11, 1949, serve as control. Leads V_1 and V_2 show tall R waves and inverted T waves, indicative of right ventricular hypertrophy. The S waves are larger than the R waves in Leads V_3 and V_4. Lead V_5 again shows larger R than S waves, and an inverted T wave, indicating that left ventricular potentials are now recorded. The transitional zone then lies to the right of Lead V_5. The second set of tracings, recorded June 23, 1949, when the patient was in acute failure with severe dyspnea and tachypnea, again show deep S_1 and S_2 and inverted T waves over the precordium. However, since these changes were already present when the patient was compensated, they cannot be adduced as evidence of acute cor pulmonale. However, at this time the transitional zone lay to the left of V_6, for left ventricular potentials are not recorded in the usual six precordial leads. This was the only electrocardiographic clue to acute cor pulmonale. The patient was a 26-year-old man with rheumatic heart disease, in congestive heart failure. Postmortem examination showed that the heart weighed 780 gm. Mitral stenosis and insufficiency, aortic stenosis, right and, to a lesser extent, left ventricular hypertrophy, and multiple pulmonary emboli of varying age, were detected.

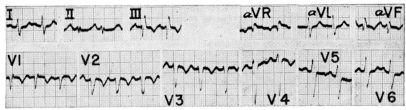

FIG. 177. *Inverted T Waves over Right Ventricle in Acute Cor Pulmonale.* The patient was a 74-year-old man with increasing dyspnea for two months and an episode of substernal tightness lasting two hours one week previously, admitted because of cyanosis, dyspnea, tachycardia (P 100–120), and tachypnea (R 30). Examination showed distant heart sounds, pulsus paradoxus, hepatomegaly, very little orthopnea and clear lungs, and varicosities but no calf tenderness. X-ray showed an enlarged heart and several areas of fuzzy density in the right lung fields. The electrocardiograms reproduced above show smartly inverted T waves in Leads V_1 to V_4. The S wave is prominent in Lead I. There is a late intrinsicoid deflection in Lead V_1. Shortly after admission the patient suddenly went into shock with cyanosis; blood pressure fell to 70–80 systolic, he became much more cyanotic, the neck veins became markedly distended, and cardiac action ceased. Postmortem examination showed massive pulmonary embolism obstructing both main stem arteries, and bilateral popliteal and tibial vein thrombosis. The heart weighed 580 gm. and showed scattered myocardial fibrosis and coronary artery narrowing without occlusion. In this case the inverted T waves and the tachycardia were the chief electrocardiographic clues to acute cor pulmonale.

monary artery branch is occluded and only an inconspicuous cone of pulmonary tissue is actually infarcted. Thus the electrocardiogram and roentgen ray may supplement one another as diagnostic procedures. However, pulmonary infarction or acute cor pulmonale may be present with a normal electrocardiogram or with normal roentgen ray findings.

The changes which may be recorded are: (1) *The development of a prominent S_1 and Q_3* (Figs. 173 to 175), which is probably related to rotation of the heart on its own longitudinal axis in a clockwise direction so that right instead of left ventricular potentials are transmitted to the left shoulder. The small R and deep S at Lead aVL are recorded unchanged in Lead I, thus deepening S_1. The small R and deep S at Lead aVL are recorded at Lead III as a small Q and tall R, thus tending to produce a Q_3. At the same time left ventricular potentials (qR) are transmitted to the left leg (aVF) and are therefore recorded unchanged in Lead III. This, therefore, contributes further to the development of a Q_3. (2) *Shift of the transitional zone to the left* may result from the chance variations in the heart's position resulting from its normal mobility. However, conspicuous leftward migration of this zone toward the axilla (Figs. 175, 176), especially if it is not otherwise explicable, is very suggestive of acute cor pulmonale. This change is probably related to clockwise rotation of the heart on its longitudinal axis and posterior displacement of the apex of the heart, both probably brought about by ballooning out of the overburdened right ventricle, thereby displacing the cardiac mass to the left. In Figure 175 the preoperative electrocardiogram showed the transitional zone between Leads V_2 and V_3; the second tracing, taken two weeks after operation, shortly after the onset of shock and tachypnea, showed the transitional zone to the left of V_4. (3) *Inversion of the T waves over the right ventricle* (Fig. 177) is probably related to a change in the repolarization process in the right ventricle (so-called "right ventricular strain"), and may occur as an isolated finding without changes in the conventional or unipolar limb leads. This change may help in the differential diagnosis from acute posterior myocardial infarction in which the T waves over the precordium are apt rather to be tall and upright. (4) *Depression of the RS-T segments* in certain limb or chest leads (Figs. 173 to 175) is probably related to subendocardial ischemia. Since RS-T segments in Leads I and II may be depressed and in Lead III may be elevated, and Q_3 may become prominent, the reason for confusion with acute posterior myocardial infarction becomes apparent. It has been claimed that in acute cor pulmonale a prominent Q_3 is not associated with a significant Q_{aVF}; while this is theoretically sound, in actual experience it is not a thoroughly reliable differentiating point. (5) *The development of incomplete right bundle branch block* (Fig. 178) can also occur as a transient phenomenon in acute myocardial infarction. In acute cor pulmonale it may be related to the increase in right ventricular pressure delaying the passage of the impulse along the right bundle branch.

The changes that occur in acute cor pulmonale disappear when re-

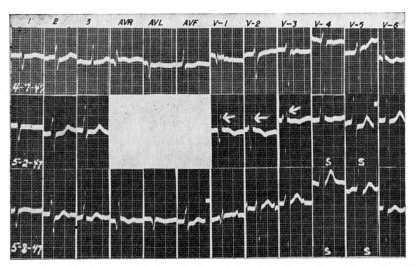

FIG. 178.   *Incomplete Right Bundle Branch Block in Acute Cor Pulmonale.* The patient was a 58-year-old man in congestive heart failure with rheumatic heart disease involving the mitral and aortic valves. The upper tracing shows right axis deviation and a late intrinsicoid deflection in Lead V_1. The second tracing, taken during a spell of acute dyspnea, shows incomplete right bundle branch block. Note RR′ complexes with late intrinsicoid deflections in Leads V_1 to V_3. The QRS complex measures 0.10 second in duration. The lower tracing recorded six days later shows return toward the original form. Postmortem examination showed multiple recent and old pulmonary infarcts.

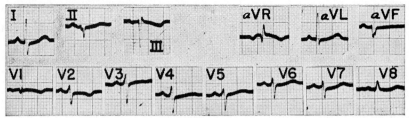

FIG. 179. *Normal Heart in Unusual Electrical Position.* The resemblance between Lead aVL and Lead |V₈ on the one hand and between Lead aVF and Lead V₁ on the other indicates that the heart is in a horizontal electrical position. The presence of S₁ and Q₃ indicates clockwise rotation (as viewed from the apex) of the heart on its longitudinal axis. And the presence of deep S waves across the precordium and of a prominent R wave in Lead aVF suggests that the apex points posteriorly. The displacement of the transitional zone to the left of Lead V₇ probably results from the last two factors. Inverted T waves may be present over the right ventricle in women without heart disease. All of the changes present may therefore be attributed to an unusual position of the heart. The patient was an 82-year-old woman, who had inoperable carcinoma of the pancreas and a large incisional hernia of the left upper abdomen with marked abdominal distention. Roentgen ray examination showed that the left leaf of the diaphragm was at the same level as the right. Note that left ventricular potentials are not recorded until Lead V₈ is reached.

covery takes place. They may persist for days or weeks but often are present over only a very few hours, hence the need for frequent electrocardiograms during the few days following an episode suspected of being acute cor pulmonale. In some cases several of the changes described may be recorded in combination; in a few cases a decision may have to be made upon the basis of a single change. It should be emphasized that any of the changes described as occurring in acute cor pulmonale may develop or be present in other conditions. The T waves may be inverted over the right ventricle as a normal finding, in hypokalemia, in pericarditis, in myocardial ischemia, and in other conditions. Incomplete right bundle branch block may occur in otherwise normal hearts, in certain forms of congenital heart disease or during acute myocardial infarction. The heart may rotate in a clockwise direction and point its apex posteriorly for other reasons than acute distention of the right ventricle. In Figure 179, for example, are shown the tracings obtained from a woman of 82 whose heart occupied a most unusual electrical position in the chest. She had a tremendous incisional abdominal hernia with a high left diaphragm, displacing her heart upward. It may be said, however, that the findings are of particular value if they have been observed to develop during the clinical episode under suspicion, and especially after abdominal operations or after injuries to the legs.

VENTRICULAR COMPLEXES RESULTING FROM DIGITALIS

In any consideration of the significance of an abnormal ventricular complex due regard must be paid to the possible influence of digitalis. This drug produces three main effects. It lengthens the P-R interval, depresses the R-T segment, and, in the absence of opposing effects, tends to shorten the Q-T interval (Fig. 180). Figure 181 shows the gradual changes in the T wave resulting from a full dose of digitalis. It will be noted that the T wave, particularly in Lead II, gradually becomes depressed and finally inverted. The R-T segment attains a U-shaped inversion with an upward concavity rather than the upward convexity which characterizes the coronary form of the T wave. In certain leads, particularly those over the right precordium, the RS-T segment may be elevated and present a convex-upward mirror image of the cupped-depressed segments observed over the left ventricle (Fig. 180); in other cases, RS-T segment depressions of the same general configuration may also be seen over the right precordium. In some cases, par-

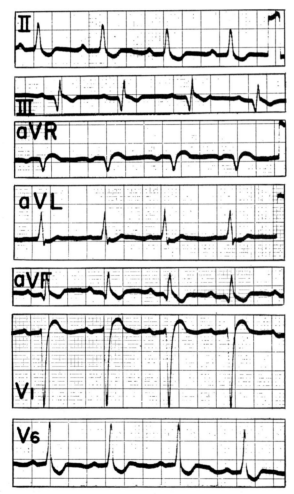

FIG. 180. *Digitalis T Waves.* The Q-T interval is shortened, the RS-T segment cupped depressed, and the T wave inverted in leads related to the left ventricle; the RS-T segment is elevated and the T waves elevated in leads related to the right ventricle. The RS-T contour over the right precordium is a mirror image of that over the left precordium and is not indicative of a "current of injury."

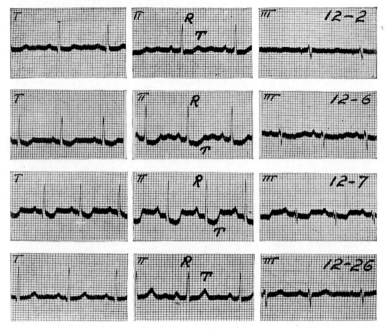

FIG. 181. *Digitalis Effect.* One and five-tenths gram of digitalis leaf was given between the first and third tracings. Note the gradual inversion of the T waves in all leads and the return to normal in three weeks. The RS-T interval becomes convex downward (cupped depressed), unlike the upward convexity in coronary thrombosis. The Q-T interval is shortened. (Author's article in Oxford Loose-Leaf Medicine, vol. II.)

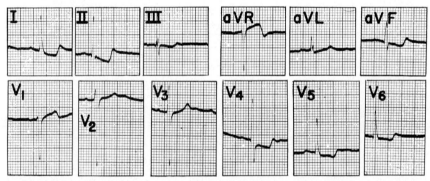

FIG. 182. *Digitalis T Waves.* The gradual straight downstroke, the rapid change in direction, and the more abrupt straight upstroke are suggestive of the jutting, stubborn, and aggressive chin of Dick Tracy. This appearance is probably a composite effect of digitalis and other factors.

ticularly when its effect is combined with that of left ventricular hypertrophy, digitalis tends to produce a slight RS-T depression and an inverted T wave with a straight gradual downstroke breaking sharply to a straight abrupt upstroke. The resulting appearance has been likened to Dick Tracy's chin (Fig. 182).

Digitalis effects on the T wave are not always seen and do not appear with small doses. They do not represent a toxic action of the drug, as they appear when full therapeutic doses are given. It requires two to three weeks for these effects to disappear after the drug is omitted.

The electrocardiographic changes described above indicate digitalis absorption and not digitalis poisoning. The full-fledged changes generally occur when the patient has been adequately digitalized, but it is wiser to depend upon clinical evidence to make the decision regarding adequate digitalization. In general, the tracings are more helpful in telling whether the patient has received any digitalis at all. Similar changes may be produced by other conditions but, in our experience, when this finding of digitalis T waves is at variance with the statement of the patient or his family, his physician much more often than not confirms the fact of recent digitalis administration.

On the other hand, certain arrhythmias and conduction disturbances may indicate or suggest that the patient has received too much digitalis. It is to be remembered at the outset that there is a drug factor and a myocardial factor in digitalis poisoning. Certain damaged hearts seem to be particularly prone to develop evidence of overdosage with the drug, showing abnormalities on a dose which has no toxic effects in other hearts. The characteristic change noted is some evidence of increased irritability of the ventricles. These include ventricular premature beats, idioventricular rhythm (nodal tachycardia), or ventricular tachycardia. Coupled ventricular beats (bigeminal rhythm), sustained or periodic, are very suggestive of digitalis overdosage but may develop in patients not receiving digitalis. Multiform ventricular premature beats generally indicate a marked degree of increased ventricular excitability. This abnormal rhythm may be seen in grave myocardial disease, but much more often than not denotes digitalis poisoning.

If the auricles are beating normally digitalis intoxication may be manifested by the various grades of auriculoventricular block. With complete heart block the ventricular rate, though more rapid than the rate in complete heart block due to most other causes, is slower than the auricular rate. The ventricles and auricles may beat independently of one another, not because of block between the auricles and ventricles, but for another reason, namely enhanced irritability of the ventricles. In this case the ventricular pacemaker, be it in the auriculoventricular node or located lower in the specialized tissues of the ventricles or in ventricular muscle proper, takes on control of the ventricular rhythm because, although conduction between auricles and ventricles may still be intact, the auriculoventricular node or other ventricular pacemaker develops an enhanced automaticity and, so to speak, gets its "punches in sooner" than the impulses coming down from the auricles. This is referred to as auriculoventricular dissociation. It is characteristic of this condition that the ventricular rate is more rapid than the auricular rate. That the junctional tissues may still conduct the beat from auricles to ventricles may be demonstrated if there is a waxing in the

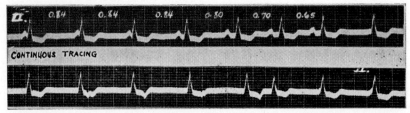

FIG. 183.   *Auriculoventricular Dissociation and Reciprocal Beating in Digitoxin Overdosage.*   The first four QRS complexes are separated by intervals of 0.84 second. Although preceded by P waves, the latter occur at too short an interval to be conducted. The auricles and ventricles during that period are beating independently of one another, the ventricles faster than the auricles. This is auriculoventricular dissociation. With the speeding up of the auricles the sixth auricular beat is conducted through to the ventricles, causing them to beat a little earlier. This repeats itself in the next beat. Thus the R-R intervals between the fifth and sixth and between the sixth and seventh QRS complexes are 0.70 and 0.65 second, respectively. This is ventricular capture (partial auriculoventricular dissociation). Beginning with the second beat in the lower strip the ventricular beats are conducted back to the auricles (retrograde beats; note inverted P waves following QRS complexes). The fifth beat is conducted back to the auricles, then, some of the ventricular fibers having lost their refractoriness, again back to the ventricles. This is true reciprocal beating. The sixth (re-conducted) QRS complex is slightly aberrant. The patient was a 58-year-old man with hypertensive cardiovascular-renal disease who had received digitoxin in the dose of 0.4 mg. daily for two or three months. When digitoxin was withheld normal sinus rhythm was restored.

automaticity of the auricular pacemaker. Under such circumstances (Fig. 183), a beat may slip through and be conducted to the ventricles, thus breaking up the ventricular rhythm. This phenomenon is referred to as "ventricular capture." The resultant arrhythmia is then designated partial auriculoventricular dissociation. Although this rhythm may be observed in other conditions, it is an important clue to digitalis poisoning.

When, on the other hand, the auricles are fibrillating, digitalis poisoning may be manifested by the development of a slow regular rhythm; this represents complete heart block. This slow regular rhythm (Fig. 89) may be detected on careful auscultation or electrocardiographic examination, even if ventricular premature beats or coupled rhythm is present. On the other hand, as when coordinate auricular activity persists, the ventricles may become regular and rapid (idioventricular rhythm). The clue to the inception of either of these changes is the sudden regularization of a previously irregular heart. It is true that normal sinus rhythm may be restored in patients with auricular fibrillation while receiving digitalis, apparently as a result of improvement in the circulation to the heart, but it should be remembered that the fundamental pharmacologic effect of digitalis is the perpetuation rather than the abolition of auricular fibrillation. Hence one should, in such cases, hesitate to ascribe the development of regular rhythm to a return to normal sinus rhythm until this has been proved electrocardiographically.

A rising ventricular rate may thus indicate the development of digitalis intoxication. It may also signal a worsening of the underlying disease process. It is sometimes exceedingly difficult to tell which. In such cases it is necessary to marshal all available clinical and laboratory evidence and make a decision, or even, at times, a gamble, one way or the other. At times it may be justifiable to take what seems a more promising course, changing tack after hours or days if and as it becomes obvious that the selected course is wrong. When prompt decision is imperative, however, an experience that may normally encompass several days may be compressed into a period of less than an hour. To this end, under careful electrocardiographic control, one may undertake the intravenous injection of potassium (p. 492) or a digitalis tolerance test with acetyl-strophanthidin, the ultra-rapid acting synthetic ester of the cardiac aglycone, strophanthidin. This test should not be undertaken lightly. In the long run it is probably best that one physician in an institution, group, or team become familiar with this technique. For details of the procedure the reader is referred to the monograph, "Current Concepts in Digitalis Therapy," by Lown and Levine.

Reference has already been made to the fact that many instances of auricular premature beats (p. 481) and the majority of bouts of paroxysmal auricular tachycardia with block (p. 492) are, in one way or another, related to digitalis intoxication.

The ventricular tachycardia which develops as an evidence of digitalis overdosage differs in no striking regard from that due to other causes. One exception to this is the inception of a peculiar and rare type

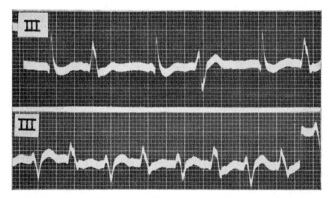

FIG. 184. *Bidirectional Paroxysmal Ventricular Tachycardia.* The upper tracing shows auricular fibrillation with ventricular premature beats in bigeminal rhythm. The ventricular rate was 110. The lower tracing taken later the same day shows paroxysmal ventricular tachycardia with bidirectional complexes. The ventricular rate was 160. Note that the second and sixth (premature) complexes in the upper strip resemble the second, fourth, sixth, and eighth complexes in the lower strip, whereas the fourth complex in the upper strip resembles the first, third, fifth, and seventh complexes of the lower strip. In short, the two ectopic ventricular foci of the upper strip have usurped and share the ventricular rhythm in the lower tracing. This rhythm is pathognomonic of digitalis overdosage. The patient was a 56-year-old man with rheumatic heart disease on digitoxin therapy for congestive heart failure. On discontinuing digitoxin for five days these toxic rhythms disappeared.

of ventricular tachycardia with alternating ventricular complexes, the so-called bidirectional paroxysmal ventricular tachycardia (Fig. 184). This rhythm is pathognomonic of digitalis intoxication.

Pericarditis

During acute pericarditis the electrocardiogram shows slight elevation of the RS-T segment. The leads in which this change is recorded vary with the area of dissemination of the pericarditis. In some cases these changes may be localized to one or two leads, e.g., Leads aVL and I; in others they may be present in two or more limb leads and all or some of the precordial leads. Not uncommonly all three conventional leads show RS-T segment elevation (Fig. 185). If Lead aVR faces the endocardial aspect of an area whose epicardium shows RS-T segment elevation, then RS-T segment depression will be recorded there (Fig. 186). Although RS-T segment depression elsewhere is unusual, and in fact may lead one to favor the diagnosis of myocardial infarction over that of pericarditis, any lead which happens to lie in relation to the endocardial aspect of a portion of the ventricular wall involved in the pericarditic reaction may show RS-T segment depression.

At this very early stage of pericarditis the T wave itself may be upright and even rather tall and peaked. By the time electrocardiography is performed on these patients, however, there is generally observed, coincident with the elevation of the RS-T segment or during its subsidence, a smart inversion of the T wave. The RS-T and T-wave changes then have a contour identical with or closely resembling that frequently seen during acute myocardial infarction and not uncommonly confused with it. Attention to three points may help in the differentiation of these two conditions: (1) In acute pericarditis a broad prominent Q wave does not develop since pericarditis does not lead to transmural myocardial damage and cavity potential is not transmitted to the epicardium. A "septal" Q wave may be present, but this is due merely to the fact that the electrode faces the left side of a normally activated septum. The issue may theoretically be confused by the presence of a broad QS or QR wave residual from a previous infarct, but this situation is more a hypothetical than a real one. The electrocardiographic diagnosis of acute pericarditis complicating acute myocardial infarction is little more than a guess; it may be suspected, however, from a temporary reversal or interruption in the characteristic sequence of electrocardiographic changes usually seen in myocardial infarction, or from the presence of RS-T segment elevations at locations not showing QRS changes. (2) The changes evolve somewhat more rapidly in pericarditis than in acute myocardial infarction, return of the RS-T segment to the isoelectric line generally occurring in the first two or three days. (3) The RS-T segment displacements and T-wave inversions are usually minor in degree. Monophasic ventricular complexes or very tall or deeply inverted T waves have not been described in pericarditis.

A positive differentiation is not always possible. Some cases of myocardial infarction, especially those rare cases of intramural or purely subepicardial infarction, show only RS-T and T-wave changes. If the patient is first seen after the subsidence of the RS-T segment displacements it may be impossible to make a definite electrocardiographic diagnosis. The changes must then be regarded as nonspecific; they might be consistent with myocardial changes due to many causes.

The traumatic pericarditis which follows cardiac surgery is apt to evolve very rapidly. The RS-T segment shift differs from that seen in other varieties of acute pericarditis in being much more poorly defined. Instead of breaking abruptly with the downstroke of the R wave it

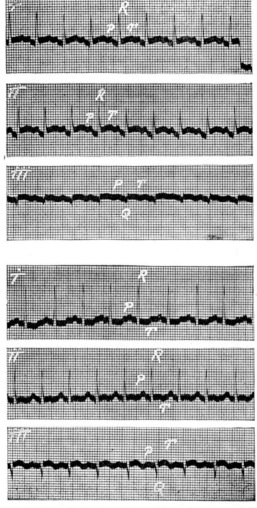

FIG. 185.   *Acute Rheumatic Pericarditis.*   Note the upward displacement of the RS-T segments in all three conventional leads (upper set) taken May 16, 1935. These changes had disappeared on June 20, 1935, when the second set was taken. The patient had acute rheumatic pericarditis with effusion.

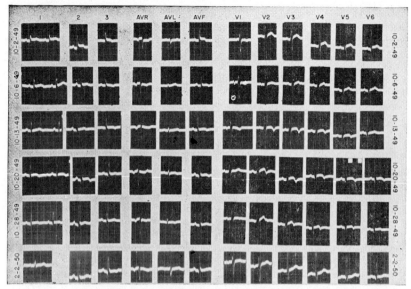

FIG. 186. *Acute Benign Pericarditis*. The initial set of tracings (10/2/49) shows elevation of the RS-T segments in all conventional limb leads and in Leads V_2 to V_6. In the second set (10/6/49) the RS-T segments have partially returned to the isoelectric line and the T waves are notched. In the third set (10/13/49) the RS-T segments are practically isoelectric and the T waves upwardly bowed and inverted, resembling "coronary" T waves. In the following set (10/20/49) the combination of minimal RS-T and T wave changes is quite characteristic. Clinical improvement coincided (10/28/49) with partial regression of these changes. Follow-up tracings three months later (2/2/50) show a normal electrocardiogram. Note the failure of broad, prominent Q waves to develop, the slight degree of RS-T segment elevation, and the lack of development of reciprocal RS-T segment changes except in leads oriented toward the endocardium (Leads aVR and V_1). The patient was a 25-year-old man with sweats, nausea, malaise, and pain in the back of the neck, first suspected of having preparalytic poliomyelitis. A pericardial friction rub, Ewart's sign, pulsus paradoxus, and reflux distention of the cervical veins on hepatic compression were present. He improved on penicillin and Aureomycin therapy, and was discharged well.

begins as a slow, smooth, ill-defined shading-off of the downstroke of the R wave into an inverted T wave (Fig. 187). This makes it difficult to identify the actual end of the R wave and thus to measure the QRS interval.

T wave inversion may persist for weeks or, in rare cases, as long as two or three months, but eventually the electrocardiogram resumes a normal appearance. If the pericarditis is complicated by pericardial effusion the voltage of the QRS complexes may decrease, apparently, as in pleural effusions or ascites, because of local short-circuiting.

Shifts of the P-R segment, presumably due to inflammation of the auricular epicardium, may occasionally be observed in acute pericarditis. And at times a striking presystolic shuffle may be heard either in the presence or absence of this electrocardiographic change, particularly in postoperative cases.

It is generally considered that the electrocardiographic changes of acute pericarditis are due to subepicardial myocarditis. Certainly the electrical changes recorded at the epicardium must have their origin in changes produced in or on the surface of heart muscle cells, and it must be very difficult, if not impossible, either clinically or experimentally, to demonstrate restriction of injury to the pericardium and not involving the underlying myocardium. Since the lesion may have progressed to a biochemical and not an anatomic stage, failure to demonstrate changes under the microscope would not exclude injury. On the other hand, the fact that isolated injury of the epicardium is unlikely and that the ultimate origin of these electrical properties is in the myocardial cell does not disprove the theoretical possibility that "pure" pericardial injury might be associated with similar electrical changes.

Patients with chronic constrictive pericarditis often show low voltage QRS complexes with or without T wave inversions (Fig. 188). The first of these changes may be due to the myocardial atrophy which so often develops in this condition, the second is possibly related to the

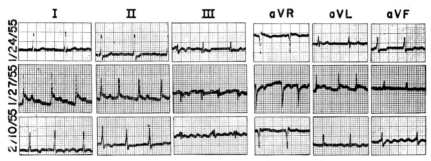

FIG. 187.   *Postoperative Pericarditis.*   The patient was a 46-year-old man with mitral stenosis, auricular fibrillation, and recurrent embolisms. Mitral valvuloplasty was carried out on January 26, 1955. On the following day the electrocardiogram showed a smooth shading-off of the downstroke of the QRS complex into an elevated RS-T segment. At this time the T waves were upright. These changes are seen in Leads I, II, and aVL. Chest leads were not recorded because of presence of the surgical dressing. Such changes are generally short-lived. The post-operative course was benign.

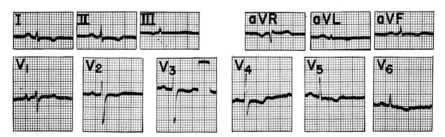

FIG. 188.   *Chronic Calcific Constrictive Pericarditis.*   The important findings are low electromotive force and inversion of the T waves. Pericardiectomy partially relieved the symptoms of congestive heart failure and the patient, a 48-year-old man, lived six years. Myocardial fibrosis was a factor limiting his improvement.

pressure of the pericardial eschar. Recent experience with chronic constrictive pericarditis, proved at surgery or autopsy, has disclosed a considerable number of patients whose tracings exhibited features characteristic of or compatible with old myocardial infarction. These changes may be the effect of intramyocardial extension of the epicardial eschar. These observations supplement the clinical and physiological observation that there is an important myocardial component in chronic constrictive pericarditis which constitutes a limiting factor in the amenability of these patients to surgery and in their prognosis following surgery. The surprising electrocardiographic finding is that these patients showed QS or QR complexes. Chronic constrictive pericarditis is primarily an epicardial process which may extend into the subjacent myocardium. If the traditional view regarding activation of the free ventricular wall (p. 587) is valid, one would expect merely a decrease in the voltage of the QRS complex. If, on the other hand, Prinzmetal's views are valid, the extension of the fibrotic process into the inner shell of the myocardium should produce QS deflections. In the present experience then the low-voltage QRS complexes are compatible with the traditional view and the complexes suggesting myocardial infarction with the new views regarding activation of the ventricular wall.

A number of patients with pericardial constriction show broad, notched P waves resembling but not quite so broad or prominent as those seen in mitral valve disease. This may be due to involvement of the auricular myocardium in the pericardial process. A considerable number also exhibit auricular fibrillation. These findings add to the difficulty in distinguishing these patients from those with rheumatic mitral valve disease.

The Electrocardiogram in Cerebrovascular Accidents

It is well known that in neurocirculatory asthenia the T waves may be inverted in certain leads and even that a so-called "false" positive Master test may be recorded. We don't know just how these effects of the central nervous system or its autonomic division come to bear on the heart. Some recent observations may bring us nearer to a solution of this problem. Occasionally there are observed, in connection with cerebrovascular accidents such as subarachnoid or intracranial hemorrhage, and in the presence or absence of heart disease, very deeply inverted and prolonged T waves and occasionally prominent U waves. These changes may resemble those seen in myocardial ischemia or infarction or electrolyte imbalance. Figure 189 shows successive sets of tracings recorded in a 69-year-old woman who was admitted in coma. The first strip shows deep inversion of the T waves resembling those seen in experimental coronary artery compression. The second set shows elevation of the RS-T segments and slightly more prominent Q waves in the same leads which originally showed the inverted T waves. An electrocardiographic diagnosis of acute myocardial infarction was rendered. At

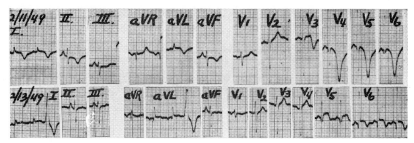

FIG. 189. *"Ischemic" T Waves in Subarachnoid Hemorrhage.* RS-T and T wave changes without infarction. The patient was a 69-year-old woman who was admitted in coma February 9, 1949, and died February 16, 1949. In the initial set of tracings obtained on February 11, 1949, the T waves in Leads I, II, aVL, aVF, and V_3 to V_6 have a characteristic "coronary" contour. In Leads V_3 to V_6 the T waves have a waterfall appearance often seen during the early days or weeks of an acute myocardial infarction or in the very earliest stages of experimental coronary artery ligature. The tracings obtained on February 13, 1949, show elevation of the RS-T segments in Leads I, aVL, and V_4 to V_6, with much less pronounced late inversion of the T waves in these same leads. Although Q waves were recorded in Leads V_4 to V_6 they are very narrow and very inconspicuous relative to the R waves in the same leads. The patient remained in coma and died two days later. Postmortem examination showed a ruptured aneurysm of the circle of Willis but no evidence of myocardial infarction or pericarditis on meticulous microscopic examination.

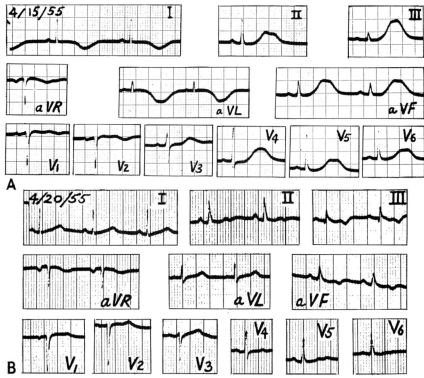

FIG. 190. *Subarachnoid Hemorrhage.* Upper set of tracings made during acute episode show bizarre prolonged Q-T interval and inverted T waves. No evidence of heart disease or electrolyte imbalance was demonstrable. The second set of tracings, made five days later, show reversion toward normal on recovery. The significance of this change has not been determined.

609

postmortem examination the heart was perfectly normal. There was a ruptured aneurysm of the circle of Willis. During an acute subarachnoid hemorrhage another patient showed changes (Fig. 190, *A*) resembling those observed in patients with electrolyte imbalance, but she demonstrated no such electrolyte abnormalities. On recovery the electrocardiogram (Fig. 190, *B*) was practically normal. At no time did this patient present evidence of heart disease. The cause of these electrocardiographic phenomena has not been established. They could be related to some disturbance in the hypothalamus or perhaps to the subendocardial hemorrhages which have recently been demonstrated in association with various intracranial diseases.

Electrolyte Imbalance and the Electrocardiogram

Changes in the chemical environment of the heart muscle cell may also produce changes in the electrocardiogram. Indeed, differences in electrolyte concentration between that on the inner and on the outer aspects of the semipermeable membrane constituting the surface of the cell account largely for the normal difference in potential across the normal resting cell. We know little, except by inference, about the effect of variations in intracellular electrolyte composition, but we know a good deal more about the effect of changes in extracellular electrolytes upon the electrocardiogram.

Hypocalcemia characteristically produces a prolongation of electrical systole manifested by a prolonged Q-T interval. Mechanical systole may or may not show a concomitant lengthening. This emphasizes the disparity between electrical and mechanical events and the danger of drawing mechanical implications from the electrocardiogram. Prolongation of the Q-T interval is often observed in advanced renal disease with phosphate retention and reciprocal depression of the serum calcium level, and in spontaneous or postoperative hypoparathyroidism (Fig. 191). Prolongation of the Q-T interval may also occur in alkalosis. This change is probably referable to concomitant changes in extracellular ionized calcium, but its development in the hypochloremia of vomiting suggests a possible relationship to changes in intracellular potassium.

The electrocardiogram may thus offer the first indication of a lowering of the serum calcium level. Although in a few reported instances the opposite chemical finding, namely hypercalcemia, has been manifested by a shortening of the Q-T interval (Fig. 192), two recent cases of multiple myeloma with high serum calcium levels showed rather a prolongation of the Q-T interval and of the QRS complex, and depression of the RS-T segments.

The deviation from the normal Q-T interval can be determined from the formula: $K = \dfrac{Q\text{-}T}{\sqrt{R\text{-}R}}$. The normal figures for K are 0.39 for men and 0.44 for women. It is generally unwise to report this as increased unless K exceeds 0.45. This figure is inaccurate at very slow and very rapid rates; in these instances the standards of Ashman should be consulted.

The kidneys retain their ability to excrete potassium until relatively late, but in anuria, from whatever cause, toxic accumulations of potassium may occur in the blood serum. By virtue of the capacity of elevated serum potassium level to paralyze the heart, this change may be a fatal complication of renal disease. This development may be foreshadowed by taking frequent electrocardiograms in anuric patients, thus providing the signal for timely and appropriate therapy. The earliest change is the development of tall, pointed, and narrow T waves (Fig. 193). Later the Q-T interval, the QRS interval (Fig. 46), and the P-R interval become prolonged. At the same time the P waves become smaller, the R waves decrease, the S waves increase in magnitude, and the RS-T segments become depressed. Eventually the RS-T segment forms an almost continuous line from the nadir of the S wave to the apex of the T wave and the P waves become unrecognizable (Fig. 46). With further accumulations of potassium the rhythm may become grossly irregular and, on further disintegration of the ventricular complex, the electrocardiogram may show the baseline to form a continuous sine wave. Ectopic rhythms, such as ventricular premature or escape beats and ventricular tachy-

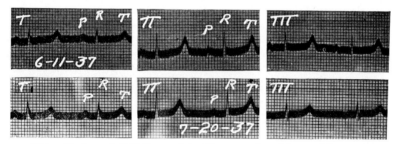

FIG. 191. *Prolonged Q-T Interval in Hypoparathyroidism.* The patient was a 68-year-old man with hypoparathyroidism. Blood calcium on June 11, 1937, was 4.7 mg. per 100 cc., and on July 20, 1937, it was 9.3 mg. per 100 cc. The Q-T interval, despite very slight slowing of the heart, decreased from 0.48 to 0.40 second. The improvement occurred as a result of dihydrotachysterol.

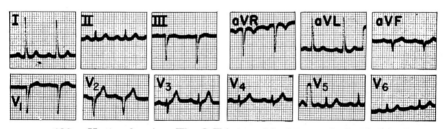

FIG. 192. *Hypercalcemia.* The Q-T interval is shortened, closely hugging the QRS complex. The patient had chronic pyelonephritis and uremia. The serum calcium level was 7.7 (normal 5), sodium 131, potassium 5.4, and phosphorus 1.4 milliequivalents per liter. The serum CO_2 content was 23.6 millimols per liter. Similar tracings may be recorded in hyperparathyroidism.

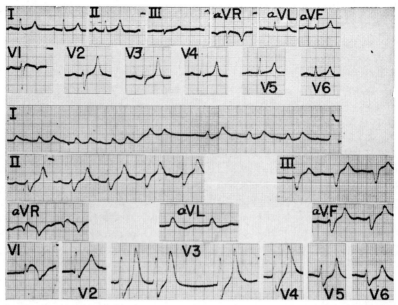

FIG. 193. *Potassium Intoxication.* The patient was a 35-year-old woman with anuria following premature separation of the placenta. The first set of tracings showed first degree heart block and tall narrow pointed T waves, the first clue to the existence of a high blood potassium level. The second set of curves, recorded five hours later, shows much more pronounced changes, including decreased height of the R waves, increased depth of the S waves, first degree heart block, intraventricular block, smooth slanting RS-T segments, and tall pointed T waves, most strikingly exhibited in the precordial leads. Sinus arrhythmia and cardiac slowing are apparent in Lead I. The serum potassium level at the time this second set of tracings was taken was 9.5 milliequivalents per liter. The patient recovered following treatment by the artificial kidney and showed normal electrocardiograms at time of discharge.

cardia, may develop at this time. The terminal mechanism in these cases may be ventricular standstill or ventricular fibrillation. Although the intraventricular block developing in these cases is generally a diffuse affair, affecting the ventricular myocardium and specialized tissues alike, in a few cases bundle branch block has been recorded. Some degree of elevation of the serum potassium level above the normal value of 4 to 5 milliequivalents per liter is generally necessary before any of these changes develop, but the parallelism between electrocardiographic appearance and the serum potassium level is only approximate. Among other possible factors affecting this relationship is the serum sodium or calcium level. An elevated serum sodium level antagonizes, while a depressed serum sodium or calcium level enhances, these characteristic effects of potassium. The effect upon potassium intoxication of variations in other ions has not as yet been clearly demonstrated.

Potassium depletion may result from excessive elimination of potassium in vomiting, nasogastric suction, gastrointestinal fistulae, intestinal intubation, diarrhea, "potassium-losing" nephritis, or from copious diuresis; from inadequate intake of potassium in starvation or during the intravenous infusion of fluids with inadequate potassium content; or from conditions associated with abnormal transfers of potassium in periodic paralysis, in insulin-treated diabetic acidosis, and in Addison's disease being treated with desoxycorticosterone acetate. The electrocardiographic effects of this electrolyte derangement consist of lowering, flattening, or inversion of the T waves (Fig. 194, A), depression of the RS-T segment (Fig. 194, B, C, E, F, and G), lengthening of the Q-T interval (Fig. 194, A, B), appearance of broader and taller U waves

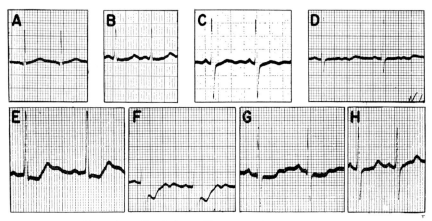

FIG. 194. *Potassium Depletion.* Electrocardiographic tracings showing the panorama of changes. The Q-T interval may be prolonged (A, B, H), the T waves low (A), notched (C, D), flattened (D), or inverted (F, G, H), the RS-T segments depressed (C, E, G, H), and the U waves prominent (C, D, E, F, G) or predominant (H). These changes may occur alone or in combination.

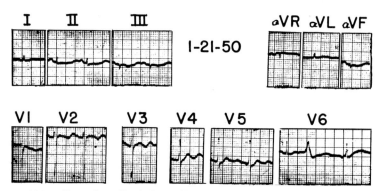

FIG. 195. *Potassium Depletion.* The patient was a 67-year-old spinster who had had a sigmoid resection for carcinoma 28 years earlier and a transabdominal total gastrectomy, partial pancreatectomy, and splenectomy on January 3, 1950. Her postoperative course was complicated by paralytic ileus and diarrhea, and she presented a most difficult problem in the regulation of her electrolyte balance and maintenance of nutrition. On January 22 the serum potassium level was 1.6 (normal 3.8–5.0) and the chloride level 95 (normal 100) milliequivalents per liter. Note the flattening or lowering of T waves, depression of RS-T segment, and presence of U waves. With subsequent return of serum potassium to normal levels the electrocardiograms became normal.

(Fig. 194, *D*, *E*, *F*, *H*), and, in a few instances, of first degree heart block and tall, sharp P waves. The T waves may become notched (Fig. 194, *C*); in association with a prominent U wave a triple-notched repolarization complex may thus be produced (Fig. 194, *D*, *E*). These changes may occur independently or in combination (Fig. 195). Nodal rhythm has been observed in a few cases. Various arrhythmias, especially supraventricular tachycardia, may develop during potassium loss, independent of prior digitalization, and be eliminated when potassium loss is corrected. The precipitation of digitalis intoxication by potassium losses has been discussed above (p. 492). The electrocardiogram may suggest potassium depletion when the serum potassium level is normal; the serum potassium level may be lowered when the electrocardiogram is normal; occasionally both parameters will indicate the defect. The concurrent use of both techniques will detect more instances of potassium depletion than use of either alone.

Wolff-Parkinson-White Syndrome (Anomalous Auriculoventricular Excitation; Pre-excitation; Accelerated Conduction)

There is one peculiar type of electrocardiogram that occurs in a small group of individuals who, in about 50 per cent of the cases, are prone to have attacks of rapid heart action of one type or another (Figs. 196 to 198). Although a few authorities have been willing to broaden the criteria upon which the diagnosis may be made, these patients generally have a shortened P-R interval, measuring 0.10 second or less, and a QRS complex broadened to 0.11 second or longer. The mechanism of this disturbance is still debated but, following the lead of Wolferth, it is widely held that this phenomenon is due to conduction over an aberrant bundle of heart muscle, such as the bundle of Kent, connecting auricles and ventricles and by-passing the normal auriculoventricular bundle. Since this tract has no junctional tissue the impulse is not delayed. In anomalous impulses activation of the ventricles is initiated over the aberrant route, probably in a direction from the epicardium toward the endocardium, but conduction down the normal pathway continues somewhat later. Activation of the ventricles generally is completed over the normal route. Thus the interval from the beginning of the P wave to the end of the QRS complex is generally unchanged. An adequate series of histologic studies in individuals with and without this mechanism is not as yet available to establish this anatomic mechanism. It has been suggested that actual protoplasmic continuity of auricular and ventricular muscle need not be necessary; mere contiguity of auricular and ventricular muscle may be adequate to establish the mechanism.

A variant explanation is that the aberration in the Wolff-Parkinson-White syndrome depends upon the integrity of the normal auriculoventricular conduction system. Although the normal beats are conducted at the usual rate through the auriculoventricular node and bundle, there exists within the structure of the auriculoventricular conduction system a sort of "express highway" capable of transmitting the impulse at an abnormally rapid rate ("accelerated conduction") into the ventricles.

An anatomical explanation for the Wolff-Parkinson-White syndrome has not been universally accepted. Complexes interpreted as identical with those of the Wolff-Parkinson-White syndrome have been recorded during cardiac catheterization on contact of the catheter with the interventricular septum. It has been suggested that a hyperexcitable ventricular focus may respond to the electrical or mechanical stimulation of auricular activation, producing isolated anomalous complexes or salvos of rapid heart action.

A few cases have been reported in which patients without organic heart disease have died as a result of the tachycardia which may complicate this syndrome. However, by and large these individuals carry on normally and have no organic heart disease. Although most of these patients have paroxysms of auricular tachycardia, I have seen instances in which the attacks of rapid heart action were auricular flutter (Fig. 198) or fibrillation (Fig. 197). The type of ventricular complex seen in the paroxysm may be normal, in which event one might postulate conduction down the normal auriculoventricular node and bundle, or it may be anomalous, in which event the individual ventricular complexes re-

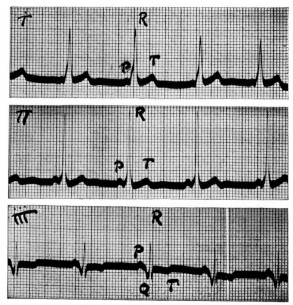

FIG. 196. *Wolff-Parkinson-White Syndrome.* Note that the P-R interval is very short (0.08 second) and the QRS complex is slurred and broadened (0.11 second). The broadening of the QRS complex is apparent only at the base, producing a characteristic "Eiffel Tower" effect. The initial or slow component of the QRS complex corresponds to activation of the ventricles over the hypothetical aberrant bundle. Because the upper part of the QRS complex possesses a normal thinness the characteristic appearance may be missed in a cursory examination. Peculiar curves of this type are seen in some individuals who have paroxysms of tachycardia but are otherwise well.

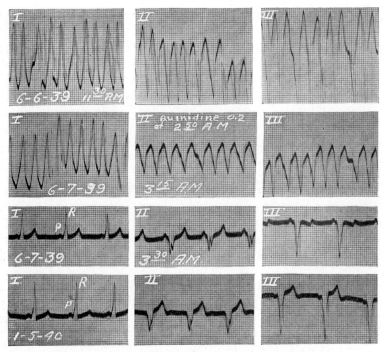

FIG. 197.   *Wolff-Parkinson-White Syndrome, with Anomalous Complexes During Paroxysmal Rapid Heart Action.*   The lower two sets of curves show typical short P-R interval (0.10 second) and long QRS interval (0.12 second). The upper two sets of curves show a paroxysm of rapid heart action in which the individual ventricular complexes are similar to those recorded out of an attack. The irregularity of the ventricles is probably due to auricular fibrillation. During auricular fibrillation the impulses apparently invade the ventricles over the aberrant pathway. These tracings simulate, and were originally published as, paroxysmal ventricular tachycardia. The heart rate at first was 292; after 0.2 gm. of quinidine it slowed to 231, and in less than one hour the rhythm was normal.

semble the aberrant complexes observed without tachycardia. If one accepts the anatomic hypothesis, the latter type of paroxysm might indicate that the impulse enters the ventricle over the aberrant pathway. It has been suggested that it is those patients who show both normal and anomalous complexes who are prone to have attacks of rapid heart action. Quinidine, probably by virtue of its predominant effect in delaying conduction over the anomalous bundle, tends to favor conduction over the normal auriculoventricular node and bundle. Exercise, by its predominant effect in decreasing vagal tone, and frequently atropine, by paralyzing vagal nerve endings, enhance conduction over the auriculoventricular node and bundle. Vagal stimulation by its predominant effect in slowing conduction in the auriculoventricular node favors earlier conduction down the aberrant bundle. There are undoubtedly concealed instances of anomalous conduction which may be brought to light by various physiologic or pharmacologic procedures such as those just enumerated. There is a different group of individuals who show a short

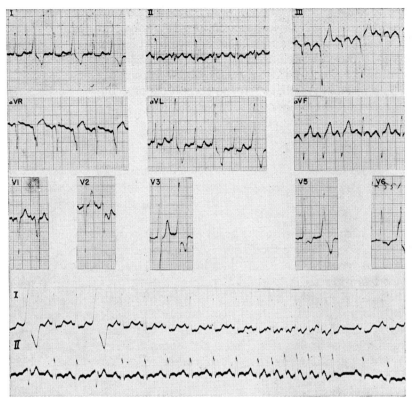

FIG. 198. *Wolff-Parkinson-White Syndrome.* Anomalous atrioventricular excitation alternating with normal atrioventricular conduction. Note that (with the
exception of Lead aVF) the first, third, and fifth complexes show normal P-R intervals and normal QRS complexes and are characteristic of left ventricular hypertrophy. The second, fourth, and sixth complexes in these leads show a short P-R
interval and a lengthened QRS duration. The slow initial portion of the QRS complex contributes to the characteristic "Eiffel Tower" effect. If the anatomic explanation for this condition is accepted it would seem that, for the most part, every other
beat is conducted earlier down the aberrant pathway than down the normal pathway, whereas alternate beats start down the normal pathway earlier. Note that the
normal complexes in Lead aVF do not show a broad or prominent Q wave. This is
evidence against the suggestion of old posterior myocardial infarction raised by the
prominent Q and QS waves in the normal and abnormal complexes respectively in
Lead III and by the broad QS waves of the abnormal complexes in Lead aVF. The
direction of the QRS complexes is downward in Leads III, aVR, aVF, V$_1$, and V$_2$,
upward in Leads I, aVL, and Leads V$_3$ to V$_6$, and equiphasic in Lead II. This suggests
that the general direction of abnormal excitation is from the right posterolateral to
the left anterolateral aspect of the heart and toward the left shoulder at right angles
to the Lead II line. During the simultaneous recording of Leads I and II on a later
occasion (lower sets), a short paroxysm of auricular flutter is recorded at a rate of
215 with 1:1 auriculoventricular response. There is no important deviation of the
spatial ventricular gradient between normal and anomalous complexes. This accords
with the hypothesis that the change from normal to anomalous complexes is merely
one in the direction of invasion of the ventricles with no local changes in the responsiveness of the ventricles.

P-R interval (about 0.12 sec.) with *normal* QRS duration who also are prone to paroxysmal rapid heart action. It is important not to be misled into the diagnosis of anomalous atrioventricular excitation when the short P-R interval–prolonged QRS complex is mimicked by a ventricular premature beat occurring only very slightly prematurely.

The resemblance between the complexes of Wolff-Parkinson-White syndrome and those characterizing myocardial infarction is only superficial. It should be remembered that paroxysmal rapid heart action, from whatever cause, may be associated with chest pain. It should not be concluded because rapid heart action and chest pain occur together that myocardial infarction is present. When myocardial infarction complicates the Wolff-Parkinson-White syndrome the electrocardiographic changes of infarction may be totally or partly lacking. With anomalous conduction the impulse proceeds from the epicardium to the endocardium, making the ventricular cavity initially positive; thus a Q wave will be lacking at an electrode overlying a transmural infarct. The situation is analogous to that in left bundle branch block in which the impulse travels from the right to the left side of the septum, similarly making the left ventricular cavity initially positive. Since ventricular activation may be completed in a normal manner, RS-T and T-wave changes may be detected in the anomalous complexes. Be that as it may, examination of spontaneous or induced "normal" complexes may reveal decisive QRS, RS-T, and T-wave changes of infarction.

Ventricular Complexes in Other Conditions

There are numerous other conditions in which the ventricular complex alters its form. In many the changes are not sufficiently characteristic or uniform to be diagnostic. Further study will be necessary before such data can be standardized and before decisive conclusions can be drawn. In the meantime it is important to be familiar with some of the peculiarities that may arise. Reference has already been made to the fact that inversion of T waves may be associated, among other conditions, with ventricular hypertrophy or with electrolyte imbalance. Frequently a definite cause for the inversion of the T waves cannot be established, yet one may be sure that they represent a pathologic state of the heart muscle. In such cases it seems wise to refer to them as abnormal nonspecific change. Markedly inverted T waves in all leads indicate a poor prognosis. Some of these markedly abnormal ventricular complexes probably represent multiple areas of healed myocardial infarctions, some of which cases have been described pathologically as fibrous myocarditis.

Flattening of the T waves and decrease in the height of the QRS complexes also occur in constrictive pericarditis (Fig. 188), marked anemia, beriberi heart (Fig. 199), emphysema (Fig. 201), myxedema (Figs. 144 and 200, *A*) and Addison's disease (Fig. 200, *B*). In pulmonary emphysema low voltage in the limb leads may or may not be associated with low voltage in the precordial leads. In pulmonary disease in general and emphysema in particular the T wave may be inverted in Lead I, but generally in these cases the T wave is upright in Leads V_5 and V_6. By contrast, inversion of the T wave in Lead I resulting from antero-lateral ischemia is generally associated with T wave inversion over the

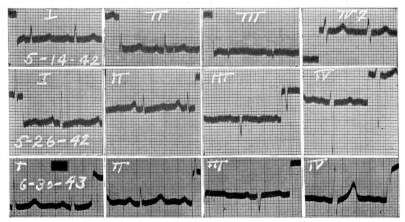

FIG. 199.   *Abnormal Form of Ventricular Complex (Low Voltage in Beriberi Heart).*   The patient was a 33-year-old man who had been drinking heavily and eating very little. He complained of weakness, shortness of breath, swelling of the legs, and pains in the limbs. He showed marked dilatation of the heart, pulmonary congestion, and some peripheral edema. A control period of digitalis caused no improvement. On a course of thiamine therapy the heart returned to normal size and all congestion disappeared. The first set of tracings (before thiamine) shows very low QRS complexes, which even in twelve days returned to normal.

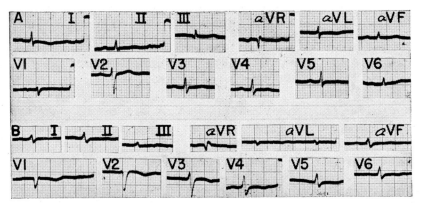

FIG. 200.   *Low Voltage Electrocardiograms in Endocrinopathies.*   The upper set of tracings (A) was obtained from a 35-year-old woman with severe myxedema. Note that low voltage is recorded here in the chest as well as in the limb leads. T_1 is inverted. These changes are reversible on thyroid therapy. The lower set of tracings (B) was obtained from a 24-year-old man with Addison's disease associated with hypothyroidism. Note the low voltage in limb and chest leads, and the prolonged Q-T interval and inverted T waves in the precordial leads. These changes resemble those observed in hypokalemia. These changes may be reversible on cortisone therapy.

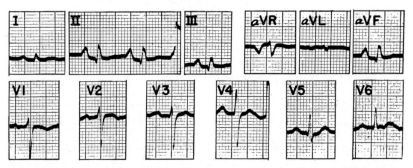

FIG. 201.   *Chronic Cor Pulmonale, Associated with Pulmonary Emphysema and Fibrosis.*   The tracings show low voltage in the limb leads and prominent P waves in Leads II, III, and aVF ("P pulmonale"). Note that while T_1 is low, almost flat, the T waves are upright over the left precordium; this is evidence against "ischemic" anterolateral myocardial changes and more consonant with pulmonary disease. The patient was a 59-year-old man with long-standing bronchial asthma, bronchiectasis, pulmonary emphysema, and recent right-sided heart failure. The presence of low voltage in the limb leads suggests, among other causes, pulmonary emphysema.

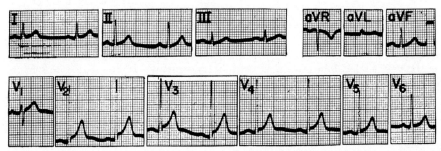

FIG. 202.   *Normal Variation in RS-T Segment.*   RS-T segment elevation of 2 mm. as normal variation. The same changes were present over many months of observation. The patient presented no evidence of heart disease. There was slight recession of these shifts on acceleration of the heart produced by exercise. This change is of dubious significance, but similar changes may be observed in the earliest phases of acute pericarditis or infarction.

left ventricle. Examples of low electromotive force in myxedema and in Addison's disease associated with myxedema are given in Figure 200.

A number of normal individuals show slight (1–2 mm.) or moderate (3 mm.) elevations of the RS-T segments in a number of the leads with upright T waves (Fig. 202). A similar elevation may be recorded as the earliest change in acute pericarditis or myocardial infarction. Repeated electrocardiograms may be necessary to establish whether this change is a normal variant for a particular individual or represents an early "current of injury." Chronic alcoholics frequently exhibit a "brisk" electrocardiogram resembling that just described. This consists of slightly elevated RS-T segments, an upright and characteristically sharp T wave, and a shortened Q-T interval (Fig. 203). The possible metabolic significance of this finding has not been determined.

Changes in the electrocardiograms are not rare during diphtheria.

Younger patients are more apt to show prolongation of the P-R interval and more advanced stages of heart block, while the older more frequently show alterations in the RS-T interval such as depression of the RS-T segment or inversion of the T wave.

Inversion of the T wave in Lead I or Lead II is not normal, and yet its presence must not always be regarded too seriously. When the inversion has the peculiar form described under myocardial infarction it may have important significance. It should be remembered, however, that T waves of this type may be recorded in intracranial disease in the absence of heart disease. Inversion of the T waves and prolongation of the Q-T interval resembling those associated with coronary artery disease may also be seen in left ventricular hypertrophy. In general, as the R wave becomes taller and greater in area the T wave becomes smaller and inverted. It is hoped that the study of the ventricular gradient in cases of this type might clarify the significance of these changes. Moreover, the T waves can be diphasic or slightly inverted in neurocirculatory asthenia. Cooling the apex of the heart by drinking cold water can produce inversion of the T wave. Nitroglycerin or amyl nitrite can temporarily correct an inverted T wave in disease of the coronary arteries,

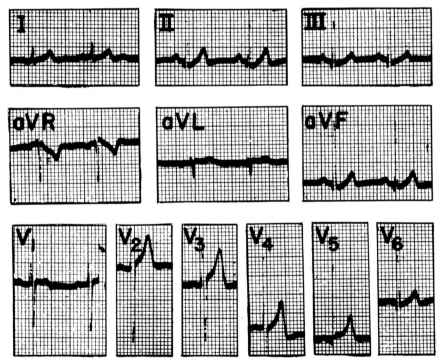

FIG. 203.   *"Brisk" Electrocardiogram of Chronic Alcoholism.*   The Q-T interval is shortened, the RS-T segments are slightly elevated, and the T waves are sharp. Such changes are frequently encountered in patients with chronic alcoholism. The possible metabolic significance of this change has not been established.

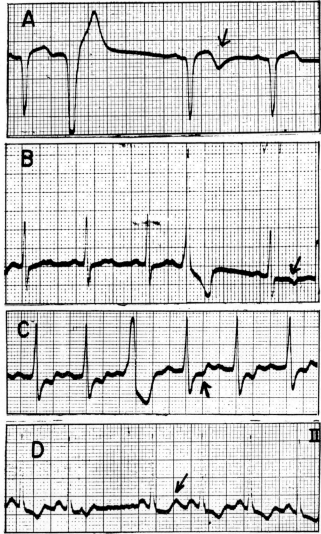

FIG. 204.   *Post-extrasystolic T-Wave Changes.*   *A*, pronounced change in direction of T wave of beat following pause, while QRS remains unchanged. The patient, a 58-year-old man, had angina pectoris and had suffered an acute anteroseptal infarct. In *B*, notching, itself an abnormal finding, was already present; the post-extrasystolic inversion of the T waves confirms this abnormality. *C*, similar T wave changes induced on a substrate of right bundle branch block. In *D*, similar "primary" T wave changes follow a pause occurring after a non-conducted auricular premature beat. Post-extrasystolic or post-pausal T wave changes signify myocardial impairment, generally myocardial ischemia.

and attacks of angina pectoris or a simple muscular effort may bring about inversion of the T waves in certain individuals.

Reference has already been made to the significance of localized T wave changes as possibly denoting myocardial ischemia (Fig. 145). Another helpful clue to myocardial impairment is the detection of post-extrasystolic T wave changes. If the QRS complex of the beat following a pause set up by a premature beat is identical with the QRS complex of all other complexes in that lead while the T wave differs strikingly from the T waves indigenous to that lead, the inference of myocardial ischemia is generally justified. The same may be said of similar T wave changes or, for that matter, U wave changes, following any pause, however induced. The first strip (A) in Figure 204 is a classic example of post-extrasystolic T wave changes in a patient with angina pectoris who had suffered a previous anteroseptal myocardial infarct. The second strip (B) reveals the same phenomenon in a lead showing notched T waves in the regular beats and confirms their abnormality. The third strip (C) shows the same type of change in a patient with severe coronary artery disease and right bundle branch block. The final strip (D) shows prominent T-wave changes after the pause following a non-conducted auricular premature beat. Here the regular T waves were inverted and the post-extrasystolic T wave was partly upright.

Electrocardiographic Interpretation

Before leaving the subject of electrocardiography, it is necessary to express a word of caution against trying to read too much into the results of this examination. Too often physicians attach significance to minor abnormalities. It must be remembered that variations among normal hearts are very great. Slight notching of QRS complexes, differences in amplitude of curves, left and right axis deviation, and even flattened diphasic or slightly inverted T waves occur without organic heart disease. Little clinical meaning is to be attached to the fact that a tracing at one time satisfies the criteria for left ventricular hypertrophy and at another time does not. Furthermore, even when certain curves are diagnostic of myocardial disease they may serve no further purpose in prognosis. In a case of typical acute coronary thrombosis the curves may show very little abnormality or may be returning to a normal configuration and yet the patient may be doing poorly or may suddenly die. It is generally idle to say that "the electrocardiograms are getting better." It is more important to know what the patient is doing clinically than to know what further changes are going on in his tracings. Hence, once the clinical diagnosis of acute myocardial infarction has been confirmed by the electrocardiogram little purpose is served by recording repeated tracings. The electrocardiogram is disappointing as an indicator of extension of an infarct. With advent of the newer knowledge regarding the electrical position of the heart an exaggerated importance has unfortunately been attributed to minor changes in this position. Too many reports contain meaningless statements that the heart has shown a "clockwise" or "counterclockwise" rotation. The implication of acute cor pulmonale from clockwise rotation of the heart is rarely justified unless this shift is pronounced and there is a concomitant tachycardia.

Although, in general, patients with inverted T waves in Lead I have a poor prognosis, there are a great many who live for years, and in fact there are some who have no clinical evidence of either angina or heart failure. In the extensive use of electrocardiography there is a danger of prostituting the entire subject. Attempts to interpret curves have been made when the leads were incorrectly applied or when the tracings were pasted upside down or wrong end to. Artefacts are being interpreted as pathologic changes, and many similar gross errors are being made. Despite all this, with care and intelligence, electrocardiography can be a most valuable aid in the management of patients with heart disease.

Pulsus Alternans

There is one disturbance in the mechanism of the heart beat that is not truly within the scope of electrocardiography because it is not diagnosed by this means. However, it needs to be considered for it is important and can easily be recognized. This condition is *pulsus alternans*, by which is meant an alternation in the strength of the beat when the rhythm is regular (Fig. 205). In this condition the impulses of the heart arise regularly in the normal pacemaker and travel through the normal pathways. The electrocardiogram is therefore normal. Every other beat, however, is stronger than the previous one. It must be clearly differentiated from a pseudo-alternation due to prematurity of each second beat. In bigeminy due to extrasystoles every second beat is also small, but this results because the contractions occur slightly ahead of time and the ventricles contain less blood. In true alternation the intervals between beats are equal and the weaker contractions are thought to be due to fatigue of the heart muscle or to impaired contractility. It has been hypothesized that isolated bits of ventricular fibers here and there do not enter into systole because of fatigue, so that each alternate systole is less effective than the preceding one.

Pulsus alternans can be recognized if a pulse tracing is taken from one of the peripheral arteries. It can be felt at the radial pulse, where every other beat will be weak. Unless this sign is looked for or unless it is very marked, it is generally overlooked. Changes in the volume of the peripheral pulse produced by different phases of respiration often interfere with and obscure the regularity of the alternation. At times the same alternation can be detected in the heart itself by noting an alternation in the intensity of the first heart sound or of an accompanying systolic murmur, or even in the force of the apex impulse. In other words, the alternation may be seen, heard, or felt. The simplest and most sensitive way of diagnosing pulsus alternans is with the sphygmomanometer. While taking the blood pressure one should listen carefully and try to detect alternation of the sounds as the pressure falls and is just approaching the systolic level. When the sounds first appear the pressure should be prevented from falling for several seconds. If alternation is present, either the sounds will alternate in intensity or only the stronger beats will be heard. If the latter occurs, then both sounds will become audible at a pressure 5 or 10 mm. lower but will still alternate in intensity. This method is more sensitive and just as reliable as the pulse tracing in the diagnosis of pulsus alternans. This anomaly should be sought for as a routine procedure in all patients with definite or suspected heart disease.

In some patients pulsus alternans only appears for several seconds after a premature beat and then disappears. Following the compensatory pause the first beat is always exaggerated, but now the second beat is markedly diminished, the third is increased, and so on for several cycles. The extrasystole brings to the surface the tendency to alternation. This has the same general significance as the more permanent form of alternation. It also may appear during the very rapid rate of paroxysmal tachycardia in a patient without organic heart disease in whom no alternation is present while the rate is slow. (It then has no prognostic significance.)

Generally the electrocardiogram fails to show abnormalities that correspond with the pulse abnormalities. Occasionally electrical alternation takes place, the QRS complex being alternately large and small (cf. Fig. 210). Such alternation is supposed to have the same bearing on prognosis as that of the peripheral pulse. Alternation of the P wave has also been noted during the rapid rate of auricular flutter.

Pulsus alternans occurring in regularly beating hearts, apart from paroxysmal tachycardia, indicates heart muscle disease of a serious degree. It is not seen in normal hearts. It is most common in association with hypertensive heart disease and with disease of the coronary arteries but occasionally is found in valvular cases. It is generally present when the rate is over 90 and may disappear as the rate falls to about 70. In fact, it is very rare when the heart is beating slowly. Its importance lies in its prognostic significance. The length of life after this sign is elicited is often not more than a year or two, although occasionally there is an exceptional patient who carries on quite satisfactorily for more than five years.

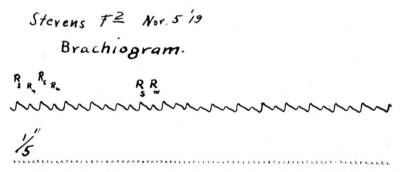

FIG. 205. *Pulsus Alternans.* Tracing taken from the brachial artery which shows a regular pulse but waves alternating in strength; R is larger than R$_w$. (Author's article in Oxford Loose-Leaf Medicine, vol. II.)

Phonocardiography

Just as electrical instruments were devised to register the action currents in the heart, similarly apparatus is now available to record graphically the heart sounds and murmurs. These instruments are called *phonocardiographs* or *stethocardiographs*. They are coming into use more and more, and it seems appropriate to touch upon the subject of phonocardiography rather briefly.

Heart sounds and murmurs can be augmented in intensity many fold so that they can become audible in an amphitheater or they can be picked up by many listeners by means of appropriate electrical wiring and ear pieces. In fact, heart sounds can be transmitted long distances. These various procedures are used very rarely, but the future may see many developments little thought of at present. What concerns us here is the photographic registration of the heart sounds as commonly obtained by the simple phonocardiographs in use.

At the outset one might inquire as to what use phonocardiography might have at present. If the physician is hard of hearing, the heart sounds can be intensified so that he may be able to detect sounds that he otherwise would not discover. If hearing is normal, it is doubtful whether any clinical interpretation of significance can be made from eliciting with the phonocardiograph faint sounds that are inaudible with the ordinary stethoscope. There are instances, however, when even the expertly trained ear finds it difficult or even impossible to time accurately a sound or murmur in the cardiac cycle. This is particularly true of the third heart sound producing a gallop rhythm. Occasionally all physicians have erroneously called a murmur systolic in time instead of diastolic, or vice versa. The simultaneous registration of heart sounds and electrocardiograms obviates any such difficulties, for it makes possible the placement of any of the auscultatory phenomena in their exact portion of the cardiac cycle.

The significance and composition of the heart sounds are being elaborately investigated by many students and will not be discussed in any detail here. Suffice it to say that the first heart sound ("lub") is made primarily by closure of the mitral and tricuspid valves. It is generally thought that it is partly muscular in origin, although some doubt this. The second heart sound ("dub") is made by closure of the aortic and pulmonary valves. The interval between "lub" and "dub" is systole, and that between "dub" and "lub" is diastole. In some normal hearts, especially in young persons in whom the rate is slow, a normal third heart sound may be heard in diastole. The auricular contraction may produce a sound that is rarely audible, although it may be present in phonocardiographic tracings. When abnormal sounds or murmurs are heard it is obviously important to place them correctly in one part or another of the cardiac cycle.

Figure 206 is an example of the normal heart sounds obtained in a regular, normal heart. It should be noted that the first heart sound comes directly after the QRS complex, and the second sound at the very end of the T wave. Figure 207 shows the character of the heart sounds in a grossly irregular heart (auricular fibrillation). The height of the vibrations is some indication of the loudness of the sounds. Figure

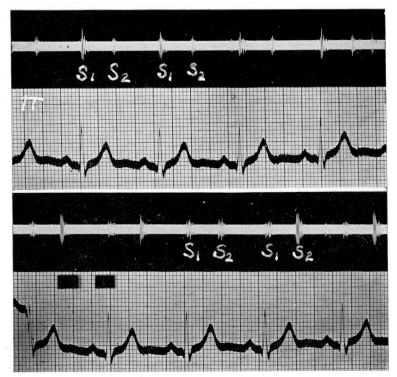

FIG. 206.   *Normal Heart Sounds.*   Simultaneous phonocardiograms and electrocardiograms of a normal man, 29 years old. The upper sound curves were taken from the apex, and the lower from the pulmonary area. Note that the first sound (S_1) is louder at the apex and fainter at the base than the second sound (S_2). The relative intensity of the two sounds varies in both normal and abnormal hearts.

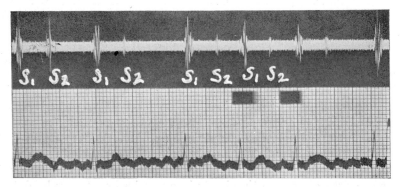

FIG. 207.   *Irregular Sounds of Auricular Fibrillation.*   Note the gross irregularity of the rhythm. Systole (S_1 to S_2) is fairly constant but diastole (S_2 to S_1) varies from cycle to cycle. The patient was a woman, 56 years of age, with thyrotoxicosis.

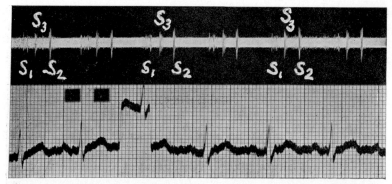

FIG. 208. *Normal Midsystolic Gallop.* Note that between the normal first heart sound (S₁) and the normal second sound (S₂) there is a definite third sound (S₃), which is even louder than the first sound. The patient was a 35-year-old woman with rheumatoid arthritis but with no heart disease.

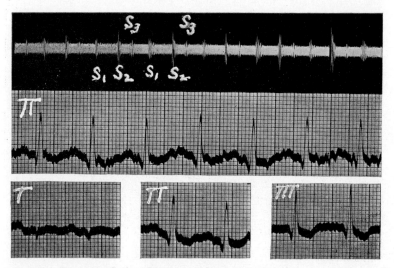

FIG. 209. *Diastolic Gallop Rhythm.* Note that the extra or third sound (S₃) occurs in diastole, i.e., between the second and first sound. This is almost invariably pathologic. The patient was a 60-year-old man who had severe congestive heart failure following an acute coronary thrombosis.

208 is a clear example of a so-called "normal" midsystolic gallop rhythm. The extra or abnormal sound occurs in midsystole, i.e., between the normal first and second heart sounds. This must be clearly differentiated from a diastolic gallop, which almost always indicates a pathologic state, in which the third or abnormal sound occurs somewhere between the second and the following first heart sound (Fig. 209).

Pulsus alternans, which has been discussed previously, is detected in the peripheral pulse. Occasionally, however, the alternating quality of the strength of consecutive beats in a regular heart may be detected in the alternate intensity of the heart sounds. This is well displayed in Figure 210. In the upper tracing the alternation in the heart sounds is accompanied by alternation in the form of the electrocardiogram. There probably is 2:1 defective intraventricular conduction. The lower tracing shows that the auscultatory alternation is still present when the electrocardiograms remain of the same form throughout. This alternation in the loudness of the heart sounds was first detected on routine physical examination. Murmurs, if present, may alternate in intensity and the apex impulse may be seen or felt to alternate in strength.

The character and intensity of the first heart sound is a matter of some importance in clinical auscultation. We know it is accentuated in mitral stenosis, hyperthyroidism, and in some nervous and other states. It may be diminished in intensity in emphysema, pericardial effusion, and acute coronary thrombosis, and, in fact, in some normal, healthy individuals. Among the various factors that determine the intensity of the first heart sound, one that is most important is the P-R interval of that beat. It has been shown that when the auriculoventricular conduction time varies in different cycles (normally 0.14 to 0.2 second) the first heart sound will be loudest in those cycles with a P-R interval of about 0.04 to 0.08 second and that as the interval becomes longer the

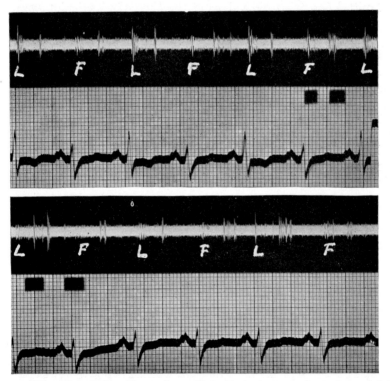

FIG. 210. *Ventricular Alternation.* Note that alternate beats have faint (F) and loud (L) sounds. In the upper strip the ventricular complexes also alternate, but in the lower set the electrocardiograms are of constant type. The alternation in the heart sounds was audible with the stethoscope, and there was also pulsus alternans in the radial artery. This man was 73 years old and had serious hypertensive and coronary artery disease.

sound becomes more distant. It follows that with intervals shorter than normal the sound is louder and with intervals longer than normal the sound becomes fainter than the normal first heart sound.

This method, although not easily applicable, is in fact the only bedside method available in judging abnormalities in the relation between the time of auricular and ventricular contractions. It may aid in the diagnosis of first, second, and third degree heart block, nodal premature beats, and paroxysmal ventricular tachycardia. There is reason to believe that the changes in the intensity of the first heart sound in these conditions result because of differences in actual position of the auriculoventricular leaflets (mitral and tricuspid) at the moment the ventricles contract. As the ventricles fill in diastole the valve leaflets gradually float upward and then the auricles contract, pushing them deeper into the ventricular cavity, or at least to a different position. The exact position these leaflets will obtain will necessarily be different when the ventricles contract immediately after this alteration resulting from auricular contraction and when a longer interval intervenes between auricular and ventricular contractions. In other words, it seems that the exact position of the mitral and tricuspid valves at the time of ventricular systole determines the loudness of the first heart sound. The character of the snap when it comes from a low position will differ from that heard when it comes from a high position. This changing intensity of the first heart sound, while the ventricle is beating quite regularly, is the pathognomonic auscultatory sign of complete heart block and is clearly illustrated in Figure 211. Note that when the P waves come very close to the QRS complex the first heart sound is very loud, and when the P-R interval is long the sound is diminished.

Numerous other illustrations can be given showing the application of phonocardiography to the study of heart sounds. Much of it is still in the developmental stage. The above cases were examples in which the ordinary ear with a simple stethoscope was able to detect significant abnormalities and make correct diagnoses, which were merely confirmed by the phonocardiograph. Possibly much more valuable data will be obtained as such studies continue.

Phonocardiography also affords a simple means of registering cardiac murmurs. With the present methods of amplifying sounds it is an easy matter to transform a faint murmur into a loud roar. That does not help the practicing physician, for he will remain dependent for the most part on what he can detect with the ear and a simple stethoscope. He will not be carrying a complicated machine like the present stethocardiograph around from house to house, although he may want to use it on occasions for special purposes or for investigative work. Furthermore, the quality of the sounds is not quite the same when electrical apparatus is introduced. Finally, most murmurs that will have any significance or of which any intelligent interpretation can be made will be audible with a stethoscope without electrical amplification. If an extremely faint systolic murmur can only be detected with special apparatus it would have no clinical importance, because even slightly louder systolic murmurs (grade I or I minus) can be heard with the ear and yet often have no pathologic meaning. However, we do know that a diastolic murmur that is diagnostic of mitral stenosis may become so faint that one observer may and another may not hear it, and, in fact, it may not be present at all. Under such circumstances amplification and registration of sounds may be valuable clinically. Exploration of such problems is much in need at present.

In a previous discussion (Chap. 17) the significance of systolic murmurs was taken up. At this point it seems appropriate to illustrate graphically one or two points concerning murmurs and to comment about their method of transmission. I have long been convinced that there was something fallacious in the prevailing teaching concerning heart murmurs. It is generally thought that murmurs are transmitted *with* the blood stream. A loud basal systolic murmur, if heard in the carotid area, is supposed to be indicative of aortic stenosis, and an apical systolic murmur, if transmitted to the axilla, indicative of mitral insufficiency. These diagnoses have been made with greater assurance when such transmission was present than when it was not. The point I should like to make is that transmission is dependent mainly, if not entirely, on the loudness of the murmur, and that transmission takes place from the point of maximal intensity (wherever the origin may be) in all directions.

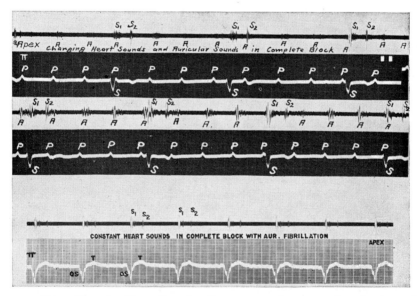

FIG. 211. *Changing Heart Sounds.* In upper tracing, note changing intensity of heart sounds, especially first sound (S_1) in different cycles. Very loud sounds occur with very short P-R intervals. When P and QRS occur simultaneously, the first sound is not increased. Also note audible auricular sounds (A). Male, age 75 years, had Adams-Stokes disease. In lower tracing, a case of complete block with auricular fibrillation shows no change in first sound. The auricles are not contracting and thus there is no P-R alteration.

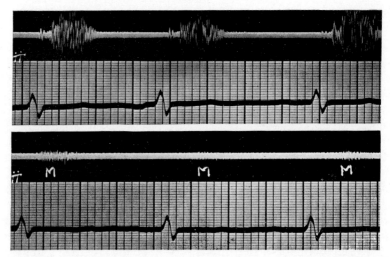

FIG. 212. *Loud Diamond-Shaped Systolic Murmur of Aortic Stenosis Trans-mitted to Elbow.* The upper tracing shows very loud systolic murmur (grade VI) in the aortic area. The lower sound tracing was taken from the right olecranon process while the blood-pressure cuff was inflated above the systolic pressure. Note that the systolic murmur is still detectable (M). The patient was a 45-year-old woman with aortic stenosis and angina pectoris.

Furthermore, there is evidence now available to show that transmission through bone is most likely of primary importance.

Loud murmurs over the aortic area are often heard in the neck because they are near the neck, and loud apical murmurs are heard in the axilla because they are near the axilla. There is no physical reason to explain the transmission of a murmur with the blood stream, because the speed of transmission of sound is a great deal faster than the velocity of blood flow. A murmur may be transmitted *in* but not *with* the blood stream. It is not likely even that the transmission in the fluid media is important, as will be seen from the following. Figure 212 shows a loud systolic murmur, heard in the aortic area in a patient with marked aortic stenosis. It was also present over the carotid arteries but was also readily heard at the right olecranon process, even when the blood pressure cuff was inflated to 220 mm. of mercury (far above the systolic pressure of the patient). This means that the systolic murmur was transmitted through the bones of the arm, for the blood supply to the elbow was entirely cut off.

The fact that the loudness rather than the site of origin determines the transmission of a murmur is shown by Figure 213. Here a very loud systolic murmur (grade VI) was heard all over the precordium, best in the third left interspace. The patient had congenital ventricular septal defect. This murmur was therefore made within the heart itself, and the current of blood producing the murmur flowed from left ventricle to right ventricle. Despite this the murmur was heard in the carotid artery and also at the left elbow while the arterial supply was cut off. This

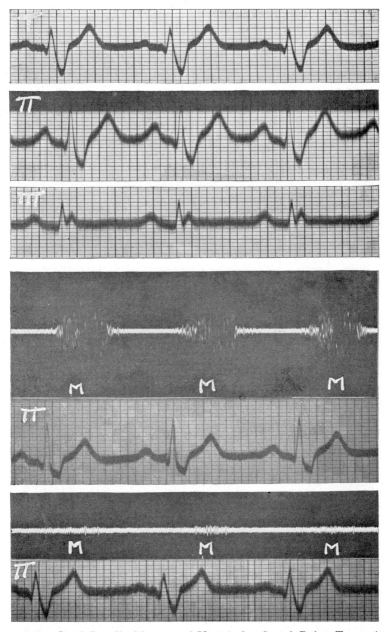

FIG. 213. *Loud Systolic Murmur of Ventricular Septal Defect Transmitted to Elbow.* The upper three strips are the three electrocardiographic leads. The middle set shows a loud systolic murmur from the third left sternal border. The lowest set shows that the murmur (M) is audible at the left olecranon process with the blood-pressure cuff inflated above the systolic pressure. The patient was a 21-year-old man, in good health, showing definite evidence of congenital ventricular septal defect.

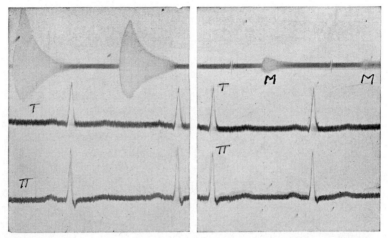

FIG. 214.   *Loud Aortic Diastolic Murmur Transmitted to Elbow.*   The left set of curves shows loud musical aortic diastolic murmur taken simultaneously with Leads I and II. The right set shows that the diastolic murmur (M) was audible over the right olecranon process with the arterial pressure occluded to that arm. The patient was a man, about 50 years old, who had aortic insufficiency, probably traumatic in origin.

murmur also must have been transmitted through bone and not the blood stream. Additional evidence that murmurs are well transmitted through bone is apparent in Figure 214. Here a loud, musical, aortic diastolic murmur was readily audible on top of the head and over the bones of the arms. It is well shown in the phonocardiogram obtained from the right olecranon process.

In general it may be stated that loud murmurs are transmitted in all directions from their maximum point of origin, and that bone is probably the main pathway of peripheral conduction. This explains why the systolic murmur of coarctation of the aorta is well heard in the interscapular region, for the site of formation of the murmur is deep in the chest and near the spine. It follows that any murmur that is loud enough, no matter what its origin, may be audible over the carotid artery or even over the bones of the arms.

Apart from the intensity of murmurs one derives very little of diagnostic value from the quality of murmurs. At times, however, the peculiar quality is of some interest. This is particularly true of the continuous machinery murmur of patent ductus arteriosus. This murmur often seems to envelop the heart sounds, becoming a little louder as the second heart sound approaches and continuing uninterruptedly after the second sound. In this way it differs from the systolic and diastolic murmurs of aortic stenosis and insufficiency, in which there appears to be two separate components. Figure 215 shows the disappearance of such a continuous murmur in a case of patent ductus arteriosus after a successful surgical division of the duct.

One or two more simple observations may be appropriate at this

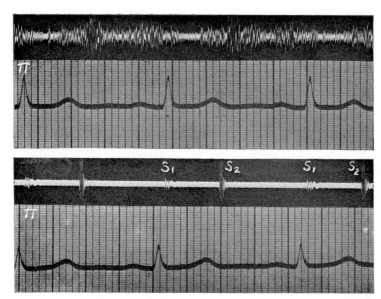

FIG. 215. *Continuous Machinery Murmur of Patent Ductus Arteriosus.* The upper set shows a coarse continuous murmur increasing in intensity on approaching the second heart sound and again in the presystole, obtained from the pulmonary area. The lower tracings show normal first and second sounds (S_1 and S_2) without any murmurs, following successful surgical division of the ductus. The patient was a 24-year-old woman with congenital patent ductus arteriosus, who was later cured.

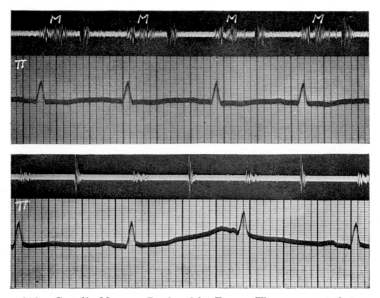

FIG. 216. *Systolic Murmur Produced by Fever.* The upper set shows systolic murmur (M) in the pulmonary area while the patient's temperature was 104° F. The lower set shows no murmur when the patient's temperature was 99.2° F. This patient had general paresis but no heart disease, and was receiving malaria therapy.

time. It has been mentioned in Chapter 17 that slight systolic murmurs may result from anemia, fever, hyperthyroidism, physical exercise, emotion, and other noncardiac causes. Figure 216 is a simple example of the production of a systolic murmur by fever. This patient had no evidence of heart disease and showed no murmurs whatever. She had general paresis and was receiving malaria therapy. A distinct basal systolic murmur present during the height of the fever (temperature 104° F.) disappeared entirely as the temperature returned to normal. Finally, it is well to bear in mind that the disappearance of a murmur with inspiration does not necessarily mean that it has no clinical significance. Many faint systolic murmurs will vary in intensity with respiration and some will disappear with a deep inspiration. However, a faint diastolic murmur that is diagnostic of organic valvular disease may also disappear after a deep breath. The procedure obviously decreases the intensity of some murmurs and the very faint ones may therefore become inaudible.

More could be discussed concerning murmurs and other sounds that may be registered by phonocardiography. This subject is growing in importance and those interested now have available complete treatises on this topic.

Index

ABDOMINAL aortic aneurysm, rupture of, coronary thrombosis confused with, 145
belt in angina pectoris, 126
in chronic cor pulmonale, 311
pain in congestive heart failure, 348
in rheumatic fever, 11
Aberrant ventricular conduction, premature auricular beats and, 478, Fig. 58
Abortion, indications for, in cardiacs, 333, 334
Acetyl digitoxin. See Digitalis
Acetyl-strophanthidin, test for digitalis toxicity, 370, 493, 603
ACTH. See Adrenal steroids
Acute bacterial endocarditis. See Bacterial endocarditis, acute
cor pulmonale. See Cor pulmonale
infections, heart in, 185
myocarditis and, 185
nephritis. See Nephritis, acute
surgical abdomen, coronary thrombosis confused with, 136, 141, 327
Adams-Stokes disease, Adrenalin for, 149, 290
cardiac pacemaker for, 291
cholecystectomy and, 291
coronary thrombosis and, 135, 138
Fiedler's myocarditis and, 541
gallbladder disease and, 291
Isuprel for, 290
normal rhythm and, 549, Fig. 136
prognosis in, 344
sarcoid and, 541
sinus pauses and, 474, 476
sodium lactate for, 290
syncope in, 290
treatment of, 290
ventricular fibrillation and, 533, Fig. 115
flutter in, 531, Fig. 113
Addison's disease, 184
electrocardiogram in, 556, 618, 619, Fig. 200
heart size in, 184
hyperthyroidism and, 195
sodium retention treatment of, 184
ventricular complex voltage in, 556
Adrenal steroids, in coronary thrombosis, 149

Adrenal steroids, in lupus erythematosus disseminatus, 184
in rheumatic fever, 17, 18
in rheumatic pericarditis, 68
in scleroderma heart, 181
tumors, hypertension and, 165
Adrenalin, for Adams-Stokes disease, 149, 290
angina pectoris and, 103
in congestive heart failure, 373
in coronary thrombosis, 147, 148
test, in angina pectoris, 110
Age at death, in aortic stenosis, 62
in mitral stenosis, 62
in tricuspid stenosis, 62
Air embolism, 300
Albumin for peripheral circulatory failure, 347
Alcohol in angina pectoris, 119
Alcoholism, chronic, electrocardiogram and, 620, Fig. 203
Allergic state in rheumatic fever, 7
Alpha-lobeline, for velocity of blood flow determination, 353
Aminophylline, for acute pulmonary edema, 174
for angina pectoris, 123
in Cheyne-Stokes respiration, 357
in congestive heart failure, 375
in coronary thrombosis, 151
in paroxysmal dyspnea, 296
Amyl nitrite, second degree heart block and, 544
test for presystolic murmur, 37
Amyloid heart disease, 186
angina pectoris and, 132
Anemia, angina pectoris and, 90, 101
dilatation of the heart in, 32
dyspnea in, 312
electrocardiogram and, 556
pericarditis and, 73
in rheumatic fever, 15
subacute bacterial endocarditis and, 215
systolic murmur and, 320
velocity of blood flow in, 352
Anesthetics, in surgery, 329–330
Aneurysm, abdominal aortic, rupture of, confused with coronary thrombosis, 144
of aorta, in Marfan's syndrome, 188

637

Morphine, for paroxysmal auricular tachycardia, 487
Mortality in coronary thrombosis, 139
Multiform premature beats, 517, 519, Fig. 102
Mumps, myocarditis and, 186
Mural thrombi, in auricular fibrillation, 387
 in coronary thrombosis, 138, 159
Murmur, in aortic insufficiency, 634, Fig. 214
 in congenital heart disease, 228
 diastolic, significance of, 636
 fever and, 635, 636, Fig. 216
 in hypertension, 172, 173
 transmission of, 631, 632, 633, Figs. 212, 213
 in tricuspid stenosis, 62
Muscular dystrophy, myocardium in, 187
Myocardial fibrosis, constrictive pericarditis and, 608
 infarction. See Coronary thrombosis
 ischemia, temporary, 146
Myocarditis, chronic. See Chronic "myocarditis"
 diphtheria and, 185
 mitral stenosis and, 398
 mumps and, 186
 paroxysmal auricular tachycardia with block and, 541
 poliomyelitis and, 187
 pregnancy associated with, 335
 rheumatic pericarditis, 67
 therapy of, 186
 virus pneumonia and, 186
Myxedema, 179
 angina pectoris and, 100, 179
 cardiac dilatation in, 179
 clinical findings in, 179
 congestive heart failure and, 395
 electrocardiogram in, 179
 low voltage of ventricular complexes in, 556, 559, Fig. 144
 pericardial effusion in, 179
 pericarditis in, 73
 thyroid medication for, 179
Myxoma of left auricle, 182, 183
 of right auricle, 182, 183

Nausea, in coronary thrombosis, 134
Neohydrin, in heart failure, 374
Neostigmine in paroxysmal auricular tachycardia, 272
Neosynephrine, for coronary thrombosis, 148
 for paroxysmal auricular tachycardia, 488
Nephrectomy, hypertension and, 166
Nephritis, acute, electrocardiogram in, 181
 heart failure in, 181, 342
 hypertension and, 165
 rheumatic fever and, 24
 chronic, auricular flutter in, 501

Nephritis, chronic, heart failure confused with, 352, 359
 hypertension and, 166, 169
 pericarditis and, 72
 prognosis in, 342
 surgery and, 328
Nervous excitement, systolic murmur and, 320
"Nervous heart." See Functional heart disease
Neurasthenic state in coronary thrombosis, 162
Neurocirculatory asthenia, 262–265. See also Functional heart disease
 constitutional factor in, 262
 electrocardiogram in, 263, 608
 military considerations of, 262, 264
 physical findings in, 263
 prognosis in, 265
 subacute bacterial endocarditis confused with, 214
 symptoms of, 263
 trauma and, 304
 treatment of, 264
Nitrol ointment for angina pectoris, 124
Nocturnal dyspnea, hypertension and, 170
Nodal beats. See Ectopic beats, nodal
 rhythm, 511, Figs. 90, 91
 auricular standstill differentiated from, 477
 rheumatic carditis and, 511, Fig. 90
Nonbacterial endocarditis, 208
 verrucous endocarditis. See Lupus erythematosus disseminatus
Norepinephrine (Levophed), coronary thrombosis and, 148
 peripheral circulatory failure and, 348
Novocain, in coronary thrombosis, 147
Nutritional state, in rheumatic fever, 21

Obesity, angina pectoris and, 117
 dyspnea and, 340
Obstetrics, cardiac disease and, 330–336. See also Pregnancy
Ocular pressure, auricular tachycardia and, 269, 271, 487
 ventricular tachycardia and, 528
Oliguria in coronary thrombosis, 136
Omentopexy for angina pectoris, 129
Opening snap, gallop rhythm, differentiation from, 172
 in mitral stenosis, 37
Ostium primum. See Atrial septal defect
 secundum. See Atrial septal defect
Ouabain, 368. See also Digitalis
Oxygen, coronary thrombosis and, 147
 heart failure and, 383
 peripheral circulatory failure and, 347

Pacemaker, disturbances of, 472–477
Paget's disease and angina pectoris, 100

Pulmonary vascular disease, in atrial septal
    defect, 230
  obstruction syndrome, 251–252
  veins, anomalous, 554
  wedge pressure, 400
    in mitral stenosis, 45
Pulmonic stenosis, electrocardiogram and,
    552, Fig. 44
  incomplete bundle branch block and,
    467, Fig. 44
Pulsating veins, in tricuspid insufficiency,
    60, 61
Pulse, in mitral stenosis, 42
  deficit, in auricular fibrillation, 39
    digitalis effect on, 362
  pressure, in aortic insufficiency, 52
    in arteriovenous fistula, 179
    in beriberi heart disease, 180
Pulsus alternans, 624–625, Fig. 205
  bigeminy, differentiated from, 624
  bundle branch block and, 469
  in congestive heart failure, 347, 359
  detection of, 171
  following ectopic beats, 625
  gallop rhythm and, 469
  heart sounds in, 628, 629, Fig. 210
  hypertension and, 171
  paroxysmal tachycardia and, 625
  prognosis in, 341–342
  significance of, 625
  paradoxus, in constrictive pericarditis, 80
    in nonconstrictive pericarditis, 86
    pericardial effusion and, 75
Pyelitis, acute, coronary thrombosis dis-
    tinguished from, 298
Pyelonephritis, hypertension and, 166

Q-M₁ interval, in mitral stenosis, 44
Q-T interval, digitalis effect on, 360
Quadruple rhythm, in Ebstein's anomaly,
    253
Quinidine, 385–393
  aberrant ventricular conduction and,
    523, Fig. 105
  for angina pectoris, 123
  anticoagulant therapy and, 391
  for auricular fibrillation, 385, 387, 389,
      392, 503, 505, 506, 509, Figs. 83,
      86, 87
    prevention of, 392
  for auricular flutter, 386, 498, 500, 501,
      526, Figs. 80, 108
  complete heart block and, 551
  contraindications for, 530
  dosage schedule for, 391
  for ectopic beats, 260, 392
  electrocardiographic effects of, 386
  emboli and, 388, 389
  in hypertensive heart disease, 390
  indications for, 389
  maintenance dose of, 391
  mechanism of action of, 386, 509

Quinidine, in mitral stenosis, 390
  for paroxysmal auricular fibrillation, 280,
    281
  for paroxysmal auricular flutter, 279
  for paroxysmal auricular tachycardia,
    488–490
    with block, 272, 493
  for paroxysmal ventricular tachycardia,
    150, 284, 285, 392, 527–530, Figs. 110,
    112
  in premature auricular beats, 481
  in premature ventricular beats, 521
  respiratory arrest and, 388, 529
  risks of, 530
  toxicity of, 386, 388, 392, 477, Fig. 56
  in ventricular fibrillation, 292
  vital capacity and, 388
  for Wolff-Parkinson-White syndrome,
    616

RADIOACTIVE iodine, for angina pectoris,
    128, 396
  for heart failure, 396
  for paroxysmal auricular fibrillation,
    282
  thyrotoxic heart disease and, 194, 195
Rauwolfia, in hypertension, 176, 177
Recumbency, circulatory dynamics in, 155
  harmful effects of, in cardiacs, 154, 155
  hypertensive heart disease and, 155
  paroxysmal nocturnal dyspnea and, 154
Reflexes from the heart, hypertension and,
    165
Regitine test, in hypertension, 175
Renal artery thrombosis, hypertension and,
    165, 166
  function, diuretics and, 380
  infarcts in coronary thrombosis, 138
  insufficiency, 342
    subacute bacterial endocarditis and,
    214
  ischemia (Goldblatt mechanism), hyper-
    tension and, 166
Respiration, electrical axis of heart and,
    435, 438, Fig. 18
Respiratory arrest, quinidine and, 388, 529
  infections and rheumatic fever, 23
Rest in treatment of coronary thrombosis,
    147, 153
Retinal changes in hypertension, 167
Rheumatic activity, assessment of, 33
  carditis, 29–34
    aortic diastolic murmur in, 32
    Aschoff nodule in, 31, 33
    electrocardiographic changes in, 30, 31
    first heart sound in, 31
    gallop rhythm in, 31, 171
    heart block in, 30, 538–543, Figs. 120,
      122, 123, 126
    mitral diastolic murmurs in, 33
      stenosis confused with, 33
    nodal rhythm in, 511, Fig. 90